The **BIOMEDICAL ENGINEERING** Series

Series Editor Michael Neuman

SIGNALS *and* SYSTEMS ANALYSIS *in* BIOMEDICAL ENGINEERING

Robert B. Northrop

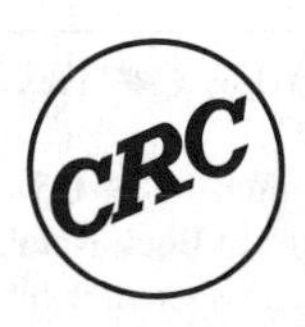

CRC PRESS

Boca Raton London New York Washington, D.C.

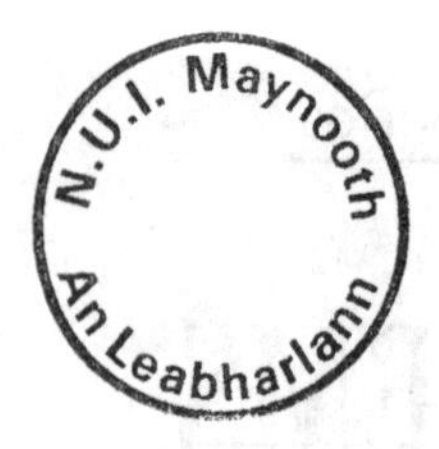

Library of Congress Cataloging-in-Publication Data

Northrop, Robert B.
Signals and systems analysis in biomedical engineering / Robert B. Northrop.
p. cm.
Includes bibliographical references and index.
ISBN 0-8493-1557-3 (alk. paper)
1. Biomedical engineering. 2. System analysis. I. Title.

R856.N58 2003
610′.28—dc21 2002191167
CIP

Direct all inquiries to CRC Press LLC, 2000 N.W. Corporate Blvd., Boca Raton, Florida 33431.

International Standard Book Number 0-8493-1557-3
Library of Congress Card Number 2002191167
Printed in the United States of America 1 2 3 4 5 6 7 8 9 0
Printed on acid-free paper

Dedication

I dedicate this text to my wife, Adelaide, whose encouragement catalyzes my inspiration.

Preface

This text is intended for use in a classroom course on signals and systems analysis in biomedical engineering taken by undergraduate students specializing in biomedical engineering. It will also serve as a reference book for biophysics and medical students interested in the topics. Readers are assumed to have had introductory core courses up to the junior level in engineering mathematics, including complex algebra, calculus and introductory differential equations. They also should have taken introductory human (medical) physiology and biomedical engineering. After taking these courses, readers should be familiar with systems block diagrams, the concepts of frequency response and transfer functions, and should be able to solve simple, linear, ordinary differential equations and do basic manipulations in linear algebra. It is also important to have an understanding of how the physiological signals and systems being characterized figure in human health.

The interdisciplinary field of biomedical engineering is demanding in that it requires its followers to know and master not only certain engineering skills (electronic, materials, mechanical and photonic), but also a diversity of material in the biological sciences (anatomy, biochemistry, molecular biology, genomics, physiology etc.). Tying these diverse disciplines together is a common reticulum of mathematical skills characterized by both breadth and specialization. This text was written to aid undergraduate biomedical engineering students by helping them to strengthen and understand this common network of applied mathematics, as well as to provide a ready source of information on the specialized mathematical tools and techniques most useful in describing and analyzing biomedical signals (including, but not limited to: ECG, EEG, EMG, ERG, heart sounds, breath sounds, blood pressure, tomographic images etc.). Of particular interest is the description of signals from nonstationary sources using the many algorithms for computing joint time-frequency spectrograms.

The text presents the traditional systems mathematics used to characterize linear, time-invariant (LTI) systems, and, given inputs, to find their outputs. The relations between impulse response, real convolution, transfer functions and frequency response functions are explained. Also, some specialized mathematical techniques used to characterize and model nonlinear systems are reviewed.

It is the very nature of living organisms that signals derived from them are *noisy* and *nonstationary*. That is, the parameters of the nonlinear systems giving rise to the signals change with time. There are many causes for nonstationary signals in biomedical systems: One is circadian rhythm, another is the action of drugs, another involves inherent periodic rhythms such as those associated with breathing or the heart's beating, and still other nonstationarity can be associated with natural processes such as the digestion of food or locomotion. Because nature has implemented many physiological systems with parallel architectures for redundancy and reliability, when recording from one "channel" of one system, one is likely to pick up the "cross-talk" from other channels as noise (e.g., in EMG recording). Also, many bioelectric signals are in the microvolt range, so electrode, amplifier and environmental noises are often significant compared with the signal level. This text introduces the basic mathematical tools used to describe noise and how it propagates through LTI and NLTI systems. It also describes at a basic level how signal-to-noise ratio can be improved by signal averaging and linear and nonlinear filtering.

Bandwidths associated with endogenous (natural) biomedical signals range from dc (e.g., hormone concentrations or dc potentials on the body surface) to hundreds of kilohertz (bat ultrasound). Exogenous signals associated with certain noninvasive imaging modalities (e.g., ultrasound, MRI) can reach into the 10s of MHz.

It is axiomatic that the large physiological systems are nonlinear and nonstationary, although early workers avoided their complexity by characterizing them as linear and stationary. Nonstationarity can generally be ignored if it is slow compared with the time epoch over which data is acquired. Nonlinearity can arise from the concatenated chemical reactions underlying physiological system function (there are no negative concentrations). The coupled ODEs of mass-action kinetics are generally nonlinear, which makes system characterization a challenge. Other nonlinearities arise in the signal processing properties of the nervous system. By considering the system behavior in a limited parameter space around an operating point, some systems can be linearized. Such piecewise linearization is often an over-simplification that obscures the detailed understanding of the system. It is important to eschew reductionism when analyzing and describing physiological and biochemical systems.

The text was written based on both the author's experience in teaching EE 202 Signals and Systems, EE 232 Systems Analysis, EE 271 Physiological Control Systems, and EE 372, Communications and Control in Physiological Systems for over 30 years in the Electrical and Computer Engineering Department at the University of Connecticut, and on his personal research in biomedical instrumentation and on certain neurosensory systems.

Signals and Systems Analysis in Biomedical Engineering is organized into 10 chapters, plus an Index, a wide-ranging Bibliography and four Appendices. Extensive chapter examples based on problems in biomedical engineering are given. The chapter contents are summarized below:

- Chapter 1, Introduction to Biomedical Signals and Systems, sets forth the general characteristics of biomedical signals and the general properties of physiological systems, including nonlinearity and nonstationarity, are examined. Also reviewed are the various means of modulating (and demodulating) signals from physiological systems. Discrete signals and systems are also introduced.

- Chapter 2, Review of Linear Systems Theory, formally presents the concepts of linearity, causality and stationarity. Linear time-invariant (LTI) dynamic analog systems are introduced and shown to be described by sets of ordinary differential equations (ODEs). General solutions of first- and second-order linear ODEs are covered. The basics of linear algebra are introduced and the solution of sets of simultaneous ODEs by the state variable method is presented. In characterizing LTI systems, the concepts of system impulse response, real convolution, general transient response, and steady-state sinusoidal frequency response are covered, including Bode and Nyquist plots. Chapter 2 also treats discrete systems and signals, including difference equations and the use of the z-transform and discrete state equations. Finally, the factors that affect the stability of systems and review certain stability tests are described.

- In Chapter 3, The Laplace Transform and Its Applications, the Laplace transform is defined and its mathematical properties are presented. Many examples are given of finding the Laplace transforms of transient signals, including causal LTI system impulse responses. Examples of the use of the Laplace transform to find the transient output of a causal LTI system given a transient input are given and the inverse Laplace transform is introduced. Real convolution of a system's impulse response with its input to find its output, y(t), in the time domain is shown to be equivalent to the Laplace transform of the output, Y(s), being equal to the product of the Laplace transforms of the input and the impulse response. The partial fraction expansion is shown to be an effective method for finding y(t), given Y(s). Solution of state equations in the frequency domain using the Laplace transform method is given.

- Chapter 4, Fourier Series Analysis of Periodic Signals, defines the real and complex forms of the Fourier series (FS) and the mathematical properties of the FS are presented. Gibbs phenomena are shown to persist even as the number of harmonic terms $\rightarrow \infty$, but their area $\rightarrow 0$. Several examples of finding the FS of periodic waveforms are given.

- The Continuous Fourier Transform is derived from the FS in Chapter 5. The (CFT) is seen to be equivalent to the Laplace transform for many applications, but the radian frequency ω is real, while s is complex. The properties of the CFT are presented and the IFT is introduced. Several applications of the CFT are given; the periodic spectrum of a sampled analog signal is derived in the Poisson sum form, and the sampling theorem is presented. Next, the generation of the analytical signal is derived using the Hilbert transform and applications are given. Finally, the modulation transfer function (MTF) is defined as the normalized spatial frequency response of an imaging system. Properties of the MTF are explored, as well as its significance in image resolution. The relation of the contrast transfer function (CTF) for a 1-D square-wave object to the MTF is discussed. In addition, Section 5.4 describes the analytical signal and the Hilbert transform and some of its biomedical applications.

- In Chapter 6, *The Discrete Fourier Transform,* the DFT and IDFT are compared with the CFT and the ICFT and their properties are described. Data window functions for finite sampled data sets are introduced and how they affect spectral resolution is demonstrated. Finally, the computational advantages of the FFT are described and several examples are given of FFT implementation.

- Chapter 7, *Introduction to Time-Frequency Analysis of Physiological Signals,* introduces the important method of TFA to characterize nonstationary signals. The case for TFA of physiological signals, such as heart and breath sounds, and EEG voltages is made. Many of the diverse methods of finding TF spectrograms are presented with their pros and cons. These include the short-term Fourier transform (STFT), the Gabor and adaptive Gabor transforms, the Wigner-Ville and pseudo-W-V transforms, Cohen's general class of reduced interference TF transforms, and finally, TF transforms based on wavelets. In addition, this chapter also examines applications of TF analysis to such signals as heart sounds, EEG waveforms, postural balance forces, etc. Software currently available for TFA is also described. A comprehensive introduction to time-frequency analysis, and the mathematical tools that have been evolving to realize high-resolution time-frequency spectrograms, including the use of wavelets is presented.

- In Chapter 8, Introduction to the Analysis of Stationary Noise and Signals Contaminated with Noise, some of the mathematical tools used to describe noise in signals and systems are introduced. These include:

  The probability density function

  Autocorrelation

  Cross-correlation

  The continuous auto- and cross-power density spectrums

  Propagation of noise through stationary causal LTI continuous systems

  Propagation of noise through stationary causal LTI discrete systems

  Characteristic functions of random variables

  Price's theorem and applications

  Quantization noise

  An introduction to "data scrubbing" by nonlinear discrete filters

  Also covered in this chapter are calculation of noise descriptors with finite discrete data, signal averaging and filtering for signal-to-noise ratio improvement. A final unique section has an introduction to the application of statistics and information theory to genomics. This section includes a review of DNA biology; RNAs and the basics of protein synthesis; introduction to statistics; introduction to information theory and an introduction to hidden Markov models in genomics. Section 8.5 also introduces the application to genomics of statistics and information theory.

- Chapter 9, Basic Mathematical Tools Used in the Characterization of Physiological Systems, again reviews the general properties of physiological systems, including the properties of nonlinear systems. The physical factors determining the dynamic behavior of physiological systems, including diffusion dynamics and biochemical systems and mass-action kinetics, are described. Some means of analyzing nonlinear physiological systems, including describing functions and the stability of closed-loop nonlinear systems, and the use of Gaussian noise-based techniques to characterize physiological systems are presented. Mathematical tools for the description of non-linear systems are also given.

- Chapter 10, Introduction to the Mathematics of Tomographic Imaging, does not cover medical imaging modalities per se, but rather the common mathematical transforms and techniques necessary to do tomographic imaging. These include algebraic reconstruction; the radon transform; the Fourier slice theorem; and the filtered back-projection algorithm (FBPA). The mathematics of tomographic imaging (the radon transform, the Fourier slice theorem and the filtered back-projection algorithm) are described at an understandable level.

The Appendices include:

A. Cramer's Rule

B. Signal Flow Graphs and Mason's Rule

C. Bode (Frequency Response) Plots

D. Computational Tools for Biomedical Signal Processing and Systems Analysis

In addition, a comprehensive Bibliography and References present entries from periodicals, the Internet and texts.

Robert B. Northrop
Storrs, CT

Author

Robert B. Northrop was born in White Plains, New York. He majored in electrical engineering at MIT, graduating with a bachelor's degree. At the University of Connecticut, he received a master's degree in control engineering, and, doing research on the neuromuscular physiology of molluscan catch muscles, received his Ph.D. in physiology from UConn.

He was hired as an Assistant Professor of EE in 1964 and, in collaboration with his Ph.D. advisor, Dr. Edward G. Boettiger, secured a 5-year training grant from NIGMS (NIH), and started one of the first interdisciplinary Biomedical Engineering graduate training programs in New England. UCONN currently awards M.S. and Ph.D. degrees in this field of study.

Throughout his career, Dr. Northrop's areas of research, while broad and interdisciplinary, have been centered around biomedical engineering. He has done sponsored research on the neurophysiology of insect vision and theoretical models for visual neural signal processing. He also did sponsored research on electrofishing and developed, in collaboration with Northeast Utilities, effective working systems for fish guidance and control in hydroelectric plant waterways on the Connecticut River using underwater electric fields.

Still another area of his sponsored research has been in the design and simulation of nonlinear adaptive digital controllers to regulate *in vivo* drug concentrations or physiological parameters, such as pain, blood pressure or blood glucose, in diabetics. An outgrowth of this research led to his development of mathematical models for the dynamics of the human immune system that were used to investigate theoretical therapies for autoimmune diseases, cancer and HIV infection.

Biomedical instrumentation has also been an active research area. An NIH grant supported studies on the use of the ocular pulse to detect obstructions in the carotid arteries. Minute pulsations of the cornea from arterial circulation in the eyeball were sensed using a no-touch phase-locked ultrasound technique. Ocular pulse waveforms were shown to be related to cerebral blood flow in rabbits and humans.

Most recently, Dr. Northrop has been addressing the problem of noninvasive blood glucose measurement for diabetics. Starting with a Phase I SBIR grant, he developed a means of estimating blood glucose by reflecting a beam of polarized light off the front surface of the lens of the eye and measuring the very small optical rotation resulting from glucose in the aqueous humor, which, in turn, is proportional to blood glucose. As an offshoot of techniques developed in micropolarimetry, he developed a magnetic sample chamber for glucose measurement in biotechnology applications. The water solvent was used as the Faraday optical medium.

He has written five textbooks, with subject matter that ranges from analog electronic circuits, instrumentation and measurements to physiological control systems, neural modeling, and instrumentation and measurements in noninvasive medical diagnosis.

Dr. Northrop was a member of the Electrical and Computer Engineering faculty at UCONN until his retirement in June, 1997. Throughout this time, he was program director of the Biomedical Engineering Graduate Program. As Emeritus Professor, he still teaches courses in Biomedical Engineering, writes texts, sails and travels. He lives in Chaplin, Connecticut, with his wife, a cat and a smooth fox terrier.

List of Figures

Contents

1

Introduction to Biomedical Signals and Systems

1.1 General Characteristics of Biomedical Signals

1.1.1 Introduction

This introductory chapter will introduce key definitions and concepts about biomedical signals and systems. The concepts of signal bandwidth, stationarity, nonstationarity and the diversity of biomedical and physiological signal modalities are presented. Section 1.1.6 introduces descriptors of signals including the mean, the sample mean, the mean-squared value, the root-mean-squared value, etc. A number of important schemes for modulation and demodulation of exogenous biomedical signals is introduced. *System* is defined for our purposes in Section 1.2.1. The concepts of system linearity, nonlinearity, and stationarity are set forth in Section 1.2.2. The general properties of physiological systems are enumerated in Section 1.2.3 and discrete signals and systems are described in Sections 1.1.4 and 1.2.4, respectively.

Intuitively, we think of a *biomedical signal* as some natural (endogenous) or man-made (exogenous), continuous, time-varying record that carries information about the internal functioning of a biomedical *system* (system is defined below). A signal can be a system input, or a system output as the result of one or more inputs, or carry information about a system state variable. In physiological systems, a signal can be an electrical potential, a force, a torque, a length or pressure, or a chemical concentration of ions or of molecules including hormones or cytokines. A signal can also be in the form of nerve impulses that lead to the contraction of muscles or the release of neurotransmitters or hormones. In an optical system, a signal can vary with position (x, y, z) as well as with time, t, and wavelength, λ.

A biomedical signal is generally acquired by a *sensor,* a *transducer,* or an *electrode,* and is converted to a proportional voltage or current for processing and storage. Naturally acquired, endogenous signals are continuous (analog) because nature viewed on a macroscale is continuous. One example of a biomedical signal is an ECG waveform recorded from the body surface; another example is blood velocity in an artery measured by Doppler ultrasound. Biomedical signals are invariably noisy because of interfering signals from the body, noise picked up from the environment, noise arising in electrodes and from signal conditioning amplifiers.

As mentioned above, hormones are a type of physiological signal. A hormone is generally quantified by its *concentration* in a *compartment,* such as the blood or extracellular fluid. Hormones are usually used as control substances as part of a closed-loop physiological regulatory system. For example, the protein hormone insulin, secreted by the pancreatic beta cells, acts on cells carrying insulin receptor molecules on their cell membranes to increase the rate of diffusion of glucose from the blood or extracellular fluid into those cells. Insulin also causes the liver to uptake glucose and store it intracellularly as the polymer glycogen [Northrop, 2000].

After initial acquisition and conditioning, an analog biomedical signal may be converted to *discrete form* by periodic analog-to-digital conversion. In discrete form, a signal can be more easily stored and can be further processed numerically by discrete filtering or other nonlinear discrete transforms. Discrete signals are very important because of the ability of digital signal processing (DSP) algorithms to reveal their properties in the time, frequency and joint time-frequency domains.

Both continuous and discrete signals can be characterized by a number of functions that will be described in later sections of this text. For example, if the signal is random in nature, the *probability density function,* the *joint probability density function* and the *auto-* and *cross-correlation functions* may serve as descriptors. In the frequency domain, we have the *auto-* and *cross-power density spectra* and *time-frequency spectrograms*. Deterministic continuous and discrete signals can be characterized by certain *transforms: Fourier, Laplace, Hilbert, Radon, Wigner,* etc., that will be described in this text.

Because biomedical signals are generally contaminated with noise; their signal-to-noise ratios (SNRs) can often be improved by filtering by analog or discrete filters or by signal averaging. How filtering and averaging can improve the SNRs will be explored in Section 8.4.

1.1.2 Signals from physiological systems

Endogenous biomedical signals from physiological systems are acquired for a number of reasons:

For purposes of diagnosis

For postsurgical intensive care monitoring

For neonatal monitoring

To guide therapy and for research

Such signals include, but certainly are not limited to, ECG, EEG, EMG, nerve action potentials, muscle force, blood pressure, temperature, respiration, hemoglobin psO_2, blood pCO_2, blood glucose concentration, the concentrations of various hormones and ions in body fluids, heart sounds, breath sounds, otoacoustic emissions etc. Signals can also be rates or frequencies derived from other signals; e.g., heart rate and respiratory rate.

In general, the bandwidths (equivalent frequency content) of endogenous physiological signals range from nearly dc (ca. 1.2×10^{-5} Hz or 12 μHz, a period of 24 h) to several kHz. This apparent low bandwidth is offset in many cases by massively parallel and redundant signal pathways in the body (as in the case of motor neurons innervating muscles).

Signals from physiological systems have another property will be encountered throughout this text, namely they are *nonstationary* (NS). This means that the physical, biochemical and physiological processes that contribute to their origins change in time. Take, for example, the arterial blood pressure (ABP). The ABP has a waveform with the almost-periodic rhythm of the heartbeat. However, many physiological factors affect the heart rate and the heart's stroke volume; the body's vasomotor tone is under control by the autonomic nervous system. The time of day (diurnal rhythm), emotional state, blood concentration of hormones such as epinephrine and norepinephrine, blood pH, exercise, respiratory rate, diet, drugs, blood volume and water intake all affect the ABP. Over a short interval of several minutes, the ABP waveform is relatively invariant in shape and period and can be said to be *short-term stationary* (STS). In fact, many physiological signals can be treated as STS; others change so rapidly that the STS assumption is not valid. For example, certain breath sounds which change from breath to breath should be treated as NS.

1.1.3 Signals from man-made instruments

In a number of instances, energy (photons, sound, radioactivity) is put into the body to measure physiological parameters and structures. For example, CW Doppler ultrasound, used to estimate blood velocity in arteries and veins, generally operates from 5 to 10 MHz. Thus, the transducers, filters, amplifiers, mixers, etc., used in a CW Doppler system must operate in the 5 to 10 MHz range. The blood velocity Doppler signal itself lies in the audio frequency range [Northrop, 2002].

An example of a prototype medical measurement system uses angle-modulated, *linearly polarized light* (LPL) to measure the optical rotation caused by glucose in the aqueous humor (AH) of the eye. Typical wavelength of the LPL is 512 nm; the angle modulation is done by a *Faraday rotator* at ca. 2 kHz. The glucose concentration in the aqueous humor (AH) follows the blood glucose concentration, which varies slowly over a 24-h period. I estimate its bandwidth to be from dc to c. 6 cycles/h (1.7 milliHz) [Northrop, 2002]. AH glucose concentration is an example of a very important physiological signal with a very low bandwidth. Indeed, many hormonal systems in the body, such as that controlling the secretion rate of the hormone melatonin, have diurnal (24-h) periods, as do parameters such as body temperature and the concentrations of certain ions in the blood, etc. Clearly, living systems have slow rhythms as well as fast.

In certain imaging systems, the radioactive decay of radioisotopes provides the signals that are processed to form a tomographic (slice) image. Tens of thousands of *random decay events/sec* can be processed to form a positron emission tomography (PET) image over a counting period of tens of minutes. The times of individual decay events are completely random, however, generally following a Poisson probability distribution.

In all medical imaging systems, it is appropriate to describe image resolution in terms of the *spatial frequency response* of the system. The spatial frequency response describes how an imaging system reproduces an object that is a 1-D spatial sinusoid in intensity as a 1-D spatial sinusoidal image. The normalized 1-D spatial frequency response is called the *modulation transfer function* (MTF) [Spring and Davidson, 2001]. The higher the cutoff frequency of the MTF, the greater the object's detail that is visible in the image. (The MTF is treated in detail in Section 5.5 of this text.)

1.1.4 Discrete signals

A discrete signal can be formed by *periodically sampling* an analog signal, $x(t)$, and converting each sample to a (digital) number, $x^*(kT)$. The sequence of numbers (samples) is considered to exist only at the sampling instants and thus can be represented by a periodic train of impulses or delta functions, each with an area equal to the value of $x(t)$ at the sampling instant, $x(kT)$. Mathematically, this can be stated as:

$$x^*(kT) = \sum_{k=0}^{\infty} x(t)\delta(t-kT) \tag{1.1}$$

Here, T is the sampling period, and $\delta(\mu)$ only exists for zero argument. Note that the sampling and A/D process is equivalent to *impulse modulation,* i.e., multiplication of the analog signal, $x(t)$, by a train of unit impulses occurring at a frequency $f_s = 1/T$. The properties of $x^*(kT)$ in the frequency domain will be treated in detail in Section 4.6. Note that other notations exist for the members of a sequence of sampled data; for example, $x(k)$ or x_k (k denotes the kth sample from a local time origin).

1.1.5 Some ways to describe signals

There are many ways to characterize one- and two-dimensional signals, i.e., signals that vary as a function of time, or spatial dimensions x and y. A signal can be described in terms of its statistical amplitude properties, its frequency properties and, if non-stationary, its time-frequency properties. To begin this section, consider a stationary continuous signal, $u(t)$. In fact, let us collect an ensemble of N signals, $\{u_k(t)\}$, all recorded from the same source under identical conditions, but at different times. The signal itself can be a voltage (e.g., an ECG record), a chemical concentration (e.g., calcium ions in the blood), a fluid pressure (e.g., blood pressure), a sound pressure (e.g., the first heart sound), etc.

Many descriptors can be applied to a signal that will characterize it quantitatively. For example, the signal's mean value, $\bar{u}$. $\bar{u}$ can be estimated by the finite time average of one, typical ensemble member:

$$\bar{u} = \frac{1}{T}\int_0^T u(t)\,dt \tag{1.2}$$

In the limit as $\mathrm{T} \to \infty$, $\overline{\mathrm{u}} \to <\mathrm{u}>$, the "true" mean of u, also known as its *expected value.* Suppose the ensemble consists of N responses to a sensory stimulus given repetitively to an animal. We can the pick a time $\mathrm{t_1}$ following each stimulus and find the *sample mean of the ensemble,* $\{\mathrm{u_k(t_1)}\}$:

$$\overline{\mathrm{u(t_1)}} = \frac{1}{\mathrm{N}} \sum_{\mathrm{k=1}}^{\mathrm{N}} \mathrm{u_k(t_1)} \tag{1.3}$$

As you will see in Section 8.4, the ensemble average shown in Equation 1.3, with $0 \leq \mathrm{t_1} \leq \mathrm{T}$, is a way of extracting a consistent evoked response signal from additive random noise with zero mean.

Another measure of a 1-D signal is its *intensity*. Definitions of intensity can vary, depending on the type of signal. For example, both sound intensity and light intensity have the units of power (Watts) per unit area ($\mathrm{m^2}$). The power can be *instantaneous power* or *average power.*

For sound, the average intensity is given by:

$$\mathrm{I} = \overline{\mathrm{p^2}}/(\rho \mathrm{c}) = \overline{\mathrm{pu}} = \rho\mathrm{c}\overline{\mathrm{u^2}} \quad \mathrm{W/m^2} \tag{1.4}$$

Where p is $\mathrm{p(t)}$, the sound pressure in Newtons/$\mathrm{m^2}$ (=Pascals) over atmospheric pressure, $\mathrm{u(t)}$ is the particle velocity in m/sec, ρ is the density of the medium in kg/$\mathrm{m^3}$ and c is the velocity of propagation in m/sec. That is, I is proportional to the mean squared (ms) sound pressure.

When $\mathrm{p(t)} = \mathrm{P_o} \sin(2\pi \mathrm{ft})$, it is easy to show that the ms sound pressure is $\mathrm{P_o^2}/2$, i.e., $1/2$ the peak pressure squared. For light, *radiant intensity* is also called the *irradiance,* with units of Watts/$\mathrm{m^2}$ incident on a surface.

A voltage signal such as an EEG recording can be described by its *average power,* given by its *mean squared voltage* divided by $\mathrm{R} = 1$ ohm:

$$\overline{\mathrm{P}} = \lim_{\mathrm{T} \to \infty} \frac{1}{\mathrm{T}} \int_0^{\mathrm{T}} \mathrm{v^2(t)\,dt} \quad \mathrm{Watts} \tag{1.5}$$

As you will see in Chapter 8, many statistical parameters can be attributed to signals, in addition to their sample means. These include the signal's *probability density function* and statistical measures such as its *variance*. Another important measure of a signal is its *frequency spectrum,* aka *power density spectrum,* with units of mean-squared volts (ms units) per Hz. A signal's *root power spectrum* is also used to describe noisy signals; it has the units of root-mean-squared volts per root Hz. The root power spectrum is simply the square root of the power density spectrum. The power spectrum describes the contribution to the total power of $\mathrm{u(t)}$ at each incremental frequency. It implies a superposition of spectral power.

Chapter 7 will show that nonstationary signals can be characterized by joint time-frequency plots. Special transforms are used to decompose a signal, $\mathrm{u(t)}$, into its spectral components as a function of time. A JTF spectrogram gives signal mean-squared volts (or rms volts) as a function of time and frequency, creating a 2- or 3-D display.

1.1.6 Introduction to modulation and demodulation of physiological signals

In general, modulation is a process whereby a signal of interest is combined mathematically with a high-frequency carrier wave to form a *modulated carrier* suitable for transmission to a receiver/demodulator where the signal is recovered.

Recorded physiological signals are modulated for two major reasons:

1. For robust transmission by wire or coaxial cable, fiber optic cable, or radio (telemetry by electromagnetic waves) from the recording site to the site where the signal will be processed and stored.
2. For effective data storage, for example, in *biotelemetry,* physiological signals such as the ECG and blood pressure modulate a carrier that is sent as an FM radio signal to a remote receiver where the signals are demodulated, digitized, filtered, analyzed and stored.

Modulation generally involves encoding a high-frequency *carrier wave,* which can be a continuous sine wave or a square wave (logic signal). There are *five* major types of modulation involving sinusoidal carrier waves:

1. Amplitude modulation (AM)
2. Single-sideband AM (SSBAM)
3. Frequency modulation (FM)
4. Phase modulation (PhM)
5. Double-sideband suppressed-carrier modulation (DSBSCM).

Modulation can also be done using a square wave (or TTL) carrier and can involve FM, PhM, delta modulation, or can use pulse position or pulse width at constant frequency. AM, FM and DSBSCM are expressed mathematically below for a sinusoidal carrier. $m(t)$ is the *normalized modulating signal,* in each case. $v_m(t)$ is the actual physiological signal. The maximum frequency of $m(t)$ must be $<< \omega_c$, the carrier frequency. $m(t)$ is defined by:

$$m(t) = \frac{v_m(t)}{V_{mmax}}, \quad 0 \le |m(t)| \le 1 \qquad \text{Normalized modulating signal} \quad (1.6A)$$

$$y_m(t) = A[1 + m(t)]\cos(\omega_c t) \qquad \text{AM} \quad (1.6B)$$

$$y_m(t) = A\cos\left[\omega_c t + K_f \int^t m(t)\,dt\right] \qquad \text{FM} \quad (1.6C)$$

$$y_m(t) = A\cos[\omega_c t + K_p m(t)] \qquad \text{PhM} \quad (1.6D)$$

$$y_m(t) = A\,m(t)\cos(\omega_c t) \qquad \text{DSBSCM} \quad (1.6E)$$

It is interesting to examine the frequency spectrums of the modulated signals. For illustrative purposes, let $m(t)$ be a pure cosine wave, $[m_o \cos(\omega_m t)]$, $0 < m_o \le 1$.

Thus, by trig identity, the AM signal can be rewritten:

$$y_m(t) = A\cos(\omega_c t) + (A\,m_o/2)[\cos((\omega_c + \omega_m)t) + \cos((\omega_c - \omega_m)t)] \quad (1.7)$$

Thus the AM signal has a carrier component and two *sidebands,* each spaced by the amount of the modulating frequency above and below the carrier frequency. In SSBAM, a sharp cut-off filter is used to eliminate either the upper or lower sideband; the information in both sidebands is redundant, so removing one means less bandwith is required to transmit the SSBAM signal.

FM and PhM are subsets of *angle modulation.* FM can be further classified as *broadband* or *narrowband FM* (NBFM). In FM, $K_f \equiv 2\pi f_d$, where f_d is called the frequency deviation constant. In NBFM, $f_d/f_{mmax} << 1$; (f_{mmax} is the highest expected frequency in $m(t)$, which is bandwidth-limited). Unlike AM, the frequency spectrum of an FM carrier is horrific to derive. Using $m(t) = m_o\cos(\omega_m t)$, we can write the FM carrier as:

$$y_m(t) = A\cos[\overset{\alpha}{\omega_c t} + \overset{\beta}{(K_f/\omega_m)m_o\sin(\omega_m t)}] \quad (1.8)$$

Using the trig identity, $\cos(\alpha+\beta) = \cos(\alpha)\cos(\beta) - \sin(\alpha)\sin(\beta)$, Equation 1.8 can be written as:

$$\begin{aligned} y_m(t) = {} & A\cos(\omega_c t)\cos[(K_f/\omega_m)m_o\sin(\omega_m t)] \\ & - A\sin(\omega_c t)\sin[(K_f/\omega_m)m_o\sin(\omega_m t)] \end{aligned} \quad (1.9)$$

Now the $\cos[(K_f/\omega_m)m_o\sin(\omega_m t)]$ and $\sin[(K_f/\omega_m)m_o\sin(\omega_m t)]$ terms can be expressed as two Fourier series whose coefficients are ordinary Bessel functions of the first kind and argument β [Clarke and Hess, 1971]; note that $\beta \equiv m_o 2\pi f_d/\omega_m$:

$$\cos[\beta\sin(\omega_m t)] = J_0(\beta) + 2\sum_{n=1}^{\infty} J_{2n}(\beta)\cos(2n\omega_m t) \quad (1.10A)$$

$$\sin[\beta\sin(\omega_m t)] = 2\sum_{n=0}^{\infty} J_{2n+1}(\beta)\sin[2(n+1)\omega_m t] \quad (1.10B)$$

The two Bessel sum relations for $\cos[\beta\sin(\omega_m t)]$ and $\sin[\beta\sin(\omega_m t)]$ can be recombined with Equation 1.9 using the trig identities, $\cos x\cos y = 1/2[\cos(x+y) + \cos(x-y)]$, and $\sin x\sin y = 1/2[\cos(x-y) - \cos(x+y)]$, and we can finally write for the FM carrier spectrum, letting $m_o = 1$:

$$\begin{aligned} y_m(t) = A\{ & J_0(\beta)\cos(\omega_c t) + J_1(\beta)[\cos((\omega_c+\omega_m)t) - \cos((\omega_c-\omega_m)t)] \\ & + J_2(\beta)[\cos((\omega_c+2\omega_m)t) + \cos((\omega_c-2\omega_m)t)] \\ & + J_3(\beta)[\cos((\omega_c+3\omega_m)t) - \cos((\omega_c-3\omega_m)t)] \\ & + J_4(\beta)[\cos((\omega_c+4\omega_m)t) + \cos((\omega_c-4\omega_m)t)] \\ & + J_5(\beta)[\cos((\omega_c+5\omega_m)t) - \cos((\omega_c-5\omega_m)t)] + \cdots\} \end{aligned} \quad (1.11)$$

At first inspection, this result appears quite messy. However, it is evident that the numerical values of the Bessel terms tend to zero as n becomes large. For example, let $\beta = 2\pi f_d/\omega_m = 1$, then $J_0(1) = 0.7852$, $J_1(1) = 0.4401$, $J_2(1) = 0.1149$, $J_3(1) = 0.01956$, $J_4(1) = 0.002477$, $J_5(1) = 0.0002498$, $J_6(1) = 0.00002094$, etc. Bessel constants $J_n(1)$ for $n \geq 4$ contribute less than 1% each to the $y_m(t)$ spectrum, so we can neglect them. Thus, the practical bandwidth of the FM carrier, $y_m(t)$, for $\beta = 1$ is $\pm 3\omega_m$ around the carrier frequency, ω_c. In general, as β increases, so does the effective bandwidth of the FM $y_m(t)$. For example, when $\beta = 5$, the bandwidth becomes $\pm 8\omega_m$ around ω_c, and when $\beta = 10$, the bandwidth required is $\pm 14\omega_m$ around ω_c [Clarke and Hess, 1971].

In the case of NBFM, $\beta << 1$. Thus, the modulated carrier can be written:

$$y_m(t) = A\cos[\overset{\alpha}{\omega_c t} + \overset{\beta}{(K_f/\omega_m)}\sin(\omega_m t)] \tag{1.12A}$$

$$\downarrow$$

$$\begin{aligned} y_m(t) &= A\{\cos(\omega_c t)\cos[\beta\sin(\omega_m t)] - \sin(\omega_c t)\sin[\beta\sin(\omega_m t)]\} \\ &\cong A\{\cos(\omega_c t)(1) - \sin(\omega_c t)[\beta\sin(\omega_m t)]\} \\ &= A\{\cos(\omega_c t) - (\beta/2)[\cos((\omega_c - \omega_m)t) - \cos((\omega_c + \omega_m)t)]\} \end{aligned} \tag{1.12B}$$

With the exception of signs of the sideband terms, the NBFM spectrum is very similar to the spectrum of an AM carrier [Zeimer and Tranter, 1990]; sum and difference frequency sidebands are produced around a central carrier.

The spectrum of a DSBSCM signal is given by:

$$\begin{aligned} y_m(t) = A\,m_o\cos(\omega_m t)\cos(\omega_c t) = (A\,m_o/2)[\cos((\omega_c + \omega_m)t) \\ + \cos((\omega_c - \omega_m)t)] \end{aligned} \tag{1.13}$$

That is, the information is contained in the two sidebands; there is no carrier. DSBSCM is widely used in instrumentation and measurement systems. For example, it is the natural result when a light beam is chopped in a photonic instrument such as a spectrophotometer, and also results when a Wheatstone bridge is given ac (carrier) excitation and nulled, then one (or more) arm resistances is slowly varied in time around its null value. DSBSCM is also present at the output of an LVDT (linear variable differential transformer) length sensor as the core is moved in and out [Northrop, 1997].

Of equal importance in the discussion of modulation is the process of *demodulation* or *detection,* in which the modulating signal, $v_m(t)$, is recovered from $y_m(t)$. There are generally several ways to modulate a given type of modulated signal and several ways to demodulate it. In the case of AM (or single-sideband AM), the signal recovery process is called *detection.*

There are several practical means of AM detection [Clarke and Hess, Chapter 10, 1971]. One simple form of AM detection is to rectify and low-pass filter $y_m(t)$. Another form of AM detection passes $y_m(t)$ through a square-law nonlinearity followed by a low-pass filter. However, the square-law detector suffers from the disadvantage of generating a second harmonic component of the recovered modulating signal. A third way to demodulate an AM carrier of the form given by Equation 1.6B is to mix it (multiply it) by a sinusoidal signal of the same frequency and phase as the carrier component of the $y_m(t)$. A phase-locked loop can be used for this purpose [Northrop, 1990]. Mathematically, we form the product:

$$y_{md}(t) = B\cos(\omega_c t)\{A\cos(\omega_c t) + (A m_o/2)[\cos((\omega_c + \omega_m)t) + \cos((\omega_c - \omega_m)t)]\} \tag{1.14}$$

By trig identity, we have:

$$y_{md}(t) = AB/2[1 + \cos(2\omega_c t)] + (AB m_o/4)[\cos(\omega_m t) + \cos((2\omega_c + \omega_m)t)] + (AB m_o/4)[\cos(-\omega_m t) + \cos((2\omega_c - \omega_m)t)] \tag{1.15}$$

After band-pass filtering to remove the dc term and the double carrier frequency terms and noting that $\cos(^*)$ is an even function, we obtain:

$$y_{mdBP}(t) = (AB/2)[m_o \cos(\omega_m t)] \tag{1.16}$$

Thus, we recover the normalized modulating signal, $[m_o \cos(\omega_m t)]$, times a scaling constant.

A fourth kind of AM demodulation can be done by finding the magnitude of the modulated signal's *analytical signal* (see Section 5.4).

Let us examine the widely used, rectifier + lowpass filter (average envelope) AM detector. Figure 1.1a illustrates a low-frequency modulating signal, $m(t)$ Figure 1.1b shows the amplitude-modulated carrier (the sinusoidal carrier is drawn with straight lines for simplicity). Figure 1.1c illustrates the block diagram of a simple half-wave rectifier circuit followed by a band-pass filter to exclude dc and terms of carrier frequency and higher. The half-wave rectification process can be thought of as multiplying the AM $y_m(t)$ by a 0, 1 switching function, $Sq(t)$, in phase with the carrier. Mathematically, this can be stated as:

$$y_{mr}(t) = A[1 + m\cos(\omega_m t)]\cos(\omega_c t)Sq(t) = A\cos(\omega_c t)Sq(t) + A m_o \cos(\omega_m t)\cos(\omega_c t)Sq(t) \tag{1.17}$$

$Sq(t)$ can be written as a *Fourier series* (see Chapter 4):

$$Sq(t) = 1/2 + (2/\pi)\sum_{n=1}^{\infty}(-1)^{n+1}\frac{\cos[(2n-1)\omega_c t]}{(2n-1)}$$
$$\downarrow$$
$$Sq(t) = 1/2 + (2/\pi)\{\cos(\omega_c t) - \frac{1}{3}\cos(3\omega_c t) + \frac{1}{5}\cos(5\omega_c t) - \ldots\} \tag{1.18}$$

Now we multiply the Fourier series by the terms of Equation 1.17:

$$y_d(t) = 1/2 A\cos(\omega_c t) + (2/\pi)A\{\cos^2(\omega_c t) - \frac{1}{3}\cos(\omega_c t)\cos(3\omega_c t) + \frac{1}{5}\cos(\omega_c t)\cos(5\omega_c t) - \ldots\} + 1/2 A m_o \cos(\omega_m t)\cos(\omega_c t)$$

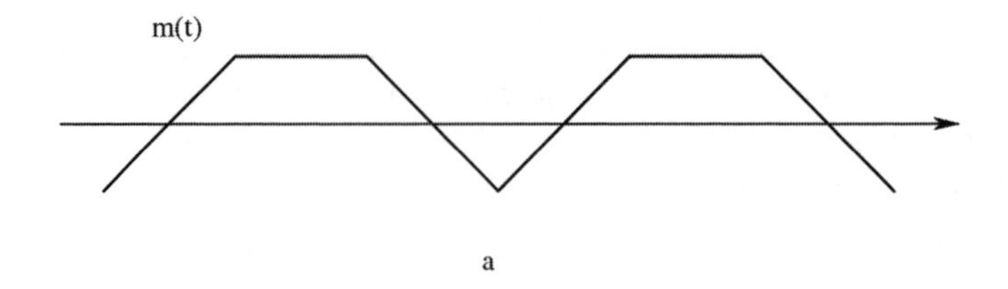

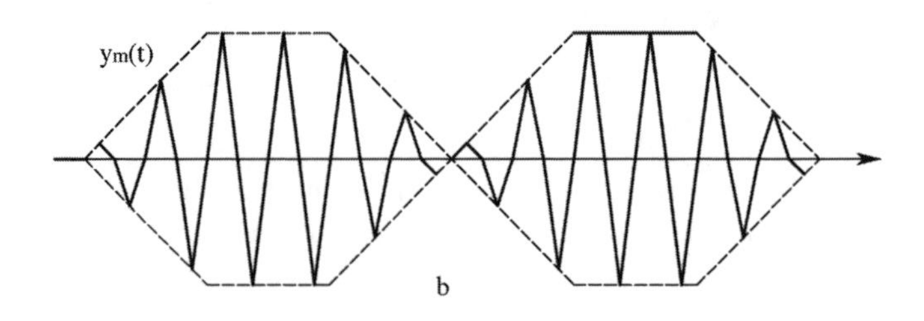

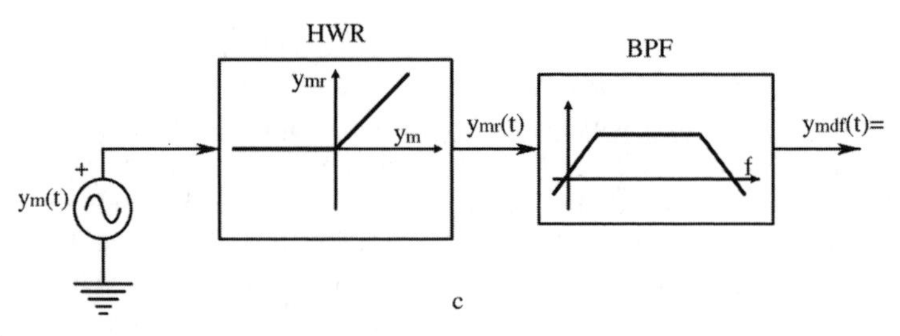

FIGURE 1.1
Detection of an AM carrier by a rectifier-band-pass filter. (a) The modulating signal. (b) The modulated carrier. (c) A simple, half-wave rectifier-BPF demodulator.

$$+(2\mathrm{A}\,\mathrm{m_o}/\pi)\cos(\omega_\mathrm{m}\,\mathrm{t})\cos^2(\omega_\mathrm{c}\,\mathrm{t}) - (2\mathrm{A}\,\mathrm{m_o}/3\pi)\cos(\omega_\mathrm{m}\,\mathrm{t})$$
$$\times\cos(\omega_\mathrm{c}\,\mathrm{t})\cos(3\omega_\mathrm{c}\,\mathrm{t}) + (2\mathrm{A}\,\mathrm{m_o}/5\pi)\cos(\omega_\mathrm{m}\,\mathrm{t})\cos(\omega_\mathrm{c}\,\mathrm{t})\cos(5\omega_\mathrm{c}\,\mathrm{t})$$
$$-(2\mathrm{A}\,\mathrm{m_o}/7\pi)\cos(\omega_\mathrm{m}\,\mathrm{t})\cos(\omega_\mathrm{c}\,\mathrm{t})\cos(7\omega_\mathrm{c}\,\mathrm{t}) + \ldots \tag{1.19}$$

Now let us examine what happens when we pass the terms of Equation 1.19 through a bandpass filter that attenuates to zero dc and all terms at above $(\omega_\mathrm{c} - \omega_\mathrm{m})$. Trig expansions of the form $\cos(\mathrm{x})\cos(\mathrm{y}) = \frac{1}{2}[\cos(\mathrm{x}+\mathrm{y}) + \cos(\mathrm{x}-\mathrm{y})]$ are used. Let the BPF's output be $\mathrm{y_{mdf}(t)}$:

$$\mathrm{y_{mdf}(t)} = (\mathrm{A}/\pi) + (\mathrm{A}/\pi)[\mathrm{m_o}\cos(\omega_\mathrm{m}\,\mathrm{t})] \tag{1.20}$$

The BPF output contains a *dc term* plus a term proportional to the desired $\mathrm{m_o}$ $\cos(\omega_m t)$. Because AM radio is usually used to transmit audio signals that do not extend to zero frequency, the *bandpass filter* blocks the dc but passes modulating signal frequencies. Thus, $\mathrm{y_{mdf}(t)} \propto \mathrm{m_o}\cos(\omega_\mathrm{m}\,\mathrm{t})$. Several other AM detection schemes exist, including *peak envelope detection* and *phase locked loops;* the interested reader can find a good description of these modes of AM detection in Clarke and Hess (1971).

When it is desired to modulate and transmit signals with a dc component, FM is the desired modulation scheme because a dc signal, V_m, produces a fixed frequency deviation from the carrier at ω_c given by:

$$\Delta\omega = (2\pi f_d)V_m \quad r/s \tag{1.21}$$

As in the case of AM, FM demodulation can be done by several means: The first step in any FM demodulation is to *limit the received signal.* Mathematically, limiting can be represented as passing the FM $y_m(t)$ through a signum function (symmetrical clipper). Mathematically, the clipper output is a square wave of peak height, $y_{mcl}(t) = B\,\mathrm{sgn}[y_m(t)]$. (The $\mathrm{sgn}(y_m)$ function is 1 for $y_m \geq 0$, and -1 for $y_m < 0$.) Clipping removes any unwanted amplitude modulation including noise on the received $y_m(t)$, one reason FM radio is noise free compared to AM. The frequency argument of $y_{mcl}(t)$ is the same as for the FM sinusoidal carrier, i.e., $\omega_{FM} = \omega_c + K_f v_m(t)$. Once limited, there are several means of FM demodulation, including the *phase-shift discriminator,* the *Foster-Seely discriminator,* the *ratio detector, pulse averaging,* and the *phase-locked loop* [Chirlian, 1981; Northrop, 1989]. It is beyond the scope of this text to describe all of these FM demodulation circuits in detail, so we will examine the simple pulse averaging discriminator. In this FM demodulation means, the limited signal is fed into a one-shot multivibrator that triggers on the rising edge of each cycle of $y_{mcl}(t)$, producing a train of standard TTL pulses, each of fixed width $\delta = \pi/\omega_c$ sec. For simplicity, assume the peak height of each pulse is 5 V and low is 0 V. Now the average pulse voltage is $v_{av}(t)$:

$$v_{av}(t) = \frac{1}{T}\int_0^{\delta} 5\,dt = \frac{\omega_c + K_f v_m}{\pi}\int_0^{\pi/\omega_c} 5\,dt = \frac{5}{2}(1 + K_f v_m/\omega_c) \tag{1.22}$$

Thus recovery of $v_m(t)$, even a dc v_m, requires:

$$v_m(t) = \left[\frac{2}{5}v_{av}(t) - 1\right](\omega_c/K_f) \tag{1.23}$$

In practice, the averaging is done by a low-pass filter with break frequency $\omega_{mmax} << \omega_f << \omega_c$.

In *phase modulation,* the modulated carrier is given by:

$$y_m(t) = A\cos[\omega_c t + K_p v_m(t)] \tag{1.24}$$

Because the frequency of the PhM carrier is the derivative of its phase, we have:

$$\omega_{PhM} = \omega_c + K_p \dot{v}_m(t) \tag{1.25}$$

PhM carriers can be both generated and demodulated using phase-locked loops [Northrop, 1989].

The demodulation of DSBSCM carriers is generally done by a phase-sensitive rectifier, (also known as a synchronous rectifier) followed by a low-pass filter. Another means of demodulating a DSBSC signal is by an *analog multiplier.* In the latter means, the multiplier output voltage, z(t), is the product of a *reference carrier* and the DSBSCM signal:

$$z(t) = (0.1)B\cos(\omega_c t) \times (A m_o/2)[\cos((\omega_c + \omega_m)t) + \cos((\omega_c - \omega_m)t)] \tag{1.26}$$

By trig identity, noting that $\cos\theta$ is an even function, the multiplier output can be written:

$$z(t) = (0.1)(A m_o B/4)[\cos((2\omega_c + \omega_m)t) + \cos(\omega_m t)] \tag{1.27}$$

After unity-gain low-pass filtering, we have:

$$\overline{z(t)} = (0.1)(AB/4)m_o \cos(\omega_m t) \tag{1.28}$$

which is certainly proportional to $v_m(t)$.

TTL FM carriers can be modulated using *voltage-to-frequency converter* integrated circuits.

The frequency output of such an IC is given by:

$$f_o = k_1 + K_v v_m(t) \quad \text{Hz.} \tag{1.29}$$

Obviously, $k_1 = f_c$, the unmodulated carrier frequency. Many VCO ICs will give simultaneous TTL, triangle and sinusoidal wave outputs over a sub-Hz to over 10 MHz range.

One way to produce a TTL wave whose *duty cycle is modulated* by $v_m(t)$ is to begin with a constant frequency, zero mean, symmetrical triangle wave, $v_T(t)$, as shown in Figure 1.2. $v_T(t)$ is one input to an analog comparator with TTL output. The other input is $v_m(t)$. As $v_m(t)$ approaches the peak voltage of the triangle wave, V_p, the duty cycle, η, of the TTL wave approaches unity; similarly, as $v_m(t) \to -V_p$, $\eta \to 0$. Mathematically, the duty cycle is defined as the positive pulse width, δ, divided by the triangle wave period, T. In other words, the comparator TTL output is HI for $v_m(t) > v_T(t)$. From the foregoing, it is easy to derive the TTL wave's duty cycle:

$$\eta = \delta/T = \tfrac{1}{2}[1 + v_m(t)/V_p] \tag{1.30}$$

Here we assume $v_m(t)$ is changing slowly enough to be considered to be constant over $T/2$.

Demodulation of a pulse-width-modulated TTL carrier is done by averaging the TTL pulse train and subtracting out the dc component present when $v_m = 0$.

Let us now consider *delta modulation* (DM) and *demodulation.* A delta modulator is also known as a 1-bit, *differential pulse code modulator* (DPCM). The output of a delta modulator is a clocked (periodic) train of TTL pulses with amplitudes that are either HI or LO depending on the state of the comparator output shown in Figure 1.3. The DM output basically tracks the derivative of the input signal. The comparator output is TTL HI if $e(t) = [v_m(t) - v_r'(t)] > 0$, and LO if $e < 0$. The D flip-flop's (DFF) complimentary output ($\overline{Q} = V_o$) is LO if the comparator output is HI at a positive transition of the TTL clock signal. The LO output of the DFF remains LO until the next positive transition of the clock signal. Then, if the comparator output has gone LO, V_o goes high for one clock period (T_c), etc. $v_r'(t)$ is the output of the analog integrator offset by V_{bias}, which is one half the maximum v_r ramp height over one clock period. V_{bias} can be shown to be $1.1T_c/(RC)$ volts. With this V_{bias}, when $v_m(t) = 0$, $v_r'(t)$ will oscillate around zero with a triangle wave with zero mean and peak height $1.1T_c/(RC)$ volts. Note that the $\overline{Q}$ output of the

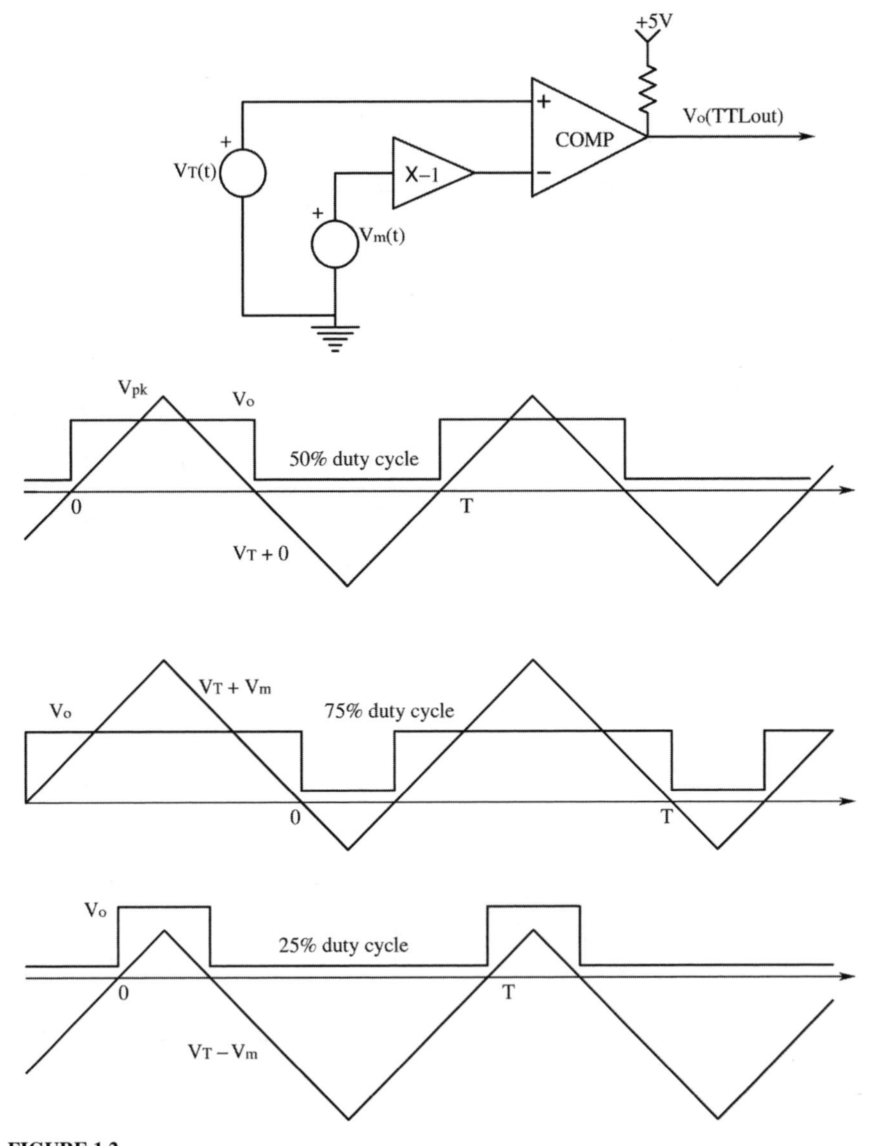

FIGURE 1.2
System to make a duty-cycle-modulated TTL wave of constant frequency. A low-frequency modulating signal, $-V_m(t)$ is added to a symmetrical triangle wave at the input of an analog comparator.

DFF must be used because the integrator gain is negative (i.e., $-1/RC$). That is, a HI V_o will cause v_r' to go negative and a low V_o will make v_r' go positive. Note that $v_r'(t)$ is *slew rate limited* at $\pm$ (2.2V/RC) volts/sec and if the slope of $v_m(t)$ exceeds this value, a large error will accumulate in the demodulation operation of the DM signal. (Slew rate is simply the magnitude of the first derivative of a signal, i.e., its

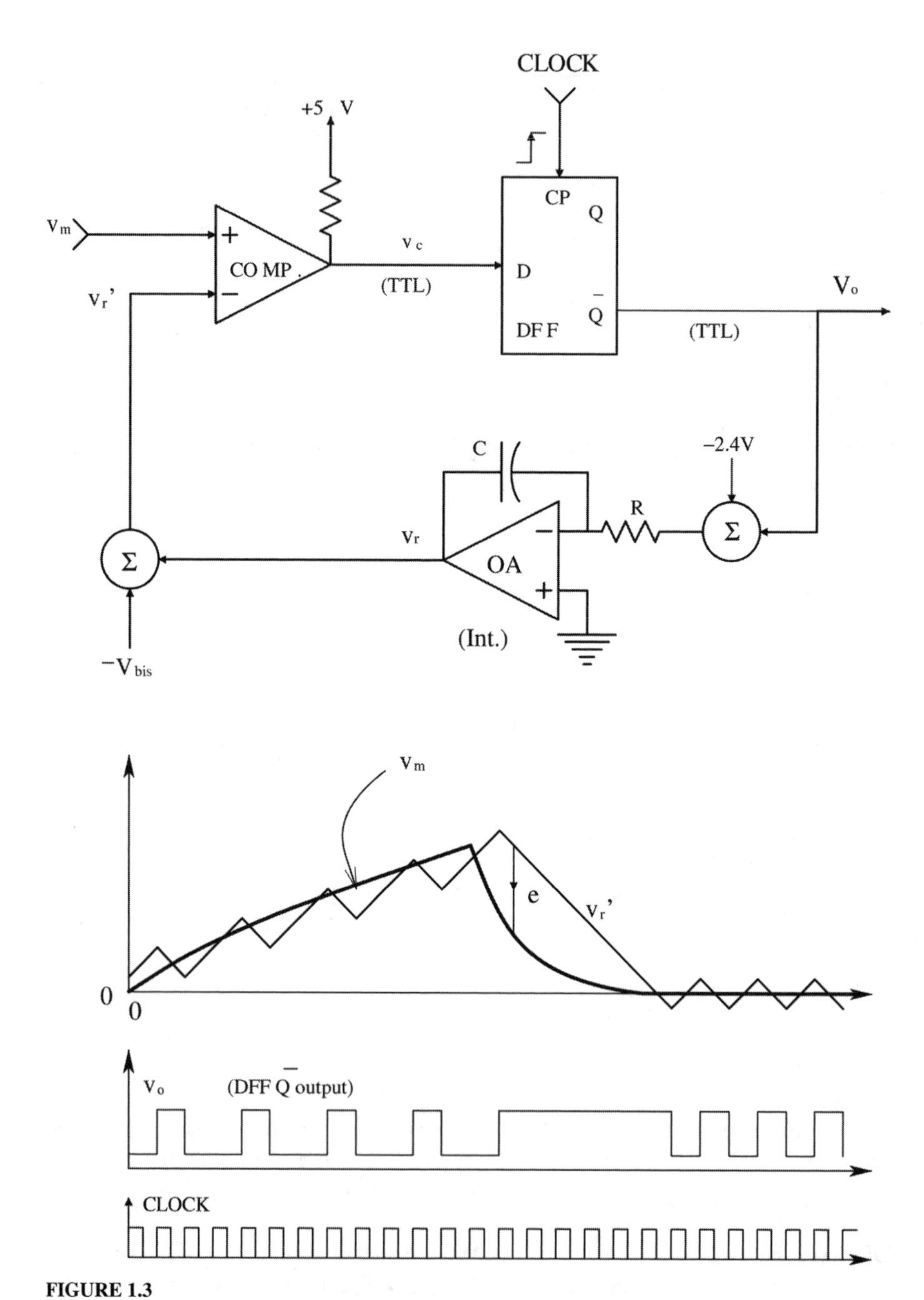

FIGURE 1.3

Top: Circuit of a delta modulator. Bottom: The associated waveforms of the delta modulator.

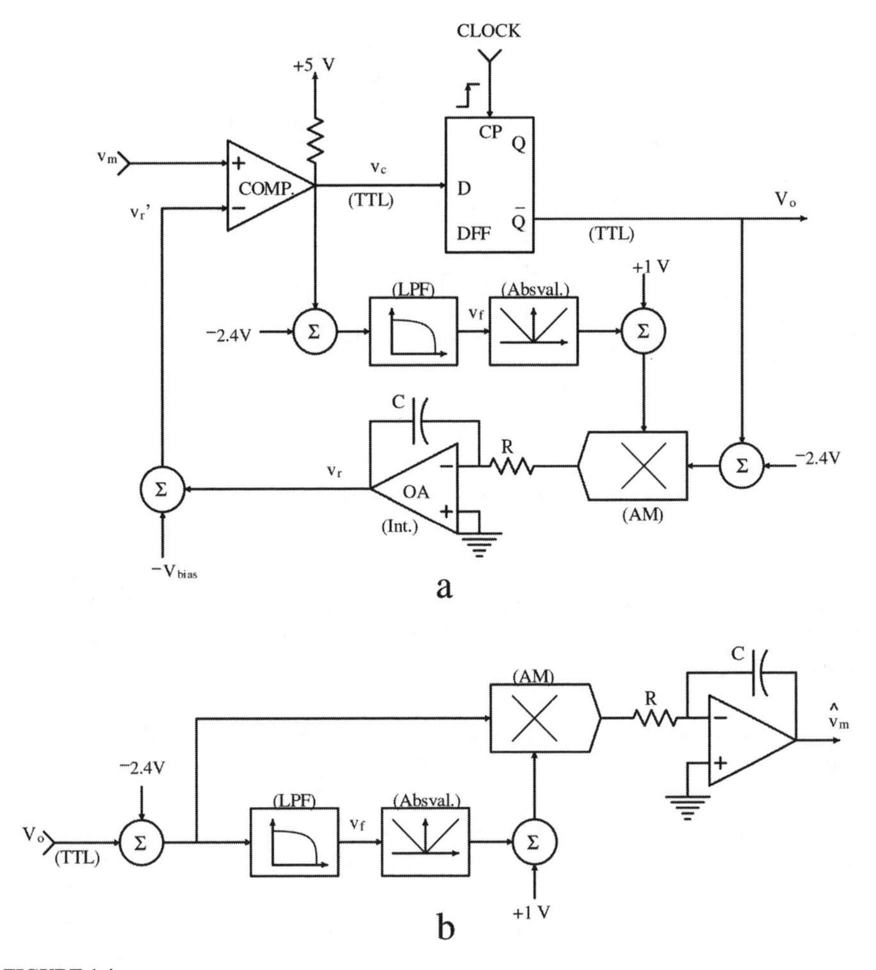

FIGURE 1.4
(a) Circuit for an adaptive delta modulator. (b) Demodulator for a ADM TTL signal.

slope.) When a DM system is tracking $v_m = 0$, $v_r'(t)$ oscillates around zero and the DM output is a periodic square wave, 1-bit "noise".

In *adaptive delta modulation* (ADM), the magnitude of the error is used to adjust the effective gain of the integrator to increase the slew rate of $v_r'(t)$ to better track rapidly changing $v_m(t)$. One version of an ADM system is shown along with pertinent waveforms in Figure 1.4. Note that, ideally, the comparator should perform the signum operation, hence we must subtract out the dc value (mean) of the TTL wave before it is filtered, absval'd and used to modulate the size of the square wave input to the integrator. A conventional analog multiplier is used as a modulator. If a large error occurs as a result of poor tracking due to low slew rate in $v_r'(t)$, the comparator output will remain HI (or LO) for a number of clock cycles. This condition produces a nonzero signal at v_f, which, in turn, increases the amplitude of the symmetrical pulse

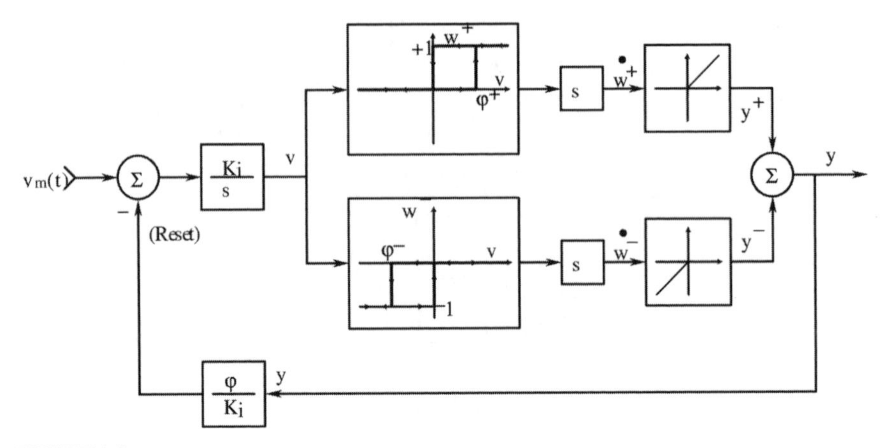

FIGURE 1.5
A two-sided, integral pulse frequency modulation (IPFM) system. Positive or negative unit impulses are emitted, depending on the polarity of $v_m(t)$.

input to the integrator. When the ADM is tracking well so that $v_r'(t)$ oscillates around a nearly constant v_m level, then $v_f \to 0$ and the peak amplitude of the error remains small. In summary, the ADM acts to minimize the mean squared error between $v_m(t)$ and $v_r'(t)$.

Besides the one shown above, there are other variations on DM, such as sigma-delta modulation, and other types of nonlinear adaptive DM designs. Much of the interest in efficient, simple, low-noise modulation schemes has been driven by the need to transmit sound and pictures over the Internet. Medical signals such as ECG and EEG also benefit from this development, because of the need to transmit them from the site of the patient to a diagnostician. Biotelemetry is an important technology in the wireless monitoring of internal physiological states, sports medicine, emergency medicine and in ecological studies.

Finally, let us consider *integral-* and *relaxation-pulse frequency modulation* (IPFM and RPFM). A systems model for a two-sided IPFM system is shown in Figure 1.5. A positive modulating signal, v_m, is integrated; the integrator output, v, goes to two threshold nonlinearities. When v reaches the positive threshold, φ_+, the nonlinearity's output, w^+, jumps to $+1$. This step is differentiated to make a positive unit impulse at time t_k, $\delta(t-t_k)$. This impulse is fed back, given a weight of φ/K_i and subtracted from the input to form $e(t_k) = v_m(t_k) - (\varphi/K_i)\delta(t-t_k)$. When integrated, this $e(t_k)$ resets the integrator output to zero and the process repeats. If $v_m < 0$, v approaches the negative threshold, φ^-. When φ^- is reached, the output from the two-sided IPFM system is a negative unit impulse. The net output from the IPFM system can be written as:

$$y(t) = \sum_{k=1}^{\infty} \delta(t-t_k) - \sum_{j=1}^{\infty} \delta(t-t_j) \tag{1.31}$$

where $\{t_k\}$ are the times that $+$ pulses are emitted and $\{t_j\}$ are the times that negative pulses occur. Many low-frequency physiological signals such as body temperature and blood pressure are positive, so the negative pulse channel on the IPFM system can be deleted. Note that a one-sided IPFM system behaves like a classical pulse FM system with a positive modulating signal and zero carrier frequency. If the modulating signal is small, the output pulse rate will be low and the IPFM system will be poor at following high-frequency perturbations superimposed on $v_m > 0$. IPFM and RPFM, described below, have been used to emulate nerve impulse generation in neural modeling studies [Northrop, 2001].

One-sided IPFM can be described mathematically by a set of integral equations:

$$v = \int K_i e(t)\, dt \tag{1.32}$$

$$\varphi = \int_{tk-1}^{tk} K_i e(t)\, dt, \quad k = 2, 3, \ldots, \infty \tag{1.33}$$

Where: K_i is the integrator gain. $e(t)$ is its input; $e(t) = v_m(t)$ for $t_{k-1} < t < t_k$. t_k is the time the kth pulse is emitted. $v(t_{k-1}) = 0$ due to resetting. Equation 1.33 can be rewritten as:

$$r_k = \frac{1}{t_k - t_{k-1}} = \frac{K_i}{\varphi} \frac{1}{t_k - t_{k-1}} \int_{t_{k-1}}^{t_k} e(t)\, dt, \quad k = 2, 3 \ldots \tag{1.34}$$

Here r_k is the kth *element of instantaneous frequency,* defined as the reciprocal of the interval between the kth and $(k-1)^{th}$ output pulses, $\tau_k = (t_k - t_{k-1})$. So the kth element of instantaneous (pulse) frequency is given by:

$$r_k \equiv 1/\tau_k = (K_i/\varphi)\overline{\{e\}}_{\tau k} \tag{1.35}$$

Thus, if v_m is constant and $v_m \geq 0$, $r = (K_i/\varphi)v_m$ pps. That is, the IPFM output frequency is proportional to the input signal amplitude.

As an example of finding the pulse emission times for a one-sided IPFM system, consider the input, $v_m(t) = 4e^{-7t}U(t)$, the threshold $\varphi = 0.025$ V and $K_i = 1$. The first pulse is emitted at t_1, which is found from the definite integral:

$$\begin{aligned} \varphi &= \int_0^{t1} v_m(t)\, dt \rightarrow 0.025 = \int_0^{t1} \frac{4e^{-7t}(-7)\, dt}{(-7)} \rightarrow \frac{-7 \times 0.025}{4} \\ &= (e^{-7t_1} - 1) \rightarrow \\ e^{-7t_1} &= (1 - 4.3750\text{E} - 2) \rightarrow -7t_1 = -4.4736\text{E} - 2 \\ &\rightarrow t_1 = 6.3908\text{E} - 3 \text{ sec.} \end{aligned} \tag{1.36}$$

The general pulse emission time, t_k, is found by recursion. For example, once t_1 is known, t_2 is found by solving:

$$\varphi = \int_{t1}^{t2} v_m(t)\, dt \tag{1.37}$$

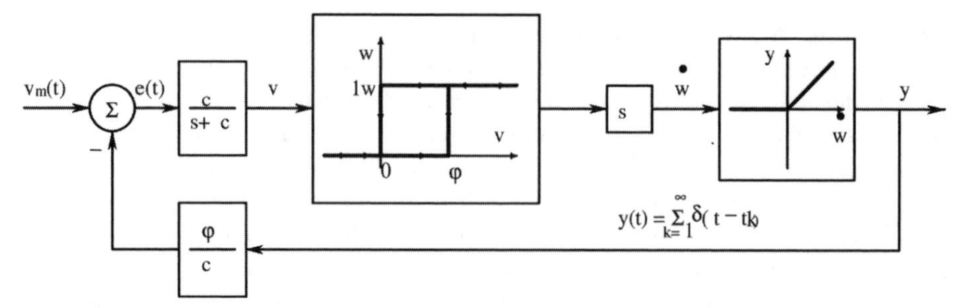

FIGURE 1.6
A one-sided, relaxation pulse frequency modulation (RPFM) system. The simple low-pass filter has finite "memory".

In this simple case it is found that $t_2 = 13.081\,E{-}3$ sec. A general formula for t_k is found for this problem by induction:

$$t_k = -\frac{1}{7}\ln\left[1 - \frac{k \times 7 \times 0.025}{4}\right] \tag{1.38}$$

From Equation 1.38, we see that t_k is only defined for a positive $\ln[*]$ argument. That is, for

$$k \leq \frac{4}{7 \times 0.025} = 22.875 \tag{1.39}$$

Thus $k_{max} = 22$; only 22 pulses are emitted.

RPFM differs from IPFM in that the integrator is replaced by a simple real-pole lowpass filter as shown in Figure 1.6. Resetting the low-pass filter output to zero is accomplished in the same manner as with IPFM by the output pulses. RPFM makes a better model for neuron spike generation because it has a finite "memory" to inputs; i.e., $v \to 0$ if $v_m = 0$.

As an example of finding the output times of pulses from a one-sided RPFM system, consider the RPFM system illustrated in Figure 1.6. Let the input be the same as for the one-sided IPFM system described above, $v_m(t) = 4e^{-7t}U(t)$, with the threshold $\varphi = 0.001$ V. The RPFM low-pass filter has natural frequency $c = 100$ r/s. When the input is first applied at $t = 0$, the filter output v rises from zero toward the threshold, φ, which it crosses at $t = t_1$. Simultaneously, a unit impulse is emitted from the RPFM system, and that impulse causes v to go abruptly from φ to 0. The process repeats itself until there is not enough amplitude left in $v_m(t)$ to cause v to reach φ. The RPFM low-pass filter has the impulse response,

$$h(t) = ce^{-ct}, \quad t \geq 0 \tag{1.40}$$

The general equation for pulse emission times involves the recursive solution of an integral equation based on *real convolution* [see Section 2.4.3]:

$$\varphi = \int_{t_{k-1}}^{t_k} 4e^{-7\mu}ce^{-c(t-\mu)}\,d\mu, \quad k = 1, 2, \ldots, t_0 = 0 \tag{1.41}$$

While simple in appearance, solution of Equation 1.41 for t_k requires the solution of a transcendental equation having the difference of two exponential terms, and must be done by trial and error on paper. It is much better to solve for the $\{t_k\}$ by computer [Northrop, 2001].

Demodulation of IPFM and RPFM positive pulse trains can be done by passing the pulses through a low-pass filter, or actually calculating the pulse train's instantaneous frequency by taking the reciprocal of the time interval between any two pulses and holding that value until the next pulse $[(k+1)^{th}]$ occurs in the sequence, then repeating the operation. Stated mathematically, instantaneous pulse frequency demodulation (IPFD) can be written:

$$\hat{v}_m(t) = \sum_{k=2}^{\infty} r_k\{U(t-t_k) - U(t-t_{k+1})\} \quad (1.42)$$

where

$$r_k \equiv 1/\tau_k = \frac{1}{t_k - t_{k-1}}, \quad k = 2, 3, \ldots \quad (1.43)$$

Note that two pulses $(k = 2)$ are required to define the first pulse interval. $\hat{v}_m(t)$ is a series of steps, the height of each being the (previous) r_k. Note that IPFD is not limited to the demodulation of IPFM and RPFM, it has been experimentally applied as a descriptor to actual neural spike signals [Northrop, 2001].

In discussing the instantaneous frequency of sinusoidal waveforms such as $y_m(t) = A\cos[\theta(t)]$, the IF $\varphi(t)$ is generally given as:

$$\varphi(t) = d\theta(t)/dt \quad r/sec. \quad (1.44)$$

That is, the IF is the derivative of the trig function's phase argument in radians.

1.2 General Properties of Physiological Systems

1.2.1 Introduction

First, let us consider the meaning of the term system. In practice, system is used in a fuzzy manner; every dictionary and engineering text contains a broad range of definitions for it. In biology and medicine, many systems can be identified. These include but are not limited to: the nervous system, musculoskeletal, respiratory, circulatory, immune, digestive, reproductive, auditory, visual, olfactory, glucoregulatory and gustatory systems etc. It is important to realize that none of these systems is isolated; all physiological systems are interconnected to some degree. Each system has identifiable components which interact. Each also has one or more inputs (excitations or commands) and one or more parameters which can be considered to be outputs (responses). Some of these inputs and outputs are *observable signals,* others are *unobservable.*

Obviously, "system" is also used in a broader context than physiology; for example, we have economic systems, the solar system, ecosystems, electromechanical systems, refrigeration systems, heating systems, ignition systems, computer systems, etc. *The common feature of all systems is that each one is formed from a collection of interconnected, interacting, interdependent, dynamic elements.* The elements can be physical entities such as neurons, mechanical components (springs, masses, dashpots), electronic circuits (resistors, capacitors, op amps, etc.), or be abstract, causal relations such as those found in economics. A system can be *continuous* (i.e., analog) or *discrete* (i.e., digital). First, we will describe analog systems.

1.2.2 Analog systems

Analog systems can be formed from elements which obey different physical laws; i.e., diffusion, chemical mass-action, Newton's second law, Kirchoff's laws, Boyle's law, Maxwell's equations, etc. If the analog system is linear, then it can be modeled or described mathematically by a set of linear *ordinary differential equations* (ODEs). A linear system's ODEs can be put on the form of a set of n first-order, ODEs, written in *state variable form* as:

$$\dot{\mathbf{x}} = \mathbf{x}\mathbf{A} + \mathbf{B}\mathbf{u} \tag{1.45}$$

Here **x** in an nth order column vector of the states, $\mathrm{x_1, x_2, \ldots x_n}$, $\dot{\mathbf{x}}$ is the nth order column vector of the state derivatives, $\dot{\mathrm{x}}_1, \dot{\mathrm{x}}_2, \ldots, \dot{\mathrm{x}}_\mathrm{n}$, **A** is the $n \times n$ system coefficient matrix **B** is the $n \times b$ input coefficient matrix, and **u** is the b inputs' column vector. When the elements of the **A** and **B** matrices are constant, the system is said to be *linear time-invariant* (LTI). (LTI systems are stationary, but not all stationary systems are linear.) If one or more elements in **A** and **B** vary in time, the system is said to be linear time-variable (LTV). These equations can be solved for the n states, **x**, given ICs and **u** for $\mathrm{t} \geq 0$. More on the solutions later. Note that system states, or functions of states, can be signals. Some states can be observable (measurable), others cannot be measured; they must be calculated.

1.2.3 Physiological systems

Physiology is the study of living systems. Certain living systems are legendary in their complexity; e.g., the CNS and the immune system, and defy attempts at modeling. Other physiological systems, such as the glucoregulatory system, have fewer states (n is smaller) and have been modeled more successfully by various workers [Northrop, 2000].

Below we list some general properties of physiological systems (PSs). These are *bulk properties,* i.e., they apply to entire systems. Some properties may seem rather obvious, others are not.

1. *PSs are generally multiple-input, multiple output (MIMO) systems. They generally have cross-coupling and interactions with related PSs.* Cross-coupling can arise from shared nervous system pathways, shared effector organs, such as the kidneys, or a hormone affecting more than one class of target cells (*pleiotropy*) *in different ways.*

2. *PSs often have transport lags (dead time) between their nodes.* Such lags can arise from the time it takes a hormone to activate a multistep biosynthetic pathway, as well as the finite time it takes nerve impulses to propagate down an axon and reach the target organ (muscle, gland, etc.). Transport lags can create stability problems in closed-loop control systems. Endogenous PRCs seldom have stability problems because their loop gains are generally low.

3. *All PSs are nonlinear.* This is not surprising because there are no negative concentrations or hormone release rates. Nonlinearities also enter PRCs from mass-action kinetics, saturation of a finite number of cell membrane receptors with a hormone, and intrinsic biochemical regulatory mechanisms that regulate biosynthesis. Fortunately, many PSs can be linearized around an operating point to expedite analysis and modeling.

4. *PSs are massively parallel systems.* Every organ is composed of hundreds of thousands of cells that have similar functions and each cell or functional group of cells may receive inputs in parallel, e.g., from nerve fibers serving a common purpose, or a hormone that affects all the cells simultaneously. Such redundant parallel architecture ensures robust behavior under conditions of injury or infection.

1.2.4 Discrete systems

No discrete systems in nature; discrete systems are man-made. Do not confuse a discrete system with one made up from many, parallel, closely-related or redundant components, such as the central nervous system. One example of a *discrete system* is a digital filter used to condition a sampled signal. The filter's I/O characteristics can be described by a set of *difference equations.* In general, The numerical outputs, $\mathbf{y}(\mathrm{k})$, of a discrete system are functions of present and past states and present and past inputs. In general, time-domain, matrix notation:

$$\mathbf{x}(\mathrm{k}+1) = \mathbf{Ax}(\mathrm{k}) + \mathbf{Bu}(\mathrm{k}) \tag{1.46A}$$

$$\mathbf{y}(\mathrm{k}) = \mathbf{Cx}(\mathrm{k}) + \mathbf{Du}(\mathrm{k}) \tag{1.46B}$$

Where $\mathbf{x}(\mathrm{k}+1)$ is an $\mathrm{n} \times 1$ (column) matrix of the discrete states at the next, $(\mathrm{k}+1)^{\mathrm{th}}$ sampling instant, $\mathbf{x}(\mathrm{k})$ is the state column matrix at the (present) k^{th} sampling instant, $\mathbf{A}$ is the $\mathrm{n} \times \mathrm{n}$, discrete state transition matrix. There are m inputs described at the kth instant by the $\mathrm{m} \times 1$, $\mathbf{u}(\mathrm{k})$ matrix. There are p outputs described by the $\mathrm{p} \times 1$, $\mathbf{y}(\mathrm{k})$ matrix. $\mathbf{B}$ is of order $\mathrm{n} \times \mathrm{m}$, $\mathbf{C}$ is of order $\mathrm{p} \times \mathrm{n}$, and $\mathbf{D}$ is of order $\mathrm{p} \times \mathrm{m}$.

In a stationary, time-invariant, discrete system, the elements of the **A**, **B**, **C** and **D** matrices are constant, i.e., they do not change with k.

An example of a simple, discrete, model for an economic system given by Rugh 1996 allows estimation of the national income, $y(k)$ in year k. $y(k)$ is the sum of *consumer expenditure,* $c(k)$, plus *government expenditure,* $g(k)$, plus *private investment,* $p(k)$. These parameters are assumed to be interrelated by the following models: First, consumer expenditure in year $k+1$ is assumed to be proportional to the national income in year k, i.e., $c(k+1) = \mu y(k)$. μ is called the *marginal propensity to consume.* Next, private investment in year k is assumed to be proportional to the increase in consumer expenditure from year k to year $k+1$. That is, $p(k+1) = \rho[c(k+1) - c(k)]$. (Note that $[c(k+1) - c(k)]$ is used as a simple approximation to $\dot{c}(t)$.)

From these model assumptions, the two difference equations can be written:

$$c(k+1) = \mu[c(k) + p(k) + g(k)] \tag{1.47A}$$

$$p(k+1) = (\rho\mu - \rho)c(k) + \rho\mu p(k) + \rho\mu g(k) \tag{1.47B}$$

We now define the state variables as $x_1(k) \equiv c(k)$ and $x_2(k) \equiv p(k)$, $y(k)$ is the output, and government expenditure, $g(k)$ is considered to be the input. The system's discrete state equations can finally be written:

$$\mathbf{x}(k+1) = \begin{vmatrix} \mu & \mu \\ \rho(\mu - 1) & \rho\mu \end{vmatrix} \mathbf{x}(k) + \begin{vmatrix} \mu \\ \rho\mu \end{vmatrix} g(k) \tag{1.48A}$$

$$\mathbf{y}(k) = [1\,1]\mathbf{x}(k) + g(k), \quad k = 0, 1, 2, 3, \ldots \tag{1.48B}$$

Other examples of discrete systems are given in Section 2.5. There attention is given to the use of the delay operator, $z^{-1} \equiv e^{-sT}$ and the use of the z-transform in solving discrete system equations.

1.3 Summary

In this introductory chapter, we have introduced, with examples, the key concepts of analog and discrete signals and analog and discrete systems. The properties system of linearity and stationarity were also described, as well as signal nonstationarity. Linear, stationary, analog and discrete systems were seen to be describable in terms of sets of linear, time-invariant, ordinary differential equations, or difference equations, respectively. Various ways to modulate and demodulate exogenous biomedical signals were also given.

Problems

1.1 A step of voltage is the input to the IPFM system illustrated in text Figure 1.5 in which $K_i = 1$ and $\varphi = 0.1$ The step input is:

$$v_m(t) = A\,U(t)$$

Find an expression for the output instantaneous frequency as a function of A.

1.2 An RPFM spike generator system (SGS) is described by the system:

$$v_m(t) = A\sum_{k=0}^{\infty}\delta(t-kT)$$
$$\tau\dot{v}+v = v_m - (\varphi\tau)\delta(v-\varphi)$$
$$y = \delta(v-\varphi)$$

Where: The system input is a train of impulses of area A occurring with period T. The RPFM system output is y and its time constant is τ. $A = 0.5$, $\varphi = 1.3$, $\tau = 0.667$ sec.

a. Draw a functional block diagram of the system.

b. Find the T value above which the RPFM SGS will never fire.

c. Now assume the SGS input is only two impulses: $v_m = A\delta(t) + A\delta(t-\delta)$. Find the range of instantaneous frequency, $r = \delta^{-1}$, over which a single output pulse is produced.

Note: Parts b and c can be solved analytically or by simulation.

1.3 Naturally occurring physiological signals recorded from the human body generally require signal conditioning before digitizing and recording. For the signals listed below, give the typical range of amplitudes where applicable and the frequency band limits (low and high break frequencies) required to faithfully amplify the signals. Note: a direct-coupled amplifier may be required in some cases. (Use the internet, a physiology text, Northrop (2002), Webster (1992), etc.)

a. Lead II ECG.

b. EEG recorded from scalp.

c. EMG of a contracting muscle recorded from the skin surface.

d. Electroretinogram (ERG).

e. Electrocochleogram (ECoG).

f. Foetal ECG recorded from mother's abdomen.

g. Nerve action potentials recorded with an intracellular microelectrode.

h. Respiratory sounds recorded with a microphone on the chest surface.

i. Heart sounds recorded with a broad-band microphone on the chest surface.

j. Blood pressure measured in the femoral artery by an electronic transducer in a catheter.

k. Blood glucose concentration measured by an electrochemical sensor in a catheter.

1.4 Figure P1.4 illustrates a DSBSC modulation/demodulation system. The carrier is delayed δ seconds in transmission to demodulator multiplier, D. The signal is $\mathrm{m(t)} = \mathrm{M_o}\cos(\omega_\mathrm{m}\mathrm{t})$, the carrier is $\mathrm{c(t)} = \mathrm{C}\cos(\omega_\mathrm{c}\mathrm{t})$. Note that $\omega_\mathrm{m} << \omega_\mathrm{c}$, and the low-pass filter blocks frequencies above $\omega_\mathrm{c}/2$. The trig identities for $(\cos\alpha\cos\beta)$ and $(\cos\alpha + \cos\beta)$ will be helpful. Find expressions for:

a. $\mathrm{w(t)}$.

b. $\mathrm{c}_\delta(\mathrm{t})$.

c. $\mathrm{z(t)}$.

d. $\overline{\mathrm{z(t)}}$. Comment on the effect of the delay, δ.

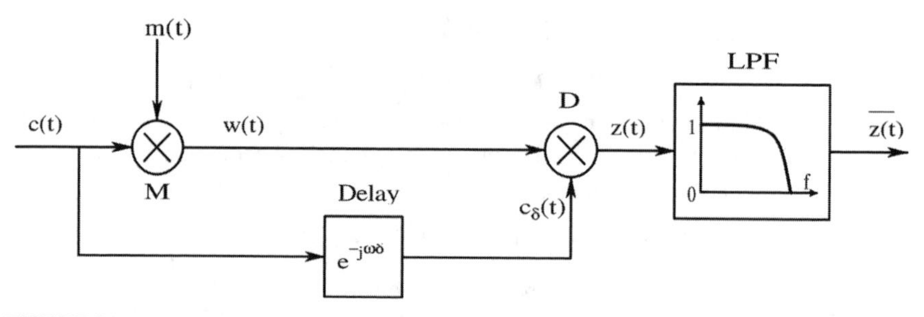

FIGURE P1.4

1.5 A DSBSC signal is modulated by multiplication by a square wave as shown in Figure P1.5. The signum function, $\mathrm{y} = \mathrm{sgn(x)}$, returns $\mathrm{y} = 1$ for $\mathrm{x} > 0$, $\mathrm{y} = 0$ for $\mathrm{x} = 0$ and $\mathrm{y} = -1$ for $\mathrm{x} < 0$. The carrier is $\mathrm{c(t)} = \cos(\omega_\mathrm{c}\mathrm{t})$. Let $\mathrm{m(t)} = 5[1+\cos(\omega_\mathrm{m}\mathrm{t})]$, with $\omega_\mathrm{c} = 10\omega_\mathrm{m} = 10\ \mathrm{r/sec}$. Sketch and dimension $\mathrm{c(t)}$, $\mathrm{sgn(c)}$, $\mathrm{w(t)}$, and $\mathrm{z(t)}$.

1.6 An RPFM (leaky integrator) SGS is used to model a nerve spike generator. It is described by the equations:

$$\tau\dot{\mathrm{v}} + \mathrm{v} = \mathrm{v_m(t)} - (\varphi\tau)\delta(\mathrm{v} - \varphi)$$
$$\mathrm{y} = \delta(\mathrm{v} - \varphi)$$

Where $\mathrm{v_m(t)} = 4\mathrm{e}^{-7\mathrm{t}}\mathrm{U(t)}$, $\varphi = 0.025$, and $\tau = 0.01$ sec.

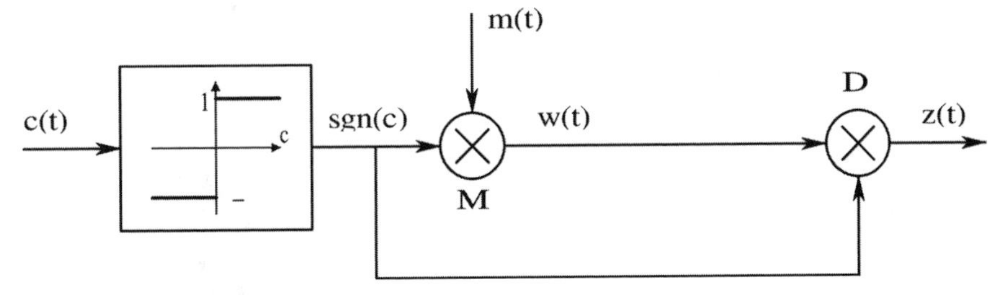

FIGURE P1.5

a. Find a general expression for t_k, the time of the kth output pulse.

b. How many output pulses occur?

c. Find the maximum instantaneous pulse frequency output.

d. Find the range of peak input voltage at $t = 0$ for which only one output pulse will occur.

1.7 Find an algebraic expression for the mean value of a full-wave rectified sine wave, $x(t) = X_o|\sin(\omega_o t)|$. Note that the average over all time for a periodic function is equal to the average over one period, T. Also, $\omega_o \equiv 2\pi/T$.

1.8 Find the root-mean-squared (rms) value of $x(t) = X_o \cos(\omega_o t)$.

1.9 Find an expression for the mean squared value of $x(t) = X_o[\sin(\omega_o t) + 1]$.

1.10 Find an expression for the mean squared value of $x(t) = X_o|\sin(\omega_o t)|$.

1.11 Find the rms value of the cosine square wave, Sq(t):

$$\mathrm{Sq}(t) = X_o \mathrm{sgn}[\cos(\omega_o t)]$$

Note: $\mathrm{sgn}(x) = 1$ for $x > 1, = 0$ for $x = 0, = -1$ for $x < 0$.

2

Review of Linear Systems Theory

2.1 Linearity, Causality and Stationarity

This chapter describes the important attributes of linear time-invariant (LTI) systems. The art of solving the ordinary differential equations (ODEs) that describe the input/output behavior of continuous LTI systems is introduced. Matrix algebra and matrix operations are covered in Section 2.3 and the state variable formalism for describing the behavior of high-order continuous dynamic systems is introduced in Section 2.3.4. Section 2.4 treats the mathematical tools used to characterize LTI systems. Introduced are the concepts of *system impulse response, real convolution, transient response* and *steady-state sinusoidal frequency response,* including *Bode* and *Nyquist plots.* Section 2.5 treats LTI *discrete (numerical) systems.* Difference equations are seen to replace ODEs in describing system behavior in the time domain and use of the z transform is introduced as a means of solving discrete state equations. Finally, Section 2.5 considers factors affecting the stability of LTI systems.

Even though the real world is fraught with thousands of examples of nonlinear systems, engineers and applied mathematicians have devoted their attention almost exclusively to developing mathematical tools to describe and analyze *linear systems.* Some reasons for this specialization appear to be that certain mechanical systems and electrical circuits can be treated as linear systems. Most electronic circuits can be easily linearized and thus the mathematical tools of linear systems analysis are easy to apply. A system is said to be linear if it obeys all of the following properties [Northrop, 2000]: By logical exclusion, *nonlinear systems do not obey one or more of the following properties:* (Here $x(t)$ is the input, $y(t)$ is the output and $h(t)$ is the LS impulse response or weighting function of the system.)

$$x_1 \rightarrow \{LS\} \rightarrow y_1 = x_1 \otimes h \qquad \textit{real convolution} \qquad (2.1A)$$

$$\begin{array}{l} \text{if} \\ \text{then} \end{array} \; \xrightarrow[a_2 x_2]{x_2} \{LS\} \xrightarrow[y_2' = a_2(x_2 \otimes h)]{y_2 = x_2 \otimes h} \qquad \textit{scaling} \qquad (2.1B)$$

$$\xrightarrow{a_1 x_1 + a_2 x_2} \{LS\} \xrightarrow{y = a_1 y_1 + a_2 y_2} \qquad \textit{superposition} \qquad (2.1C)$$

$$\xrightarrow[+x_2(t-t_2)]{x_1(t-t_1)} \{LS\} \xrightarrow[+y_2(t-t_2)]{y = y_1(t-t_1)} \qquad \textit{shift invariance} \qquad (2.1D)$$

Note that a dynamic system can still be linear and have time-variable (TV) coefficients in its describing ODEs. That is:

$$\dot{\mathbf{x}} = \mathbf{A}(t)\mathbf{x} + \mathbf{B}(t)\mathbf{u} \tag{2.2}$$

Where: $\dot{\mathbf{x}}$ is an n-element column matrix of the time derivates of the system's states, $\mathbf{x}$ is a column matrix of the system's n dependent variables, $\mathbf{u}$ is a column vector of p independent inputs, $\mathbf{A}(t)$ is a square, $n \times n$ matrix of the system's time-variable coefficients and $\mathbf{B}(t)$ is an $n \times p$ matrix of the time-variable coefficients describing how the p inputs $\mathbf{u}$ enter the system. Solution of such TV linear systems is tedious and best done by simulation. Most of the systems described in this text are *linear time-invariant* (LTI) in nature.

Causality is a property of reality. A non-causal system can respond to an input before it occurs in time. Probably the only time you will encounter non-causal systems is in the derivation and implementation of *matched filters* and *Wiener filters* for time signals. In these cases, they must be approximated by causal filters [Schwartz, 1959].

Stationarity is a term generally used to describe random processes and noise, but it can be extended to the description of linear systems as well. In describing noise, we say a noisy voltage (or parameter) is nonstationary if the underlying physical processes generating it are changing in time. These changes cause the noise statistics to change in time (e.g., probability density function, auto-power spectrum, etc.). A system is said to be nonstationary if it is time-variable and can be characterized by matrices, $\mathbf{A}(t)$ and $\mathbf{B}(t)$, as in Equation 2.2 above. A signal is generally nonstationary if it arises from a nonstationary system.

Sadly, physiological systems are all nonlinear and nonstationary. They are causal, however. We still can use linear system theory to analyze and describe certain of them under appropriate limiting conditions, using linearization strategies and assuming short-term stationarity.

2.2 Analog Systems

2.2.1 SISO and MIMO systems

SISO means *single input-single output.* Such linear system architecture is ideal for learning the basic mathematics of linear systems analysis, but is seldom encountered in physiology, where systems are generally *multiple input-multiple output* (MIMO) and are cross-coupled to other systems. In a linear, MIMO system, the kth input, in general, has an effect on the jth output. That is, there is a cross-coupling transfer function, $H_{jk}(s)$, defined for each causal path that relates output y_j to input u_k.

2.2.2 Introduction to ODEs and their solutions

Many dynamic physical and chemical processes that govern the behavior of linear systems can be described by *linear ordinary differential equations* (ODEs) with constant

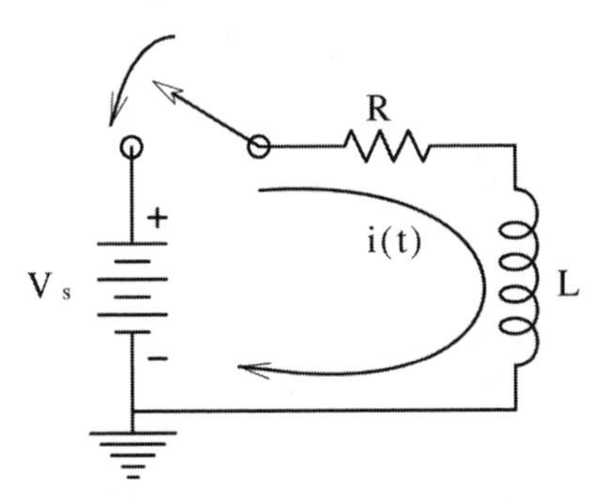

FIGURE 2.1
A simple series R-L circuit connected to a switched dc source.

coefficients. The calculus solution of an ODE has *two parts:* the *natural* or *transient solution* and a *forced solution.* The natural solution is derived from the roots of the *characteristic equation* of the ODE; the forced solution is the result of the forcing function, u, that is considered to be the input to the system described by the ODE. An ODE can have zero forcing and exhibit a natural solution from initial conditions on its states.

A simple first example of a first-order ODE describes the current flow in an inductor connected to a resistor from a dc voltage source, as shown in Figure 2.1. By *Kirchoff's voltage law,* when the switch is closed, the voltages around the loop are given by:

$$\begin{aligned} &\mathrm{V_s(t) = i(t)R + L(di/dt), \quad t \geq 0} \\ &\downarrow \\ &\mathrm{di/dt + i(t)(R/L) = V_s(t)/L} \end{aligned} \tag{2.3}$$

This is a first-order linear ODE of the form:

$$\dot{x} = -x\omega_o + bF \tag{2.4}$$

(Here and hereafter we use the familiar dot notation, $\dot{x} \equiv dx/dt$.) For a step input, Equation 2.4 has the general solution:

$$x(t) = x_{ss} + [x(0) - x_{ss}]\exp(-\omega_o t) \tag{2.5}$$

Where: $x(0)$ is the initial value of x at $t = 0+$ and x_{ss} is x at $t = \infty$ (when $\dot{x} \to 0$). For the simple R-L circuit, $x(t) = i(t)$, $x_{ss} = bF/\omega_o = V_s/R$ amps, $b = 1/L$, $\omega_o = R/L$ r/sec, and $V_s = F$. Thus, given $x(0) = 0$, the solution is:

$$i(t) = (V_s/R)[1 - \exp(-\omega_o t)] \tag{2.6}$$

Thus, $i(t)$ begins at 0 and rises exponentially to V_s/R amps in the steady-state.

A second example of a first-order LTI system is taken from *compartmental pharmacokinetics* (CPKs). A drug is injected into the blood stream by a continuous IV drip, starting at $t = 0$. It is known that the drug is removed from the circulatory system by the liver at a rate proportional to its concentration. The drug's blood concentration, [D], is in μg/l volume of the circulatory system. Thus we can write the ODE:

$$[\dot{D}] = -K_L[D] + (R_D/V_c)U(t) \quad (\mu g/l)/min \tag{2.7}$$

Where: $U(t)$ is the unit step function, K_L is the drug loss rate, V_c is the volume of the circulatory system in liters (here assumed to be constant), R_D is the rate of drug input in μg/min and $[\dot{D}]$ is the rate of increase of the drug concentration in (μg/l)/min. Using the solution format of the first example, we can write the general time-domain solution:

$$[D](t) = [D]_{ss} + \{[D]_{(0)} - [D]_{ss}\} \exp(-K_L t) \quad \mu g/l \tag{2.8}$$

If we let the initial drug concentration be zero ($[D]_{(0)} = 0$), the steady-state value can be found from the ODE by setting $[\dot{D}] \to 0$. Thus $[D]_{ss} = R_D/(K_L V_c)$ μg/l and

$$[D](t) = R_D/(K_L V_c)[1 - \exp(-K_L t)] \quad \mu g/l \tag{2.9}$$

For a third example, consider the simple physical example of a second-order linear system consisting of the simple mass-spring-friction mechanical system is shown in Figure 2.2. By Newton's second law we can sum the forces acting on the mass:

$$0 = M\ddot{x} + B\dot{x} + Kx - F(t) \tag{2.10}$$

$F(t)$ is the input (force) acting on the mass for $t \geq 0$. This ODE can be put in the form:

$$\ddot{x} + \dot{x}(B/M) + x(K/M) = F(t)/M \tag{2.11}$$

This ODE is of the general form:

$$\ddot{x} + b\dot{x} + cx = f(t) \tag{2.12}$$

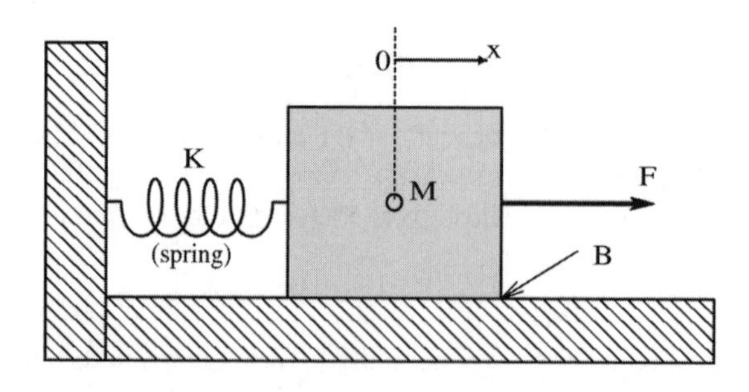

FIGURE 2.2
A second-order, LTI mechanical system, consisting of a mass and a spring effectively in parallel with a dashpot having viscous friction, B, Newtons/(m/sec).

Where $a = (B/M)$, $b = (K/M)$ and $f(t) = F(t)/M$. If we use the *operator notation* for the derivative In which $p[x] = \dot{x}$ and $p^2[x] = \ddot{x}$, Equation 2.12 can thus be written in the form:

$$x\{p^2 + pb + c\} = f(t) \tag{2.13}$$

The form of the natural response of Equation 2.12 depends on the form of the two roots of the *quadratic characteristic equation* in p given in Equation 2.14.

$$\{p^2 + pb + c\} = 0 \tag{2.14}$$

For a simple passive mechanical system, the roots can be *unequal real* and *negative, equal real* and *negative* or *complex conjugate with a negative real part.* In general, the constants b and c are positive and the roots are given by the well-known quadratic formula:

$$p_1, p_2 = -b/2 \pm {}^1\!/_2\sqrt{b^2 - 4c} \tag{2.15}$$

For the roots to be real, negative and unequal, b and c must be > 0 and $b > 2\sqrt{c}$. The general solution of Equation 2.12 for any root's form is:

$$x(t) = C_1 \exp(\mathbf{p_2}t) + C_2 \exp(\mathbf{p_1}t) \tag{2.16}$$

In Equation 2.16 and the following expressions, C_1 and C_2 are constants that must be evaluated from initial and final conditions.

The roots are negative, real and equal when $b = 2\sqrt{c}$ i.e., $p_1 = p_2 = -b/2$. The solution then has the form:

$$x(t) = C_1 t \exp[-(b/2)t] + C_2 \tag{2.17}$$

For the roots to be complex-conjugate, $b < 2\sqrt{c}$. Now $\mathbf{p_1}, \mathbf{p_2} = -b/2 \pm j{}^1\!/_2\sqrt{4c - b^2} = \alpha \pm j\beta$, where $\alpha = -b/2$ and $\beta = \sqrt{4c - b^2} > 0$. Now the natural response solution can be written in the general exponential form:

$$x(t) = C_1 \exp[(\alpha + j\beta)t] + C_2 \exp[(\alpha - j\beta)t] \tag{2.18}$$

By using the Euler relation:

$$\exp[\pm j\theta] = \cos(\theta) \pm j\sin(\theta) \tag{2.19}$$

Equation 2.18 can be written:

$$x(t) = e^{\alpha t}\{C_1[\cos(\beta t) + j\sin(\beta t)] + C_2[\cos(\beta t) - j\sin(\beta t)]\} \tag{2.20A}$$

$$\downarrow$$

$$x(t) = e^{\alpha t}[(C_1 + C_2)\cos(\beta t) + j(C_1 - C_2)\sin(\beta t)] \tag{2.20B}$$

$$\downarrow$$

$$x(t) = e^{\alpha t}\sqrt{(C_1 + C_2)^2 + (C_1 - C_2)^2}\cos(\beta t - \theta) \tag{2.20C}$$

and

$$\theta = \tan^{-1}\left(\frac{C_1 - C_2}{C_1 + C_2}\right) \tag{2.20D}$$

In terms of the original mechanical parameters: $b = B/M$, $c = K/M$, hence $\alpha = -B/(2M)$ and

$$\beta = \sqrt{(K/M) - 4(B/M)^2} \tag{2.21}$$

The underdamped quadratic ODE can also be expressed in terms of a *standard form* given by:

$$\{p^2 + p(2\xi\omega_n) + \omega_n^2\} = 0 \tag{2.22}$$

From the foregoing, $\omega_n^2 = c = K/M\,(r/sec)^2$ is the squared, *undamped natural frequency* of the system. That is, $\omega_n = \sqrt{(K/M)}\,r/sec$. ξ is the damped quadratic system's *damping factor;* $0 \le \xi \le 1$. Since $2\xi\omega_n = b = B/M$, it follows that $\xi = B/(2\sqrt{KM})$. Similarly it can be shown that $\alpha = -\omega_n\xi$ and $\beta = \omega_n\sqrt{1-\xi^2}$. Figure 2.3 shows the position of the roots of the characteristic equation, Equation 2.22,

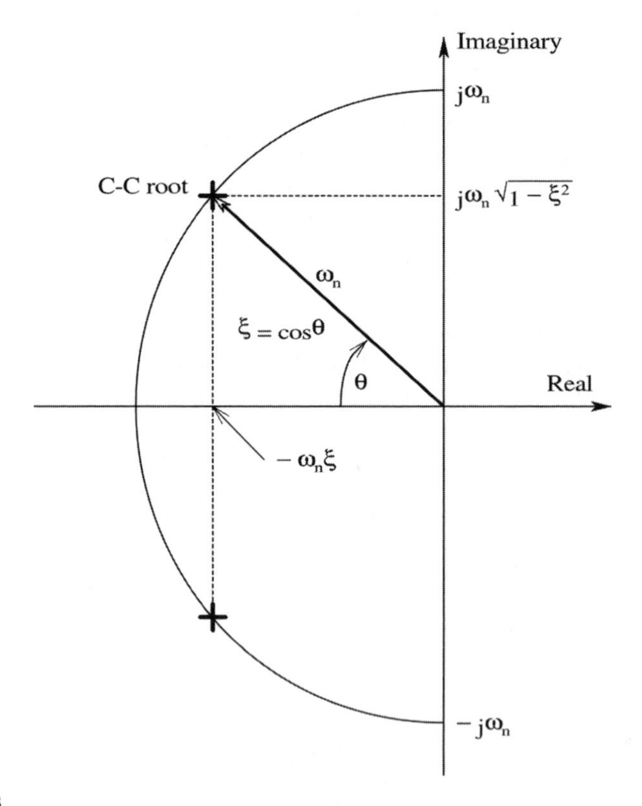

FIGURE 2.3
Location of the complex-conjugate roots of the quadratic characteristic equation, Equation 2.22. See text for discussion.

as a function of ξ and ω_n for $0 \leq \xi \leq 1$. The CC roots lie on the dotted semicircle, their position determined by ξ. In all the above discussion of natural responses of ODE systems, the constants C_1 and C_2 are evaluated from a knowledge of initial and steady-state conditions.

Let us now examine a fourth example of a *complete solution* to an overdamped, second-order system with forcing, f(t):

$$\ddot{x} + 4\dot{x} + 3x = f(t) = 4\exp(-2t), \quad t \geq 0 \tag{2.23}$$

Now the solution consists of the natural response plus the forced response. The system's characteristic equation is:

$$\{p^2 + 4p + 3\} = 0 \tag{2.24}$$

which has the negative real roots: $p_1, p_2 = -\frac{4}{2} \pm {}^1\!/_2\sqrt{16 - 12} = -2 \pm 1 = -3, -1$. Thus, the general form of the solution can be written:

$$x(t) = C_1 e^{-t} + C_2 e^{-3t} + C_3 e^{-2t} \tag{2.25}$$

For this example, we are given the initial conditions, $x(0) \equiv 2 = C_1 + C_2 + C_3$ and $\dot{x}(0) \equiv 4 = -C_1 - 3C_2 - 2C_3$. These two algebraic equations do not allow us to find the three constants. We must also use the fact that $C_3 e^{-2t}$ must satisfy the ODE. That is:

$$4e^{-2t} = C_3 e^{-2t}(-2)^2 + 4C_3(-2)e^{-2t} + 3C_3 e^{-2t} \tag{2.26}$$

The e^{-2t} terms cancel and simple algebra yields $C_3 = -4$. This C_3 value can be substituted into the two initial condition equations and C_1 and C_2 can be solved for using Cramer's rule:

$$2 = C_1 + C_2 + (-4) \rightarrow 6 = C_1 + C_2 \tag{2.27A}$$

$$4 = -C_1 - 3C_2 - 2(-4) \rightarrow -4 = -C_1 - 3C_2 \tag{2.27B}$$

From the simultaneous equations in C_1 and C_2 we find $C_1 = 7$ and $C_2 = -1$. So the complete solution of the ODE Equation 2.23 is:

$$x(t) = 7e^{-t} - 1e^{-3t} - 4e^{-2t} \tag{2.28}$$

As a fifth example, consider the same system used in the first example, with different ICs. Now let the input forcing be a ramp function: $f(t) \equiv 9t$, for $t \geq 0$. Now the general solution is of the form:

$$x(t) = C_1 e^{p_1 t} + C_2 e^{p_2 t} + C_3 t + C_4 \tag{2.29}$$

As before, the roots of the characteristic equations are: $p_1 = -1$ and $p_2 = -3$. From the ICs:

$$x(0) \equiv 2 = C_1 + C_2 + C_4 \tag{2.30A}$$

$$\dot{x}(0) \equiv 4 = -C_1 - 3C_2 + C_3 \tag{2.30B}$$

Also, the forced solution, $C_3 t + C_4$, must satisfy the ODE. Thus:

$$9t = 0 + 4C_3 + 3(C_3 t + C_4) \tag{2.31}$$

Comparing like terms, we see that $9t = 3C_3 t$, so $C_3 = 3$. Also, $0 = 4C_3 + 3C_4$, so $C_4 = -4$. Now when C_3 and C_4 are substituted into Equation 2.30A above, we can again use Cramer's rule to solve for $C_1 = 9.5$ and $C_2 = -3.5$. Thus the final solution is:

$$x(t) = 9.5e^{-t} - 3.5e^{-3t} + 3t - 4 \tag{2.32}$$

It is also important to examine the response of a second-order linear system to a *sinusoidal input* applied for $t \geq 0$. In this sixth example, $y(t)$ is the system's output and $x(t) = A\sin(\omega t)U(t)$ is its input. Thus, in general:

$$\ddot{y} + b\dot{y} + cy = A\sin(\omega t)U(t), \quad t \geq 0 \tag{2.33}$$

The general form of the solution, as before, is composed of a natural plus a forced component:

$$y(t) = \{C_1 e^{p_1 t} + C_2 e^{p_2 t}\} + C_3 \sin(\omega t) + C_4 \cos(\omega t) \tag{2.34}$$

The complete solution of the ODE is very involved, especially for an underdamped second-order system. For expediency, we will consider the solution for large $t >> 1/p_1$ and $1/p_2$. Thus, the transient, natural solution can be assumed to have gone to zero, leaving the forced solution:

$$y_{ss}(t) = \{0\} + C_3 \sin(\omega t) + C_4 \cos(\omega t) = \sqrt{C_3^2 + C_4^2}\sin(\omega t + \psi) \tag{2.35}$$

Where: $\psi = \tan^{-1}(C_4/C_3)$. This solution must be a solution to the ODE:

$$\begin{aligned} A\sin(\omega t) = {} & c[C_3 \sin(\omega t) + C_4 \cos(\omega t)] + b[C_3 \omega \cos(\omega t) - C_4 \omega \sin(\omega t)] \\ & + [-C_3 \omega^2 \sin(\omega t) - C_4 \omega^2 \cos(\omega t)] \end{aligned} \tag{2.36}$$

When we compare terms:

$$A\sin(\omega t) = \sin(\omega t)[cC_3 - bC_4\omega - C_3\omega^2] \tag{2.37A}$$

$$0 = \cos(\omega t)[cC_4 + bC_3\omega - C_4\omega^2] \tag{2.37B}$$

From which we can write simultaneous equations for C_3 and C_4:

$$A = C_3(c - \omega^2) - C_4 b\omega \tag{2.38A}$$

$$0 = C_3 b\omega + C_4(c - \omega^2) \tag{2.38B}$$

Solving with Cramer's rule (see Appendix A), we find:

$$\Delta = (c - \omega^2)^2 + b^2\omega^2 \tag{2.39A}$$

$$C_3 = A(c-\omega^2)/\Delta \tag{2.39B}$$

$$C_4 = -Ab\omega/\Delta \tag{2.39C}$$

$$\sqrt{C_3^2+C_4^2} = \frac{A}{\sqrt{(c-\omega^2)^2+b^2\omega^2}} \tag{2.39D}$$

Thus the solution, Equation 2.35, can be written:

$$y_{ss}(t) = \frac{A}{\sqrt{(c-\omega^2)^2+b^2\omega^2}}\sin(\omega t+\psi) \tag{2.40}$$

In other words, the system's *steady-state frequency response magnitude* is simply the peak magnitude of the output sinusoid divided by the input peak magnitude, A. That is,

$$\frac{|Y|}{|A|} = \frac{1}{\sqrt{(c-\omega^2)^2+b^2\omega^2}} = |\mathbf{H}(\omega)| \tag{2.41}$$

Note that this function has a peak at $\omega = \sqrt{c}$. As you will see in Section 2.4.4, there are simpler ways to find a system's frequency response than by solving the ODE for the forced solution in the steady state.

The *phase angle* of the response is given by:

$$\psi = \tan^{-1}\frac{C_4}{C_3} = \tan^{-1}\frac{-Ab\omega/\Delta}{A(c-\omega^2)/\Delta} = \tan^{-1}\frac{-b\omega}{(c-\omega^2)} \tag{2.42}$$

Note that at $\omega = 0$, $\psi = 0$; as ω increases, ψ goes negative (a phase lag). $\psi \to -90°$ at $\omega = \sqrt{c}$, and flips to $+90°$ for $\omega = \sqrt{c+}$. As $\omega \to \infty$, $\psi \to 0+$.

2.3 Systems Described by Sets of ODEs

2.3.1 Introduction

Multicompartmental pharmacokinetic (PK) systems [Godfrey, 1983; Northrop, 2000] are an excellent example of a class of biomedical systems that are generally describable by sets of coupled first-order linear ODEs. If N compartments are interconnected, there will, in general, be N ODEs and N roots in the overall system's characteristic equation. The roots will generally be real and negative.

As a first example, consider the linear second-order system:

$$\ddot{x} + \dot{x}b + xc = u \tag{2.43}$$

To express this second-order system as two interconnected first-order systems, we now define *two state variables:* $x_1 \equiv x$ and $x_2 \equiv \dot{x}_1 = \dot{x}$. Now the ODE of Equation 2.44 can be rewritten as:

$$\dot{x}_1 = x_2 \tag{2.44A}$$

$$\dot{x}_2 = -x_1 c - x_2 b + u \tag{2.44B}$$

As you will see in the next section, these two first-order ODEs can be put in state variable form using vector matrix notation.

As a second example, consider a general n^{th} order system with one input:

$$\frac{dx^n}{dt^n} + a_{n-1}\frac{dx^{n-1}}{dt^{n-1}} + \cdots + a_1\frac{dx}{dt} + a_0 x = b_0 u(t) \tag{2.45}$$

As above, we define $x_1 \equiv x$, $x_2 \equiv \dot{x} = \dot{x}_1$, $x_3 \equiv \dot{x}_2, \ldots, x_n \equiv \dot{x}_{n-1}$, from which we can find the set of n first-order ODEs:

$$\begin{aligned}
\dot{x}_1 &= x_2 \\
\dot{x}_2 &= x_3 \\
\dot{x}_3 &= x_4 \\
&\vdots \\
\dot{x}_{n-1} &= x_n \\
\dot{x}_n &= -a_0 x_1 - a_1 x_2 - a_2 x_3 \ldots - a_{n-2} x_{n-1} - a_{n-1} x_n + b_n u(t)
\end{aligned} \tag{2.46}$$

PK systems with $N \geq 3$ can give sets of equations with considerable complexity [Godfrey, 1983]. Solution of these ODEs is made easier by the state variable formalism and, in some cases, by using signal flow graphs to describe the system. When solving a system with pencil and paper, *Mason's rule* (see Appendix B) can be easily used with signal flow graphs to find a high-order PK system's transfer function without the need for *matrix inversion.* Once the transfer function is known, its outputs can be readily found, given its inputs.

2.3.2 Introduction to matrix algebra

Before describing *state variables* we will review some basic properties of *matrices.* A matrix is simply a collection of numbers or algebraic *elements* arranged in a rectangular or square array of rows and columns. The elements can be the coefficients of a set of simultaneous linear algebraic equations. A matrix can have one row, one column or n rows and m columns or be square with n rows and n columns. A matrix is said to be of *order* (n,m) if it has n rows of elements and m columns of elements. A matrix is not a *determinant,* although a determinant can be calculated from the elements of a square $(n \times n)$ matrix. A square, 3×3 matrix is shown below in Equation 2.47.

$$\mathbf{A} = \begin{bmatrix} a_{11} & a_{12} & a_{13} \\ a_{21} & a_{22} & a_{23} \\ a_{31} & a_{32} & a_{33} \end{bmatrix} \tag{2.47}$$

The determinant of **A** is a number or algebraic quantity:

$$\det \mathbf{A} = a_{11}(a_{22}a_{33} - a_{32}a_{23}) - a_{21}(a_{13}a_{33} - a_{32}a_{13}) + a_{31}(a_{12}a_{23} - a_{22}a_{13}) \quad (2.48A)$$

or

$$\det \mathbf{A} = a_{11}(a_{22}a_{33} - a_{32}a_{23}) - a_{12}(a_{21}a_{33} - a_{31}a_{23}) + a_{13}(a_{21}a_{32} - a_{31}a_{22}) \quad (2.48B)$$

and so forth.

A *diagonal matrix* is a square matrix in which the diagonal elements, a_{kk}, are nonzero, and all the other a_{jk} elements ($j \neq k$) are zero. A *unit* or *identity matrix,* **I**, is defined as a diagonal matrix in which all $a_{kk} = 1$.

A *singular matrix* is a square matrix whose determinant$= 0$. Singularity is the result of nonindependence of the n simultaneous equations from which the matrix elements were derived.

For example, consider the three simple linear algebraic equations below:

$$x_1 + 2x_2 + 3x_3 = 0 \quad (2.49A)$$

$$8x_1 - x_2 - x_3 = 0 \quad (2.49B)$$

$$7x_1 - 3x_2 - 4x_3 = 0 \quad (2.49C)$$

In matrix form, these equations can be written:

$$\mathbf{Ax} = 0 = \begin{bmatrix} 1 & 2 & 3 \\ 8 & -1 & -1 \\ 7 & -3 & -4 \end{bmatrix} \mathbf{x} \quad (2.50)$$

The determinant of **A** is $\det \mathbf{A} = 1(4-3) - 8(-8+9) + 7(-2+3) = 0$. Singularity was the result of the third equation's being derived by subtracting the top equation from the middle equation, causing it not to be independent.

2.3.3 Some matrix operations

The *transpose of a matrix* is found by exchanging its columns for rows. For example, $\mathbf{B^T}$ is the transpose of **B**. Let

$$\mathbf{B} = \begin{bmatrix} 1 & 4 \\ 2 & 5 \\ 3 & 6 \end{bmatrix}, \quad \text{then} \quad \mathbf{B^T} = \begin{bmatrix} 1 & 2 & 3 \\ & & \\ 4 & 5 & 6 \end{bmatrix} \quad (2.51)$$

The *adjoint matrix* of the square matrix **A** is $\operatorname{adj} \mathbf{A} = (\operatorname{cof} \mathbf{A})^{\mathbf{T}}$. That is, it is the transpose of the *cofactor matrix* of **A**. These operations are best shown by example. Given a square **A**:

$$\mathbf{A} = \begin{bmatrix} a_{11} & a_{12} & a_{13} \\ a_{21} & a_{22} & a_{23} \\ a_{31} & a_{32} & a_{33} \end{bmatrix} \quad (2.52)$$

$$\text{cof}\,\mathbf{A} = \begin{bmatrix} (a_{22}a_{33} - a_{32}a_{23}) & -(a_{21}a_{33} - a_{31}a_{23}) & (a_{21}a_{32} - a_{31}a_{22}) \\ -(a_{12}a_{33} - a_{32}a_{13}) & (a_{11}a_{33} - a_{31}a_{13}) & -(a_{11}a_{32} - a_{31}a_{12}) \\ (a_{12}a_{23} - a_{22}a_{13}) & -(a_{11}a_{23} - a_{21}a_{13}) & (a_{11}a_{22} - a_{21}a_{12}) \end{bmatrix} \quad (2.53)$$

Now the transpose of cof **A** gives the desired adj **A**:

$$\text{adj}\,\mathbf{A} = \begin{bmatrix} (a_{22}a_{33} - a_{32}a_{23}) & -(a_{12}a_{33} - a_{32}a_{13}) & (a_{12}a_{23} - a_{22}a_{13}) \\ -(a_{21}a_{33} - a_{31}a_{23}) & (a_{11}a_{33} - a_{31}a_{13}) & -(a_{11}a_{23} - a_{21}a_{13}) \\ (a_{21}a_{32} - a_{31}a_{22}) & -(a_{11}a_{32} - a_{31}a_{12}) & (a_{11}a_{22} - a_{21}a_{12}) \end{bmatrix} \quad (2.54)$$

Matrix addition: Two matrices can be added algebraically if they are of the same $(n \times m)$ order. Sic:

$$\mathbf{A} + \mathbf{B} = \mathbf{D} \quad (2.55)$$

The associative and commutative laws of addition and subtraction of real numbers holds for matrices of equal order. That is:

$$(\mathbf{A} + \mathbf{B}) + \mathbf{C} = \mathbf{A} + (\mathbf{B} + \mathbf{C}) \quad \text{(Associative law)} \quad (2.56)$$

$$\mathbf{A} + \mathbf{B} + \mathbf{C} = \mathbf{B} + \mathbf{C} + \mathbf{A} = \mathbf{C} + \mathbf{A} + \mathbf{B} \quad \text{(Distributive law)} \quad (2.57)$$

Matrix multiplication: A necessary condition to multiply two matrices together is that they be *conformable.* That is, the number of columns of **A** must equal the number of rows of **B**. Equation 2.58 below illustrates how matrix multiplication is done for a 3×2 times a 2×3 matrix:

$$\mathbf{AB} = \begin{bmatrix} a_{11} & a_{12} & a_{13} \\ \\ a_{21} & a_{22} & a_{23} \end{bmatrix} \begin{bmatrix} b_{11} & b_{12} \\ b_{21} & b_{22} \\ b_{31} & b_{32} \end{bmatrix} = \mathbf{C}$$

$$= \begin{bmatrix} c_{11} & c_{12} \\ (a_{11}b_{11} + a_{12}b_{21} + a_{13}b_{31}) & (a_{11}b_{12} + a_{12}b_{22} + a_{13}b_{32}) \\ \\ (a_{21}b_{11} + a_{22}b_{21} + a_{23}b_{31}) & (a_{21}b_{12} + a_{22}b_{22} + a_{23}b_{32}) \\ c_{21} & c_{22} \end{bmatrix} \quad (2.58)$$

Note that each element in the left-hand matrix's top row is multiplied by the corresponding element in the right-hand matrix's first (left-hand) column and the products of elements are added together to form the c_{11} element of the product matrix, **C**. Next, each element of the top row of **A** is multiplied by the corresponding element of the right-hand column of **B** and the element products are added together to form c_{12} of **C**.

Now observe what happens when the order of multiplication is reversed:

$$\mathbf{BA} = \begin{bmatrix} b_{11} & b_{12} \\ b_{21} & b_{22} \\ b_{31} & b_{32} \end{bmatrix} \begin{bmatrix} a_{11} & a_{12} & a_{13} \\ \\ a_{21} & a_{22} & a_{23} \end{bmatrix} = \mathbf{D}$$

$$= \begin{bmatrix} (b_{11}a_{11}+b_{12}a_{21}) & (b_{11}a_{12}+b_{12}a_{22}) & (b_{11}a_{13}+b_{12}a_{22}) \\ (b_{21}a_{11}+b_{22}a_{21}) & (b_{21}a_{12}+b_{22}a_{22}) & (b_{21}a_{13}+b_{22}a_{23}) \\ (b_{31}a_{11}+b_{32}a_{21}) & (b_{31}a_{12}+b_{32}a_{22}) & (b_{31}a_{13}+b_{32}a_{23}) \end{bmatrix} \quad (2.59)$$

It is clear that $\mathbf{AB} \neq \mathbf{BA}$ and, except for some special cases, matrix multiplication is not commutative. That is, matrix multiplication is order-dependent. For example:

$$(\mathbf{A}+\mathbf{B})\mathbf{C} = \mathbf{AC}+\mathbf{BC} \quad (2.60A)$$

and

$$\mathbf{C}(\mathbf{A}+\mathbf{B}) = \mathbf{CA}+\mathbf{CB} \quad (2.60B)$$

As a final example of matrix multiplication, consider the product:

$$[2\ 1\ 3]\begin{bmatrix} 2 \\ 1 \\ 5 \end{bmatrix} = [20] \quad (2.61)$$

An *identity matrix,* **I** is a (square) diagonal matrix in which all the a_{kk} elements are 1s and all the other ($a_{jk}, j \neq k$) elements are zeros. Note that an exception to the $\mathbf{AB} \neq \mathbf{BA}$ rule is:

$$\mathbf{AI} = \mathbf{IA} = \mathbf{A} \quad (2.62)$$

Note that the order of **A** must agree with that of **I** for this to happen. That is, the number of elements in the rows of the left-hand matrix must equal the number of elements in the columns of the right hand matrix. As an example, let

$$\mathbf{A} = \begin{bmatrix} a_{11} & a_{12} \\ a_{21} & a_{22} \\ a_{31} & a_{32} \end{bmatrix} \quad (2.63)$$

Then

$$\mathbf{AI} = \begin{bmatrix} a_{11} & a_{12} \\ a_{21} & a_{22} \\ a_{31} & a_{32} \end{bmatrix} \begin{bmatrix} 1 & 0 \\ 0 & 1 \end{bmatrix} = \begin{bmatrix} a_{11} & a_{12} \\ a_{21} & a_{22} \\ a_{31} & a_{32} \end{bmatrix} = \mathbf{A} \quad (2.64)$$

Also:

$$\mathbf{IA} = \begin{bmatrix} 1 & 0 & 0 \\ 0 & 1 & 0 \\ 0 & 0 & 1 \end{bmatrix} \begin{bmatrix} a_{11} & a_{12} \\ a_{21} & a_{22} \\ a_{31} & a_{32} \end{bmatrix} = \begin{bmatrix} a_{11} & a_{12} \\ a_{21} & a_{22} \\ a_{31} & a_{32} \end{bmatrix} = \mathbf{A} \quad (2.65)$$

In Equation 2.64, a 2×2 identity matrix is required for conformity, in Equation 2.64, a 3×3 **I** matrix is used.

The *inverse of a (square) matrix* is another important matrix operation. It is written as:

$$\mathbf{A}^{-1} = \text{adj}\,\mathbf{A}/\det\mathbf{A} \quad (2.66)$$

That is, $\mathbf{A}^{-1}$ is the adjoint matrix of $\mathbf{A}$, each element of which is divided by the determinant of $\mathbf{A}$. Consider the example of the 3×3 matrix $\mathbf{A}$:

$$\mathbf{A} = \begin{bmatrix} 2 & 1 & 1 \\ 1 & 2 & 3 \\ 3 & 2 & 1 \end{bmatrix} \tag{2.67}$$

It is easy to find the determinant of $\mathbf{A}$:

$$\begin{aligned} \det \mathbf{A} &= 2(2\times 1 - 2\times 3) - 1(1\times 1 - 2\times 1) + 3(1\times 3 - 2\times 1) \\ &= -8 + 1 + 3 = -4 \end{aligned} \tag{2.68}$$

Now the elements of the adjoint of $\mathbf{A}$ can be found: $A_{11} = (2\times 1 - 2\times 3) = -4$, $A_{12} = -(1\times 1 - 3\times 3) = +8$, $A_{13} = (1\times 2 - 3\times 2) = -4$. Similarly, the other six adj $\mathbf{A}$ elements are found from the cofactors of $\mathbf{A}$: $A_{21} = 1$, $A_{22} = -1$, $A_{23} = -1$, $A_{31} = 1$, $A_{32} = -1$, $A_{33} = 3$. Finally, we can write the inverse of $\mathbf{A}$ as:

$$\mathbf{A}^{-1} = \frac{1}{-4} \begin{bmatrix} -4 & 1 & 1 \\ 8 & -1 & -5 \\ -4 & -1 & 3 \end{bmatrix} \tag{2.69}$$

Other properties of inverse matrices are [Lathi, 1974]:

$$\mathbf{A}^{-1}\mathbf{A} = \mathbf{A}\mathbf{A}^{-1} = \mathbf{I} \tag{2.70}$$

and

$$(\mathbf{A}^{-1})^{-1} = \mathbf{A} \tag{2.71}$$

Inverting a large matrix is tedious pencil and paper work, best done by a computer using Matlab™. You will see that inverse matrices are used when solving sets of simultaneous equations. For example:

$$y_1 = a_{11}x_1 + a_{12}x_2 + a_{13}x_3 \tag{2.72A}$$

$$y_2 = a_{21}x_1 + a_{22}x_2 + a_{23}x_3 \tag{2.72B}$$

$$y_3 = a_{31}x_1 + a_{32}x_2 + a_{33}x_3 \tag{2.72C}$$

Where $\mathbf{x}$ are the unknowns, $\mathbf{y}$ and $\mathbf{A}$ are given. In matrix notation, $\mathbf{y} = \mathbf{A}\mathbf{x}$, and the unknowns are found from [Lathi, 1974]:

$$\mathbf{x} = \mathbf{A}^{-1}\mathbf{y} \tag{2.73}$$

When a matrix is *time variable,* i.e., describes a nonstationary system, some or all of its elements are functions of time. Such a matrix is generally written as $\mathbf{A}(t)$. The time derivative of $\mathbf{A}(t)$ is a matrix formed from the time derivatives of each of its elements. For example:

$$\mathbf{A}(t) = \begin{bmatrix} a_{11}e^{-bt} & a_{12}U(t) & a_{13}\sin(\omega t) \\ a_{21} & a_{22}[1+\cos(ct)] & a_{23} \\ a_{31} & a_{32}t & a_{33}e^{\nu t} \end{bmatrix} \tag{2.74}$$

$$\dot{\mathbf{A}}(t) = \begin{bmatrix} -ba_{11}e^{-bt} & a_{12}\delta(t) & a_{13}\omega\cos(\omega t) \\ 0 & -a_{22}c\sin(ct) & 0 \\ 0 & a_{32} & a_{33}\nu e^{\nu t} \end{bmatrix} \tag{2.75}$$

Matrix algebra contains many other theorems and identities. For examples, see the venerable texts by (Guillemin (1949), Kuo (1967), and Lathi (1974)].

2.3.4 Introduction to state variables

The state-variable (SV) formality provides a powerful, compact, mathematical means for characterizing dynamic linear systems. Many physiological and pharmacokinetic systems can be linearized and therefore analyzed using the state equation approach. Many others, however, are frankly nonlinear and can be solved easily and directly by simulation by a specialized computer program such as Simnon^{TM}. Linear state variable systems are easily simulated with Matlab^{TM}, but can also be solved by Simnon^{TM}.

Any linear system describable by a one or more linked, high-order ODEs can be reduced to state variable form as we did for Equation 2.46. A general notation for an nth order, linear, stationary, dynamic SV system is shown below:

$$\dot{\mathbf{x}} = \mathbf{Ax} + \mathbf{Bu} \tag{2.76A}$$

$$\mathbf{y} = \mathbf{Cx} + \mathbf{Du} \tag{2.76B}$$

Where: $\dot{\mathbf{x}}$ and $\mathbf{x}$ are n-element column matrices (x_j is the jth system state). $\mathbf{A}$ is the $n \times n$ *system matrix,* $\mathbf{B}$ is the $n \times b$ *input matrix,* $\mathbf{u}$ is a column vector of *b inputs,* $\mathbf{y}$ is an p-element column matrix of *system outputs* derived from the n states and the b inputs. $\mathbf{C}$ is a $p \times n$ element matrix and $\mathbf{D}$ is a $p \times b$ element matrix. Note that, in the simplest case, the system can be SISO, so $\mathbf{y} = c_1x_1$, $\mathbf{u} = u_n$ and

$$\mathbf{D} = \begin{bmatrix} 0 \\ 0 \\ 1 \end{bmatrix} \tag{2.77}$$

for $n = 3$.

In the *first example,* consider an LS described by a third-order linear ODE. Following the approach we used in Equations 2.45 and 2.46, we write:

$$\frac{d^3x}{dt^3} + 4\frac{d^2x}{dt^2} + 3\frac{dx}{dt} + 2x = u(t) \tag{2.78}$$

As in the example of Equation 2.46, we let $x_1 = x$, $x_2 = \dot{x}_1$ and $x_3 = \dot{x}_2$. Thus, the matrices are:

$$\mathbf{x} = \begin{bmatrix} x_1 \\ x_2 \\ x_3 \end{bmatrix}, \quad \mathbf{A} = \begin{bmatrix} 0 & 1 & 0 \\ 0 & 0 & 1 \\ -2 & -3 & -4 \end{bmatrix}, \quad \mathbf{B} = \begin{bmatrix} 0 \\ 0 \\ 1 \end{bmatrix}, \quad \mathbf{u} = u(t) \tag{2.79}$$

If the output is $y = x_1 + 7u$, then the output state equation is written:

$$\mathbf{y} = \mathbf{Cx} + \mathbf{Du}, \tag{2.80}$$

where

$$\mathbf{C} = [1\ 0\ 0], \quad \mathbf{D} = [0\ 0\ 7] \text{ and } \mathbf{u} = \begin{bmatrix} 0 \\ 0 \\ u \end{bmatrix}. \tag{2.81}$$

A very important case is when the right-hand side of the ODE includes derivatives of the input, u. In general, the order of the highest derivative on the right-hand side will be $\leq n$, the order of the highest derivative of x. Starting with a second-order, SISO system example:

$$\frac{d^2x}{dt^2} + a_1\frac{dx}{dt} + a_2x = b_0\frac{d^2u}{dt^2} + b_1\frac{du}{dt} + b_2u \tag{2.82}$$

The goal is to eliminate the input derivative terms from the ODE [Kuo, 1967]. One way to do this is to first define state $x_1 \equiv (x - b_0u)$. Now $x = x_1 + b_0u$. When this latter equation is substituted into Equation 2.82, we can write:

$$\frac{d^2x_1}{dt^2} + b_0\frac{d^2u}{dt^2} + a_1\frac{dx_1}{dt} + a_1b_0\frac{du}{dt} + a_2x_1 + a_2b_0u = b_0\frac{d^2u}{dt^2} + b_1\frac{du}{dt} + b_2u$$

$$\downarrow$$

$$\frac{d^2x_1}{dt^2} + a_1\frac{dx_1}{dt} + a_2x_1 = \frac{du}{dt}(b_1 - a_1b_0) + u(b_2 - a_2b_0) \tag{2.83}$$

We next define state $x_2 \equiv \dot{x}_1 - (b_1 - a_1b_0)u$, or

$$\dot{x}_1 = x_2 + (b_1 - a_1b_0)u \tag{2.84}$$

Equation 2.84 is substituted into Equation 2.83. After simplifying, we obtain the state equation:

$$\dot{x}_2 + (b_1 - a_1b_0)\dot{u} + a_1[x_2 + (b_1 - a_1b_0)u] + a_2x_1 = \dot{u}(b_1 - a_1b_0) + u(b_2 - a_2b_0)$$

$$\downarrow$$

$$\dot{x}_2 = -a_2x_1 - a_1x_2 + [(b_2 - a_2b_0) - a_1(b_1 - a_1b_0)]u \tag{2.85}$$

To summarize, the state equations are:

$$\dot{x}_1 = x_2 + (b_1 - a_1b_0)u \tag{2.86A}$$

$$\dot{x}_2 = -a_2x_1 - a_1x_2 + [(b_2 - a_2b_0) - a_1(b_1 - a_1b_0)]u \tag{2.86B}$$

In SV form:

$$\dot{\mathbf{x}} = \overset{\mathbf{A}}{\begin{bmatrix} 0 & 1 \\ -a_2 & -a_1 \end{bmatrix}} \mathbf{x} + \overset{\mathbf{B}}{\begin{bmatrix} (b_1 - a_1b_0) \\ (b_2 - a_2b_0) - a_1(b_1 - a_1b_0) \end{bmatrix}} u(t) \tag{2.87}$$

Kuo (1967) gave a general form for resolving n^{th} order ODEs with input derivatives to standard SV form. The nth order ODE is:

$$\overset{\cdot n}{x} + a_1 \overset{\cdot(n-1)}{x} + a_2 \overset{\cdot(n-2)}{x} + \cdots + a_{n-1}x + a_n \dot{x} = b_0 u + b_1 \overset{\cdot n}{u} + \cdots + b_{n-1} \overset{\cdot(n-1)}{u} + b_n \dot{u} \tag{2.88}$$

Kuo shows that the general form of the **A** matrix is, starting with $x = (x_1 + b_0 u)$:

$$\mathbf{A} = \begin{bmatrix} 0 & 1 & 0 & 0 & \dots & 0 \\ 0 & 0 & 1 & 0 & \dots & 0 \\ 0 & 0 & 0 & 1 & \dots & 0 \\ \cdot & \cdot & \cdot & \cdot & \cdot & \cdot \\ 0 & 0 & 0 & \dots & 0 & 1 \\ -a_n & -a_{n-1} & -a_{n-2} & \dots & -a_2 & -a_1 \end{bmatrix} \tag{2.89}$$

The n elements of the **B** (column) matrix are then:

$$\begin{aligned} \beta_1 &= (b_1 - a_1 b_0) \\ \beta_2 &= (b_2 - a_2 b_0) - a_1 \beta_1 \\ \beta_3 &= (b_3 - a_3 b_0) - a_2 \beta_1 - a_1 \beta_2 \\ &\cdot \\ &\cdot \\ &\cdot \\ \beta_n &= (b_n - a_n b_0) - a_{n-1}\beta_1 - a_{n-2}\beta_2 - \cdots - a_2 \beta_{n-1} - a_1 \beta_n \end{aligned} \tag{2.90}$$

Another way to eliminate the input derivative terms in Equation 2.88. is to use signal flow graphs. Laplace transforms are described in Chapter 3. Mason's rule is covered in Appendix B.

Solution of a set of state equations in the time domain is first approached by considering the general solution of Equation 2.76A when $u = 0$, i.e., the solution of the homogeneous state equation, $\dot{\mathbf{x}} = \mathbf{Ax}$, with initial conditions. A simple ODE of the form

$$\dot{x} = a x(t) \tag{2.91}$$

can be rewritten as:

$$\frac{dx(t)}{dx} = a\,dt \tag{2.92}$$

Which is easily integrated to:

$$\ln[x(t)] = at + C_1 \tag{2.93}$$

Let $C_1 = \ln[k]$, now Equation 2.93 can be rewritten as:

$$\ln[x(t)] = \ln[e^{at}] + \ln[k] \rightarrow x(t) = k e^{at} \tag{2.94}$$

The constant k is simply $x(0)$, the initial value of x. For any initial time $t = t_o$, the initial value of x by definition is $x(t_o)$. From Equation 2.95 we can write:

$$x(0) = e^{-at}x(t_o) \tag{2.95}$$

Now substituting Equation 2.95 into Equation 2.94 we find:

$$x(t) = e^{a(t-t_o)}x(t_o) \tag{2.96}$$

which is the solution of the ODE Equation 2.91 for any IC, $x(t_o)$.

By inference from the above development it is reasonable to assume that the solution of the homogeneous state equation, $\dot{\mathbf{x}} = \mathbf{A}\mathbf{x}$, is of the form:

$$x(t) = e^{\mathbf{A}(t-t_o)}\mathbf{x}(t_o) \tag{2.97}$$

Note that the exponential function of matrix **A** is given by:

$$e^{\mathbf{A}(t-t_o)} = \exp[\mathbf{A}(t-t_o)] = \mathbf{I} + \mathbf{A}(t-t_o) + \frac{\mathbf{A}^2(t-t_o)^2}{2!} + \cdots + \frac{\mathbf{A}^k(t-t_o)^k}{k!} + \cdots \tag{2.98A}$$

or:

$$e^{\mathbf{A}(t-t_o)} = \sum_{n=0}^{\infty} \mathbf{A}^n \frac{(t-t_o)^n}{n!} \tag{2.98B}$$

The *state-transition matrix* or *fundamental matrix* of **A** is defined as:

$$\Phi(t) \equiv e^{\mathbf{A}t} \tag{2.99}$$

Thus the solution of the homogeneous equation can finally be written as:

$$x(t) = \Phi(t-t_o)\mathbf{x}(t_o) \tag{2.100}$$

Kuo gives the following properties of $\Phi(t)$ with proofs:

$$\Phi(0) = \mathbf{I} \quad \text{(identity matrix)} \tag{2.101A}$$

$$\Phi(t_2 - t_1)\Phi(t_1 - t_o) = \Phi(t_2 - t_o) \tag{2.101B}$$

$$\Phi(t_1 - t_o) = [\Phi(t_o - t_1)]^{-1} \quad \text{or} \quad [\Phi(t)]^{-1} = \Phi(-t) \tag{2.101C}$$

Solution of the homogeneous set of state equations in the time domain is formidable as a pencil and paper project. My best advice is to avoid it at whatever cost. The same comment is emphatically underscored when solving state equations with many inputs **u** (forcing). That is:

$$\dot{\mathbf{x}} = \mathbf{A}\mathbf{x} + \mathbf{B}\mathbf{u} \tag{2.102}$$

Kuo shows that the general time-domain solution can be written as:

$$\mathbf{x}(t) = \Phi(t - t_o)\mathbf{x}(t_o) + \int_{t_o}^{t} \Phi(t - \tau)\mathbf{B}\mathbf{u}(\tau)\,d\tau, \quad t \geq t_o \geq 0 \qquad (2.103)$$

Thus, the complete solution for the states, $\mathbf{x}(t)$, consists of the homogeneous solution independent from the solution due to specific inputs, $\mathbf{u}$. Although the use of IC time, $t_o > 0$, is more general, in most cases, we assume the solution starts at $t = 0$ and we take the ICs at $t_o = 0$.

Thus Equation 2.103 becomes:

$$\mathbf{x}(t) = \Phi(t)\mathbf{x}(0) + \int_{0}^{t} \Phi(t - \tau)\mathbf{B}\mathbf{u}(\tau)\,d\tau, \quad t \geq 0 \qquad (2.104)$$

Frequency-domain solutions are, in general, a much easier approach to the solution of state variable systems. They are considered in detail in Chapter 3.

2.4 Linear System Characterization

2.4.1 Introduction

We listed the properties of linear systems in Section 2.1. Probably the most important property is that of *superposition.* From superposition follows convolution and application of frequency domain transforms such as Laplace, Fourier and Hilbert. The *impulse response* is introduced below as a unique descriptor of a linear system. From the impulse response we can calculate the system's time-domain output given an input, using real convolution. It can also be used to find the system's transfer function and steady-state sinusoidal frequency response.

2.4.2 System impulse response

A *unit impulse,* $\delta(t)$, is also called a *delta function;* it has some interesting properties, as shown below:

$$\delta(t) = 0, \quad t \neq 0$$

$$\int_{-\infty}^{\infty} \delta(t)\,dt = \int_{-\varepsilon}^{\varepsilon} \delta(t)\,dt = 1 \qquad (2.105A)$$

$$\int_{-\infty}^{\infty} f(t)\delta(t - t_o)\,dt = \int_{p}^{q} f(t)\delta(t - t_o)\,dt = f(t_o), \quad p < 0 < q \qquad (2.105B)$$

$$\int_{-\infty}^{\infty} f(x - t)\delta(t - t_o)\,dt = f(x - t_o) \qquad (2.105C)$$

Relations 2.105b and 2.105c illustrate the important *sifting* or *sampling property* of the impulse function, which only exists at a point for $\delta(0)$. A unit impulse can be visualized as what happens to a narrow rectangular pulse of width ε and height $1/\varepsilon$ in the limit as $\varepsilon \to 0$. The pulse's height $\to \infty$ and its width $\to 0$ so that its area remains unity. In fact, two parameters describe an impulse function; its area and the point at which it occurs is when its argument$= 0$.

We also have the property that the derivative of a unit step function is a unit impulse, sic:

$$\dot{\mathrm{U}}(\mathrm{t}-\mathrm{t_o}) \equiv \delta(\mathrm{t}-\mathrm{t_o}) \tag{2.106}$$

Conversely, the integral of an impulse is a unit step beginning at the origin of the impulse:

$$\int_{-\infty}^{\mathrm{t}} \delta(\tau-\mathrm{t_o})\,\mathrm{d}\tau = \mathrm{U}(\mathrm{t}-\mathrm{t_o}), \quad \mathrm{t} > \mathrm{t_o} \tag{2.107}$$

Another important use of the unit impulse is to characterize linear systems. When a unit impulse is the input to a system, the resulting output is called the *impulse response* or *weighting function* of the system. As you will see below, the Laplace transform of the system's impulse response gives the system's *transfer function;* its Fourier transform yields the system's *frequency response function.*

2.4.3 Real convolution

Real convolution is a direct result of the property of superposition. Real convolution allows us to calculate the output of an LTI system at some time $\mathrm{t_1} > 0$, given the system's continuous input $\mathrm{x(t)}$ for $\mathrm{t} \geq 0$ and the system's impulse response, $\mathrm{h(t)}$.

To derive the real convolution integral, let the system's input be a continuous function, $\mathrm{x(t)}$, defined for $\mathrm{t} \geq 0$. This input signal is approximated by a continuous train of rectangular pulses, as shown in Figure 2.4. That is, each pulse has a height

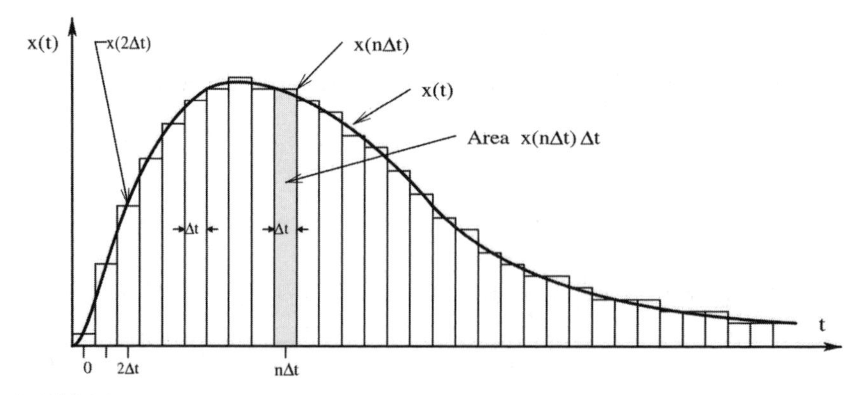

FIGURE 2.4
The continuous function, $\mathrm{x(t)}$ is approximated by a continuous train of rectangular pulses. This figure is important in the derivation of the real convolution integral.

$x(n\Delta t)$ and occurs at time $t = n\Delta t$, $n = 0, 1, 2, \ldots \infty$. Thus, each rectangular pulse has an area of $[x(n\Delta t)\Delta t]$. If we let $\Delta t \to 0$ in the limit, the nth pulse produces an *impulse response* given by:

$$y(n\Delta t) = \lim_{\Delta t \to 0} [x(n\Delta t)\Delta t] h(t - n\Delta t), \quad t \geq n\Delta t \tag{2.108}$$

That is, $y(n\Delta t)$ is the impulse response to an (approximate) impulse of area $[x(n\Delta t)\Delta t]$ occurring at time $t = n\Delta t$. At a particular time, $t_1 > n\Delta t$, this response to a single input impulse is:

$$y_1(n\Delta t) = \lim_{\Delta t \to 0} [x(n\Delta t)\Delta t] h(t_1 - n\Delta t), \quad t_1 \geq n\Delta t \tag{2.109}$$

Now by superposition, the *total response* at time t_1 is given by the sum of the responses to each component (equivalent) impulse making up the input approximation, $x(n\Delta t)$:

$$y(t_1) = \lim_{\Delta t \to 0} \sum_{n=0}^{n\Delta t = t_1} [x(n\Delta t)\Delta t] h(t_1 - n\Delta t) \tag{2.110}$$

Because the system is causal, input pulses occurring beyond $t = t_1$ have no effect on the response at t_1. In the limit, the discrete summation becomes the real convolution an integral:

$$y(t_1) = \int_0^{t_1} x(t) h(t_1 - t)\, dt \tag{2.111}$$

It is less confusing to replace the time variable of integration in Equation 2.111 with τ and to replace t_1 with a general time, t, at which we view the output. Thus, we have the general form for *real convolution:*

$$y(t) = \int_0^{t} x(\tau) h(t - \tau)\, d\tau \tag{2.112}$$

Some properties of real convolution:

1. *Real convolution is commutative.* That is,

$$f_1(t) \otimes f_2(t) = f_2(t) \otimes f_1(t) \tag{2.113A}$$

This can be proven by writing:

$$f_1(t) \otimes f_2(t) = \int_{-\infty}^{\infty} f_1(\tau) f_2(t - \tau)\, d\tau \tag{2.113B}$$

Now let us substitute $t - \mu$ for τ. We can now write:

$$f_1(t) \otimes f_2(t) = \int_{-\infty}^{\infty} f_2(\mu) f_1(t - \mu)\, d\mu = f_2(t) \otimes f_1(t) \tag{2.113C}$$

For a linear system with input x and output y, this means that:

$$y(t) = x(t) \otimes h(t) = h(t) \otimes x(t) \tag{2.113D}$$

2. Convolution is also *distributive.* That is:

$$f_1(t) \otimes [f_2(t) + f_3(t)] = f_1(t) \otimes f_2(t) + f_1(t) \otimes f_3(t) \tag{2.113E}$$

3. It is also *associative,* sic:

$$f_1(t) \otimes [f_2(t) \otimes f_3(t)] = [f_1(t) \otimes f_2(t)] \otimes f_3(t) \tag{2.113F}$$

A *first example* of a graphical interpretation of the convolution process helpful in understanding the abstract notation given by Equation 2.112 is shown in Figure 2.5. In this example, the system's impulse response $h(t) = B$ for $0 \le t \le 2T$, and 0 for $t < 0$ and $t > 2T$. The input, $x(t)$, is a triangular pulse of height A and duration T. Analytically, $x(t)$ can be expressed:

$$x(t) = A - (A/T)t = A(1 - t/T) \tag{2.114}$$

for $0 \le t \le T$ and 0 elsewhere. These waveforms are shown as functions of the age variable, τ. In the middle figure, $h(t - \tau)$ is plotted as $h(\tau)$ reversed in time τ and shifted to the right by $t > 0$ so that $h(t - \tau)$ overlaps the input pulse $x(\tau)$. The value of the convolution integral for a particular shift, t_1, is the integral of the product $x(\tau)h(t_1 - \tau)$, *where the functions overlap.* In this example, the integral can be divided into three regions: $0 \le t < T$, $T \le t < 2T$ and $2T \le t \le 3T$. In the first region:

$$y_1(t) = \int_0^t BA(1 - \tau/T)\, d\tau = BA(t - t^2/2T), \quad 0 \le t < T \tag{2.115}$$

In the second region, $h(t - \tau)$ overlaps the triangle, $x(\tau)$ and the integral is simply the triangle's area times B, a constant. By inspection:

$$y_2(t) = BAT/2, \quad T \le t < 2T \tag{2.116}$$

In the third region, the trailing edge of $h(t - \tau)$ sets the lower limit of the integral to $t - 2T$ and the upper limit is set by $x(\tau)$ to T, sic:

$$\begin{aligned} y_3(t) &= \int_{t-2T}^{T} BA(1 - \tau/T)\, d\tau = BA[\tau - \tau^2/2T]\Big|_{t-2T}^{T} \\ &= BA[T - T/2] - BA[(t - 2T) - (t - 2T)^2/2T] \\ &= BAT/2 - BAt + BA2T + BAt^2/2T - BA4tT/2T + BA4T^2/2T \\ &= \frac{9}{2}BAT - 3BAt + BA(t^2/2T) \end{aligned} \tag{2.117}$$

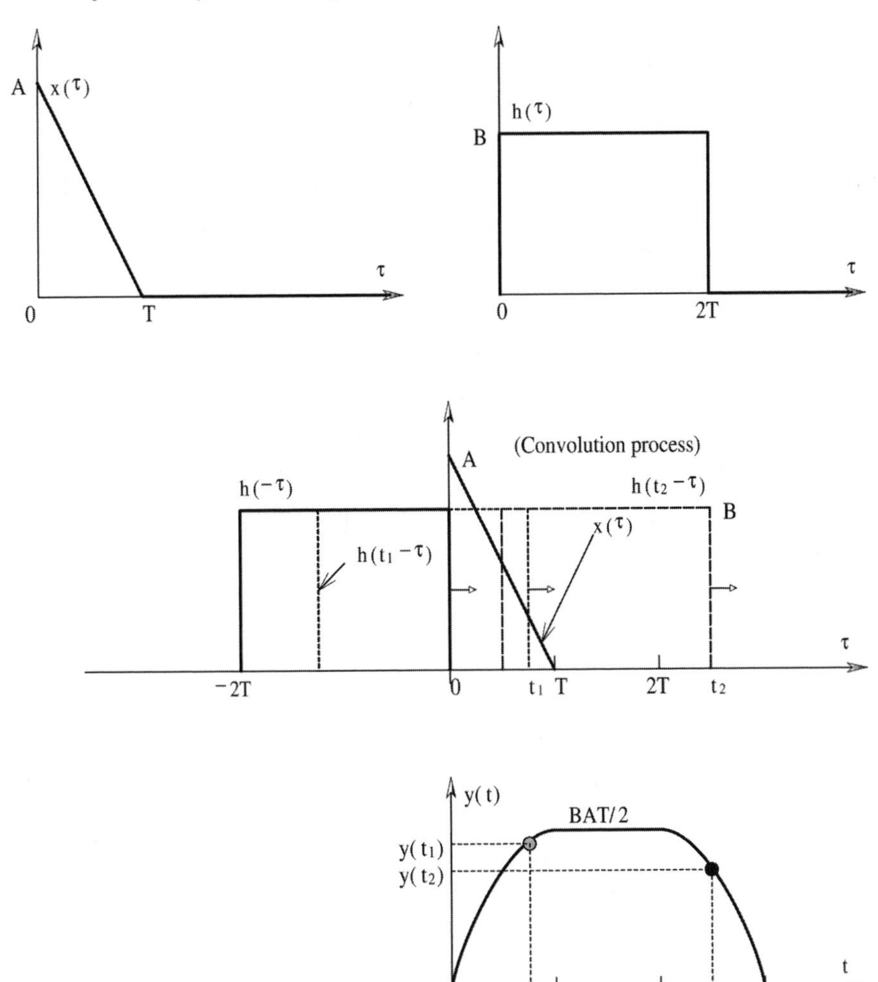

FIGURE 2.5
Steps illustrating graphically the process of continuous, real convolution between an input $x(t)$ and an LTI system with a rectangular impulse response, $h(t)$. In this example, $h(\tau)$ is reversed in time and displaced as $h(t-\tau)$ and slid past $x(\tau)$. Where $h(t-\tau)$ overlaps $x(\tau)$, their product is integrated to form the system output, $y(t)$.

When $t = 2T$, $y_3(t) = BAT/2$ and when $t \geq 3T$, $y_3(t) = 0$, which agrees with the limits seen in the figure.

For a *second graphical example* of real convolution, consider the signals shown in Figure 2.6. The input is a rectangular pulse of duration T and amplitude A. The system weighting function is $h(\tau) = Be^{-b\tau}$. In this case, the convolution integral can be

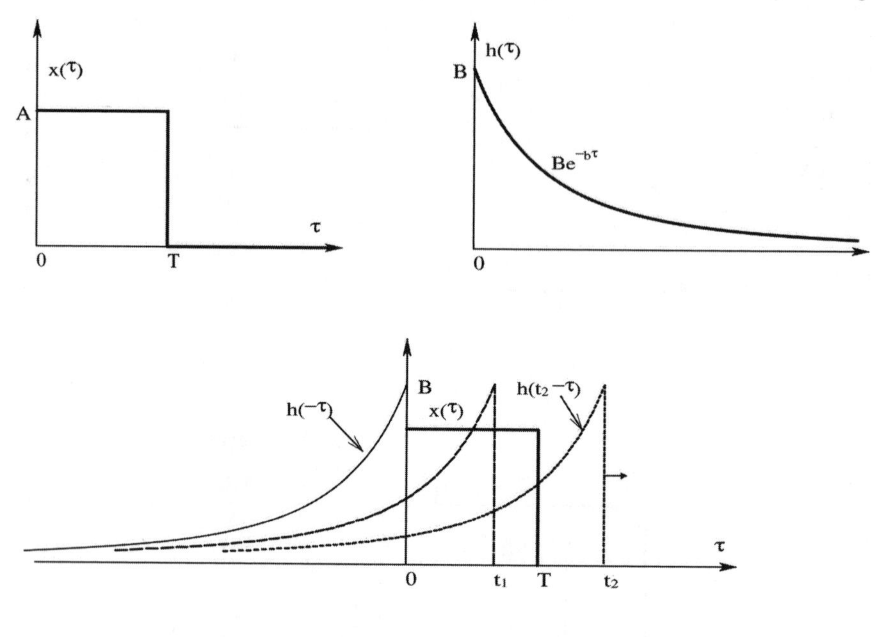

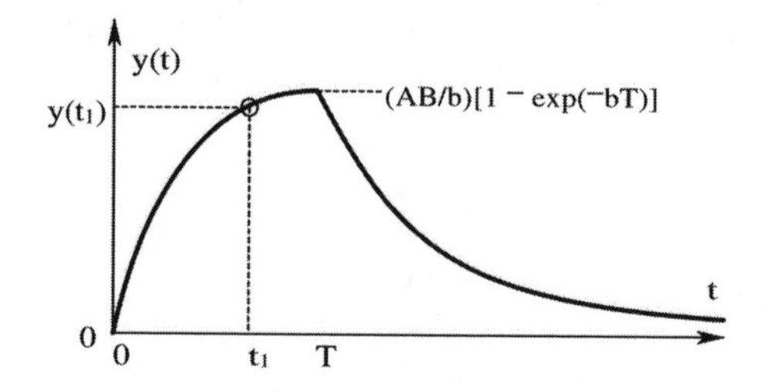

FIGURE 2.6

Another graphical example of real convolution. The system's input is a rectangular pulse; the system's weighting function is a simple exponential decay, characteristic of a first-order low-pass filter. The output $y(t)$, rises to a peak and then decays.

broken up into two regions over which $x(\tau)$ and $h(t-\tau)$ overlap to form a nonzero product.

$$
\begin{aligned}
y_1(t) &= \int_0^t AB\exp[-b(t-\tau)]\,d\tau = AB\exp(-bt)\int_0^t \exp(b\tau)\,d\tau \\
&= AB\exp(-bt)\exp(bt)/b - AB\exp(-bt)/b
\end{aligned}
$$

$$\downarrow$$

$$y_1(t) = (AB/b)[1-\exp(-bt)], \quad 0 \le t \le T \tag{2.118}$$

The second region exists for $T < t \leq \infty$. The value of the convolution integral in this region is:

$$y_2(t) = \int_0^T AB\exp[-b(t-\tau)]\,d\tau = AB\exp(-bt)\int_0^T \exp(b\tau)\,d\tau$$
$$= AB\exp(-bt)\exp(bT)/b - AB\exp(-bt)(1/b)$$
$$\downarrow$$
$$y_2(t) = (AB/b)\exp(-bt)[\exp(bT)-1], \quad T < t \leq \infty \tag{2.119}$$

Thus, the peak $y(t)$ occurs at $t = T$ and is: $y(T) = (AB/b)[1-\exp(-bT)]$.

Real convolution can also be performed on *discrete (sampled) signals.* In this case, the input is written as $x(nT)$ or $x(n)$. T is the sampling period and n is the sample number. Similarly, the system's impulse response is also expressed in numerical (sampled) form, $h(nT)$ or $h(n)$. Following the development above, we can write the discrete system output $y(nT)$ as:

$$y(n) = \sum_{k=0}^{\infty} x(k)h(n-k) = \sum_{k=0}^{\infty} h(k)x(n-k) \tag{2.120}$$

All of the properties of convolution with continuous variables apply to discrete convolution.

An important use of convolution is *deconvolution* or signal recovery. As an example, an acoustical signal, $x(t)$, (such as heart valve sounds) propagates through the lungs and chest walls where acoustic power at certain frequencies is attenuated and delayed. The sound, $y(t)$, is picked up at the chest surface. If $y(t)$ is convolved *(deconvolved)* with an *inverse* filter that essentially compensates for the effects of the propagation of $x(t)$ through tissues, then an estimate of $x(t)$ can be recovered [Widrow and Stearns, 1985].

2.4.4 Transient response of systems

Three major classifications of inputs to systems are used to characterize their input/output characteristics. These are:

1. Transient inputs (including impulses, steps and ramps)
2. Steady-state sinusoidal inputs
3. Stationary random inputs (viewed in the steady-state)

Often we are interested in the settling time of a system when it is suddenly disturbed by an input. Such *transient inputs* include the *impulse function* (practically, a pulse of known area whose duration is much less than the shortest time constant in the system's weighting function). The system's output in response to an impulse input is the LTI system's *weighting function,* which tells us something about the system's dynamic behavior. *Step functions* are also used to characterize the dynamic behavior of LTI systems. By definition, the step response of an LTI system is the integral of the system's weighting function. A *ramp* input, starting at $t = 0$, can also be used experimentally to characterize the error properties of closed-loop control systems. *Wavelets* (see Section 6.9) can also be used as transient test inputs to LTI systems.

The *inverse Laplace transform* is widely used to calculate system outputs, given the system's *transfer function* and the Laplace transform of the system's input. This process is covered in detail in Chapter 3.

If a system is described at the level of its component ODEs or state equations, it is often more expedient to simulate the system's transient response with *Matlab/ Simulink*™ or *Simnon*™ than to derive its transfer function and then use Laplace transforms.

2.4.5 Steady-state sinusoidal frequency response of LTI systems

If a sinusoidal input, $x(t) = A\sin(\omega t)$, has been applied to a linear system for time that is very long compared with the longest time constant in the system's transient response, the system is said to be in the *sinusoidal steady-state* (SSS). In the steady-state, the exponential transient terms of the homogeneous solutions to the system's ODEs have died out to zero. In sinusoidal steady-state excitation, the linear system's output will be of the same frequency as the input, but generally will have a different phase and amplitude, thus $y(t) = B\sin(2\pi ft + \phi)$. By definition, the LTI system's *frequency response function* is a 2-D vector with magnitude (B/A) and phase angle, ϕ. That is, in polar notation, $\mathbf{H}(f) = (B/A)\angle\phi$. Note that the frequency response function can be written as a function of Hz frequency, f or radian frequency, $\omega = 2\pi f$. Both (A/B) and ϕ are functions of frequency. For reasons that will be made clear in the next section, engineers and scientists generally plot $20\log_{10}|\mathbf{H}(f)|$ on a linear vertical scale vs. a logarithmic frequency scale. $\phi(f)$ is plotted on linear vs. log frequency scales, as well. Such plots are called *Bode plots*. *Polar plots* of frequency response can also be made where $|\mathbf{H}(f)|$ is plotted vs. $\phi(f)$ on polar coordinates for a set of f values.

To find a linear system's frequency response from its defining ODE, we first write the nth order system ODE in general form:

$$\overset{\cdot n}{y} + a_1 \overset{\cdot(n-1)}{y} + a_2 \overset{\cdot(n-2)}{y} + \cdots + a_{n-1}\dot{y} + a_n y = b_0 \overset{\cdot n}{u} + b_1 \overset{\cdot(n-1)}{u} + \cdots + b_{n-1}\dot{u} + b_n u \tag{2.121}$$

Next, we write the ODE in *operator notation,* where $py = \frac{dy}{dt}$, and $p^n y = \frac{d^n y}{dt^n}$, etc.

$$p^n y + p^{n-1} y a_1 + p^{n-2} y a_2 + \cdots + pya_{n-1} + ya_n = p^n ub_0 + p^{n-1} ub_1 + \cdots + pub_{n-1} + ub_n \tag{2.122}$$

This equation can also be written in a factored form:

$$y[p^n + a_1 p^{n-1} + a_2 p^{n-2} + \cdots + a_{n-1} p + a_n] = u[b_0 p^n + b_1 p^{n-1} + \cdots + b_{n-1} p + b_n] \quad (2.123)$$

It can be shown that, if we replace p by the imaginary number, $j\omega$, where ω is the radian frequency of the sinusoidal input, $u(t) = A\sin(\omega t)$, then $y(t)$ and $u(t)$ can be treated as vectors (phasors), **Y** and **U**, respectively. The angle of the input, **U**, is by definition, 0, and its magnitude is A. **Y** has magnitude B and angle ϕ. Thus, the linear n^{th} order SISO system's frequency response is given in general by the ratio of two vectors:

$$\frac{\mathbf{Y}}{\mathbf{U}}(j\omega) = \frac{\overbrace{b_0(j\omega)^n + b_1(j\omega)^{n-1} + \cdots + b_{n-2}(j\omega)^2 + b_{n-1}(j\omega) + b_n}^{\mathbf{B}}}{\underbrace{(j\omega)^n + a_1(j\omega)^{n-1} + \cdots + a_{n-2}(j\omega)^2 + a_{n-1}(j\omega) + a_n}_{\mathbf{A}}} = \mathbf{H}(j\omega) \quad (2.124)$$

Note that n = even powers of $(j\omega)$ in the numerator and denominator are $\pm$ real numbers and n = odd powers are imaginary with either $\pm j$ factors. Recall also that the ratio of two vectors can be written as:

$$\mathbf{P} = \frac{\mathbf{Q}}{\mathbf{R}} = \frac{|\mathbf{Q}|\angle\theta_q}{|\mathbf{R}|\angle\theta_r} = (Q/R)\angle\theta_q - \theta_r \quad (2.125)$$

In this case, $\phi(\omega) = \theta_q - \theta_r$ and $Q/R = A/B$. Since terms in the numerator and denominator are either real or imaginary, we can group them accordingly:

$$\mathbf{H}(j\omega) = \frac{\alpha(\omega) + j\beta(\omega)}{\gamma(\omega) + j\delta(\omega)} \quad (2.126)$$

The denominator can be made real by multiplying numerator and denominator by the *complex conjugate* of the denominator, which is $[\gamma(\omega) - j\delta(\omega)]$.

$$\mathbf{H}(j\omega) = \frac{[\alpha(\omega)\gamma(\omega) + \beta(\omega)\delta(\omega)] + \mathbf{j}[\beta(\omega)\gamma(\omega) - \alpha(\omega)\delta(\omega)]}{\gamma^2(\omega) + \delta^2(\omega)} \quad (2.127)$$

Note that

$$\phi(\omega) = \mathbf{H}(j\omega) = \tan^{-1}\left\{\frac{[\beta(\omega)\gamma(\omega) - \alpha(\omega)\delta(\omega)]}{[\alpha(\omega)\gamma(\omega) + \beta(\omega)\delta(\omega)]}\right\} \quad (2.128)$$

As a *first example,* let us find the frequency response of the pharmacokinetic system described in Section 2.2.2. Recall that this system described the rate that a drug was removed from the blood volume. [D] is the drug concentration in the blood in (μg/l), K_L is the loss rate constant (units, 1/min.), V_c is the total blood volume in l and R_D is the rate of drug injection in μg/min. The system ODE is:

$$[\dot{D}] = -K_L[D] + (R_D/V_c)U(t) \quad (\mu g/l)/\min \quad (2.129)$$

Rewriting the ODE in operator form:

$$[\mathrm{D}](\mathrm{p}+\mathrm{K_L}) = \mathrm{R_D}(\mathrm{t})/\mathrm{V_c} \tag{2.130}$$

Normally, for an IV drip, R_D is a constant (a step). Because we wish to examine the sinusoidal response of this system, it is tempting to let $R_D = R_{Do}\sin(\omega t)$. However, the sine wave is negative over half of each cycle, which is physically impossible in a PK system (there are no negative drug infusions, injections or concentrations). Thus, we must add a constant level to $R_D(t)$ so it does not go negative. Thus the input will be:

$$\mathrm{R_D}(\mathrm{t}) = \mathrm{R_{Do}}[1+\sin(\omega \mathrm{t})]\mathrm{U}(\mathrm{t}) > 0 \tag{2.131}$$

This input is actually the sum of a step and a sinusoid. By superposition, the steady-state step response is:

$$[\mathrm{D}]_{\mathrm{ss}} = \mathrm{R_{Do}}/(\mathrm{K_L V_c}) \quad \mu\mathrm{g/l} \tag{2.132}$$

To find the SS frequency response, as we have shown above, let $p \to j\omega$ in Equation 2.130. Thus:

$$\frac{\mathbf{[D]}}{\mathbf{R_D}}(\mathrm{j}\omega) = \frac{1/\mathrm{V_c}}{\mathrm{j}\omega+\mathrm{K_L}} = \frac{1/\mathrm{V_c}}{\sqrt{\omega^2+\mathrm{K_L^2}}}\angle\phi \tag{2.133A}$$

$$\phi = -\tan^{-1}(\omega/\mathrm{K_L}) \tag{2.133B}$$

Thus, the sinusoidal drug concentration in the blood lags the input injection sinusoid by ϕ degrees and falls off with frequency to reach $-90°$ (the system behaves like a first-order low-pass filter). The output sine response sits on the dc response, $R_{Do}/(K_L V_c)$, required to make $u(t)$ non-negative.

In a *second example,* we will illustrate finding the SS frequency response of a second-order time-domain SV system given by:

$$\dot{\mathbf{x}} = \mathbf{A}\mathbf{x}+\mathbf{B}\mathbf{u} \tag{2.134A}$$

$$\mathrm{y}(\mathrm{t}) = \mathrm{x_1}(\mathrm{t}) \tag{2.134B}$$

The **A** and **B** matrices are:

$$\mathbf{A} = \begin{bmatrix} 0 & 1 \\ -2 & -3 \end{bmatrix}, \quad \mathbf{B} = \begin{bmatrix} 0 \\ 1 \end{bmatrix} \tag{2.135}$$

and $u(t) = A\sin(\omega t)$. Using p as the differential operator, the SS sinusoidal frequency response of this simple linear SISO system is given by:

$$\begin{aligned} &\mathrm{p}\mathbf{x} = \mathbf{A}\mathbf{x}+\mathbf{B}\mathbf{u} \\ &\downarrow \\ &\mathrm{p}\mathbf{x} - \mathbf{A}\mathbf{x} = \mathbf{B}\mathbf{u} \\ &\downarrow \\ &(\mathrm{p}\mathbf{I} - \mathbf{A})\mathbf{x} = \mathbf{B}\mathbf{u} \end{aligned} \tag{2.136}$$

Assume $\mathbf{u} = \mathrm{u(t)} = \mathrm{A}\sin(\omega \mathrm{t})$. Replace the operator p with the imaginary number, $\mathrm{j}\omega$ and solve for the state phasors:

$$\mathbf{X} = (\mathrm{j}\omega\mathbf{I} - \mathbf{A})^{-1}\mathbf{B}\mathbf{U} \tag{2.137}$$

The inverse matrix, $\Phi(\mathrm{j}\omega) \equiv (\mathrm{j}\omega\mathbf{I} - \mathbf{A})^{-1}$ has complex elements. It is found by first calculating:

$$(\mathrm{j}\omega\mathbf{I} - \mathbf{A}) = \left(\mathrm{j}\omega \begin{bmatrix} 1 & 0 \\ 0 & 1 \end{bmatrix} - \begin{bmatrix} 0 & 1 \\ -2 & -3 \end{bmatrix} \right) = \begin{bmatrix} \mathrm{j}\omega & -1 \\ 2 & \mathrm{j}\omega + 3 \end{bmatrix} \tag{2.138}$$

The inverse of $(\mathrm{j}\omega\mathbf{I} - \mathbf{A}) \equiv \mathrm{adj}(\mathrm{j}\omega\mathbf{I} - \mathbf{A})/\det(\mathrm{j}\omega\mathbf{I} - \mathbf{A}) = \Phi(\mathrm{j}\omega)$. $\det(\mathrm{j}\omega\mathbf{I} - \mathbf{A}) = (\mathrm{j}\omega)^2 + 3\mathrm{j}\omega + 2$. The adjoint of $(\mathrm{j}\omega\mathbf{I} - \mathbf{A})$ is found to be:

$$\mathrm{adj}\,(\mathrm{j}\omega\mathbf{I} - \mathbf{A}) = \begin{bmatrix} \mathrm{j}\omega + 3 & 1 \\ -3 & \mathrm{j}\omega \end{bmatrix} \tag{2.139}$$

Thus, the $\Phi(\mathrm{j}\omega)$ is:

$$\Phi(\mathrm{j}\omega) = \frac{\begin{bmatrix} \mathrm{j}\omega + 3 & 1 \\ -3 & \mathrm{j}\omega \end{bmatrix}}{(\mathrm{j}\omega)^2 + 3\mathrm{j}\omega + 2} \tag{2.140}$$

The system output is $\mathrm{y(t)} = \mathrm{x_1(t)}$, or in phasor notation, $\mathbf{Y} = \mathbf{X_1}(\mathrm{j}\omega)$. Thus, the system's frequency response function is:

$$\mathbf{X}(\mathrm{j}\omega) = \frac{\begin{bmatrix} \mathrm{j}\omega + 3 & 1 \\ -3 & \mathrm{j}\omega \end{bmatrix} \begin{bmatrix} 0 \\ 1 \end{bmatrix} \mathbf{U}}{(\mathrm{j}\omega)^2 + 3\mathrm{j}\omega + 2} \tag{2.141}$$

and

$$\begin{aligned} \frac{\mathbf{Y}}{\mathbf{U}}(\mathrm{j}\omega) &= \frac{1}{(\mathrm{j}\omega)^2 + 3\mathrm{j}\omega + 2} = \frac{1}{(2 - \omega^2) + 3\mathrm{j}\omega} \\ &= \frac{1}{\sqrt{(2 - \omega^2)^2 + 9\omega^2}} \angle\phi \end{aligned} \tag{2.142A}$$

$$\text{Where } \phi = -\tan^{-1}\left(\frac{3\omega}{2 - \omega^2}\right) \tag{2.142B}$$

Note that there are easier pencil and paper means of finding a system's frequency response or transfer function, given its state equations. Finding $\Phi(\mathrm{j}\omega)$ for a quadratic (2×2) SV system is relatively easy, but for $\mathrm{n} \geq 3$, it becomes tedious and quite subject to algebraic errors. A simpler approach is to construct a *signal flow graph* from the state equations and reduce it using *Mason's rule* [see Appendix B], which is far more direct algebraically than crunching $\Phi(\mathrm{j}\omega)$ for $\mathrm{n} \geq 3$.

2.4.6 Bode plots

As we mentioned above, A Bode plot is a system's frequency response plot done on log-linear graph paper. The (horizontal) frequency axis is logarithmic; on the linear vertical axis is plotted $20\log_{10}|\mathbf{H}(f)|$ which has the units of decibels (dB) and the phase angle of $\mathbf{H}(f)$, which is the phase angle between the output and input sinusoids. One advantage of plotting $20\log_{10}|\mathbf{H}(f)|$ vs. f on semilog paper is that plots are made easier by the use of *asymptotes* giving the frequency response behavior relative to the system's break frequencies or natural frequencies. Also, by using a logarithmic function, products of terms appear graphically as sums. Perhaps the best way to introduce the art of Bode plotting is by example.

Example 1: A simple low-pass system

Let us assume a system is described by the first-order ODE:

$$a\dot{y} + by = cu \tag{2.143}$$

In operator notation this is:

$$a\,py + by = cu \tag{2.144}$$

Assume the input $u(t) = U(t)A\sin(\omega t)$ and the system is in the SSS. Now:

$$\mathbf{Y}[aj\omega + b] = c\mathbf{U} \tag{2.145}$$

Writing the phasors as a ratio:

$$\frac{\mathbf{Y}}{\mathbf{U}}(j\omega) = \frac{c}{aj\omega + b} \tag{2.146}$$

When doing a Bode plot, the frequency response function should be put into *time-constant form*. That is, the 0th power of ($j\omega$) is given a coefficient of 1, in both numerator and denominator:

$$\frac{\mathbf{Y}}{\mathbf{U}}(j\omega) = \frac{c/b}{j\omega(a/b) + 1} = \mathbf{H}(j\omega) \quad \text{(time-constant form)} \tag{2.147}$$

The quantity (a/b) is the system's time constant; it has the units of time. One advantage of the time-constant format is that when u is dc, $\omega = 0$ and the dc gain of the system is simply (c/b). The magnitude of the frequency response function is just:

$$|\mathbf{H}(j\omega)| = \frac{c/b}{\sqrt{\omega^2(a/b)^2 + 1}} \tag{2.148}$$

And its dB logarithmic value is:

$$\text{dB} = 20\log(c/b) - 10\log[\omega^2(a/b)^2 + 1] \tag{2.149}$$

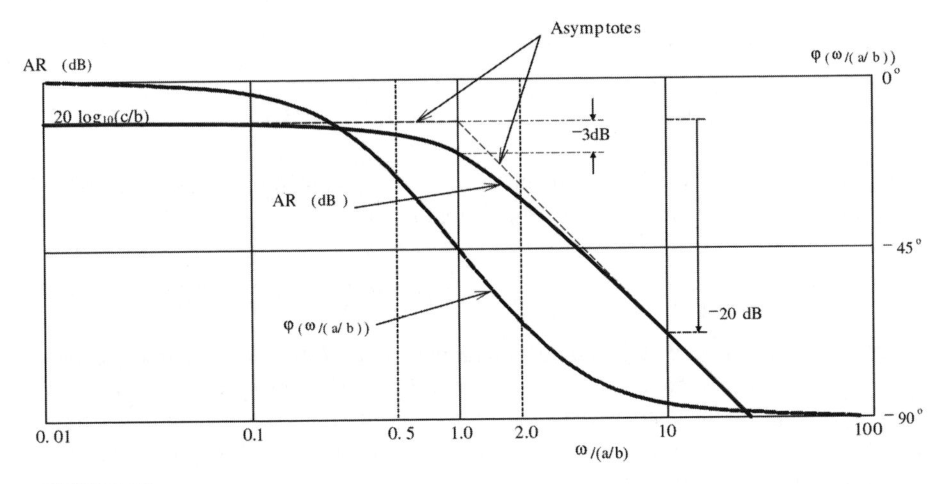

FIGURE 2.7
Bode plot (magnitude and phase) frequency response of a simple, first-order, real-pole, low-pass filter (such as described in Figure 2.6). See text for discussion.

For $\omega = 0$, $\mathrm{dB} = 20\log(\mathrm{c/b})$. For $\omega = (\mathrm{a/b})^{-1}$ r/s, $\mathrm{dB} = 20\log(\mathrm{c/b}) - 10\log[2]$ or the dc level minus 3dB. $\omega_o = (\mathrm{a/b})^{-1}$ r/s is the system's break frequency. For $\omega \geq 10\omega_0$, the amplitude response is given by:

$$\mathrm{dB} = 20\log(\mathrm{c/b}) - 20\log[\omega] - 20\log[\mathrm{a/b}] \tag{2.150}$$

From Equation 2.150, we see that the asymptote has a slope of -20 dB/decade of radian frequency, or equivalently, -6 dB/octave (doubling) of frequency. The phase of this system is given by:

$$\phi(\omega) = -\tan^{-1}(\omega \mathrm{a/b}) \tag{2.151}$$

Thus, the phase goes from $0°$ at $\omega = 0$ to $-90°$ as $\omega \to \infty$. Figure 2.7 illustrates the complete Bode plot for the simple first-order, low-pass system.

Example 2: Underdamped second-order low-pass system described by the ODE:

$$\mathrm{a}\ddot{\mathrm{y}} + \mathrm{b}\dot{\mathrm{y}} + \mathrm{cy} = \mathrm{du(t)} \tag{2.152}$$

As before, $\mathrm{u(t)} = \mathrm{U(t)A}\sin(\omega \mathrm{t})$ has been applied to the system for a long time so it is in the steady-state. Again we use operator notation:

$$\mathrm{ap^2y} + \mathrm{bpy} + \mathrm{cy} = \mathrm{dU(t)} \tag{2.153}$$

The output $\mathrm{y(t)}$ will be a sinusoid of some amplitude B and phase ϕ with respect to $\mathrm{u(t)}$ so it can be represented as a vector Y. The input can also be represented as a vector with amplitude A and zero (reference) phase. Again we let $\mathrm{p} = \mathrm{j}\omega$.

$$\mathbf{Y}[\mathrm{a(j\omega)^2} + \mathrm{b(j\omega)} + \mathrm{c}] = \mathrm{d}\mathbf{U} \tag{2.154}$$

Thus the frequency response function is:

$$\frac{\mathbf{Y}}{\mathbf{U}}(j\omega) = \frac{d}{a(j\omega)^2 + b(j\omega) + c} = \frac{B}{A}\angle\phi = \mathbf{H}(j\omega) \tag{2.155}$$

To put this frequency response function in time-constant form to facilitate Bode plotting, we must divide numerator and denominator by c:

$$\frac{\mathbf{Y}}{\mathbf{U}}(j\omega) = \frac{d/c}{(a/c)(j\omega)^2 + (b/c)(j\omega) + 1} = \frac{d/c}{(j\omega)^2/\omega_n^2 + (2\xi/\omega_n)(j\omega) + 1} \tag{2.156}$$

The constant, $c/a \equiv \omega_n^2$, the system's *undamped natural radian frequency* squared, and $b/c \equiv 2\xi/\omega_n$, where ξ is the system's *damping factor.* The system has complex-conjugate roots to the characteristic equation of its ODE if $0 < \xi < 1$. In this second example, we have assumed that the system is underdamped, i.e., $0 < \xi < 1$. Now the Bode magnitude plot is found from:

$$dB = 20\log(d/c) - 10\log\{[1 - \omega^2/\omega_n^2]^2 + [(2\xi/\omega_n)\omega]^2\} \tag{2.157}$$

At dc and $\omega << \omega_n$ and $\omega_n/2\xi$, dB $\cong 20\log(d/c)$. The undamped natural frequency is $\omega_n = \sqrt{c/a}$ r/sec. When $\omega = \omega_n$, dB $= 20\log(d/c) - 20\log[(2\xi/\omega_n)\omega_n] = 20\log(d/c) - 20\log[2\xi]$ and when $\omega >> \omega_n$, dB $= 20\log(d/c) - 40\log[\omega/\omega_n]$. Thus, for $\omega = \omega_n$ and $\xi < 0.5$, the dB curve rises to a peak above the intersection of the asymptotes. The high frequency asymptote has a slope of -40 dB/decade of radian frequency or -12 dB/octave (doubling) of radian frequency. These features are shown schematically in Figure 2.8. The phase of the second-order low-pass system can be found by inspection of the frequency response function of Equation 2.156. It is simply:

$$\phi = -\tan^{-1}\left(\frac{\omega(2\xi/\omega_n)}{1 - \omega^2/\omega_n^2}\right) \tag{2.158}$$

It can be shown [Ogata, 1970] that the magnitude of the resonant peak normalized with respect to the system's dc gain is:

$$M_r = \frac{|\mathbf{H}(j\omega)|_{max}}{|\mathbf{H}(j0)|} = \frac{1}{2\xi\sqrt{1-\xi^2}} \quad \text{for } 0.707 \geq \xi \geq 0 \tag{2.159}$$

And the frequency at which the peak AR occurs is given by:

$$\omega_p = \omega_n\sqrt{1 - 2\xi^2} \quad r/sec \tag{2.160}$$

Example 3: A lead/lag filter is described by the ODE:

$$\dot{y}/\omega_2 + y = \dot{x}/\omega_1 + x \tag{2.161}$$

Again using the derivative operator p, substituting $j\omega$ for p and treating the output and input like vectors, we can write:

$$\frac{\mathbf{Y}}{\mathbf{X}} = \frac{j\omega/\omega_1 + 1}{j\omega/\omega_2 + 1} = \mathbf{H}(j\omega), \quad \omega_2 > \omega_1 \tag{2.162}$$

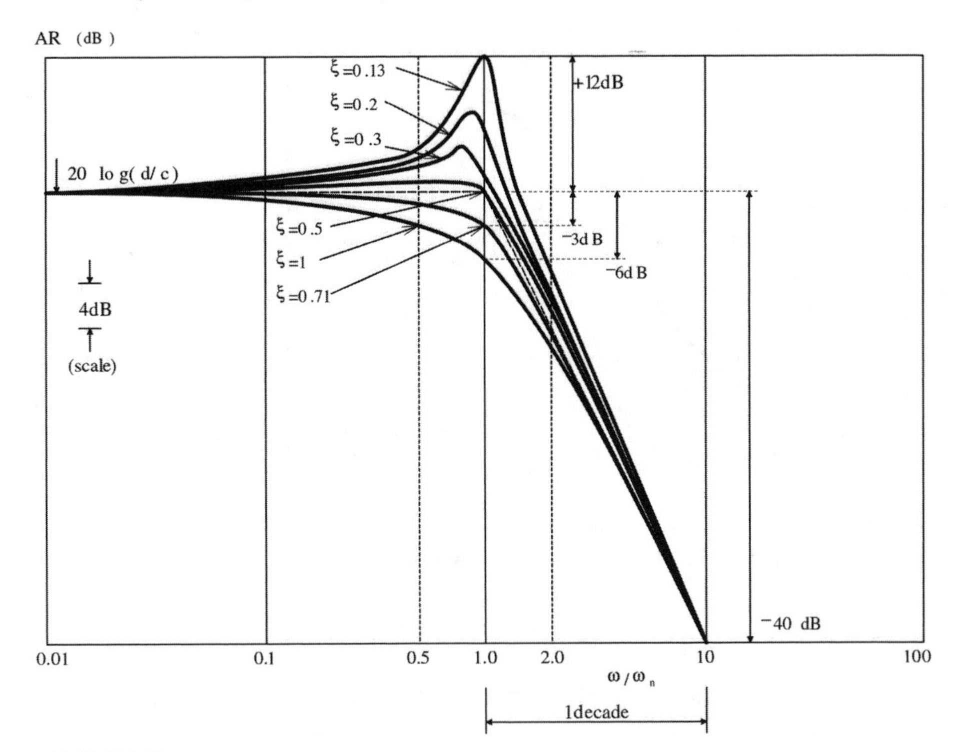

FIGURE 2.8
Bode AR plot for a general, second-order, under-damped, low-pass system. See text for analysis.

For the Bode plot, at $\omega = \text{dc}$ and $<< \omega_1, \omega_2$, $\text{dB} = 20\ \log|\mathbf{H}(j\omega)| = 0$ dB. At $\omega = \omega_1$, $\text{dB} \cong 20\ \log(\sqrt{2}) - 20\ \log(1) = +3$ dB. For $\omega >> \omega_2$, $\text{dB} \cong 20\ \log(\omega_2/\omega_1)$. The phase of the lead/lag filter is given by:

$$\phi = \tan^{-1}(\omega/\omega_1) - \tan^{-1}(\omega/\omega_2) \tag{2.163}$$

The Bode magnitude response and phase of the lead/lag filter are shown in Figure 2.9.

Because frequency response has traditionally been used as a descriptor for electronic amplifiers and feedback control systems, many texts on electronic circuits and control systems have introductory sections on this topic with examples. (See for example, Northrop, 1990; Ogata, Section 6.2, 1990; Schilling and Belove, 1989, Section 9.1.2; Nise, 1995, Chapter 10.) Modern circuit simulation software applications such as MicroCap™, SPICE and Multisim™ compute Bode plots for active and passive circuits and Matlab® and Simulink® will provide them for general linear systems described by ODEs or state equations.

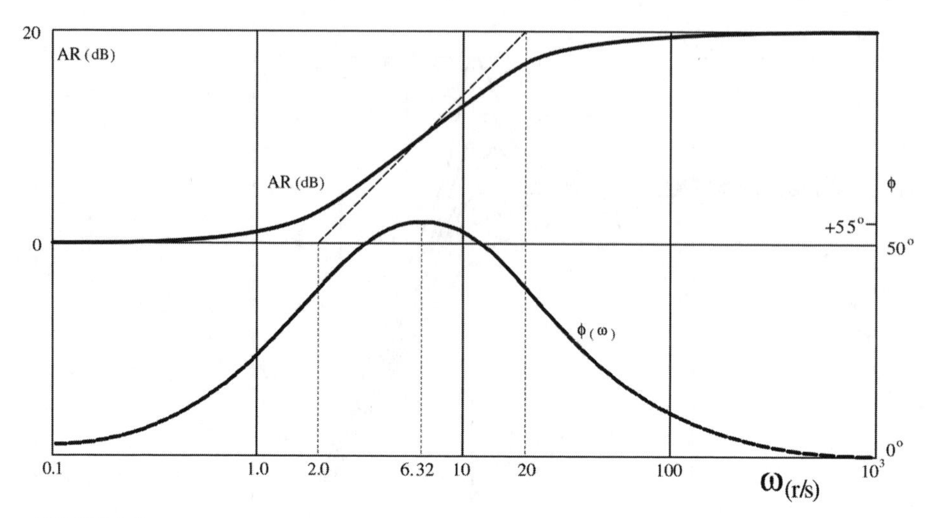

FIGURE 2.9
Bode plot (AR and phase) for a lead-lag filter. See Equation 2.162. $\omega_2 = 10\omega_1$.

2.4.7 Nyquist plots

A Nyquist plot is a *polar plot* of $|\mathbf{H}(j\omega)|$ vs. $\phi(\omega)$ for various ω values. Its primary use lies in predicting the stability of *nonlinear feedback systems* by the *Popov criterion* [Northrop, 1990] or for predicting stability, limit cycle frequency and amplitude when using the *describing function method* [Ogata, 1970] on SISO closed-loop, nonlinear control systems. In the describing function method, the nonlinear feedback system's *loop gain* is partitioned into a nonlinear function and a single-input/single-output (SISO) LTI system. Both the inverse describing function and the Nyquist plot are plotted on polar graph paper. For a *first example* of a Nyquist plot, consider the simple single time constant low pass filter:

$$\mathbf{H}(j\omega) = \frac{-1}{j\omega/\omega_o + 1} \tag{2.164}$$

What is plotted in Figure 2.10 is

$$|\mathbf{H}(j\omega)| = 1 \Big/ \left[\sqrt{\omega^2/\omega_o^2 + 1}\right] \text{ vs. } \phi = -180^\circ - \tan^{-1}(\omega/\omega_o) \tag{2.165}$$

Note that this Nyquist plot is a semicircle starting at -1 in the polar plane and ending at the origin at an angle of -270°. At $\omega = \omega_o$, $|\mathbf{H}(j\omega_o)| = 0.707$ and $\phi = -180^\circ - 45^\circ = -225^\circ$.

For a *second example* of a Nyquist plot, consider the quadratic low-pass frequency response function:

$$\mathbf{H}(j\omega) = \frac{1}{(j\omega)^2/9 + (j\omega)(0.2) + 1} \tag{2.166}$$

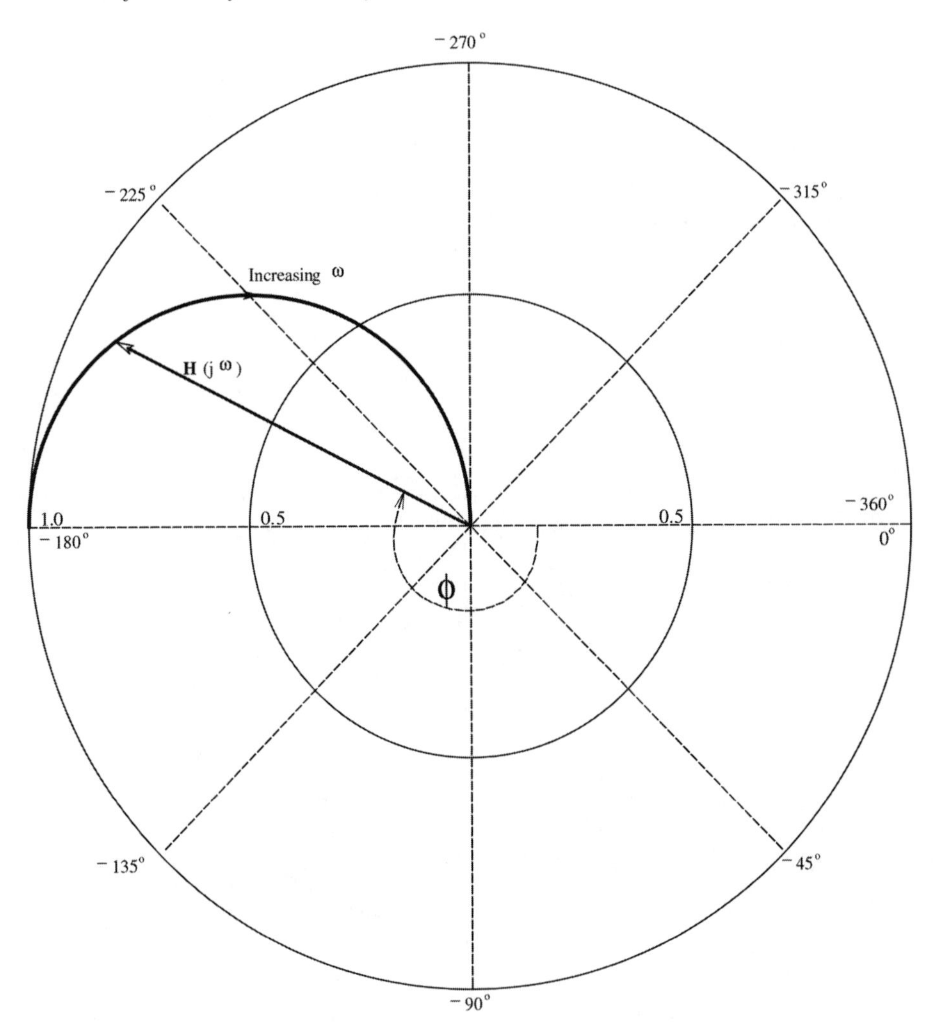

FIGURE 2.10
Nyquist (polar) plot of the frequency response of a simple, inverting, realpole, LPF given by Equation 2.164.

Here $\omega_n = 3$ r/s, $2\xi/\omega_n = 0.2$, so $\xi = 0.3$. In Figure 2.11, I have plotted:

$$|\mathbf{H}(j\omega)| = \frac{1}{\sqrt{\{[1-\omega^2/9]^2 + \omega^2(0.04)\}}} \quad \textbf{vs.} \quad \phi = -\tan^{-1}\left(\frac{0.2\omega}{1-\omega^2/9}\right) \tag{2.167}$$

At $\omega = 0$, $|\mathbf{H}(j0)| = 1$ and $\phi = 0°$. When $\omega = \omega_n$, $|\mathbf{H}(j\omega_n)| = 1.667$ and $\phi = -90°$. And as $\omega \to \infty$, $|\mathbf{H}(j\infty)| \to 0$, at an angle of $-180°$.

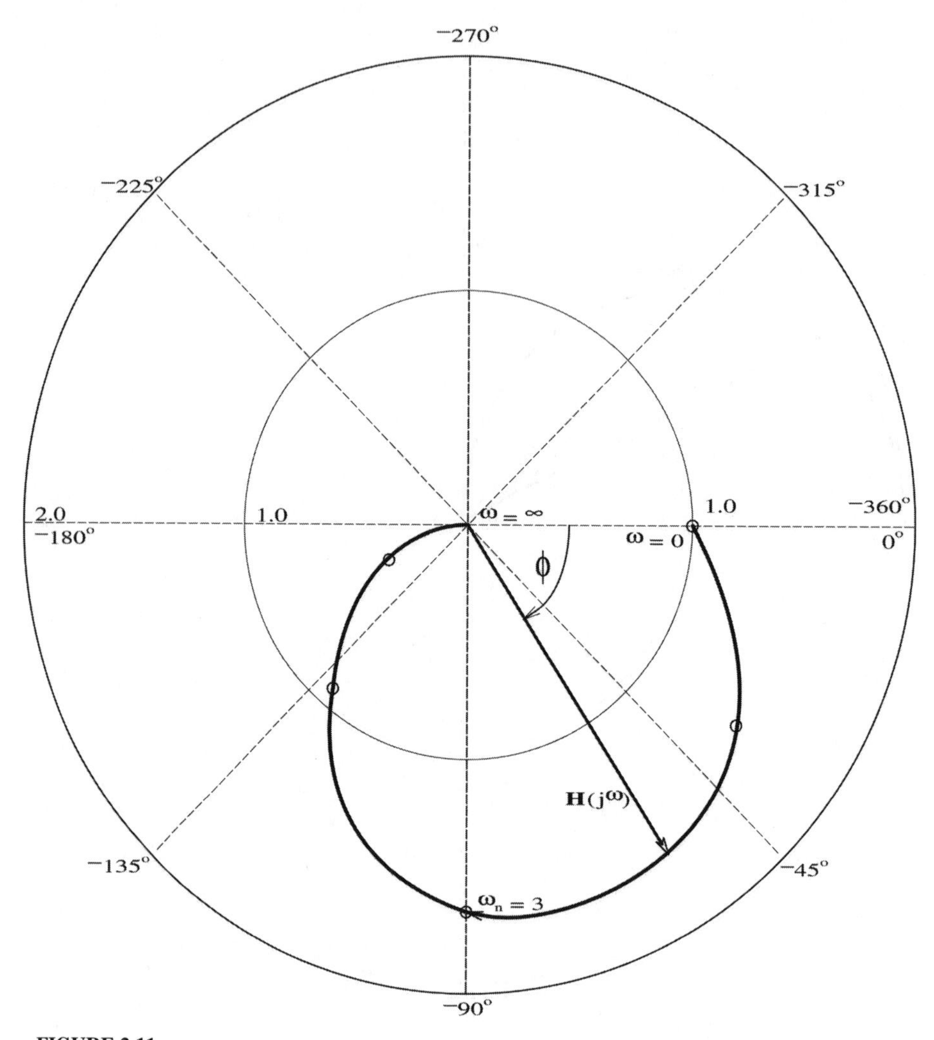

FIGURE 2.11

Nyquist plot of an underdamped, quadratic LPF in which $\omega_n = 3$ r/sec, $\xi = 0.3$ and $\mathbf{H}(0) = 1$. See Equation 2.166.

2.5 Discrete Signals and Systems

2.5.1 Introduction

Many mathematical tools to describe and process continuous, stationary analog signals are available. These include the Laplace and Fourier transform pairs and real convolution. As you have seen, LTI systems can be characterized by their responses to inputs such as transient analog signals, including the *unit impulse function*, $\delta(t)$, the *unit step function*, $U(t)$, the *ramp function*, $x(t) = at,\ t \geq 0$, the *sinusoid*, $x(t) = A\sin(\omega t),\ t \geq 0$, the *exponential*, $x(t) = Be^{-bt},\ t \geq 0$, etc. Note that *discrete systems* and *signals* also enjoy a congruent array of mathematical tools.

Discrete signals can be thought of as periodically sampled analog signals. A sampled analog signal can remain in analog form as a charge or voltage in the registers of a charge-coupled device (CCD) or be periodically converted into digital (numerical) form by an analog-to-digital converter (ADC). We will focus our attention on the latter form of discrete signals because digital signal processing (DSP) by computers uses sequentially acquired numerical samples. A general way of writing a discrete (sampled) signal is by the summed products:

$$x^*(t) = \sum_{n=-\infty}^{\infty} x(t)\delta(t - nT) = x(t) \times \delta_T(t) \tag{2.168}$$

$x^*(t)$ can be interpreted as a sequence of numbers, $\{x(kT)\}$, each spaced T seconds apart in time (T is the sampling period). Equation 2.168 also represents a process called *impulse modulation*, where a periodic train of unit impulses, $\delta_T(t)$, is multiplied by the analog signal, $x(t)$. Because $x^*(t)$ exists only at sampling instants, where $t = nT$, Equation 2.168 can be written as:

$$x^*(t) = \sum_{n=-\infty}^{\infty} x(nT)\delta(t - nT) \tag{2.169}$$

Now $\delta_T(t)$ can be written in the *frequency domain* as a sum of sequentially delayed 1s. The *Laplace delay operator*, e^{-snT}, is used. (More will be said about the delay operator in Chapter 3 and impulse modulation in Section 5.3.2.) Thus, in the frequency domain:

$$\boldsymbol{L}\{x^*(t)\} = \sum_{n=0}^{\infty} x(nT)e^{-snT} = X^*(s) \tag{2.170}$$

Now we *define* the complex variable, $\mathbf{z} \equiv e^{sT}$. Equation 2.170 becomes:

$$\mathbf{X}(z) = \boldsymbol{L}\{x^*(t)\} = \sum_{n=0}^{\infty} x(nT)z^{-n} = \sum_{n=0}^{\infty} x(n)z^{-n} \tag{2.171}$$

The right-hand expression of Equation 2.171 is the *open-form definition* of the *z transform* of $x(t)$. So

$$X(z) = \{x(0) + x(T)z^{-1} + x(2T)z^{-2} + \cdots + x(nT)z^{-n} + \cdots\} \tag{2.172}$$

Or, in terms of sample number, with sample period T understood:

$$X(z) = \{x(0) + x(1)z^{-1} + x(2)z^{-2} + \cdots + x(n)z^{-n} + \cdots\} \tag{2.173}$$

Note that a sampled unit impulse is $\delta(\mathrm{n}) = 1$ for $\mathrm{n} = 0$ and 0 for $\mathrm{n} \neq 0$; in general, $\delta(\mathrm{n}-\mathrm{p}) = 1$ for $\mathrm{n} = \mathrm{p}$ and 0 for any $\mathrm{n} \neq \mathrm{p}$. A sampled unit step is $\mathrm{U}(\mathrm{n}) = 1$ for all $\mathrm{n} \geq 0$ and 0 for $\mathrm{n} < 0$. Thus, a sampled step, $\mathrm{U}(\mathrm{t})$, can be written as its z transform in open form as:

$$\mathbf{U}(\mathrm{z}) = \{1 + 1\mathrm{z}^{-1} + 1\mathrm{z}^{-2} + \cdots + 1\mathrm{z}^{-\mathrm{n}} + \cdots\} = \sum_{\mathrm{n}=0}^{\infty} \mathrm{z}^{-\mathrm{n}} \tag{2.174}$$

By long division, the summation can be shown to be equal to:

$$\mathbf{U}(\mathrm{z}) = \frac{1}{1-\mathrm{z}^{-1}} = \frac{\mathrm{z}}{\mathrm{z}-1} \tag{2.175}$$

A discrete signal can be *delayed* by m sampling periods. That is, the input to the delay element is the sequence $\mathrm{x}(\mathrm{n})$; at the output the sequence is $\mathrm{y}(\mathrm{n}) = \mathrm{x}(\mathrm{n}-\mathrm{m})$. This means that if $\mathrm{x}(\mathrm{n}) = 0$ for $\mathrm{n} < 0$ and $\mathrm{x}(0) = 1, \mathrm{x}(1) = 2, \ldots$, then $\mathrm{y}(0) = \mathrm{y}(1) = \ldots \mathrm{y}(\mathrm{m}-1) = 0$, $\mathrm{y}(\mathrm{m}) = 1$, $\mathrm{y}(\mathrm{m}+1) = 2$, etc. The z transform of an m-unit delay is just $\mathbf{D}(\mathrm{z}) = \mathrm{z}^{-\mathrm{m}} = 1/\mathrm{z}^{\mathrm{m}}$.

The continuous operations of *differentiation* and *integration* can be approximated by a number of digital routines. The simplest form of *numerical differentiation* approximates the slope of $\mathrm{x}(\mathrm{t})$ at $\mathrm{t} = \mathrm{nT}$ by calculating the difference, $[\mathrm{x}(\mathrm{n}) - \mathrm{x}(\mathrm{n}-1)]$ and dividing it by the sample interval, T. That is, the *first-difference derivative estimate* can be written in the discrete time domain as:

$$\mathrm{y}_{1\mathrm{d}}(\mathrm{n}) = [\mathrm{x}(\mathrm{n}) - \mathrm{x}(\mathrm{n}-1)]/\mathrm{T} \cong \dot{\mathrm{x}}(\mathrm{n}) \tag{2.176}$$

This is the simple *two-point difference equation* for differentiation. Written in terms of the delay operator, z^{-1}, we have:

$$\mathrm{Y}_{1\mathrm{d}} = \mathrm{X}\left[1-\mathrm{z}^{-1}\right]/\mathrm{T} \rightarrow \frac{\mathrm{Y}_{\mathrm{d}}}{\mathrm{X}}(\mathrm{z}) = \frac{\mathrm{z}-1}{\mathrm{zT}} = \mathrm{H}_{\mathrm{d}2}(\mathrm{z}) \tag{2.177}$$

Another difference equation for estimating $\dot{\mathrm{x}}(\mathrm{t})$ is the *three-point central difference algorithm* (3PCDA). Written as a time-domain difference equation that can be implemented on a computer, this is:

$$\mathrm{y}_{3\mathrm{cd}}(\mathrm{n}) = \frac{1}{2\mathrm{T}}[\mathrm{x}(\mathrm{n}) - \mathrm{x}(\mathrm{n}-2)] \tag{2.178}$$

Again, we use the z^{-1} delay operator to find the z transform of the 3PCDA:

$$\mathrm{Y}_{3\mathrm{cd}} = \mathrm{X}\frac{1}{2\mathrm{T}}\left[1-\mathrm{z}^{-2}\right] \rightarrow \frac{\mathrm{Y}_{\mathrm{cd}}}{\mathrm{X}}(\mathrm{z}) = \frac{\mathrm{z}^2-1}{\mathrm{z}^2 2\mathrm{T}} = \mathrm{H}_{\mathrm{d}3}(\mathrm{z}) \tag{2.179}$$

Many other high-order difference equations exist for estimating $\dot{\mathrm{x}}(\mathrm{t})$. All of these routines have been designed to attenuate the high frequency components of $\mathrm{x}(\mathrm{t})$, including noise, so they will not dominate $\mathrm{y}_{\mathrm{d}}(\mathrm{k})$. Figure 2.12 illustrates the frequency response (magnitude and phase) of an ideal analog differentiator, the two-point difference and the 3PCD differentiation algorithms. For example, the frequency response

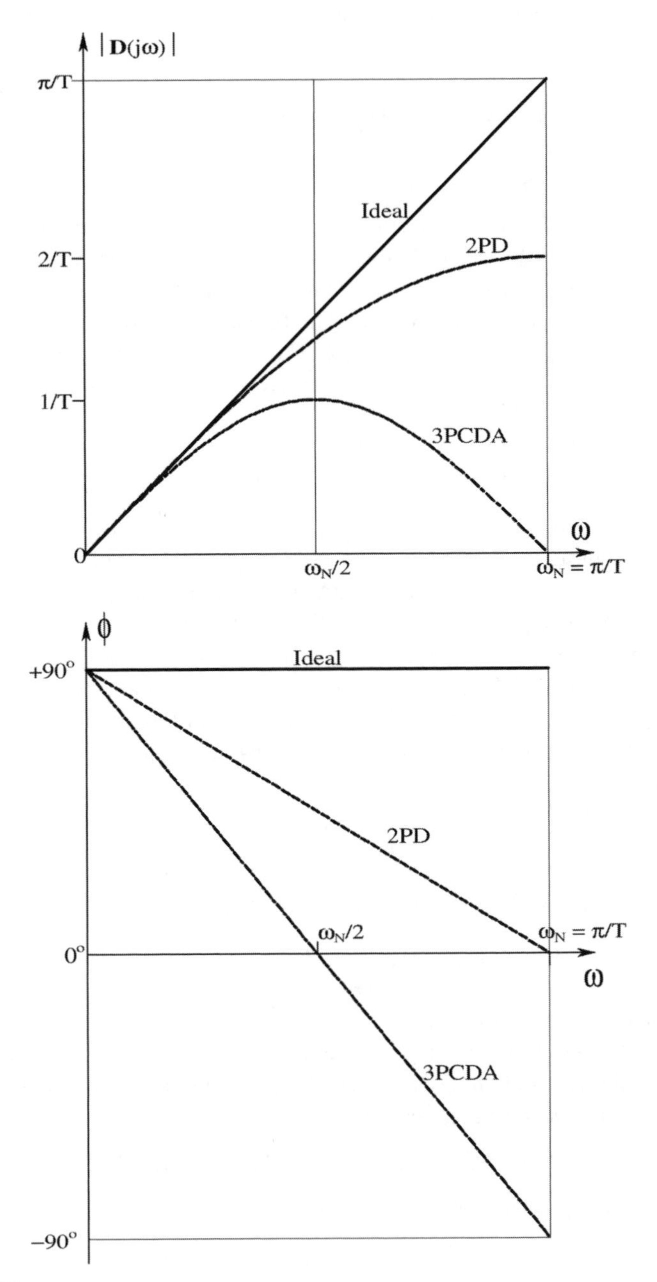

FIGURE 2.12

Frequency response (magnitude and phase) of an ideal analog differentiator, a two-point difference discrete differentiator and the 3-point central difference discrete differentiator algorithm. Note the radian frequency spans zero to the Nyquist frequency of the discrete differentiators. See text for derivations.

of the 2PD differentiator is found by substituting $e^{-j\omega T}$ for $z^{-1} = e^{-sT}$. Thus, using the Euler identity for $\sin\varphi = \frac{e^{j\varphi} - e^{-j\varphi}}{2j}$:

$$\frac{\mathbf{Y_{1d}}(j\omega)}{\mathbf{X}(j\omega)} = (1/T)\left[1 - e^{-j\omega T}\right] = \mathbf{H_{d2}}(j\omega) = (1/T)\left[e^{+j\omega T/2} - e^{-j\omega T/2}\right]e^{-j\omega T/2}$$
$$= \{(2/T)\sin(\omega T/2)\}je^{-j\omega T/2} \tag{2.180}$$

The amplitude of $\mathbf{H_{1d}}(j\omega)$ is in brackets and the angle from the mixed notation is $\theta(\omega) = (\pi/2 - \omega T/2)$ radians. (Note that $\sin(\omega T/2)$ has negative values for $2\pi/T \leq \omega \leq 4\pi/T$, $6\pi/T \leq \omega \leq 8\pi/T$, etc.) When $\sin(\omega T/2)$ goes negative, it effectively adds $-\pi$ radians to the $H_{d2}(\omega)$ phase. The frequency response of the *ideal analog differentiator* is: $\mathbf{H_{id}}(j\omega) = j\omega = \omega\angle\pi/2$. The 3PCDA has the frequency response:

$$\mathbf{H_{3cd}}(j\omega) = 1/(2T)\left[1 - e^{-j2\omega T}\right] = 1/(2T)\left[e^{+j\omega T} - e^{-j\omega T}\right]e^{-j\omega T}$$
$$= \{(1/T)\sin(\omega T)\}je^{-j\omega T}$$
$$= \{(1/T)\sin(\omega T)\}\angle(\pi/2 - \omega T) \tag{2.181}$$

Recall that the sampling period is $T = 1/f_s = 2\pi/\omega_s$ seconds. The differentiator frequency responses are plotted from 0 to $\omega = \omega_N = \omega_s/2 = \pi/T$, the Nyquist radian frequency. Both the 2PDA and the 3PCDA closely approximate $\dot{x}(t)$ for low frequencies on $x(t)$. At $\omega = \frac{3}{4}\omega_N$, the magnitude of the 3PCDA frequency response function is *decreasing* and its phase is $[\pi/2 - (3\pi/4T)T] = -\pi/4$ radians, a lag. Thus, above $\omega = \omega_N/2$, the 3PCDA behaves like a low-pass filter, not a differentiator. At very low ω, $\mathbf{H_{3cd}}(j\omega) \to \omega\angle\pi/2$, the behavior of an ideal differentiator.

The simplest form of *discrete integration* is *rectangular.* Here we wish to approximate:

$$y(t) = \int_0^t x(t)\,dt \tag{2.182}$$

The frequency response function of *ideal integration* is:

$$\mathbf{H_{ii}}(j\omega) = \frac{1}{j\omega} = (1/\omega)\angle -\pi/2 \tag{2.183}$$

Note the fixed, $-90°$ phase lag.

Numerical *integration routines* are generally *recursive,* i.e., the present output depends on the past output(s) as well as the past input(s). The output of a simple *rectangular integrator* is given by:

$$y_{ri}(n) = y_{ri}(n-1) + Tx(n-1), \quad n = 0, 1, 2, \ldots \tag{2.184}$$

Writing this process using the z^{-1} delay operator:

$$Y_{ri}\left[1 - z^{-1}\right] = T \times z^{-1} \tag{2.185}$$

Multiply both sides of Equation 2.185 by z and rearrange terms to find the transfer function in z:

$$\frac{Y_{ri}}{X}(z) = \frac{T}{z-1} = H_{ri}(z) \tag{2.186}$$

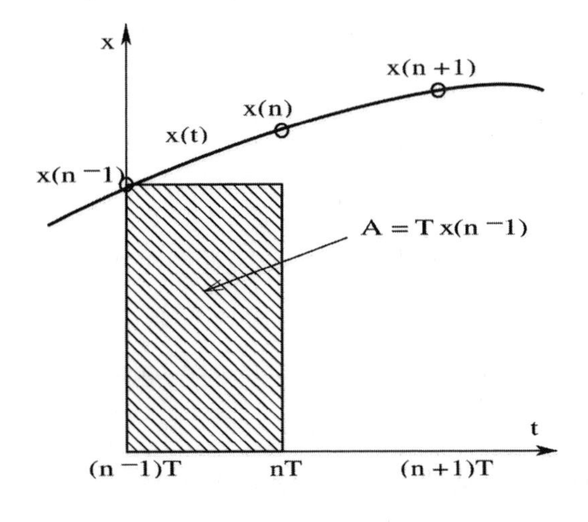

a

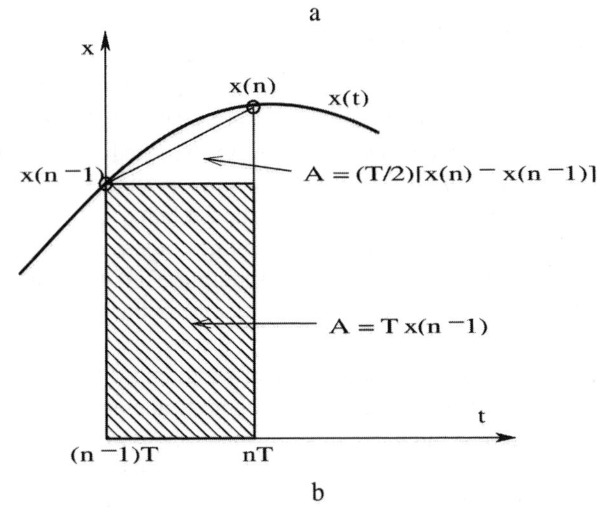

b

FIGURE 2.13
a) Illustration of simple discrete rectangular integration of a sampled analog signal, $x(nT)$. b) Illustration of trapezoidal integration. Note the extra triangular area over the basic area, $Tx(n-1)$ that more closely approximates $\int x(t)\,dt$ over $(n-1)T \le t \le nT$.

A more accurate estimator for the integral of $x(t)$ is by *trapezoidal integration.* In this routine, we include the triangular area between $x(n)$ and $x(n-1)$ (see Figure 2.13b). The difference equation for trapezoidal integration is:

$$
\begin{aligned}
y_{ti}(n) = y_{ti}(n-1) + Tx(n-1) + [x(n) - x(n-1)](T/2) = y_{tr}(n-1) \\
+(T/2)[x(n) + x(n-1)] \qquad (2.187)
\end{aligned}
$$

As for the case of rectangular integration, we use the z^{-1} delay operator to find the z-transform of the trapezoidal integrator:

$$Y_{ti}\left[1-z^{-1}\right]=(T/2)X\left[1+z^{-1}\right] \tag{2.188}$$

Again, multiplying both sides of Equation 2.188 by z, we find:

$$\frac{Y_{ti}}{X}(z)=\frac{(T/2)[z+1]}{[z-1]}=H_{ti}(z) \tag{2.189}$$

Simpson's rule integration is implemented by the difference equation:

$$y_{si}(n)=y_{si}(n-2)+(T/3)[x(n)+4x(n-1)+x(n-2)] \tag{2.190}$$

As before, we write Equation 2.190 in terms of the delay operator, z^{-m}:

$$Y_{si}\left[1-z^{-2}\right]=(T/3)X\left[1+4z^{-1}+z^{-2}\right] \tag{2.191}$$

Multiplying through by z^2, we obtain the Simpson's rule integration transfer function in z:

$$\frac{Y_{si}}{X}(z)=\frac{(T/3)[z^2+4z+1]}{z^2-1}=H_{si}(z) \tag{2.192}$$

The frequency responses of rectangular, trapezoidal and Simpson's integration routines can be found in an analogous manner to that used for the differentiators. Rectangular, trapezoidal and Simpson's rule integration routines are shown in block diagram form using unit delay operators in Figure 2.14a,b,c.

There are many other digital integration routines, some of which are adaptive in nature and which are used to solve sets of nonlinear ODEs. These include the various *Runge-Kutta* algorithms the *Gear* and *Adams* routines, all too specialized to be considered here.

In addition to simple derivative and integration programs, difference equations that will perform operations on discrete signals analogous to analog filtering operations on continuous signals can be written. That is; *low-pass, high-pass, band-pass, all-pass* and *band reject* or *notch.* Digital filtering algorithms offer the advantage that the filter coefficients can be updated every sampling period, permitting the design of adaptive filters [Widrow and Stearns, 1985].

2.5.2 Discrete convolution

If a linear discrete time-invariant system {LDTIS} is given a unit impulse input at time $t=nT$, then it will respond by its discrete weighting function at $t=nT$. That is:

$$\delta(k-n)\rightarrow\{\text{LDTIS}\}\rightarrow h(k-n),\quad k\geq n\geq 0 \tag{2.193}$$

If a discrete input x(k) is given to the system having weighting function h(k), the output y(k) is given by *discrete convolution,* which, like continuous convolution, is commutative:

$$y(n)=\sum_{p=-\infty}^{\infty}x(p)h(n-p)=\sum_{p=-\infty}^{\infty}h(p)x(n-p) \tag{2.194}$$

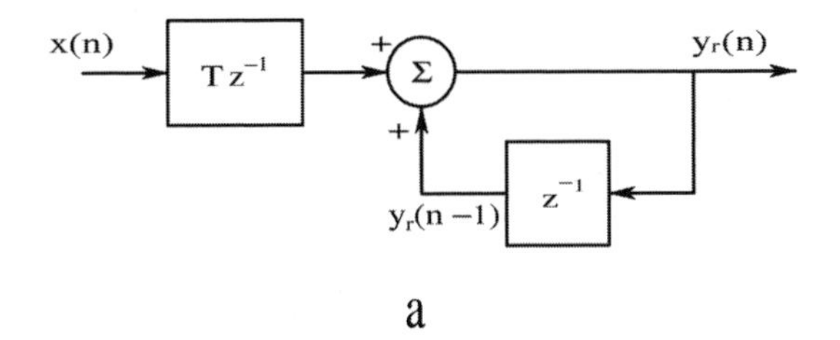

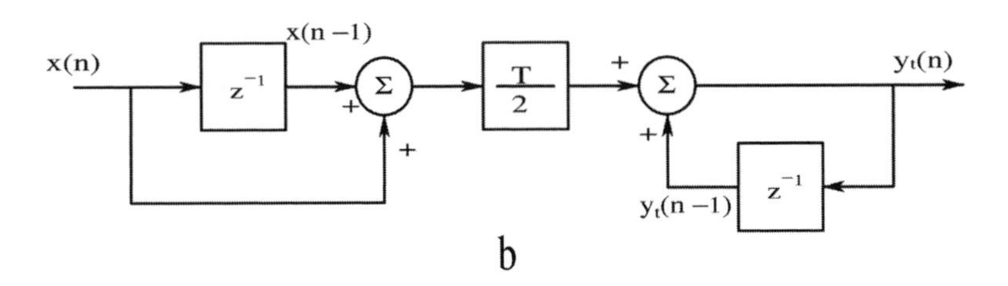

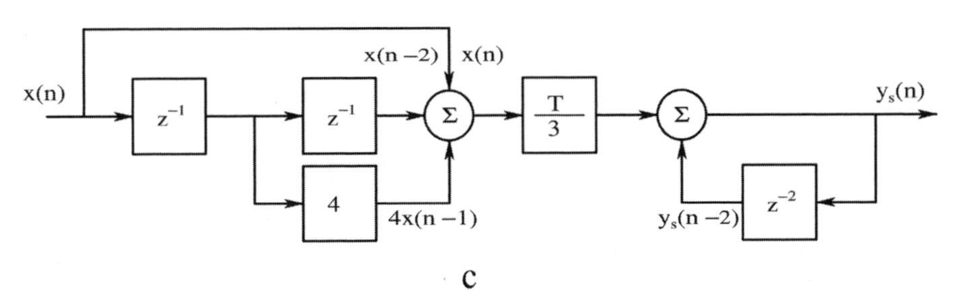

FIGURE 2.14
Block diagram implementation of three discrete integration routines in the time domain, written in terms of realizable unit delays, z^{-1} and summations. a) Rectangular integration. b) Trapezoidal integration. c) Simpson's rule integration.

As an example of discrete convolution, let $h(n) = \exp(-n)U(k)$ and $x(t) = U(n) - U(n-3)$. Thus:

$$y(n) = \sum_{p=0}^{\infty} e^{-p}x(n-p) \tag{2.195}$$

Refer to Figure 2.15 for a graphical interpretation of the process. We find: $y(0) = 1$, $y(2) = 1 + 0.36788 + 0.13534 = 1.5032$, $y(4) = 0.13534 + 0.049787 + 0.018316 = 0.20344$.

Table 2.1 summarizes the properties of discrete time-domain convolution:

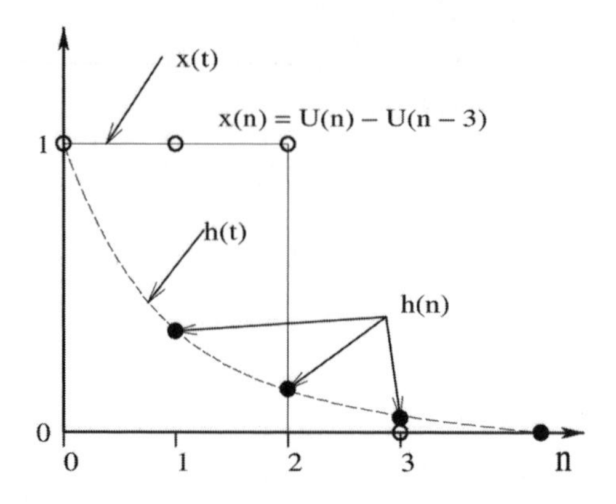

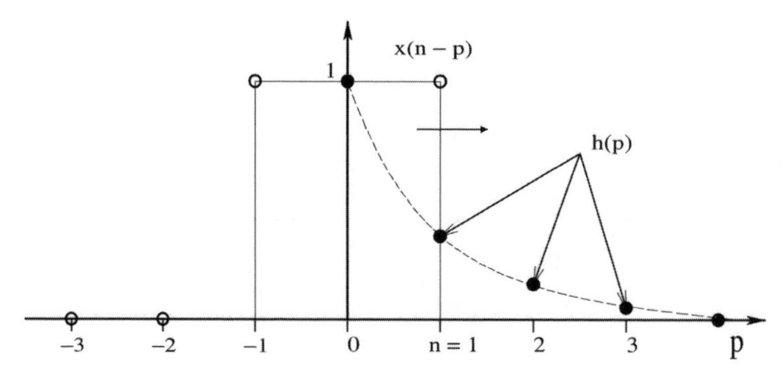

FIGURE 2.15

Illustration of discrete convolution. A sampled, rectangular pulse is the system's input; the discrete system weighting function is an exponential decay waveform. See text for a description of the process.

TABLE 2.1
Properties of discrete convolution

Property	Operation	Equivalence
Commutative property	$x(n) \rightarrow [h(n)] \rightarrow y(n)$	$h(n) \rightarrow [x(n)] \rightarrow y(n)$
	$y(n) = x(n) \otimes h(n)$	$y(n) = h(n) \otimes x(n)$
Associative property	$x(n) \rightarrow [h_1(n)] \rightarrow$	$x(n) \rightarrow [h_2(n)] \rightarrow$
	$[h_2(n)] \rightarrow y(n)$	$[h_1(n)] \rightarrow y(n)$
	$h(n) = h_1(n) \otimes h_2(n)$	$y(n) = x(n) \otimes h(n)$
Distributive property	$\rightarrow [h_1(n)] \rightarrow$	$y(n) = x(n) \otimes [h_1(n) + h_2(n)]$
	$x(n) \rightarrow \rightarrow y(n)$	$y(n) = x(n) \otimes h(n)$
	$\rightarrow [h_2(n)] \rightarrow$	$h(n) = h_1(n) + h_2(n)$

2.5.3 Discrete systems

We saw that, in the case of differential equations describing continuous systems, that the differential operator, $p = d(*)/dt$ or $px = \dot{x}$, was of considerable use in determining the system's natural frequencies and its steady-state sinusoidal (SSS) frequency response. In dealing with discrete systems, it is also expedient to define a unit delay operator, z^{-1}. You have seen above that $\mathbf{z^{-1}}$ is a complex variable given by the frequency-domain delay operator, e^{-sT}, where s is the Laplace complex variable, $\mathbf{s} = \sigma + j\omega$. In the SSS case, $s \to j\omega$. Consider the impulse response of a LDTIS; it is the number sequence

$$\begin{aligned} h(n) = \{&h(0)\delta(0) + h(1)\delta(n-1) + h(2)\delta(n-2) + \cdots \\ &+ h(k)\delta(n-k) + \cdots\} \end{aligned} \tag{2.196}$$

Each successive impulse defines the numerical value of $h(*)$ at a particular value of n. Each impulse is delayed by $t = nT$ and can be replaced by a delay operator, z^{-n}. Thus:

$$\begin{aligned} \mathbf{Z}[h(n)] &= \{h(0) + h(1)z^{-1} + h(2)z^{-2} + \cdots + h(k)z^{-k} + \cdots\} = \sum_{n=0}^{\infty} h(n)z^{-n} \\ &\equiv \mathbf{H}(z) \end{aligned} \tag{2.197}$$

Equation 2.197 is the working definition of the open form of the *unilateral* z *transform* of the sequence $h(n)$ defined for $n \geq 0$ [Papoulis, 1977]. The unilateral z transform is used in the analysis of discrete physically realizable LTI systems and signals.

Note that system weighting functions are generally written in terms of delays, z^{-k}, because delays are physically realizable. However, the z transform evolved in terms of the complex variable, $\mathbf{z} \equiv e^{\mathbf{s}T}$. We discuss the stability of discrete systems in terms of their poles relative to the unit circle in the z-plane, not the z^{-1} plane.

Some properties of Equation 2.197 are illustrated by the examples:

1. If $f(n) = \delta(n-m)$ (a delayed impulse), then $\mathbf{F}(z) = 1z^{-m}$.
2. If $f(n) = a_2\delta(n-2) + a_4\delta(n-4)$, then $\mathbf{F}(z) = a_2z^{-2} + a_4z^{-4}$.
3. If $g(n-m)$ exists, then $\mathbf{F}(z) = z^{-m}\mathbf{G}(z)$.

There are two categories of discrete (digital) filter for discrete signals: *non-recursive* and *recursive*. Nonrecursive filters are also called *finite impulse response* (FIR) filters because there are a finite number of terms in their impulse responses. For example, N terms:

$$\mathbf{H}(z) = \sum_{k=0}^{N-1} h(n)z^{-n} \tag{2.198}$$

Recursive filters are also known as *infinite impulse response* (IIR) filters because, theoretically, their impulse responses are of infinite duration. The transfer function of a general IIR filter has the form [Tompkins, 1993]:

$$\mathbf{H}(z) = \frac{\sum_{i=0}^{M} a_j z^{-i}}{1 - \sum_{i=1}^{N} b_j z^{-i}} = \frac{a_0 + a_1 z^{-1} + a_2 z^{-2} + \cdots + a_M z^{-M}}{1 - \{b_1 z^{-1} + b_2 z^{-2} + \cdots + b_N z^{-N}\}} = \frac{\mathbf{Y}(z)}{\mathbf{X}(z)} \quad (2.199)$$

To see how an IIR filter can be implemented on a computer, consider the case where $M = N = 1$. That is,

$$\frac{\mathbf{Y}(z)}{\mathbf{X}(z)} = \frac{a_0 + a_1 z^{-1}}{1 - b_1 z^{-1}} \quad (2.200)$$

In the discrete time domain,

$$\begin{aligned} &y(k) - b_1 y(k-1) = a_0 x(k) + a_1 x(k-1) \\ &\downarrow \\ &y(k) = b_1 y(k-1) + a_0 x(k) + a_1 x(k-1) \end{aligned} \quad (2.201)$$

Equation 2.201 is implemented on the computer. (Present $y(k)$ requires present input, one sample-old input and one sample-old output.)

As *a second example* of an IIR filter, consider

$$\mathbf{H}(z) = \frac{z}{z - e^{-aT}} = \frac{1}{1 - z^{-1} e^{-aT}} = \frac{\mathbf{Y}(z)}{\mathbf{X}(z)} \quad (2.202)$$

In the discrete (time) domain this can be written:

$$\begin{aligned} &x(n) = y(n) - e^{-aT} y(n-1), \quad b_1 = e^{-aT} \\ &\downarrow \\ &y(n) = x(n) + b_1 y(n-1) \end{aligned} \quad (2.203)$$

Thus, calculation of this filter's output requires the present input sample and the one sample-old output. The $H(z)$ in this example is derived from a simple continuous exponential weighting function, $h(t) = e^{-at}$.

In the general case given by Equation 2.199, we can write in the filter's implementation:

$$\begin{aligned} y(n) = &\{b_1 y(n-1) + b_2 y(n-2) + \cdots + b_N y(n-N)\} + \{a_0 x(n) + a_1 x(n-1) \\ &+ \cdots + a_M x(n-M)\} \end{aligned} \quad (2.204)$$

A block diagram illustrating how this difference equation can be implemented is shown in Figure 2.16.

Figure 2.17 illustrates a general N^{th} order *FIR filter.* In implementing this filter in software, N registers are required to store the present and past x samples. At the end of every computation cycle for $y(n)$, $x(n-N)$ is discarded, $x(n-N-1)$ is put

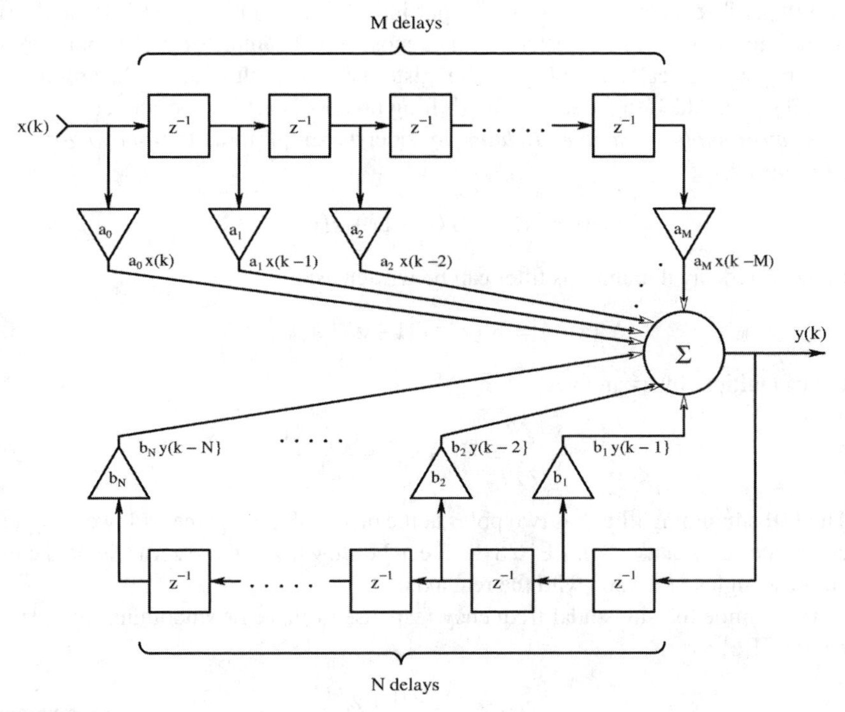

FIGURE 2.16
General form for implementing an Nth order IIR filter. The lower sequence of tapped delays with b_n coefficients represents the structure of the transfer function's denominator; the upper sequence of tapped delays with a_n coefficients forms the filter's M^{th} order numerator.

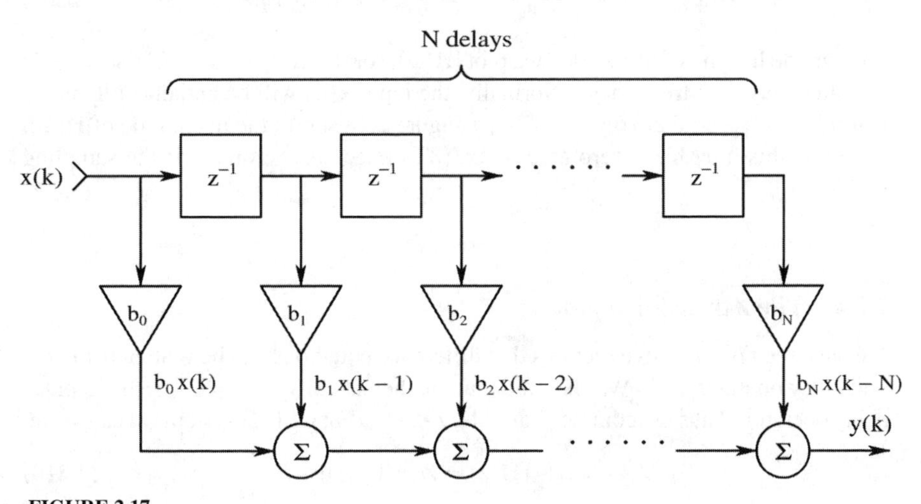

FIGURE 2.17
Implementation of an Nth order IIR filter.

into the Nth register, $x(n-N-2)$ is put into the $(N-1)^{th}$ register etc. and $x(n)$ is put into the $(n-1)^{th}$ register etc. The most recent sample of $x(t)$ is put into the $x(n)$ register. To calculate $y(n)$, each register value is multiplied by the appropriate b_n value and added together and the shifting process is again repeated, etc.

As *an example of a simple FIR filter*, consider the simple three-term *moving-average LPF* given by:

$$y(n) = [x(n) + x(n-1) + x(n-2)]/3 \tag{2.205}$$

In the z^{-1}-delay domain this filter can be written as:

$$Y\left(z^{-1}\right) = X\left(z^{-1}\right)\left[1 + z^{-1} + z^{-2}\right]/3 \tag{2.206}$$

Let us multiply by z^2 and get:

$$\frac{Y(z)}{X(z)} = H(z) = \frac{z^2 + z^1 + 1}{3z^2} \tag{2.207}$$

The FIR smoothing filter has two poles at the origin of the z-plane and two complex-conjugate zeros at $\mathbf{z} = -0.5 \pm j\sqrt{3}/2$. It can be shown that these zeros lie on the unit circle at angles of $\pm 120°$ with the real axis.

To examine the sinusoidal frequency response of this FIR smoothing filter, let us rewrite $H(z)$ as:

$$H(z) = \frac{z + 1 + z^{-1}}{3z} \tag{2.208}$$

Now we let $\mathbf{z} = e^{j\omega T}$ and use the Euler relation for $\cos(\theta)$:

$$\mathbf{H}(\omega) = \frac{e^{j\omega T} + e^{-j\omega T} + 1}{3e^{j\omega T}} = \frac{1}{3}[1 + 2\cos(\omega T)]e^{-j\omega T} \tag{2.209}$$

To examine how this filter works, we plot $|\mathbf{H}(\omega)|$ for $0 \leq \omega \leq \omega_N = \pi/T$ r/sec. ω_N is the filter's Nyquist frequency. (Normally, the input $x(n)$ will be antialias filtered so that it has no spectral energy above ω_N.) Figure 2.18 shows the magnitude of $\mathbf{H}(\omega)$. Note that this filter has a zero at $\omega = 2\pi/(3T)$ r/sec. As before, T is the sampling period.

2.5.4 The z transform pair

We have seen in the above sections that difference equations can be written using the unit delay operator, z^{-1}. We also said that, mathematically, $z^{-1} = e^{-sT}$, the Laplace delay operator. Thus the complex variable, $\mathbf{z} \equiv e^{sT}$. For a LDTI system we can write:

$$\mathbf{Y}(z) = \mathbf{X}(z)\,\mathbf{H}(z) = \mathbf{Z}\{x(k) \otimes h(k)\} \tag{2.210}$$

That is, the product of the z transforms of the system's input and its weighting function (discrete impulse response) give the z transform of its output, $\mathbf{Y}(z)$. $\mathbf{Y}(z)$ can also

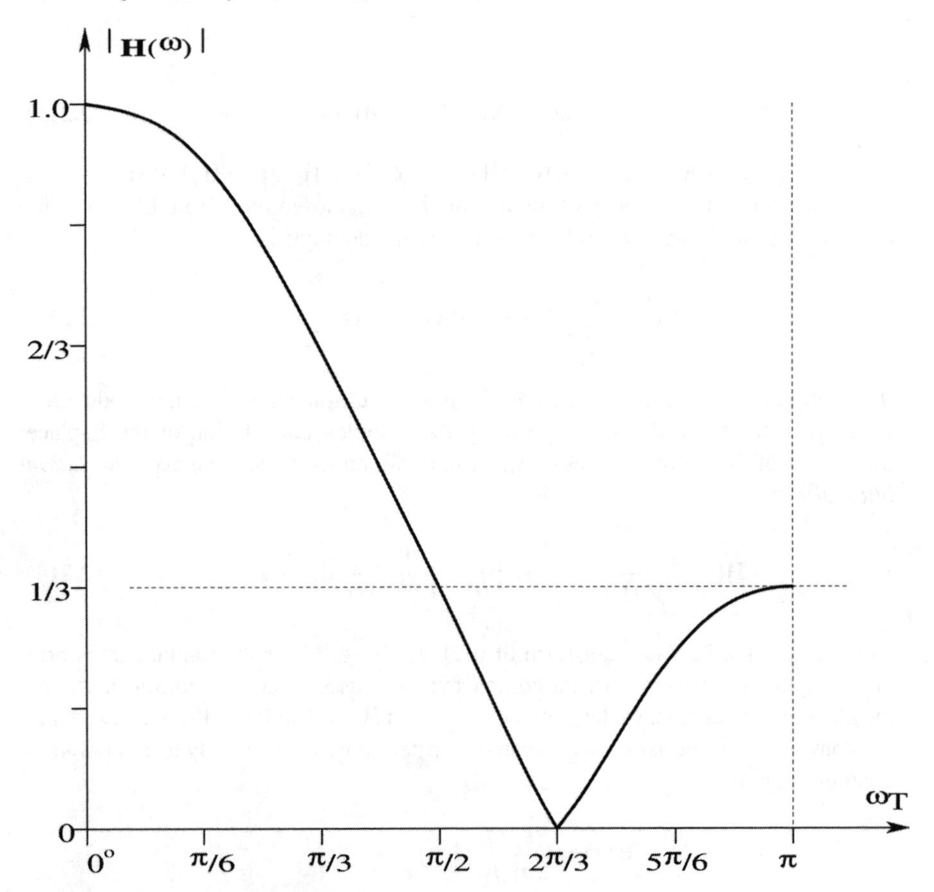

FIGURE 2.18
Frequency response, $|\mathbf{H}(\omega)|$, found from H(z) by letting $z = e^{j\omega T}$. H(z) is the transfer function of a second-order, moving-average, IIR LPF. The time-domain, computer-implemented difference equation is given by Equations 2.205–2.209. See the text for details.

be found from the z transform of the discrete real convolution of input and weighting function.

If the input to a continuous LTI system, H(s), is an impulse-modulated analog signal, $x^*(nT)$, the continuous time-domain output *at sampling instants* can be found from:

$$y(n) = y(nT) = Z^{-1}\{X(z)H(z)\} \tag{2.211}$$

Where H(z) is the z transform of H(s). If two, analog LTI systems are cascaded, the time-domain output is:

$$y(n) = \mathbf{Z}^{-1}\{X(z)Z[H_1(s)H_2(s)]\} \quad (2.212)$$

Note that it is easy to show that $H_1(z)H_2(z) \neq \mathbf{Z}[H_1(s)H_2(s)] = H_1H_2(z)$.

Another, more formal, way of finding any $\mathbf{H}(z)$ in closed form from $h(t)$ uses the basic definition of impulse modulation in the time domain:

$$h^*(t) = \sum_{n=0}^{\infty} h(t)\delta(t-nT) = h(t) \times \delta_T(t) \quad (2.213)$$

It is well known that the Laplace transform of a multiplication (i.e., the modulation process) in the time domain is given by the complex convolution of the Laplace transforms of the products. Thus, $H(z)$ can be found from the *complex convolution integral:*

$$\mathbf{H}(z) = \frac{1}{2\pi j}\int_{c-j\infty}^{c+j\infty} \mathbf{H}(p)\frac{1}{1-e^{-(s-p)T}}\,dp, \quad \mathbf{z} \equiv e^{sT} \quad (2.214)$$

Here $\mathbf{H}(s)$ is the Laplace transform of $h(t)$, $1/(1-e^{-sT})$ is the Laplace transform of the impulse train, $\delta_T(t)$, p is the complex variable used in the convolution, and once the integral is evaluated, we let $z^{-1} = e^{-sT}$ to find $\mathbf{H}(z)$. Lindorff (1965) showed that the convolution of Equation 2.214 can be written more conveniently as a (complex) contour integral:

$$\mathbf{H}(z) = \frac{1}{2\pi j}\int_C \mathbf{H}(p)\frac{z}{z-e^{pT}}\,dp \quad (2.215)$$

(Lindorff covers the process rigorously for those interested in the details of the complex variable mathematics.) Evaluation of $\mathbf{H}(z)$ by contour integration is of academic interest only. You will probably never have to do it. Instead, make use of Table 2.1 in this text or the comprehensive tables of z transforms that are found in almost every text on digital control and DSP.

There are several ways of finding the inverse z transform of $Y(z)$. That is, finding $y(k)$ from $Y(z)$. The first way uses the complex contour integral:

$$y(k) = \frac{1}{2\pi j}\int_C \mathbf{Y}(z)z^{k-1}\,dz \quad (2.216)$$

Where **C** is a counter-clockwise circular path enclosing all the poles of $\mathbf{Y}(z)z^{k-1}$. This integral can be evaluated using Cauchy's residue theorem [Kuo, 1967]. Kuo gives the example:

$$Y(z) = \frac{0.632z}{z^2 - 1.368z + 0.368} = \frac{0.632z}{(z-1)(z-0.368)} \quad (2.217)$$

Thus, the integral is:

$$y(k) = \frac{1}{2\pi j} \int_C \frac{0.632\,z^k}{(z-1)(z-0.368)}\,dz \tag{2.218}$$

From the method of residues, we can write:

$$y(n) = \sum \text{residues of } \frac{0.632\,z^n}{(z-1)(z-0.368)} \text{ at poles } z=+1 \text{ and } z=+0.368. \tag{2.219}$$

$$\downarrow$$

$$y(n) = \frac{0.632(1)^n}{1-0.368} + \frac{0.632(0.368)^n}{0.368-1} = 1-(0.368)n = 1-e^{-n} \tag{2.220}$$

The last equality on the right of Equation 2.220 is evident if we recall that $e^{-1} = 0.368$.

A second way of finding the inverse z transform uses a power series in z^{-1} by *long division.* Consider:

$$\mathbf{H}(z) = \frac{z}{z-0.4} \tag{2.221}$$

Dividing the denominator into the numerator, we find:

$$H(z) = 1 + 0.4z^{-1} + 0.16z^{-2} + 0.064z^{-3} + 0.0256z^{-4} + \cdots + (0.4)^n z^{-n} + \cdots \tag{2.222}$$

Thus, by inspection,

$$h(n) = \sum_{n=0}^{\infty} (0.4)^k \delta(k-n) \tag{2.223}$$

For example, $h(4) = 0.0256$.

In *another example* of finding $h(k)$ by long division, consider the transfer function $H(z)$:

$$\mathbf{H}(z) = \frac{0.632\,z}{z^2 - 1.368\,z + 0.368} = 0.632z^{-1} + 0.864z^{-2} + 0.95z^{-3} + 0.982z^{-4} + \cdots \tag{2.224}$$

Now it is evident that $h(0) = 0$, $h(1) = 0.632$, $h(2) = 0.864, \ldots$. A closed form for $h(n)$ is not obvious in this case.

Still another way of finding the inverse z transform of $H(z)$ when it is a rational polynomial in z, the denominator is of order N and the numerator is of order $M < N$, is to do a *partial fraction expansion* of $H(z)/z$. The denominator of $H(z)/z$ must be factored and the residues C_k found in the manner used with factored Laplace transforms.

$$\frac{H(z)}{z} = \frac{C_1}{z+a_1} + \frac{C_2}{z+a_2} + \cdots + \frac{C_N}{z+a_N} \tag{2.225}$$

Now all the terms in the PF expansion are multiplied by z to obtain $H(z)$ again, and a standard table of inverse z transforms is used to assemble the corresponding sum of discrete time functions from the expansion terms:

$$h(n) = \sum_{m=1}^{N} h_m(n) \tag{2.226}$$

As *an example* of the PF method, consider the function:

$$H(z) = \frac{z^2}{z^2 - 0.6z + 0.05} \tag{2.227}$$

We put it in the form, $H(z)/z$ and factor it:

$$H(z)/z = \frac{z}{(z-0.1)(z-0.5)} = \frac{A}{(z-0.1)} + \frac{B}{(z-0.5)} \tag{2.228A}$$

$$\underset{z\to 0.1}{A} = (z-0.1)\frac{z}{(z-0.1)(z-0.5)} = \frac{0.1}{-0.4} = -0.250 \tag{2.228B}$$

$$\underset{z\to 0.5}{B} = (z-0.5)\frac{z}{(z-0.1)(z-0.5)} = \frac{0.5}{0.4} = 1.250 \tag{2.228C}$$

Finally, we can write:

$$H(z) = \frac{-0.250z}{(z-0.1)} + \frac{1.250z}{(z-0.5)} \tag{2.229}$$

In the time domain, this is:

$$h(nT) = h(n) = -0.250(0.1)^n + 1.250(0.5)^n, \quad n = 0,1,2,\ldots \tag{2.230}$$

Two other cases occur with PF expansions with z transforms. Repeated poles of the form, $(z-b)^r$, $r \geq 2$ and complex-conjugate quadratic pole-pairs. Covering these cases is beyond the scope of this introductory chapter. The interested reader is encouraged to consult Section 3.4 in Proakis and Manolakis (1989).

As an example of using the z transform to find the discrete (sampled) output of a discrete system, consider the discrete causal LTI system with weighting function $h(n) = u(n)e^{-naT}$. This system has the discrete input, $x(n) = u(n)e^{-nbT}$ for $n = 0,1,2,\ldots$. We wish to find the discrete system's output, $y(n)$. First, we note that $Y(z) = X(z)H(z)$ and $y(n)$ can be found from z-transform tables after a partial fraction expansion. Let us express this relation in terms of z^{-1} instead of z, because of algebraic simplicity. Thus $Y(z^{-1})$ is simply:

$$Y(z^{-1}) = \frac{1}{1 - z^{-1}e^{-aT}} \frac{1}{1 - z^{-1}e^{-bT}}, \quad \text{where } b > a \tag{2.231}$$

Written as a partial fraction,

$$Y(z^{-1}) = \frac{A}{1 - z^{-1}e^{-aT}} + \frac{B}{1 - z^{-1}e^{-bT}} \tag{2.232}$$

Now we evaluate the constants A and B:

$$A = \left. \frac{(1 - z^{-1}e^{-aT})}{1 - z^{-1}e^{-aT}} \frac{1}{1 - z^{-1}e^{-bT}} \right|_{z^{-1} = e^{aT}} = \frac{e^{-aT}}{e^{-aT} - e^{-bT}} \tag{2.233A}$$

$$B = \left. \frac{(1 - z^{-1}e^{-bT})}{1 - z^{-1}e^{-bT}} \frac{1}{1 - z^{-1}e^{-aT}} \right|_{z^{-1} = e^{bT}} = \frac{-e^{-bT}}{e^{-aT} - e^{-bT}} \tag{2.233B}$$

Thus, the output transform can be written:

$$Y(z^{-1}) = \frac{1}{e^{-aT} - e^{-bT}} \left[\frac{e^{-aT}}{1 - z^{-1}e^{-aT}} - \frac{e^{-bT}}{1 - z^{-1}e^{-bT}} \right] \tag{2.234}$$

Using z transform tables and some algebra, we finally obtain:

$$y(n) = \frac{1}{(e^{-aT} - e^{-bT})} \left[e^{-a(n+1)T} u(n) - e^{-b(n+1)T} u(n) \right], \quad n = 0, 1, 2, \ldots \infty \tag{2.235}$$

In another example, a DLTI system is described by the recursive difference equation:

$$y(n) - \frac{3}{4} y(n-1) + \frac{1}{8} y(n-2) = x(n) \tag{2.236}$$

We wish to find the system's transfer function and weighting function. First, we take the z-transform of the difference equation above:

$$Y(z^{-1}) \left[1 - \frac{3}{4} z^{-1} + \frac{1}{8} z^{-2} \right] = X(z^{-1}) \tag{2.237}$$

Next, we find the transfer function, $H(z^{-1}) = \frac{Y(z^{-1})}{X(z^{-1})}$. The quadratic denominator of $H(z^{-1})$ is also factored and the partial fractions found:

$$H(z^{-1}) = \frac{1}{(1 - 1/2\, z^{-1})(1 - 1/4\, z^{-1})} = \frac{A}{(1 - 1/2\, z^{-1})} + \frac{B}{(1 - 1/4\, z^{-1})} \tag{2.238}$$

Solving for A and B:

$$A = \left.\frac{(1 - {}^1\!/_2\, z^{-1})}{(1 - {}^1\!/_2\, z^{-1})(1 - {}^1\!/_4\, z^{-1})}\right|_{z^{-1}=2} = 2 \tag{2.239A}$$

$$B = \left.\frac{(1 - {}^1\!/_4\, z^{-1})}{(1 - {}^1\!/_2\, z^{-1})(1 - {}^1\!/_4\, z^{-1})}\right|_{z^{-1}=4} = -1 \tag{2.239B}$$

Thus, the transfer function is:

$$H(z^{-1}) = \frac{2}{(1 - {}^1\!/_2\, z^{-1})} - \frac{1}{(1 - {}^1\!/_4\, z^{-1})} \tag{2.240}$$

From the z transform tables, by inspection, we have the system's weighting function sequence:

$$h(n) = 2u(n)({}^1\!/_2)^n - u(n)({}^1\!/_4)^n, \quad n = 0, 1, 2, \ldots, \infty \tag{2.241}$$

In yet another *example,* we will use the *identity:*

$$\sum_{n=0}^{N-1} \rho^n z^{-n} \equiv \frac{1 - (\rho z^{-1})^N}{1 - \rho z^{-1}} \tag{2.242}$$

For example, from

$$\sum_{n=0}^{\infty} \rho^n z^{-n} \equiv \frac{1}{1 - \rho z^{-1}} = \frac{z}{z - \rho} \tag{2.243}$$

It is clear that

$$Z\{\rho^n u(n)\} \longleftrightarrow \frac{z}{z - \rho} \tag{2.244}$$

If we differentiate Equation 2.243 above with respect to ρ, we obtain:

$$\sum_{n=0}^{\infty} n \rho^{n-1} z^{-n} = \frac{z}{(z - \rho)^2} \tag{2.245}$$

Which, by the reasoning above, leads to the z transform pair:

$$Z\{n \rho^{n-1} u(n)\} \longleftrightarrow \frac{z}{(z - \rho)^2} \tag{2.246}$$

By differentiation of Equation 2.243 m times with respect to ρ, we can generalize the transform:

$$Z\left\{\binom{n}{m}\rho^{n-m}u(n)\right\} \longleftrightarrow \frac{z}{(z-\rho)^{m+1}} \quad (2.247)$$

Below is a *table of z transforms* for common time functions. The time functions can be analog inputs or system weighting functions.

TABLE 2.2
One-Sided Causal Z Transform Pairs and Theorems

Time Function, $f(t), t \geq 0$.	**$F(z)(z \equiv e^{sT})$ (T is sampling period)**
$\delta(t)$	1
$p_a(t) = 1, 0 \leq t \leq a$, else 0, (unit pulse) $kT < a < (k+1)T$	$1 + z^{-1} + z^{-2} + \cdots + z^{-k} = \frac{z^k + z^{k-1} + \cdots + z + 1}{z^k}$
$U(t)$ (unit step)	$z/(z-1)$ or $1/(1-z^{-1})$
$tU(t)$ (unit ramp)	$Tz/(z-1)^2$
$e^{-at}U(t)$ (exponential)	$z/(z-e^{-aT})$ or $1/(1-z^{-1}e^{-aT})$
$\frac{1}{b-a}(e^{-at} - e^{-bt})$	$\frac{1}{b-a}\left(\frac{z}{z-e^{-aT}} - \frac{z}{z-e^{-bT}}\right)$
$(1/a)(1-e^{-at})U(t)$	$\frac{z(1-e^{-aT})}{a(z-1)(z-e^{-aT})}$
$te^{-at}U(t)$	$\frac{zTe^{-aT}}{(z-e^{-aT})^2}$
$\sin(\omega_o t)U(t)$	$\frac{z\sin(\omega_o T)}{z^2 - 2z\cos(\omega_o T) + 1}$
$\cos(\omega_o t)U(t)$	$\frac{z(z-\cos(\omega_o T))}{z^2 - 2z\cos(\omega_o T) + 1}$
$e^{-at}\sin(\omega_o t)U(t)$	$\frac{ze^{-aT}\sin(\omega_o T)}{z^2 - 2ze^{-aT}\cos(\omega_o T) + e^{-2aT}}$
$e^{-at}\cos(\omega_o t)U(t)$	$\frac{z(z-e^{-aT}\cos(\omega_o T))}{z^2 - 2ze^{-aT}\cos(\omega_o T) + e^{-2aT}}$

Note: Proofs of theorems can be found in Cunningham (1992). Note that the z transforms of sampled time functions, $f(nT) = f(n)$, are the same as for continuous $f(t)$ in the left-hand column. Many authors express the z transforms in the right-hand column in terms of integer powers of z^{-1}.

TABLE 2.3
Some properties of the one-sided z transform

Property	Time Domain	z-Domain
Notation	$x(n)$ $x_1(n)$ $x_2(n)$	$X(z)$ $X_1(z)$ $X_2(z)$
Superposition	$b_1 x_1(n) + b_2 x_2(n)$	$b_1 X_1(z) + b_2 X_2(z)$
Time delay	$x(n-k)$	$z^{-k}X(z)$
Time reversal	$x(-n)$	$X(z^{-1})$
Modulation	$h(t) = f(t) \times g(t)$	$H(z) = \frac{1}{2\pi j}\int_C F(\nu)G(z/\nu)\nu^{-1}\,d\nu$ (complex convolution)
Initial value theorem	$f(0)$	$\lim_{z\to\infty} F(z)$
Final value theorem	$f(\infty)$	$\lim_{z\to 1}(z-1)F(z)$
Differentiation in z domain	If $x(n) \longleftrightarrow X(z)$, then $nx(n)$	$-z\frac{dX(z)}{dz}$
Real convolution	$f(t) \otimes g(t)$	$F(z)\,G(z)$

Large factored polynomials in z can be broken up by partial fraction expansion, similar to Laplace polynomials and each additive component can be looked up in the table above to find its inverse transform in the time domain.

Some properties of the one-sided z transform are given in Table 2.3.

2.5.5 z Transform solutions of discrete state equations

Let a discrete system be described by a set of n discrete (difference) state equations:

$$\mathbf{x}(k+1) = \mathbf{A}\mathbf{x}(k) + \mathbf{B}\mathbf{u}(k) \tag{2.248A}$$

$$\mathbf{y}(k) = \mathbf{C}\mathbf{x}(k) + \mathbf{D}\mathbf{u}(k) \tag{2.248B}$$

Where $\mathbf{x}(k+1)$ is the new set of states to be used in the next iteration, $\mathbf{u}(k)$ are the p inputs, and $\mathbf{y}(k)$ are the m outputs at $t = kT$. We take the z transform of both sides of the state equation, 2.248A:

$$z\mathbf{X}(z) - z\mathbf{x}(0+) = \mathbf{A}\mathbf{X}(z) + \mathbf{B}\mathbf{U}(z) \tag{2.249}$$

Equation 2.249 is solved for $\mathbf{X}(z)$:

$$\mathbf{X}(z) = (z\mathbf{I} - \mathbf{A})^{-1} z\mathbf{x}(0+) + (z\mathbf{I} - \mathbf{A})^{-1}\mathbf{B}\mathbf{U}(z) \tag{2.250}$$

The inverse z transform of X(z) is:

$$\mathbf{x}(k) = \mathbf{Z}^{-1}\{(z\mathbf{I}-\mathbf{A})^{-1}z\}\mathbf{x}(0+) + \mathbf{Z}^{-1}\{(z\mathbf{I}-\mathbf{A})^{-1}\mathbf{B}\mathbf{U}(z)\} \tag{2.251}$$

Now we define the *discrete state transition matrix* as [Kuo, 1967]:

$$\Phi(k) = \mathbf{Z}^{-1}\{(z\mathbf{I}-\mathbf{A})^{-1}z\} = \mathbf{A}^k \tag{2.252}$$

Now the discrete state transition equation giving the present states becomes:

$$\mathbf{x}(k) = \Phi(k)\mathbf{x}(0+) + \sum_{i=0}^{k-1} \Phi(k-i-1)\mathbf{B}\mathbf{u}(i) \tag{2.253}$$

Kuo also gives the general solution for the states when the states at $t = nT$ are known ($0 \leq n < k$):

$$\mathbf{x}(k+n) = \Phi(k)\mathbf{x}(n) + \sum_{i=0}^{k-1} \Phi(k-i-1)\mathbf{B}\mathbf{u}(i+n) \tag{2.254}$$

2.5.6 Discussion

Section 2.5 has provided a rigorous treatment of discrete LTI systems and stationary discrete signals. Periodic sampling of an analog signal was shown to be equivalent to impulse modulation, which, in turn, was shown to lead to the open form of the z transform. Three examples of discrete differentiation were examined as difference equations in the time-domain transfer functions in z and in terms of sinusoidal frequency response in the interval from $\omega = 0$ to $\omega = \omega_N = \pi/T$, the Nyquist frequency. Certain discrete integration routines were examined in the same context. We also examined discrete convolution and the general form for discrete filters as *finite impulse response* (FIR) (feed-forward architecture) or *infinite impulse response* (IIR) (recursive architecture). We also considered only causal systems and signals defined for $t \geq 0$, i.e., discrete signals and systems characterized by one-sided z transforms.

The definition of the one-sided z transform by complex convolution, based on impulse modulation, was introduced. Use of a complex contour integral to find the inverse z transform of a one-sided Y(z) was shown to be avoidable by using the method of residues and partial fraction expansion of Y(z). A number of examples of finding y(n) for $n \geq 0$ from various Y(z)s were given.

Finally, we showed how the z transform can be used to find the states $\mathbf{X}(z)$, hence $\mathbf{x}(k)$, given a DLTI state system described in the time domain.

2.6 Stability of Systems

The stability of a closed-loop feedback system is not guaranteed by the use of negative feedback. Under suitable conditions, both positive and negative LTI feedback systems can be stable or become unstable. Much has been written on the design and compensation required to preserve closed-loop system stability, and several tests have been developed to predict instability before the loop is closed.

We know that if we turn on a public address system, speak into the microphone and hear a loud howl or screech that overwhelms the amplified speech, that there is audio feedback that renders the PA system useless until we either reorient the microphone with respect to the loudspeakers, or turn down the system's amplification. The howl is a form of system instability in which the system oscillates at a high audio frequency determined by a number of factors, such as the amplifier gain and frequency response and room acoustics, including the sound propagation delay time from the loudspeakers to the microphone. The feedback itself *can be positive or negative* and the instability can be the result of one or more of the factors cited above. The oscillations generally begin as soon as the speaker begins to talk into the microphone and grow exponentially in amplitude until some part of the system (loudspeaker, microphone, amplifier) saturates. Then they persist at this obnoxious level.

Another form of instability in feedback systems occurs when the system output grows without oscillation to a level where the system is saturated and useless. Fortunately, there are many tests that one can apply to the *loop gain transfer function* $(A_L(s))$ of a feedback system that will predict whether it will be unstable in the closed-loop configuration and if so, whether it will simply saturate its output or will oscillate, and at what frequency. Some tests are practical, based on experimental frequency response data, such as the *Nyquist Stability Criterion,* the *Describing Function Method* and the *Popov Criterion* for nonlinear systems. Other stability tests are mathematical, focusing on the poles, zeros and gain of the loop gain (*Routh-Hurwitz Test, Root-Locus Analysis,* the *Lyupanov* method). Figure 2.19 illustrates a single-input–single-output feedback system defining $A_L(s)$. The feedback is considered to be negative if there is a net minus sign preceding $A_L(s)$. In this text, we will examine only the venerable Nyquist test and Describing functions. The reader interested in pursuing the general topic of the prediction of system stability and compensation for system stability should consult one of the many texts on control systems, such as Nise (1995), Ogata (1990) or Rugh (1996).

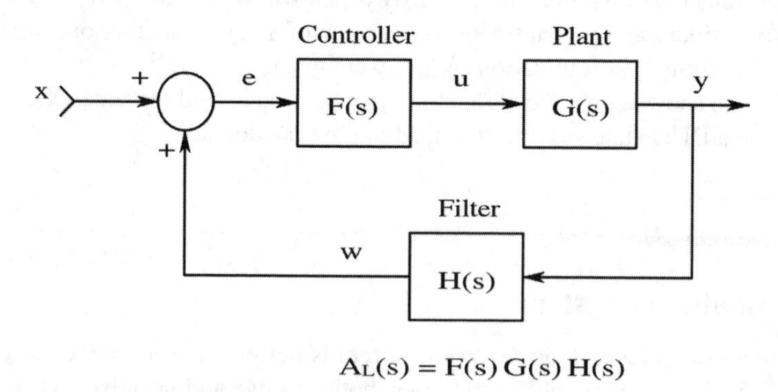

FIGURE 2.19
A SISO continuous, LTI feedback system used to define the loop gain, $A_L(s) = \frac{W}{E}(s)$.

In general, a closed-loop causal continuous, LTI system is stable if all its poles lie in the left-hand s-plane. If one pole of a continuous system's closed-loop transfer function lies in the right-half s-plane, the output will theoretically grow exponentially without bound. Practically, some element in such a system always saturates (or burns out, etc.). If a linear system has a pair of complex-conjugate poles in the right-half s-plane, the system's output will be an exponentially growing oscillation. In either case, the unstable behavior is undesirable and robust system design generally will compensate the closed-loop system so that unstable behavior cannot occur under any set of input conditions.

Note that system poles on the $j\omega$ axis in the s-plane present a special problem. Two or more poles at the origin yield an unbounded impulse response. One pole yields a constant component to the impulse response (the impulse response of an integrator). A pair of conjugate poles on the $j\omega$ axis will yield an oscillation of fixed peak amplitude and frequency dependent on initial conditions and the input. As remarked above, a pair of complex-conjugate poles must lie in the right-half s-plane to produce exponentially growing oscillations.

Likewise, a *discrete* causal LTI system is stable if all its poles lie inside the unit circle in the z-plane. Alternately, a stable, discrete, causal, LTI system's impulse response must sum absolutely to less than infinity [Oppenheim and Willsky, 1983]. That is:

$$\sum_{n=0}^{\infty} |h(n)| < \infty \qquad (2.255)$$

Discrete causal LTI system transfer function poles on the unit circle in the z-plane present the same limiting conditions as continuous causal LTI system poles on the $j\omega$ axis of the s-plane.

It is important to realize that instability is deliberately designed into certain classes of *nonlinear feedback systems.* Such systems are intended to oscillate in *bounded limit cycles* around a desired *set point.* They generally use a simple, ON/OFF type of controller. One example of limit-cycling control systems is the ubiquitous home heating (or cooling) system; another example is drug infusion control systems [Northrop, 2000]. Analysis of limit-cycling closed-loop control systems is generally done effectively with the describing function method, and is covered in Section 9.4.3.

2.7 Chapter Summary

The purpose of this chapter has been to review the basics of LTI system theory. It began by considering the system properties of linearity, causality and stationarity. Closed-loop system architecture was classified as simple-to-analyze SISO or the complex MIMO forms generally found in physiological systems. LTI analog systems were shown to be described by one or more linear time-invariant ordinary differential equations (ODEs). We examined the basics of solving first- and second-order LTI ODEs. System ODEs were shown to be reformatted in state-variable form in which all ODEs are first-order and which can be solved in the time or frequency domains by matrix algebra. Matrix algebra was reviewed.

Characterization methods for LTI systems were next examined. The impulse response of an LTI system was defined, real convolution was derived and its properties made clear. The usefulness of other transient inputs was described. The steady-state, sinusoidal frequency response of a continuous LTI system was shown to be an effective frequency-domain system descriptor. Frequency response is typically displayed as a Bode plot or a Nyquist (polar) diagram.

As summarized above, Section 2.5 has dealt with discrete systems and signals, the z transform and discrete state equations. Section 2.6 reviewed the basis for various stability tests on continuous and discrete LTI systems. For continuous systems, we employ various tests to predict or detect closed-loop system poles in the right-half s-plane; for discrete systems, we test for closed-loop poles on or outside the unit circle in the z-plane. Note that, long before a system becomes frankly unstable with an exponentially growing output, it can be useless for the purpose it was intended because its output is too oscillatory (underdamped). Good system design includes more than a theoretical test for instability. Simulation is necessary.

Problems

2.1 When a certain drug is injected intravenously (IV) into a patient to build up a concentration in the blood and then stopped, the drug's concentration is found to decrease at a rate proportional to the concentration. In terms of a simple first-order linear ODE, this can be written:

$$\dot{C} = -K_L C + R_{in}/V_B \quad (\mu g/l)/min$$

Where C is the drug concentration in the blood in μg/l, K_L is the loss rate constant in 1/min, R_{in} is the drug input rate in μg/min and V_B is the volume of blood in liters.

a. Plot and dimension $C(t)$ when $R_{in}(t) = R_o\delta(t)\mu g$, (a bolus injection at $t = 0$).

b. Plot and dimension $C(t)$ when $R_{in}(t) = R_d U(t)$ (a steady IV drip, modeled by a step function). Give the steady-state C.

2.2 An LTI system is described by the second-order ODE:

$$\ddot{y} + 7\dot{y} + 10y = x(t)$$

a. Use the p operator notation to find the roots of the characteristic equation, p_1 and p_2.

b. Assume zero initial conditions. Find an expression for $y(t)$ given $x(t) = \delta(t)$.

c. Now let $x(t) = 10U(t)$. Find the steady-state value of y.

2.3 In this problem, there are two compartments where a drug can exist in a patient: in the blood volume (V_B) and in the extracellular fluid (ECF) volume (V_E). A drug is injected IV into the blood compartment at a rate R_{in} μg/min. The drug can diffuse from the blood compartment to the ECF compartment at a rate $K_{BE}(C_B - C_E)$ μg/min, assuming $C_B > C_E$. Otherwise, the direction of diffusion is reversed if $C_B < C_E$. Drug is lost physiologically only from the blood compartment. The ECF compartment acts only for drug storage. Two linear first-order ODEs describe the system:

$$\begin{aligned} \dot{C}_B V_B &= -K_{BE}(C_B - C_E) - K_{LB} C_B + R_{in} \ \mu g/min \\ \dot{C}_E V_E &= K_{BE}(C_B - C_E) \end{aligned}$$

a. Note that in the steady-state, for $t \to \infty$, both $\dot{C}_B$ and $\dot{C}_E = 0$. Find expressions for $C_B(\infty)$ and $C_E(\infty)$, given a step infusion, $R_{in}(t) = R_d U(t)\mu g/min$.

b. Plot and dimension $C_B(t)$ and $C_E(t)$, given zero initial conditions and a bolus injection of drug, $R_{in}(t) = R_o\delta(t)\mu g$. It is best if you solve this problem by simulation (use Matlab™or Simnon™). Let $V_E = 15$ l, $V_B = 3$ l, $K_{BE} = K_{LB} = 1$ l/min.

2.4 A quadratic low-pass filter is described by the second-order ODE:

$$\ddot{y} + (2\xi\omega_n)\dot{y} + \omega_n^2 y = x(t)$$

a. The characteristic equation for this ODE in terms of the p operator has complex-conjugate roots. Find an algebraic expression for the position of the roots.

b. Let $x(t) = U(t)$ (a unit step). Find the steady-state output, y_{ss}.

c. Let $x(t) = \delta(t)$. Find, sketch and dimension $y(t)$ for $0 \leq t \leq \infty$ for $\xi = 0.5$, and $\omega_n = 1$ r/sec.

2.5 An alternate way of writing the ODE for an underdamped quadratic low-pass system is:

$$\ddot{y} + 2a\dot{y} + (b^2 + a^2)y = x(t)$$

Let $a = 0.5$, $b = 0.86603$. Repeat a, b and c in the preceding problem.

2.6 Consider a capacitor that is charged to V_{co} at $t = 0-$ and then allowed to discharge through a nonlinear conductance for which $i_{nl} = \beta V_c^2$, as shown in Figure P2.6. Thus, for $t \geq 0$, system behavior is given by the nonlinear node ODE:

$$C\dot{V}_c + \beta V_c^2 = 0$$

We are interested in finding $V_c(t)$ for this circuit for $t \geq 0$. The ODE is a form of a nonlinear ODE called *Bernoulli's equation,* which can be linearized by a change in its dependent variable. In its general form, Bernoulli's equation is:

$$\frac{dy}{dx} + P(x)y = Q(x)y^n$$

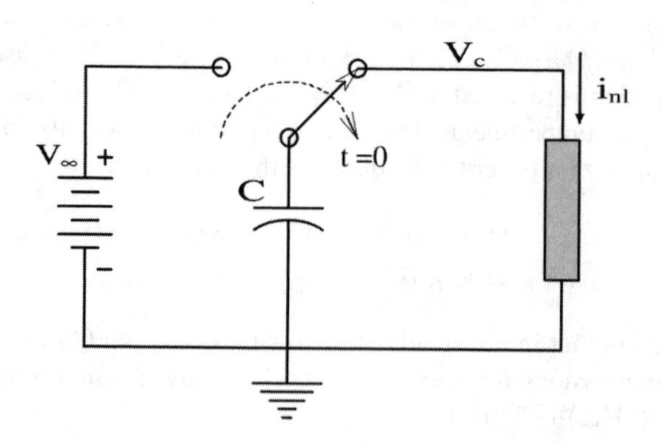

FIGURE P2.6

This equation can be linearized for solution by making the substitution, $u \equiv y^{1-n}$. Since $du/dx = (1-n)y^{-n}(dy/dx)$, this leads to the ODE linear in u:

$$\frac{1}{1-n}\frac{du}{dx} + P(x)u = Q(x)$$

Substitute $n = 2$, $P = 0$, $y = V_c$, $x = t$ and $Q = -\beta/C$ into the linearized ODE above and solve for $V_c(t)$. Plot and dimension $V_c(t)$ for $-C/(\beta V_{co}) \leq t \leq \infty$. (Hint: note that the capacitor discharge through this nonlinearity generates a hyperbola, rather than an exponential decay.)

2.7 Find the nonlinear element, $i_{nl} = f(V_c)$ that, when placed in parallel with the capacitor of Problem 2.6, will give a $V_c(t)$ of the form:

$$V_c(t) = K \log_{10}\left(\frac{1}{t+t_o}\right), t \geq 0.$$

2.8 Find the determinants of the matrices below:

$$\text{a. } \begin{bmatrix} 2 & 3 \\ -1 & 4 \end{bmatrix} \quad \text{b. } \begin{bmatrix} 1 & 0 & 0 \\ 2 & 3 & 5 \\ 4 & 1 & 3 \end{bmatrix} \quad \text{c. } \begin{bmatrix} 1 & 0 & 6 \\ 3 & 4 & 15 \\ 5 & 6 & 21 \end{bmatrix}$$

2.9 Find the adjoint matrices of the square **A** matrices below:

$$\text{a. } \begin{bmatrix} a & b \\ c & d \end{bmatrix} \quad \text{b. } \begin{bmatrix} 1 & 2 & 3 \\ 2 & 3 & 2 \\ 3 & 3 & 4 \end{bmatrix} \quad \text{c. } \begin{bmatrix} 1 & 2 & 3 \\ 1 & 3 & 4 \\ 1 & 4 & 3 \end{bmatrix}$$

d. Find $\mathbf{A} \cdot \textbf{adj } \mathbf{A}$ for the matrix of b.

2.10 We have seen that the inverse of a square matrix can be found from: $\mathbf{A}^{-1} = \textbf{adj}\mathbf{A}/\det \mathbf{A}$. Find the inverse matrices for:

$$\text{a. } \begin{bmatrix} 2 & 3 \\ 1 & 4 \end{bmatrix} \quad \text{b. } \begin{bmatrix} 1 & 2 & 3 \\ 1 & 3 & 4 \\ 1 & 4 & 3 \end{bmatrix} \quad \text{c. } \begin{bmatrix} 2 & 3 & 1 \\ 1 & 2 & 3 \\ 3 & 1 & 2 \end{bmatrix}$$

2.11 Solve the simultaneous equations using Cramer's rule:

a.
$$3x_1 - 5x_2 = 0$$
$$x_1 + x_2 = 2$$

b.
$$2x_1 + x_2 + 5x_3 + x_4 = 5$$
$$x_1 + x_2 - 3x_3 - 4x_4 = -1$$
$$3x_1 + 6x_2 - 2x_3 + x_4 = 8$$
$$2x_1 + 2x_2 + 2x_3 - 3x_4 = 2$$

2.12 A single input-single output (SISO) LIT system is described by the 2nd order ODE:

$$\ddot{y} + 5\dot{y} + 2y = r(t)$$

Let $y = x_1$, $x_2 = \dot{x}_1$. Find the **A** and **B** matrices in the state-variable form of this system:

$$\dot{\mathbf{x}} = \mathbf{A}\mathbf{x} + \mathbf{B}r(t)$$

2.13 A SISO LTIS is described by:

$$2\ddot{y} + 3\dot{y} + y = \dot{r} + 2r$$

Where $y = x_1$, $\dot{x}_1 = x_2$. Find the **A** and **B** matrices for this system.

2.14 A SISO LTIS is described by:

$$\dddot{y} + 3\dot{y} + 2y = 3\ddot{r} + 5\dot{r} + r$$

Where $y = x_1$, $\dot{x}_1 = x_2$. Find the **A** and **B** matrices for this system and the **C** and **D** matrices in the equation: $y(t) = \mathbf{C}\mathbf{x} + \mathbf{D}r(t)$.

2.15 a. Find an expression for, plot and dimension the magnitude and phase frequency response of the discrete *rectangular integration routine.* Consider $0 \leq \omega \leq \pi/T$ r/sec. π/T is the r/sec Nyquist frequency; T is the sampling period.

$$\frac{Y_r}{X}(z) = \frac{T}{z-1} = I_r(z)$$

Hint: Write the transfer function in terms of the delay operator, $z^{-1} = e^{-j\omega T}$ and use the Euler relations for $\sin\theta$ or $\cos\theta$.

b. Find an expression for, plot and dimension the magnitude and phase frequency response of the discrete *trapezoidal integration routine.* Consider $0 \leq \omega \leq \pi/T$ r/sec. π/T is the r/sec Nyquist frequency; T is the sampling period.

$$\frac{Y_t}{X}(z) = \frac{(T/2)[z+1]}{z-1} = I_t(z)$$

Hint: Write the transfer function in terms of the delay operator, $z^{-1} = e^{-j\omega T}$ and use the Euler relations for $\sin\theta$ or $\cos\theta$.

c. Repeat parts a and b for the *Simpson's rule integrator:*

$$\frac{Y_s}{X}(z) = \frac{(T/3)[z^2 + 4z + 1]}{z^2 - 1}$$

d. Plot the frequency response of an ideal (analog) integrator on the same axes as the FR of the rectangular and trapezoidal integrators.

2.16 Consider the discrete LTI system defined by the difference equation:

$$y(n) - \frac{1}{3}y(n-1) = x(n), \quad n \geq 0.$$

$y(n)$ is the output, the input is $x(n) = u(n)$, a unit step. There are zero ICs. Find an expression for and plot and dimension $y(n)$.

2.17 Find $x(n)$, $n \geq 0$, for the $X(z) = \frac{3 - \frac{5}{6}z^{-1}}{(1-\frac{1}{4}z^{-1})(1-\frac{1}{3}z^{-1})}$. Use a partial fraction expansion, and assume convergence for both poles: $|z| > 1/4$, $|z| > \frac{1}{3}$.

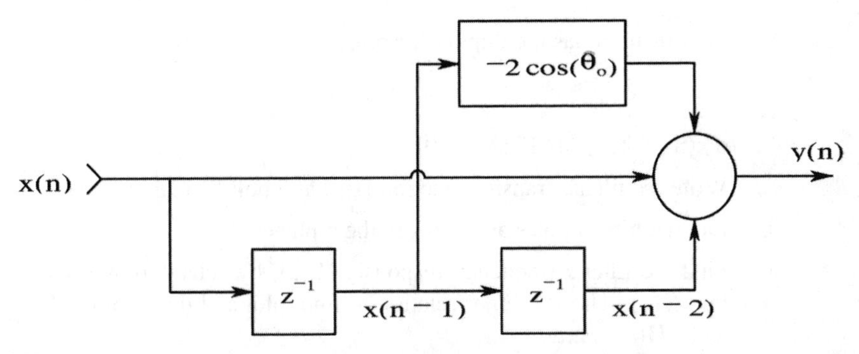

FIGURE P2.12

2.18 Use the relation, $\sum_{n=0}^{N-1} \rho^n = \frac{1-\rho^N}{1-\rho}$, to find the Z transform, G(z), of the truncated exponential decay, $g(n) = e^{-aTn}$, defined for $0 \le n \le N-1$ and zero for $n < 0$ and $n > N-1$. *Hint:* note that there is an $(N-1)^{th}$ pole at the origin of the z-plane for G(z).

2.19 Find the z transform of the discrete sequence, $x(n) = \left(\frac{1}{2}\right)^n u(n) + \left(\frac{1}{3}\right)^n u(n)$, defined for $0 \le n \le \infty$. Express X(z) as a factored, rational polynomial. Plot the poles and zeros of X(z) in the z-plane.

2.20 Consider the simple FIR filter shown in Figure P2.12=P2.20.

a. Sketch and dimension the impulse response of this filter.

b. Find the transfer function for this filter, H(z). Let $\theta_0 = \pi/4$ radians. Plot and dimension the filter's poles and zeros in the z-plane.

c. Plot and dimension both $|\mathbf{H}(\omega)|$ and $\angle\mathbf{H}(\omega)$ for the filter. Let $z^{-1} = e^{-j\omega T}$ and set $\theta_0 = \pi/2$. Find the radian frequency where $|\mathbf{H}(\omega)| \to 0$. Note that the phase has a $-\pi$ jump when $\cos(\omega T)$ goes negative.

d. The FIR filter is given a step input, $x(n) = u(n)$ at $n = 0$. Use the long division method to find y(n) in the steady-state.

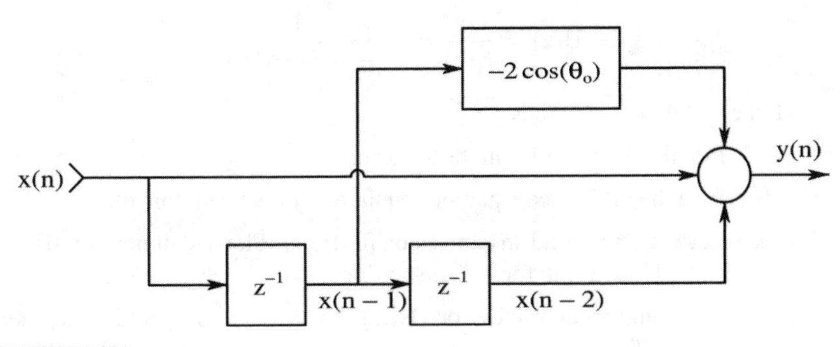

FIGURE P2.20

2.21 A causal FIR filter has the impulse response:

$$h(n) = x(n) - x(n-4)$$

Where $x(n) = \delta(0)$ (a "1" at $n = 0$).

a. Write the filter's transfer function $H(z)$ as a polynomial in z.

b. Plot the filter's poles and zeros in the z-plane.

c. Find the filter's frequency response, $\mathbf{H}(\omega)$, by substituting $z = e^{j\omega T}$ into $H(z)$. Use the Euler relation to find, plot and dimension $|\mathbf{H}(\omega)|$ and $\angle\mathbf{H}(\omega)$ vs. ω.

d. Find and plot the filter's output, $y(n)$, in response to a unit step input to the filter, $u(n)$.

2.22 Consider the difference equation for the causal recursive filter with input $x(n)$ and output $y(n)$:

$$y(n) = 1/2\, y(n-1) + x(n) + 1/2\, x(n-1)$$

a. Find the filter's transfer function, $H(z)$. Plot its pole and zero in the z-plane.

b. Use long division to find the filter's impulse response sequence, $h(n)$.

2.23 The difference equation for a causal FIR notch filter is given as:

$$y(n) = b_0 x(n) + b_1 x(n-1) + b_2 x(n-2)$$

a. Find the filter's transfer function, $H(z)$.

b. Find an expression for $\mathbf{H}(\omega)$, magnitude and phase. Let $b_0 = b_2$, and use the Euler relation for $\cos\theta$.

c. Find the b_0 and b_1 values required such that $\mathbf{H}(0) = 1\angle 0°$, and $\mathbf{H}(\pi/4T) = 0$.

2.24 Papoulis (1977) gives an example of a causal, discrete, LTI filter that has a resonant frequency response.

$$H(z) = \frac{Y(z)}{X(z)} = \frac{1}{z^2 - 2r\cos(\alpha)z + r^2}$$

Let $r = 0.9$, $\alpha = \pi/2$ rads.

a. Plot the filter's poles in the z-plane.

b. Find the difference equation required to implement this filter.

c. Let $\mathbf{z} \equiv e^{j\omega T}$. Find an expression for $H(\omega)$. Plot and dimension $|\mathbf{H}(\omega)|$ and $\angle\mathbf{H}(\omega)$ vs. ω for $0 \le \omega \le \pi/T$.

d. Give numerical values for $|\mathbf{H}(\omega)|$ for $\omega = 0$, $\omega = \alpha/T = \omega_r$, and $\omega = \pi/T$.

2.25 A certain causal digital filter has the transfer function

$$H(z) = \frac{1}{[1 - \frac{1}{3}z^{-1}][1 - \frac{1}{6}z^{-1}]}$$

a. Find the recursive difference equation that produces this $H(z)$.

b. Give the impulse response, $h(n)u(n)$, for this filter.

2.26 Find the inverse z transform of the $Y(z)$ polynomial by partial fraction expansion of the $Y(z)/z$ polynomial and using tables:

$$Y(z) = \frac{(1 - e^{-1})z}{z^2 - 1.368z + 0.3682}$$

2.27 Which of the LTI system transfer functions below are unstable? Plot their poles and zeros in the s-plane.

a. $H(s) = \dfrac{s - 8}{s^2 + 3s + 2}$

b. $H(s) = \dfrac{s + 1}{s^2 + 3s + 3}$

c. $H(s) = \dfrac{s + 1}{s^2 + 3s - 3}$

d. $H(s) = \dfrac{s + 1}{s^2 - 3s - 3}$

e. $H(s) = \dfrac{s - 1}{s^2 + 3s - 4}$

2.28 A SISO, LTI, negative feedback system is shown in Figure P2.21. Note that the plant is unstable.

a. Find the K value above which the closed-loop system is stable.

b. Can the closed-loop system be stable for any negative value of K?

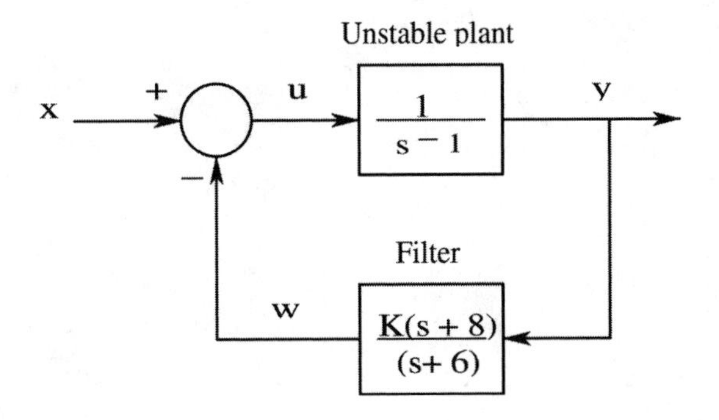

FIGURE P2.21

2.29 A certain causal discrete LTI system has the transfer function:

$$H(z) = \frac{z^2}{z^2 - z(2\rho\cos(\alpha) + \rho^2}$$

a. Plot the poles and zeros of $H(s)$ in the z-plane. Let $\alpha = \pi/4, \rho = 0.85$.

b. Find the first eight terms of this IIR system's impulse response, $h(n)$.

c. Find the range of real ρ over which this system is stable.

3

The Laplace Transform and Its Applications

3.1 Introduction

The Laplace transform was developed in the early 19th century by Pierre Simon Laplace (1749–1827), a gifted French mathematician, astronomer, cosmologist and physicist. Laplace studied many natural phenomena and invented novel mathematical tools to describe and explain his results. He is best known today for devising the concept of spherical harmonics, the concept of potential, $V(x, y, z)$ and the *Laplacian operator*, Equation 3.1,

$$\nabla^2 V = \frac{\partial^2 V}{\partial x^2} + \frac{\partial^2 V}{\partial y^2} + \frac{\partial^2 V}{\partial z^2} = 0, \tag{3.1}$$

and, of course, the transform that bears his name.

The Laplace transform allows time (or space) functions to be written as functions in the (vector) frequency domain, i.e., $f(t) \Leftrightarrow F(s)$, $t \geq 0$. You will see that one advantage of frequency-domain representation by Laplace transform is that the Laplace-transformed (LT'd) output, $Y(s)$, of an LTI system with a Laplace-transformed impulse response, $H(s)$, given an LT'd transient input, $X(s)$, is simply the complex product, $X(s)H(s)$. (Real convolution is not necessary.) $H(s)$ is also called the LTI system's *transfer function.*

The *one-sided Laplace transform* is defined by the real, definite integral:

$$L\{f(t)\} = F(s) \equiv \int_{t=0-}^{\infty} f(t)e^{-st}\,dt \tag{3.2}$$

Where: s is a *complex variable* (2-D vector); $\mathbf{s} \equiv \sigma + j\omega$; where σ is $Re\{s\}$ and ω is $Im\{s\}$. The lower limit of $0-$ allows the transforming of $f(t)$s that are discontinuous at $t = 0$, such as the exponential, $f(t) = e^{-at}U(t)$, or $f(t)$ with an impulse at the origin. Note that the Laplace transform of $f(t)$ exists only if the integral in Equation 3.2 *converges* [Kuo, 1967]. That is, for some real σ_1, we have the finite integral:

$$\int_{0-}^{\infty} |f(t)|e^{-\sigma_1 t}\,dt < \infty. \tag{3.3}$$

For example, if $|f(t)| = Ae^{\sigma_2 t}$, $0 < t < \infty$, the integral will converge if $\infty > \sigma_1 > \sigma_2 > 0$.

For a first example, let us find the Laplace transform of $f(t) = A e^{-bt} U(t)$. This is simply:

$$F(s) = \int_0^\infty f(t) e^{-st} dt = A \int_0^\infty e^{-(s+b)t} dt = -\frac{A}{s+b} e^{-(s+b)t} \Big|_0^\infty = \frac{A}{s+b} \tag{3.4}$$

As a second example, consider the Laplace transform of the *unit step function,* $x(t) = U(t)$.

$$X(s) = \int_{0-}^\infty 1 e^{-st} dt = -\frac{e^{-st}}{s} \Big|_0^\infty = -\frac{1}{s}(0-1) = \frac{1}{s} \tag{3.5}$$

This integral converges for $Re\{s\} > 0$ and $t > 0$.

Now consider $g(t) = e^{at} U(t)$. This is an *exponentially increasing* time function for $t \geq 0$. Its Laplace transform can be written:

$$G(s) = \int_{0-}^\infty e^{at} e^{-st} dt = \int_{0-}^\infty e^{-(-a+\sigma+j\omega)t} dt = -\frac{e^{-(s-a)t}}{s-a} \Big|_0^\infty = \frac{1}{s-a} \tag{3.6}$$

This integral will converge only for the real part of s, $\sigma > a$.

In a fourth example of the Laplace transform, consider $f(t) = A \sin(\omega_o t) U(t)$. Now, by the Euler relation:

$$G(s) = \int_{0-}^\infty \left[\frac{e^{j\omega_o t} - e^{-j\omega_o t}}{2j} \right] e^{-st} dt = \frac{1}{2j} \left[\frac{-e^{-(s-j\omega_o)t}}{s-j\omega_o} + \frac{-e^{-(s+j\omega_o)t}}{s+j\omega_o} \right] \Bigg|_{0-}^\infty \tag{3.7}$$

Now the integral will converge only if the real part of the complex variable, s, σ, is > 0. Therefore, the *abscissa of absolute convergence* for the sine Laplace transform is the $j\omega$ axis in the vector s-plane, (i.e., $\sigma = 0$) and the *region of absolute convergence* is the entire right half of the s-plane [Kuo, 1967]. Assuming the convergence requirements are met, we can write the well-known result (you do the algebra):

$$G(s) = \frac{1}{2j} \left[\frac{1}{s-j\omega_o} - \frac{1}{s+j\omega_o} \right] = \frac{\omega_o}{s^2 + \omega_o^2} \tag{3.8}$$

All the signals and system weighting functions we will consider in this chapter are *causal.* That is, they are defined for $0 \leq t \leq \infty$. The two-sided Laplace transform is used to characterize noncausal signals (e.g., those that have components that exist for $-\infty \leq \tau \leq 0$, such as cross- and autocorrelation functions); we will not treat the two-sided LT here.

As a fifth example of convergence properties, consider the truncated exponential decay, which can be written in two ways. The latter is simply the product of $e^{-ct} U(t)$ times a unit pulse of duration T.

$$f(t) = e^{-ct} U(t) - e^{-c(t-T)} U(t-T) = e^{-ct} [U(t) - U(t-T)] \tag{3.9}$$
$$f(t) = 0 \text{ for } t < 0 \text{ and } t > T.$$

The Laplace transform of this f(t) can be written:

$$F(s) = \int_{0-}^{\infty} e^{-ct}[U(t) - U(t-T)]e^{-st}\,dt \tag{3.10A}$$

$$F(s) = \int_{0-}^{T} e^{-ct}\,e^{-st}\,dt = \left[-\frac{1}{s+c}e^{-(s+c)t}\right]\Bigg|_{0-}^{T} = -\frac{1}{s+c}e^{-(s+c)T} + \frac{1}{s+c} \tag{3.10B}$$

$\downarrow$

$$F(s) = \frac{1 - e^{-cT}\,e^{-sT}}{s+c} \tag{3.10C}$$

The Laplace transform, Equation 3.10A, blows up at the upper limit only if $\sigma = Re\{s\} = -\infty$. Thus the *abscissa of absolute convergence* for this $F(s)$ is $\sigma = -\infty$ and the s-plane *region of convergence* is for $\sigma > -\infty$. (See Equation 3.13 below for an alternate approach to finding this $F(s)$).

3.2 Properties of the Laplace Transform

The many interesting properties of the Laplace transform are listed below. Several are based on the fact that the Laplace transform is a *linear* operation.

1. $L\{kf(t)\} = kF(s)$ (amplitude scaling theorem)
2. $L\{f_1(t) \pm f_2(t)\} = F_1(s) \pm F_2(s)$ (superposition theorem)
3. $L\{f(t-T)\} = e^{-sT}F(s)$ (time shift theorem)
4. $L\{e^{-at}f(t)\} = F(s+a)$, (complex translation theorem)
   $L\{e^{at}f(t)\} = F(s-a)$
5. $L\{f(at)\} = (1/a)F(s/a)$ (time scaling theorem)
6. $L\left\{\int_{0-}^{t} f(t)e^{-st}\,dt\right\} = \frac{F(s)}{s}$ (integration theorem)
7. $L\left\{\frac{df(t)}{dt}\right\} = sF(s) - f(0_-)$ (differentiation theorem includes initial condition on f(t).)

   and $L\left\{\frac{d^2f(t)}{dt^2}\right\} = s^2F(s) - sf(0_-) - \dot{f}(0_-)$

In general, the initial conditions on derivatives are written as:

$$L\left\{\frac{d^nf(t)}{dt^n}\right\} = s^nF(s) - \lim_{t\to 0-}[s^{(n-1)}f(t) + s^{(n-2)}\,df(t)/dt + \cdots + s^0 d^{(n-1)}f(t)/dt^{n-1}]$$

$$= s^n F(s) - [s^{(n-1)} f(0_-) + s^{(n-2)} \dot{f}(0_-) + s^{(n-3)} \ddot{f}(0_-) + \cdots + s^0 \overset{(n-1)\cdot}{f}(0_-)]$$

8. $f(\infty) = \lim_{s \to 0} sF(s)$ (final value theorem)

9. $f(0_+) = \lim_{s \to \infty} sF(s)$ (initial value theorem)

10. $L\{t^n f(t)\} = (-1)^n \frac{d^n F(s)}{ds^n}$ (multiplication by t^n)

11. $L\{f(t) \otimes g(t)\} = F(s)G(s)$ (real convolution transforms to complex multiplication)

12. $L\{f(t)g(t)\} = F(s) \otimes F(s) = \frac{1}{2\pi j} \int_{c-j\infty}^{c+j\infty} F(p)G(s-p)\,dp = \frac{1}{2\pi j} \int_{c-j\infty}^{c+j\infty} G(p)F(s-p)\,dp$ (Laplace transform of the product of two time functions is equal to the complex convolution of their transforms.)

13. $g_T(t) = g_T(t - T)$ for $t \geq 0$, i.e., $g_T(t)$ is periodic with period T, $t \geq 0$. $g(t) = g_T(t)$ for $0 \leq t < T$ and zero for all other t. $G(s) = L\{g(t)\}$.

$$L\{g_T(t)\} = \frac{G(s)}{1 - e^{-sT}}$$ (Laplace transform of a periodic function with period T.)

As an example of 13, consider an ∞ train of narrow pulses of width σ, height $= 1$ and period T. G(s) is simply $[(1/s) - (1/s)e^{-\sigma s}]$, so the Laplace transform of the impulse train is:

$$G_T(s) = \frac{1 - e^{-\sigma s}}{s(1 - e^{-sT})}. \tag{3.11}$$

The reader interested in the derivation or proof of any of the above theorems and properties of Laplace transforms should see Chapter 8 of Kuo (1967) where they are exhaustively derived. Finding the inverse Laplace transform from its defining integral and the process of complex convolution requires a knowledge of *complex variable theory,* including contour integration in the complex plane. Fortunately, for most applications, we can use Laplace transform tables which relate various $F(s) \Leftrightarrow f(t)$.

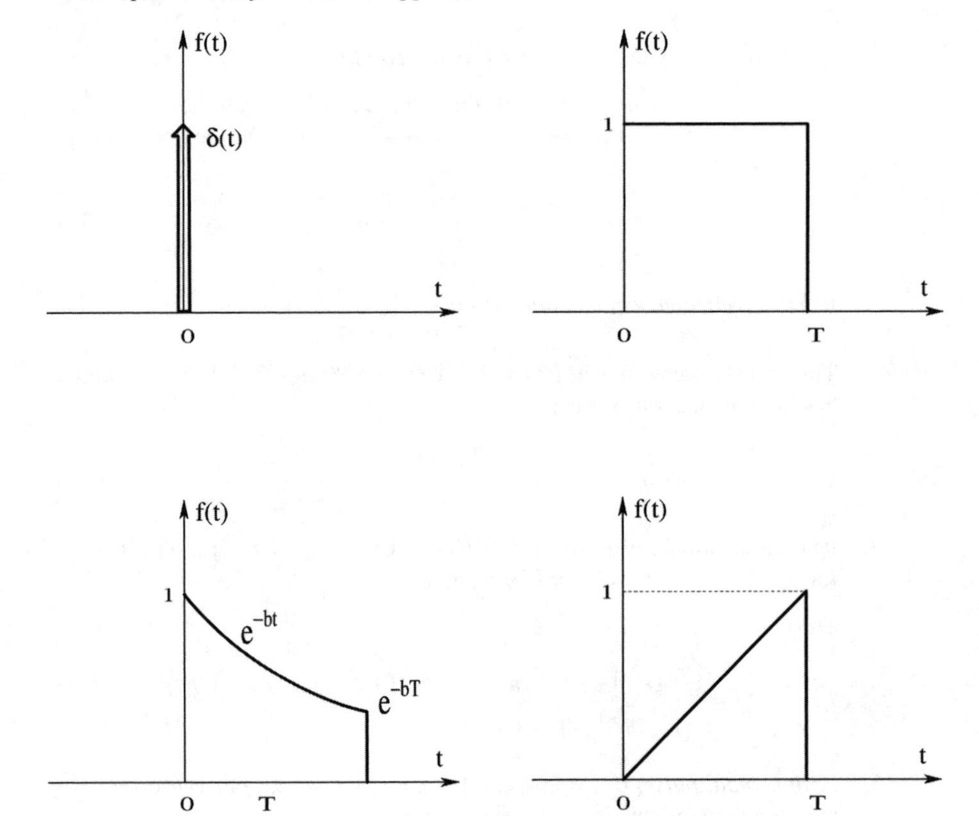

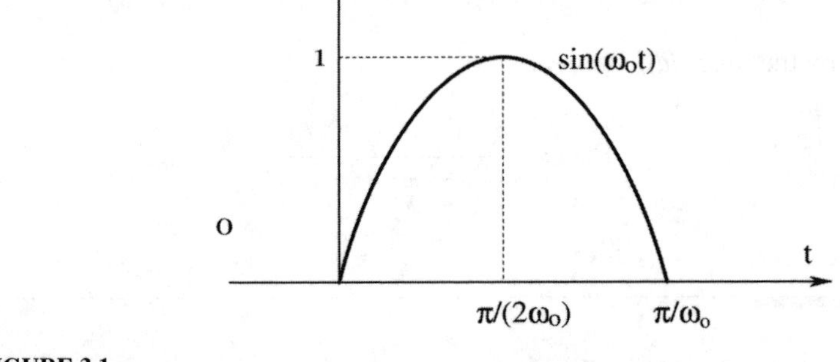

FIGURE 3.1
Transient time-domain signals used in Section 3.3 to find Laplace transforms. From top to bottom, left to right: Unit impulse at $t = 0$, unit rectangular pulse of duration T, truncated exponential decay, truncated ramp and a half-cycle of a sine wave.

3.3 Some Examples of Finding Laplace Transforms

See Figure 3.1, which illustrates the waveforms below. Note that $U(t-\sigma)$ is a unit step function beginning at $t = \sigma$; that is $U(t-\sigma) = 1$ for $t \geq \sigma$ and 0 for $t < 0$.

1. $f(t) = \delta(t)$, so by the *sifting property of delta functions,* $F(s) = 1$.

2. $f(t)$ is a *rectangular pulse* of duration T. This can be written as $f(t) = U(t) - U(t-T)$. Now using relations 2) and 3) in the previous section, we have:

$$F(s) = \frac{1}{s} - \frac{e^{-sT}}{s} = \frac{1-e^{-sT}}{s}. \tag{3.12}$$

3. $f(t)$ is a *truncated exponential.* $f(t) = e^{-bt}, \quad 0_- < t \leq T$
$f(t) = 0, \quad t > T,\ t < 0$
This can also be written as $f(t) = e^{-bt}U(t) - e^{-bT}e^{-b(t-T)}U(t-T)$ which has the Laplace transforms:

$$F(s) = \frac{1}{s+b} - \frac{e^{-bT}e^{-sT}}{s+b} = \frac{1-e^{-bT}e^{-sT}}{s+b} \tag{3.13}$$

4. $f(t)$ is a *sawtooth pulse.* $f(t) = t/T\,U(t) - U(t-T) - [(t-T)/T]U(t-T)$, for $0- \leq t \leq T$ $f(t) = 0$ for $t > T$ and $t < 0$.

Thus,

$$F(s) = [1/(Ts^2)] - e^{-sT}/s - e^{-sT}[1/(Ts^2)] = (1/T)(1/s^2) \times [1 - e^{-sT}(sT+1)]. \tag{3.14}$$

5. A *sinusoidal pulse,* $f(t) = \sin(\omega_o t)P(t)$, $0 \leq t \leq \pi/\omega_o$, otherwise zero. In the time domain, this $f(t)$ can be written as:

$$f(t) = \sin(\omega_o t)U(t) + \sin[\omega_o(t - \pi/\omega_o)t]U(t - \pi/\omega_o)$$

Thus by the *time shift theorem:*

$$F(s) = \frac{\omega_o\left[1+e^{-(\pi/\omega_o)s}\right]}{s^2+\omega_o{}^2} \tag{3.15}$$

3.4 The Inverse Laplace Transform

We have seen that finding the Laplace transform of a transformable time function is relatively easy. Basically, it involves the solution of a definite integral between limits of 0 and ∞. Finding an inverse Laplace transform often can be challenging because of the algebraic complexity of $Y(s)$. The Laplace inversion integral is a complex integral:

$$y(t) \equiv \frac{1}{2\pi j}\int_{c-j\infty}^{c+j\infty} Y(s)\,e^{st}\,ds = \mathcal{L}^{-1}\{Y(s)\} \tag{3.16}$$

That is, it is a function of the complex variable, s and is generally performed as a closed-contour integration in the s-plane to find the *residues* of Y(s). A knowledge of complex variables is required to carry out the complex inversion integral, Equation 3.16. A more common practice is to find the inverse transform of Y(s) from a *partial fraction expansion* and tables of inverse transforms.

The one-sided Laplace transforms which we have discussed above have been for causal signals and systems, i.e., those signals and system weighting functions that only exist for nonnegative time. The *two-sided Laplace transform,* not covered here, is used when signals and systems exist for negative time (or distance, x). In such cases, a time function is broken up into negative and positive time components. We will not treat two-sided transforms here.

3.5 Applications of the Laplace Transform

3.5.1 Introduction

The Laplace transform provides us with a relatively easy, pencil-and-paper means for finding the output of an LTI system in algebraic form, given the system's impulse response, h(t), or its Laplace transform, H(s), which is also called the system's *transfer function.* Often, H(s) is in the form of a rational polynomial in s, i.e., the numerator is of the form, $[b_0 s^m + b_1 s^{m-1} + \cdots + b_{m-1} s^1 + b_m]$ and the denominator looks like: $[s^n + a_1 s^{n-1} + \cdots + a_{n-1} s^1 + a_n]$, where generally, $m \leq n$. To find the inverse transform by any means, it is expedient to factor the denominator into its n roots. In a stable causal system, the real parts of all of the denominator's roots will be negative, i.e., the roots, known as *poles,* will lie in the left-half s-plane. Some poles may be complex-conjugate, others will be real and negative. One or more poles or zeros can exist at the origin of the s-plane.

If the input, x(t), to a causal LTI system is some transient waveform defined for $t \geq 0$, then the output waveform is given by:

$$y(t) = \boldsymbol{L}^{-1}\{Y(s)\} = \boldsymbol{L}^{-1}\{X(s)H(s)\} \tag{3.17}$$

This result is powerful because it allows us to find the output, given an LTI system's transfer function and any input, X(s).

Every text that describes Laplace transforms has an obligatory table of commonly used transforms to expedite inverse transforming. This text is no exception; see Table 3.1.

3.5.2 Use of partial fraction expansions to find y(t)

Let us examine several examples of using partial fractions to find y(t), given H(s) and X(s). There are two common forms for Y(s). As a rational polynomial in factored form and also in factored denominator form (assuming no poles at the origin):

TABLE 3.1
Useful Laplace transform–time function pairs

Time function, f(t), t ≥ 0	Laplace Transform, F(s)
$\delta(t)$ (unit impulse)	1
$U(t)$ (unit step function)	$1/s$
$tU(t)$ (unit ramp function)	$1/s^2$
$(t^n/n!)U(t)$	$1/s^{n+1}$
$e^{-at}U(t)$	$\frac{1}{s+a}$
$te^{-at}U(t)$	$\frac{1}{(s+a)^2}$
$\frac{1}{(n-1)!}t^{n-1}e^{-at}$	$\frac{1}{(s+a)^n}$
$\frac{e^{-at}-e^{-bt}}{b-a}U(t)$	$\frac{1}{(s+a)(s+b)}$
$(1/a)(1-e^{-at})U(t)$	$\frac{1}{s(s+a)}$
$(1/a^2)(at-1+e^{-at})U(t)$	$\frac{1}{s^2(s+a)}$
$(1/a^2)[1-(1+at)e^{-at}]U(t)$	$\frac{1}{s(s+a)^2}$
$(1/ab)\left[1-\frac{b}{b-a}e^{-at}+\frac{a}{b-a}e^{-bt}\right]U(t)$	$\frac{1}{s(s+a)(s+b)}$
$\sin(\omega_o t)U(t)$	$\frac{\omega_o}{s^2+\omega_o^2}$
$\cos(\omega_o t)U(t)$	$\frac{s}{s^2+\omega_o^2}$
$\frac{\omega_n^2}{\sqrt{1-\xi^2}}e^{-\xi\omega_n t}\sin[(\omega_n\sqrt{1-\xi^2})t]U(t)$	$\frac{\omega_n^2}{s^2+2\xi\omega_n+\omega_n^2}$
$1+\frac{1}{\sqrt{1-\xi^2}}e^{-\xi\omega_n t}\sin[(\omega_n\sqrt{1-\xi^2})t+\varphi]U(t)$ Where $\varphi=\tan^{-1}[(\sqrt{1-\xi^2})/(-\xi)]$	$\frac{\omega_n^2}{s(s^2+2\xi\omega_n+\omega_n^2)}$

Note: The denominators of stable transfer functions can be factored into terms comprising s^n (poles at the origin of the s-plane), $(s+a_k)$ (poles lying on the negative real axis of the s-plane) and $(s^2+2\xi\omega_n+\omega_n^2)$ (complex-conjugate poles with negative real parts. Such factors can be expanded by partial fractions to a sum of terms, each of which has a simple s, $(s+a_k)$, or $(s^2+2\xi\omega_n+\omega_n^2)$ in its denominator.

$$Y(s) = \frac{b_m s^m + b_{m-1}s^{m-1} + \cdots + b_1 s_1 + b_0}{[s^n + a_{n-1}s^{n-1} + \cdots + a_1 s^1 + a_0]}$$
$$= \frac{b_m s^m + b_{m-1}s^{m-1} + \cdots + b_1 s_1 + b_0}{(s - s_1)(s - s_2)\ldots(s - s_{n-1})(s - s_n)}, \quad n > m \tag{3.18}$$

By the fundamental law of algebra, an nth order denominator polynomial will have n roots, $\mathbf{s_k}$. A root is a complex value of s that when substituted into $[s^n + a_{n-1}s^{n-1} + \cdots + a_1 s^1 + a_0] = \psi$ will make ψ equal zero. When the denominator of $Y(s) = 0$, $Y(\mathbf{s_k}) \to \infty$, hence the n $\mathbf{s_k}$ values are called the *poles* of the $Y(s)$ rational polynomial. The m roots of the numerator polynomial are called the *zeros* of $Y(s)$. To do a partial fraction expansion, the denominator must be factored into its n factors. One or more pairs of factors may have complex-conjugate roots, hence can be written in the standard, underdamped quadratic form: $(s^2 + 2\xi\omega_n s + \omega_n^2)$. In the first example below, we will examine a polynomial that has only real, negative roots.

Example 1

Let $Y(s)$ be given by:

$$Y(s) = \frac{s+1}{s^2 + 5s + 6} \overset{\text{factoring}}{\Rightarrow} \frac{s+1}{(s+2)(s+3)} \tag{3.19}$$

Now the poles are at $\mathbf{s_1} = -2$, $\mathbf{s_2} = -3$. We will write $Y(s)$ in the form:

$$Y(s) = \frac{A_1}{s+2} + \frac{A_2}{s+3} \tag{3.20}$$

which is easily seen (from Table 3.1) to have the inverse Laplace transform:

$$y(t) = A_1 e^{-2t} + A_2 e^{-3t}, t \geq 0, \text{ or, } y(t) = A_1 e^{-2t} U(t) + A_2 e^{-3t} U(t) \tag{3.21}$$

Where $U(t)$ is the unit step function, defined as 1 for all $t \geq 0$ and 0 for $t < 0$.

The constants A_1 and A_2 are found systematically by *partial fraction expansion.* To find A_1, we multiply the factored rational polynomial $Y(s)$ by $(s+2)$ and let $s = -2$.

$$A_1 = (s+2)\Big|_{s \to -2} \frac{s+1}{(s+2)(s+3)} = \frac{-2+1}{-2+3} = -1 \tag{3.22A}$$

and

$$A_2 = (s+3)\Big|_{s \to -3} \frac{s+1}{(s+2)(s+3)} = \frac{-3+1}{-3+2} = +2 \tag{3.22B}$$

Thus:

$$Y(s) = \frac{-1}{s+2} + \frac{2}{s+3} \Longleftrightarrow y(t) = -1e^{-2t} + 2e^{-3t}, \ t \geq 0 \quad \text{QED} \tag{3.23}$$

A more general form of a $\mathrm{Y(s)}$ after factoring is given below:

$$\mathrm{Y(s)} = \frac{b_m s^m + b_{m-1}s^{m-1} + \cdots + b_1 s_1 + b_0}{s(s+s_1)(s+s_2)\ldots(s+s_{n-2})(s+s_{n-1})} \tag{3.24}$$

The pole at the origin can be due to a step input. The PF expansion has the same form:

$$\mathrm{Y(s)} = \frac{A_0}{s} + \frac{A_1}{s+s_1} + \frac{A_2}{s+s_2} + \cdots + \frac{A_n}{s+s_n} \tag{3.25}$$

Now the A_k constants are evaluated by:

$$A_0 = \underset{s\to 0}{s\,Y(s)} = [b_0/(s_1 s_2 s_3 \ldots s_n)] \tag{3.26A}$$

$$A_k = \underset{s\to -s_k}{(s+s_k)Y(s)} = (-s_k + s_k) \times \frac{b_m(-s_k)^m + b_{m-1}(-s_k)^{m-1} + \cdots + b_1(-s_k) + b_0}{(-s_k)(-s_k+s_1)(-s_k+s_2)\ldots(-s_k+s_k)\ldots(-s_k+s_n)} \tag{3.26B}$$

So

$$y(t) = [b_0/(s_1 s_2 s_3 \ldots s_n)]U(t) + \sum_{k=1}^{n} A_k \exp(-s_k t),\ t \geq 0 \tag{3.26C}$$

Example 2

Let $\mathrm{Y(s)}$ be:

$$\mathrm{Y(s)} = \frac{s+1}{s(s+2)(s+3)} \Rightarrow \frac{\frac{1}{6}}{s} + \frac{\frac{1}{2}}{s+2} + \frac{\frac{-2}{3}}{s+3} \tag{3.27}$$

Thus,

$$y(t) = \frac{1}{6}U(t) + \frac{3}{6}e^{-2t} + \frac{-4}{6}e^{-3t} \tag{3.28}$$

By the *initial value theorem,* $y(0+) = \underset{\lim s\to\infty}{s\,Y(s)} = \frac{\infty}{\infty\infty} \to 0$.

By the *final value theorem,* $y(\infty) = y_{ss} = \underset{\lim s\to 0}{s\,Y(s)} = \frac{1}{6}$, which agrees with the $y(t)$ found.

Example 3

In this case, we have a *repeated root* (r^{th} order) in the denominator of $\mathrm{Y(s)}$, e.g.,

$$\mathrm{Y(s)} = \frac{b_m s^m + b_{m-1}s^{m-1} + \cdots + b_1 s_1 + b_0}{(s+s_1)(s+s_2)\ldots(s+s_m)^r\ldots(s+s_{n-r})} \tag{3.29}$$

$$\downarrow$$

$$Y(s) = \frac{A_1}{(s+s_1)} + \frac{A_2}{(s+s_2)} + \cdots + \left\{ \frac{c_r}{(s+s_m)^r} + \frac{c_{r-1}}{(s+s_m)^{r-1}} + \cdots + \frac{c_1}{(s+s_m)^1} \right\} + \cdots \quad (3.30)$$

The general formula for calculating the $r\{c_k\}$ is [Ogata, 1970]:

$$c_k = \frac{1}{(r-k)!} \frac{\partial^{r-k}[(s+s_m)^r Y(s)]}{\partial s^{r-k}} \bigg|_{s=-s_m} \qquad k = 1, 2, \ldots r \quad (3.31)$$

Having described the general case for a repeated pole, let us examine a specific example in which $r = 2$:

$$Y(s) = \frac{8s+2}{(s+1)(s+4)^2} = \frac{A_1}{s+1} + \frac{c_2}{(s+4)^2} + \frac{c_1}{(s+4)} \quad (3.32)$$

Now, as before, $\dot{A}_1 = \underset{s=-1}{(s+1)Y(s)} = \frac{-8+2}{(-1+4)^2} = -(2/3)$ (3.33A)

The repeated root is of order $r = 2$. Thus c_2 is $(k = 2)$:

$$c_2 = \frac{1}{(2-2)!} \frac{\partial^0[(s+4)^2 Y(s)]}{\partial s^0} \bigg|_{s=-4} = \frac{-32+2}{-4+1} = 10 \quad (3.33B)$$

Note that $0! = 1! = 1$ and $\partial^0(*)/\partial s^0$ is no derivative at all. The second coefficient is then:

$$c_1 = \frac{1}{(2-1)!} \frac{\partial^1[(s+4)^2 Y(s)]}{\partial s^1} \bigg|_{s=-4} = \frac{(s+1)8-(8s+2)1}{(s+1)^2} \bigg|_{s=-4} = \frac{2}{3} \quad (3.33C)$$

From the Laplace tables:

$$y(t) = -\frac{2}{3}e^{-t} + 10te^{-4t} + \frac{2}{3}e^{-4t}, \ t \geq 0 \quad (3.33D)$$

Example 4

Consider a function in which the order of the denominator, n, is the same as the numerator, m. An example of such a function is the *all-pass filter:*

$$H(s) = \frac{s-b}{s+b} \quad (3.34A)$$

In this case, we divide the numerator by the denominator and get:

$$H(s) = 1 - \frac{2b}{s+b} \quad (3.34B)$$

By inspection, using the table above, this filter's impulse response is:

$$h(t) = \delta(t) - 2be^{-bt}U(t) \quad (3.34C)$$

Example 5

Finally, let us examine the inverse transform of a transfer function having a complex-conjugate pole pair. First, we factor the denominator of $Y(s)$:

$$Y(s) = \frac{1}{s(s+2)(s^2+2s+4)} = \frac{1}{s(s+2)(s+1+j\sqrt{3})(s+1-j\sqrt{3})} \quad (3.35A)$$

Partial fraction expanding:

$$Y(s) = \frac{A}{s} + \frac{B}{s+2} + \frac{\mathbf{C_1}}{(s+1+j\sqrt{3})} + \frac{\mathbf{C_2}}{(s+1-j\sqrt{3})} \quad (3.35B)$$

Note that the constants $\mathbf{C_1}$ and $\mathbf{C_2}$ are boldface because, in general, they are complex (vectors). $\mathbf{C_2}$ is generally the conjugate of $\mathbf{C_1}$. That is, $\mathbf{C_2} = \mathbf{C_1}^*$. Also, when the quadratic term is factored, the factors are complex conjugates and it is of the general form:

$$(s^2+2\xi\omega_n s+\omega_n^2) = (s+\xi\omega_n+j\omega_n\sqrt{1-\xi^2})(s+\xi\omega_n-j\omega_n\sqrt{1-\xi^2}) \quad (3.35C)$$

Let us now evaluate the constants:

$$A = sY(s)|_{s=0} = \frac{1}{8} \quad (3.35D)$$

$$B = (s+2)\,Y(s)|_{s=-2} = \frac{1}{-2(4-4+4)} = -\frac{1}{8} \quad (3.35E)$$

$$\mathbf{C_1} = (s+1+j\sqrt{3})Y(s)|_{s=-(1+j\sqrt{3})}$$

$$= \frac{1}{-(1+j\sqrt{3})(-1-j\sqrt{3}+2)(-1-j\sqrt{3}+1-j\sqrt{3})} =$$

$$\downarrow$$

$$\mathbf{C_1} = \frac{1}{-(2\angle 60°)(2\angle -60°)(-2j\sqrt{3})} = [1/(8\sqrt{3})])\angle -90° \quad (3.35F)$$

$$\mathbf{C_2} = (s+1-j\sqrt{3})Y(s)|_{s=-1+j\sqrt{3}}$$

$$= \frac{1}{(-1+j\sqrt{3})(-1+j\sqrt{3}+2)(-1+j\sqrt{3}+1+j\sqrt{3})} =$$

$$\downarrow$$

$$\mathbf{C_2} = [1/(8\sqrt{3})]\angle +90° \quad (3.35G)$$

Thus, $Y(s)$ in expanded, PF form is:

$$Y(s) = \frac{\frac{1}{8}}{s} + \frac{-\frac{1}{8}}{s+2} + \frac{[1/(8\sqrt{3})]\angle -90°}{s+1+j\sqrt{3}} + \frac{[1/(8\sqrt{3})]\angle +90°}{s+1-j\sqrt{3}} \quad (3.35H)$$

In the time domain this is:

$$y(t) = \frac{1}{8}U(t) - \frac{1}{8}e^{-2t} + [1/(8\sqrt{3})]\{e^{-(1+j\sqrt{3})t}e^{-j90} + e^{-(1-j\sqrt{3})t}e^{+j90}\}$$

$$\downarrow$$

$$y(t) = \frac{1}{8}U(t) - \frac{1}{8}e^{-2t} + [1/(8\sqrt{3})]e^{-t}\{e^{j(\sqrt{3}t+90)} + e^{-j(\sqrt{3}t+90)}\} \quad (3.35I)$$

Now, from the Euler relation, $\cos\theta = 1/2(e^{j\theta} + e^{-j\theta})$ and the trig identity that $\cos(\theta + 90°) = -\sin\theta$, we can finally write:

$$y(t) = \frac{1}{8}U(t) - \frac{1}{8}e^{-2t} - [1/(4\sqrt{3})]e^{-t}\sin(\sqrt{3}t),\ t \geq 0 \quad (3.35J)$$

In terms of the general quadratic notation, we can also write:

$$y(t) = \frac{1}{8}U(t) - \frac{1}{8}e^{-2t} - [1/(4\sqrt{3})]e^{-\xi\omega nt}\sin[(\omega_n\sqrt{1-\xi^2})t] \quad (3.35K)$$

where $\omega_n = 2$, and $\xi = 1/2$.

The example above illustrates the tedious algebra of finding the inverse Laplace transform of functions having underdamped quadratic factors in their denominators. I recommend the use of Laplace transform tables if an algebraic expression for $y(t)$ is desired, or simulation if a plot is required. Stay sane.

3.5.3 Application of the Laplace transform to continuous state systems

Recall that an nth order continuous state system is written as:

$$\dot{\mathbf{x}} = \mathbf{A}\mathbf{x} + \mathbf{B}\mathbf{u} \quad (3.36)$$

Now let us Laplace transform the state equation, Equation 3.36, including initial conditions:

$$s\mathbf{X}(s) - \mathbf{x}(0_+) = \mathbf{A}\mathbf{X}(s) + \mathbf{B}\mathbf{U}(s)$$

$$\downarrow$$

$$s\mathbf{X}(s) - \mathbf{A}\mathbf{X}(s) = \mathbf{x}(0+) + \mathbf{B}\mathbf{U}(s)$$

$$\downarrow$$

$$(s\mathbf{I} - \mathbf{A})\mathbf{X}(s) = \mathbf{x}(0+) + \mathbf{B}\mathbf{U}(s) \quad (3.37)$$

The solution of Equation 3.37 is

$$\mathbf{X}(s) = (s\mathbf{I} - \mathbf{A})^{-1}[\mathbf{x}(0+) + \mathbf{B}\mathbf{U}(s)] = \mathbf{\Phi}(s)\mathbf{x}(0+) + \mathbf{\Phi}(s)\mathbf{B}\mathbf{U}(s) \quad (3.38)$$

$(s\mathbf{I} - \mathbf{A})^{-1} \equiv \mathbf{\Phi}(s)$ is the *resolvent matrix* of the system. For $n \geq 3$, finding $\mathbf{\Phi}(s)$ on paper is a tedious waste of time, considering that more expeditious methods exist, such as Matlab™.

3.5.4 Use of signal flow graphs to find y(t) for continuous state systems

In Section 2.3.1, we saw that an nth order SISO linear system described by the ODE

$$\overset{\cdot n}{x} + a_{n-1}\overset{\cdot(n-1)}{x} + \cdots + a_1\dot{x} + a_0 x = b_0 u(t) \tag{3.39}$$

can be represented by a set of n first-order state ODEs in which $x = \dot{x}_1$ and $x_2 = \dot{x}_1 = \dot{x}$:

$$\begin{aligned}
\dot{x}_1 &= x_2 \\
\dot{x}_2 &= x_3 \\
\dot{x}_3 &= x_4 \\
&\;\vdots \\
\dot{x}_{n-1} &= x_n \\
\dot{x}_n &= -a_0 x_1 - a_1 x_2 - a_2 x_3 \ldots a_{n-1} x_n + b_0 u(t)
\end{aligned} \tag{3.40}$$

This system's **A** matrix is simply:

$$\mathbf{A} = \begin{bmatrix} 0 & 1 & 0 & 0 & \ldots & 0 \\ 0 & 0 & 1 & 0 & \ldots & 0 \\ 0 & 0 & 0 & 1 & \ldots & 0 \\ & & & & & \\ 0 & 0 & 0 & 0 & \ldots & 1 \\ -a_0 & -a_1 & -a_2 & & \ldots & -a_{n-1} \end{bmatrix} \tag{3.41}$$

Now we place these state equations in a graphical context, as shown in Figure 3.2. Following the rules for signal flow graph reduction found in Appendix A, we can write:

$$\frac{X(s)}{U(s)} = \frac{b_0\, s^{-n}}{1 - [-a_{n-1}s^{-1} - a_{n-2}s^{-2} - \cdots a_1 s^{n-1} - a_0 s^{-n}]} \tag{3.42}$$

We multiply top and bottom by s^n and obtain:

$$\frac{X(s)}{U(s)} = \frac{b_0}{s^n + a_{n-1}s^{n-1} + a_{n-2}s^{n-2} + \cdots + a_1 s^1 + a_0} = H(s) \tag{3.43}$$

The next three steps are to factor the denominator, then expand the factors by partial fractions, and finally find the inverse transform, $h(t)$ which is the system's weighting function.

As a first example, let us use the signal flow graph technique to find the output of a three-state system with zero ICs, given a unit step input. The system state equation is:

$$\dot{\mathbf{x}} = \begin{bmatrix} 0 & 1 & 0 \\ 0 & 0 & 1 \\ -6 & -11 & -6 \end{bmatrix} \mathbf{x} + \begin{bmatrix} 0 \\ 0 \\ 1 \end{bmatrix} u(t) \tag{3.44}$$

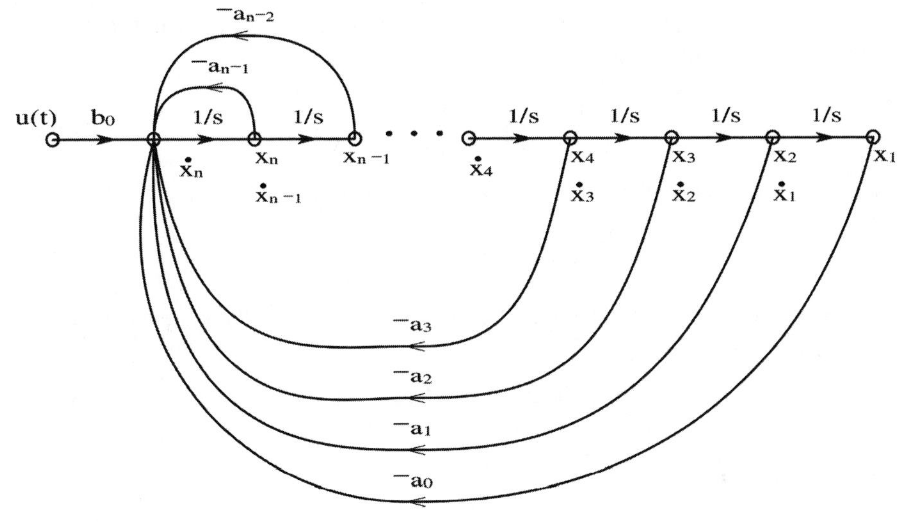

FIGURE 3.2
A signal flow graph representation of a continuous n^{th}-order SISO LTI system. Note the $n-1$ feedback loops and n integrators.

The individual ODEs are:

$$\begin{aligned}\dot{x}_1 &= x_2 \\ \dot{x}_2 &= x_3 \\ \dot{x}_3 &= -6x_1 - 11x_2 - 6x_3 + u(t)\end{aligned} \tag{3.45}$$

The output, $x = x_1$. Figure 3.3 shows the signal flow graph for the system. The transfer function is found by inspection, using Mason's rule:

$$\frac{X(s)}{U(s)} = \frac{s^{-3}}{1 - [-6s^{-1} - 11s^{-2} - 6s^{-3}]} \tag{3.46}$$

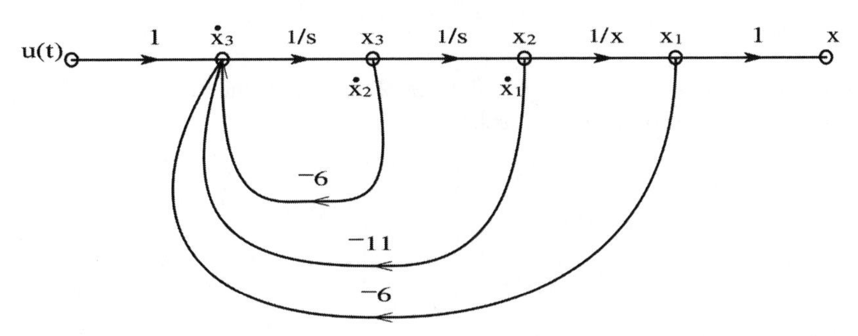

FIGURE 3.3
A third-order SFG describing the continuous LTI state system given by Equation 3.44.

Multiply numerator and denominator of Equation 3.46 by s^3 to put the transfer function in standard Laplace form:

$$\frac{X(s)}{U(s)} = \frac{1}{s^3 + 6s^2 + 11s^1 + 6} \tag{3.47}$$

The denominator is next factored (use Matlab's "roots" program):

$$\frac{X(s)}{U(s)} = \frac{1}{(s+1)(s+2)(s+3)} \tag{3.48}$$

Let the system have a unit step input. That is, $U(s) = s^{-1}$, now the system output can be written

$$X(s) = \frac{1}{s(s+1)(s+2)(s+3)} \tag{3.49}$$

Now, from the partial fraction expansion:

$$X(s) = \frac{A}{s} + \frac{B}{(s+1)} + \frac{C}{(s+2)} + \frac{D}{(s+3)} \tag{3.50A}$$

To find A: $A = s\,X_{s=0}(s) = \frac{1}{6}$. The other constants are:

$$B = (s+1)\underset{s=-1}{X(s)} = \frac{1}{(-1)(-1+2)(-1+3)} = -\frac{1}{2} \tag{3.50B}$$

$$C = (s+2)\underset{s=-2}{X(s)} = \frac{1}{(-2)(-2+1)(-2+3)} = \frac{1}{2} \tag{3.50C}$$

$$D = (s+3)\underset{s=-3}{X(s)} = \frac{1}{(-3)(-3+1)(-3+2)} = -\frac{1}{6} \tag{3.50D}$$

The time function, $x(t)$, can now be written from inspection, noting that $1/s \Leftrightarrow U(t)$ (the unit step) and $1/(s+a) \Leftrightarrow e^{-at}$. Thus:

$$x(t) = \frac{1}{6}U(t) - \frac{1}{2}e^{-t} + \frac{1}{2}e^{-2t} - \frac{1}{6}e^{-3t},\ t \geq 0. \tag{3.50E}$$

In a second example of using a signal flow graph to find the output of a two-state system, consider the quadratic system below:

$$\dot{\mathbf{x}} = \begin{bmatrix} -3 & 1 \\ -1 & -1 \end{bmatrix} \mathbf{x} + \begin{bmatrix} 0 \\ 1 \end{bmatrix} u(t) \tag{3.51}$$

$$y(t) = x_1(t)$$

The state equations for this system are:

$$\dot{x}_1 = -3x_1 + x_2$$

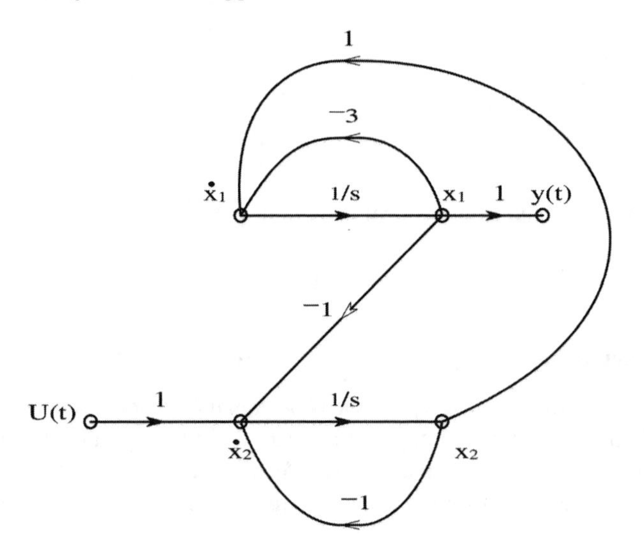

FIGURE 3.4
A second-order SFG describing the continuous LTI state system given by Equation 3.51. Note that this SFG has three loops, two of which are nontouching.

$$\dot{x}_2 = -x_1 - x_2 + u(t) \tag{3.52}$$

Figure 3.4 illustrates the SFG for this system. Note the three feedback loops. The transfer function for this system is found by applying Mason's rule:

$$\frac{Y(s)}{U(s)} = \frac{1/s^2}{1 - [-1/s - 3/s - 1/s^2] + \{(-1/s)(-3/s)\}}$$

$$\downarrow$$

$$\frac{Y(s)}{U(s)} = \frac{1}{s^2 + 4s + 4} = \frac{1}{(s+2)^2} = H(s) \tag{3.53}$$

Now let us examine the step response of this system. $U(s) = 1/s$:

$$Y(s) = \frac{1}{s(s+2)^2} = \frac{A}{s} + \frac{B}{(s+2)^2} + \frac{C}{(s+2)} \tag{3.54A}$$

The partial fraction constants are:

$$A = \underset{s=0}{s\,Y}(s) = \frac{1}{4} \tag{3.54B}$$

$$B = \underset{s=-2}{(s+2)^2}\, Y(s) = -\frac{1}{2} \tag{3.54C}$$

$$C = \left.\frac{\partial\{(s+2)^2 Y(s)\}}{\partial s}\right|_{s=-2} = \frac{-1}{s^2} = -\frac{1}{4} \tag{3.54D}$$

Thus,

$$Y(s) = \frac{(1/4)}{s} - \frac{(1/2)}{(s+2)^2} - \frac{(1/4)}{s+2} \tag{3.54E}$$

Taking the inverse Laplace transform from tables, we find:

$$y(t) = (1/4)U(t) - (1/2)te^{-2t} - (1/4)e^{-2t},\ t \geq 0. \tag{3.54F}$$

3.5.5 Discussion

The effectiveness of the above approach using signal flow graphs and Mason's rule is predicated on the fact that, on paper, it is easier to find $H(s)$ and $y(t)$ from the SFG approach than it is to invert the matrix, $(s\mathbf{I} - \mathbf{A})$ and use $(s\mathbf{I} - \mathbf{A})^{-1}$ to find $y(t)$. More on signal flow graphs, Mason's rule and examples of SFG reduction are presented in Appendix B.

3.6 Chapter Summary

In this chapter, we introduced the one-sided Laplace transform, a real, definite integral transform using the complex variable (2-D vector), $\mathbf{s} = \sigma + j\omega$. Examples were given to show that the existence of the Laplace transform of $f(t)$ depends on the value of the real component of $\mathbf{s}$, σ. Next, we summarized the properties of the Laplace transform, some of which are based on the fact that it is a linear operator. Several examples of finding Laplace transforms are given in Section 3.3 using some of the theorems and relations tabulated in Section 3.2.

The inverse Laplace transform was shown to be most expediently done using a partial fraction expansion of the rational polynomial, $Y(s)$, written with a factored denominator. Section 3.5.2 gives a number of useful examples of finding $y(t)$ from the $Y(s)$ polynomial by the method of partial fractions. The Laplace transform method is applied to the solution of time-domain state equations in Section 3.5.3, and the venerable signal flow graph method is presented in Section 3.5.4 as a shortcut to finding a state system's transfer function, $H(s)$. The LTI system's output can generally be found as $y(t) = L^{-1}[Y(s) = X(s)H(s)]$.

Problems

3.1 Slate and Sheppard (1982) used a simplified dynamic LTI model to describe the transient reduction in mean arterial pressure following an IV infusion of sodium nitroprusside (SNP).Their transfer function is:

$$\frac{\Delta MAP}{U}(s) = \frac{-K_p \exp(-s\delta_p)}{(\tau_p s + 1)} = G_p(s)$$

Where: ΔMAP is the SNP-induced change in MAP, U is the specific SNP, IV infusion rate in (mg/kg patient weight)/min. K_p is the individual patient's SS response constant (units are mmHg/[(mg/kg patient weight) /min]. δ_p is the plant's dead time in minutes (aka transport lag before a change in $u(t)$ affects the ΔMAP). τ_p is the plant's time constant in minutes. *Assume:* $K_p = 1.0$, $\tau_p = 0.75\,\text{min}$, $\delta_p = 0.5\,\text{min}$.

a. Plot and dimension the plant's impulse response (to $u(t) = \delta(t)$).

b. Plot and dimension the plant's response to a unit step of SNP infusion rate.

c. Plot and dimension the plant's steady-state, sinusoidal frequency response for an input rate of the form: $u(t) = [1 + \sin(2\pi f t)]$ for $0.01\,\text{cycles/min.} \leq f \leq 100\,\text{cycles/min.}$ Note that the "1" in $u(t)$ is so $u(t)$ is nonnegative. Make a Bode plot: $20 \log|\mathbf{G_p}(2\pi f)|$ vs. f on a log scale and $\angle \mathbf{G_p}(2\pi f)$ vs. f on the same scale. Note that $f = \omega/2\pi$.

3.2 When a bolus of SNP is infused IV, the bolus recirculates through the circulatory system until it reaches a nearly constant concentration. This effect can be incorporated into the model plant transfer function:

$$\Delta MAP = \frac{-K_p \exp(-\delta_p s)[1 + \alpha \exp(-\delta_c s)]}{\tau_p s + 1} U(s)$$

Use the same parameters as in Problem 2.1, with the addition of $\alpha = 0.25$, $\delta_c = 0.5\,\text{min}$. Repeat parts a, b and c of Problem 2.1.

3.3 Consider the transfer function in which $K = 5.263$ and the natural frequencies are in r/min:

$$H(s) = \frac{K(s + 1.9)}{(s + 10)(s + 1)}$$

a. Find $h(t)$:

b. Put the transfer function in time-constant form, then plot and dimension the complete Bode plot for the system over the range $0.01 \leq f \leq 100\,\text{cycles/min}$.

3.4 The unit impulse (bolus) response of the central compartment of a three-compartment mammillary pharmacokinetic system [Godfrey, 1983] is:

$$h_2(t) = 0.7e^{-5t} + 0.2e^{-t} + 0.1e^{-0.1t} \quad \text{concentration units}$$

a. Find the system's transfer function, $H_2(s)$, in factored, rational form (it has three poles and two zeros).

b. Find the response of this system to a unit step of drug infusion rate.

3.5 The transfer function of a system is

$$H_5(s) = 0.1\frac{s+100}{s+10}$$

a. Find, plot and dimension the system's weighting function.

b. Find, plot and dimension the system's steady-state sinusoidal frequency response (Bode plot), dB magnitude and phase for $0.1 \le f \le 10^3$ Hz.

3.6 An all-pass filter has the transfer function:

$$H_a(s) = \frac{s-6.28}{s+6.28}$$

a. Find, plot and dimension the system's weighting function.

b. Find, plot and dimension the system's steady-state sinusoidal frequency response (Bode plot), dB magnitude and phase for $0.1 \le f \le 100$ Hz.

3.7 A minimum phase filter has a Bode plot (given in Figure P3.7). Find, plot and dimension the filter's weighting function, $h_7(t)$.

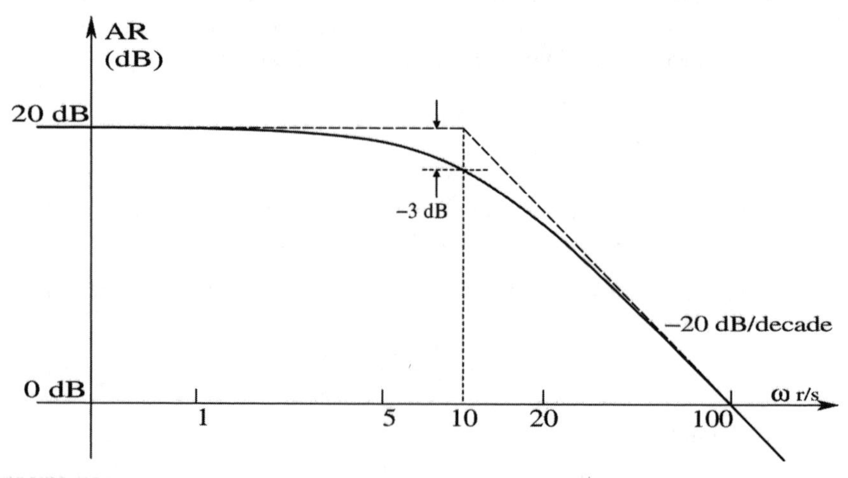

FIGURE P3.7

3.8 A minimum phase filter has a Bode plot (given in Figure P3.8). Find, plot and dimension the filter's weighting function, $h_8(t)$.

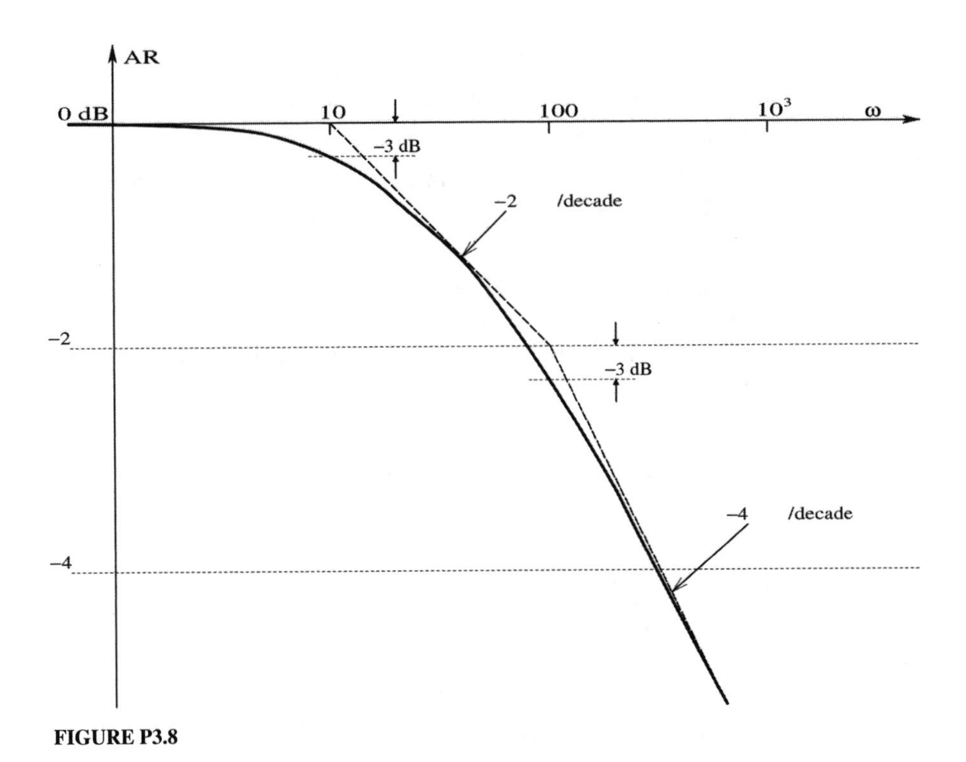

FIGURE P3.8

3.9 Digital-to-analog converters (DACs) convert digital number sequences to analog voltage or current. A simple means representing the dynamics of digital-to-analog conversion is the *zero-order hold* (ZOH) (aka boxcar hold). The input to the ZOH can be considered to be a periodic train of impulses, $x^*(t)$:

$$x^*(t) = \sum_{n=0}^{\infty} x(nT)\delta(t - nT) \qquad \text{(P3.9-1)}$$

The area of the kth impulse is $x(kT)$; T is the sampling period. The output of the ZOH, $y_o(t)$, is a train of steps of duration T; each step has height $x(nT)$. This behavior can be written in the time domain as:

$$y_o(t) = \sum_{n=0}^{\infty} x(nT)[U(t - nT) - U(t - (n+1)T)],$$

$$\text{for } nT \leq t < (n+1)T \qquad \text{(P3.9-2)}$$

The impulse response of the ZOH, $h_o(t)$, is its output given a "1" at $t = 0$ and no other input.
From Equation P3.9-2, we have:

$$h_o(t) = U(t) - U(t - T)$$

This is simply a unit pulse of duration T, beginning at $t = 0$.

a. Write the Laplace transform of $h_o(t)$.

b. By letting $s = j\omega$, find, plot and dimension the Bode frequency response of the ZOH. Hint: use the Euler relation for $\sin(\omega T/2) = [e^{j\omega T/2} - e^{-j\omega T/2}]/(2j)$.

3.10 The *first-order hold* uses the simple first-difference derivative estimate of the number sequence, $x^*(n)$, to improve hold accuracy. Its unit impulse response, $h_1(t)$, is shown in Figure P3.10. From the figure, we see that $h_1(t)$ is made up of six components:

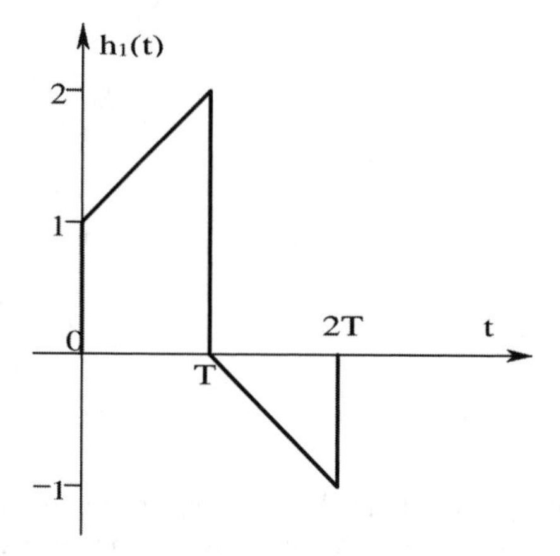

FIGURE P3.10

$$h_1(t) = U(t) + (t/T) - 2U(t - T) - \frac{2(t - T)}{T}U(t - T) + U(t - 2T) + \frac{t - 2T}{T}U(t - 2T)$$

Where T is the sampling period and the unit step function $U(t - a) = 1$ for $t \geq a$ and 0 for $t < a$.

a. Find the Laplace transform of $h_1(t)$, $H_1(s)$, in compact form. Note that the delay terms can be factored.

b. Now find the Fourier transform of $h_1(t)$ by substituting $s = j\omega$ in $H_1(s)$. As in the case of the ZOH, the Euler relation for $\sin(\omega T/2)$ should be used. Plot and dimension the Bode plot for $\mathbf{H_1}(j\omega)$ (magnitude and phase).

3.11 Proakis and Manolakis (1989, pp 429–430), describe a *linear interpolation hold* with delay. Its impulse response, $h_i(t)$, is shown in Figure P3.11. Written in the time domain, $h_i(t)$ is seen to be composed of three ramp functions:

$$h_i(t) = \frac{t}{T} - 2\frac{t-T}{T}U(t-T) + \frac{t-2T}{T}U(t-2T), \quad t \geq 0$$

a. Find $H_i(s)$ in compact form.

b. Let $s = j\omega$ in $H_i(s)$ and find $\mathbf{H}_i(j\omega)$. Again, use the Euler notation for $\sin(\omega T/2)$. Plot and dimension the Bode plot for $\mathbf{H_i}(j\omega)$ (magnitude and phase).

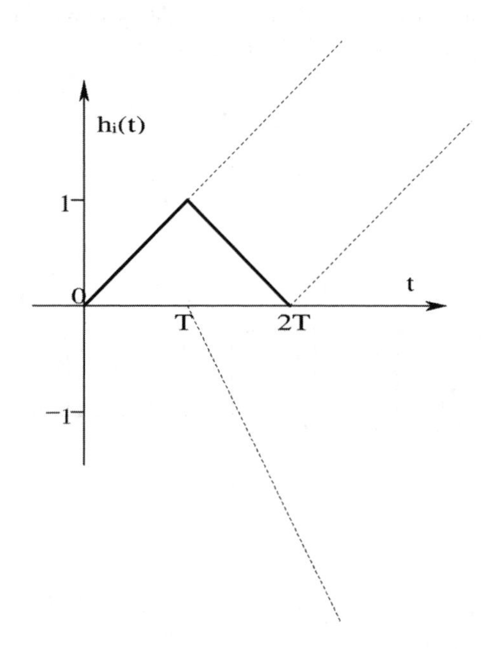

FIGURE P3.11

3.12 A causal continuous LTI system is described by the first-order ODE:

$$\dot{y} + 3y = x(t)$$

a. Find the system's transfer function, $H(s) = Y(s)/X(s)$.

b. Give the system's weighting function, $h(t)$.

c. Let $x(t) = U(t)[1 + 2e^{-t}]$. Use a partial fraction expansion to find $y(t)$.

3.13 A causal continuous LTI system is described by the second-order ODE:

$$\ddot{y} + 8\dot{y} + 15y = 5x(t)$$

a. Find the system's transfer function, $H(s)$, in partial fraction form.

b. Give the system's impulse response, $h(t)$, $t \geq 0$.

c. Let the system's input be a unit step, $x(t) = U(t)$. Find $y(t)$.

3.14 Find the Laplace transform of the infinite train of unit impulses, $P_T(t)$, in closed form. T is the period of the impulse train.

$$P_T(t) = \sum_{k=0}^{\infty} \delta(t - kT),\ t \geq 0.$$

3.15 Now consider the infinitely long square wave, $x(t)$ shown in Figure P3.15. Note that this wave can be decomposed into a sum of positive and negative delayed unit step functions. Use the identity,

$$\sum_{k=0}^{\infty} e^{-skT} = \frac{1}{1 - e^{-sT}}$$

to find $X(s)$ in closed form.

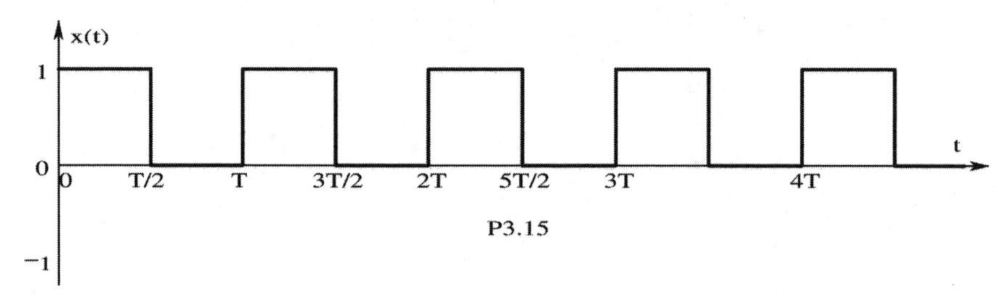

FIGURE P3.15

3.16 An infinite train of unit impulses, $x(t) = P_T(t) = \sum_{k=0}^{\infty} \delta(t - kT), t \geq 0$, is input into a low-pass filter with transfer function $H(s) = 1/(s + a)$, $a > 0$. Find a closed-form expression for the filter output, $Y(s)$.

3.17 Find the closed-form Laplace transform of the periodic sawtooth wave illustrated in Figure P3.17.

3.18 The Laplace transform of a causal, LTI system's output is:

$$Y(s) = \frac{2}{s(s^2 + 3s + 2)}$$

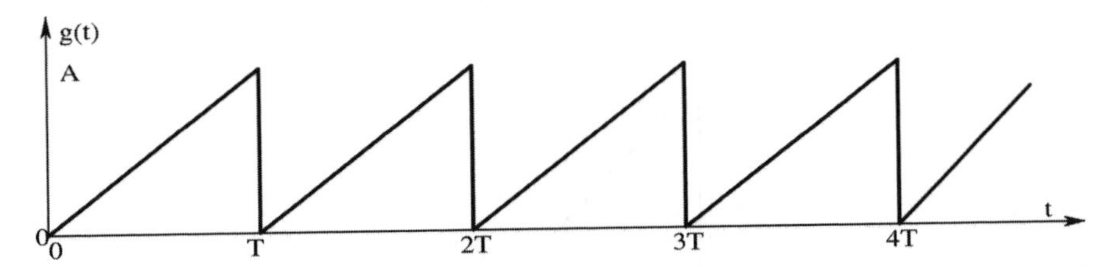

FIGURE P3.17

a. Factor the system's denominator to find its real poles.

b. Use the Laplace final value theorem to find $y(\infty)$.

c. Find $y(t)$ by partial fraction expansion and verify part b. Also find $y(0)$.

3.19 Find the Laplace transform, $X(s)$, of the transient waveform, $x(t)$, as shown in Figure P3.19.

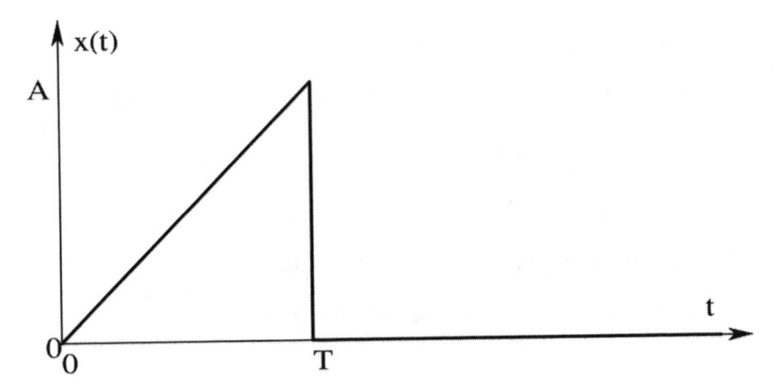

FIGURE P3.19

3.20 Find the Laplace transform, $X(s)$, of the transient waveform, $x(t)$, as shown in Figure P3.20.

3.21 Find the Laplace transform, $X(s)$, of the transient waveform, $x(t)$, as shown in Figure P3.21.

3.22 A causal, LTI system has the impulse response:

$$h(t) = \delta(t) - \frac{4}{3}e^{-t}U(t) + \frac{1}{3}e^{2t}\,U(t)$$

a. Plot and dimension $h(t)$. Is this a stable system?

b. Find $H(s)$ in PF form.

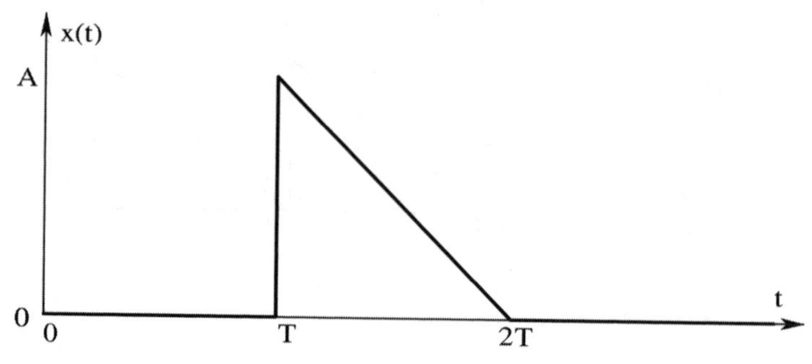

FIGURE P3.20

c. Now write H(s) as a rational polynomial. Plot its poles and zeros in the s-plane.

3.23 Find the inverse Laplace transform of the transfer function

$$H(s) = \frac{10}{(s+4)(s+2)^3}$$

by using a partial fraction expansion.

3.24 a. Sketch and dimension the waveforms of the time functions:

$$y_1(t) = e^{-ct}U(t-T), \quad c,\ T > 0$$
$$y_2(t) = e^{-c(t-T)}U(t-T)$$

b. Find the Laplace transforms for y_1 and y_2.

3.25 A second-order LPF is described by the ODE:

$$\ddot{y} + 2\dot{y} + 3y = 5r(t)$$

Let $r(t) = U(t)$ (a unit step). Use the Laplace final value theorem to find $y(\infty)$.

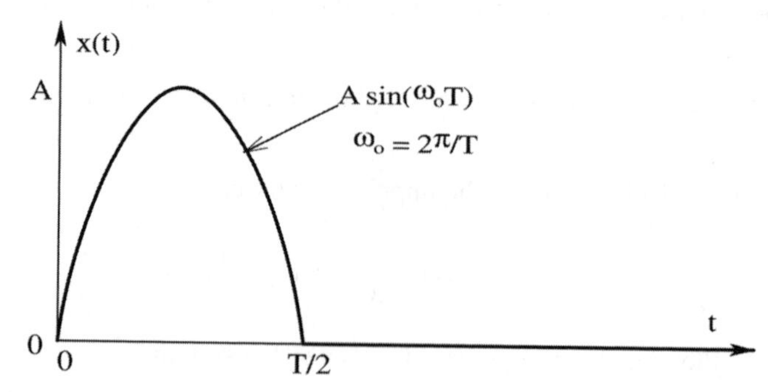

FIGURE P3.21

3.26 A causal LTI system has the transfer function:

$$\frac{Y}{R}(s) = \frac{s+3}{s^2+3s+2}$$

Let $R(s) = 1/s$ (unit step). Use the Laplace initial value theorem to find $y(0+)$.

4

Fourier Series Analysis of Periodic Signals

4.1 Introduction

This chapter introduces the Fourier series (FS) representation of periodic signals, examines the properties of Fourier series and gives examples of their use. The Fourier series may be seen as the mathematical portal to frequency-domain analysis of signals. A periodic signal that has an FS is shown to be made up of an infinite sum of sinusoidal and cosinusoidal harmonics, the amplitudes of which generally decrease as harmonic order increases. Thus, the frequency content of a periodic signal can be deduced from its FS. The Fourier transform can be viewed as a limiting case of the Fourier series (see Chapter 5).

Jean-Baptiste Joseph Fourier was one of several renowned Napoleonic-era mathematicians and physicists who left an indelible mark on modern physics and engineering. He was born in 1768 in Auxerre, France and died in 1830 in Paris. J-B. J. Fourier's career was a mixture of governmental administrative posts to which he was appointed by Napoleon, and academic positions. His research in applied mathematics was focused on describing heat flow. In 1807 he published his seminal "memoir" *On the Propagation of Heat in Solid Bodies,* which included the development of the now well-known series that bears his name. The initial reviewers of Fourier's paper were no less than Lagrange, Laplace, Monge and Lacroix. Fourier's series was introduced about a century before modern electrical engineering arose as a discipline and concepts such as the sinusoidal frequency response of a system were developed and found relevant.

Fourier showed that a *periodic function,* $f(t)$, under certain conditions, could be represented by an infinite sum of sine and cosine waves whose frequency arguments are integral multiples of the *fundamental frequency* of the periodic function. For each harmonic value, each sine and cosine wave is scaled by an amplitude coefficient which must be calculated from $f(t)$ by definite integrals.

Put mathematically, given some $f(t) = f(t + kT)$ for $-\infty \leq t \leq \infty$, and all integer k, where T is the period of $f(t)$ and $f_o = 1/T$ is the *fundamental frequency* (in Hz) of $f(t)$, it is possible to express $f(t)$ as:

$$f(t) = a_0 + \sum_{n=1}^{\infty} [a_n \cos(n2\pi t/T) + b_n \sin(n2\pi t/T)], \quad \text{(n is the harmonic number)} \tag{4.1}$$

Or, more compactly, let $\omega_o \equiv 2\pi/T$, so:

$$f(t) = a_0 + \sum_{n=1}^{\infty} [a_n \cos(n\omega_o t) + b_n \sin(n\omega_o t)] \tag{4.2}$$

Where the harmonic magnitude coefficients are given by :

$$a_0 \equiv \frac{1}{T}\int_{-T/2}^{T/2} f(t)\,dt \quad \text{(Mean value of f(t) over T.)} \tag{4.3}$$

$$a_n \equiv \frac{2}{T}\int_{-T/2}^{T/2} f(t)\cos(n\omega_o t)\,dt, \quad n = 1, 2, 3, \ldots \infty \tag{4.4}$$

$$b_n \equiv \frac{2}{T}\int_{-T/2}^{T/2} f(t)\sin(n\omega_o t)\,dt, \quad n = 1, 2, 3, \ldots \infty \tag{4.5}$$

You will see that there are several equivalent forms for expressing the Fourier series of $f(t)$. (The Fourier coefficients can also be found by integrating with respect to an angle argument, rather than time.) Of great interest in the discussion of sampling and discrete signals is the *complex form* of the Fourier series:

$$f(t) = \sum_{n=-\infty}^{\infty} c_n \exp[j(n\omega_o t)], \quad j = \sqrt{-1}. \tag{4.6}$$

$$c_n \equiv \frac{1}{T}\int_{-T/2}^{T/2} f(t)\exp[-j(n\omega_o t)]\,dt, \quad n = 0, \pm1, \pm2, \pm3, \ldots \pm\infty \tag{4.7}$$

(note range of n)

Exact representation of a continuous periodic $f(t)$ requires an infinite number of harmonic terms ($n \to \infty$), but, if a finite number of terms are used, for example to approximate an $f(t)$ with discontinuities such as square waves or sawtooth waves, a curious phenomenon is observed in the Fourier sum around the discontinuities in $f(t)$. These are the well-known *Gibbs phenomena,* shown in Figure 4.1. The Gibbs phenomena were investigated rigorously by J.W. Gibbs and reported in 1898 and 1899. As the number of terms, n, becomes larger, the frequency of the ripple increases, concentrating it around the regions of the discontinuities. Strangely, the peak heights of the ripples remain constant as $n \to \infty$. Thus, the area under the ripples $\to 0$ as $n \to \infty$. The height of the peaks relative to $f(t)$ is given by the *Wilbraham-Gibbs constant* [Finch, 2001]. For a zero-mean, equal duty cycle square wave, the largest ripple peak overshoot (and undershoot) closest to the discontinuity is 18% of the peak height of the square wave [Guillemin, 1949, Chapter 7]. Put mathematically, the mean-squared error in the Fourier series goes to zero as n approaches ∞. That is:

$$\overline{[f(t) - \{a_0 + \sum_{k=1}^{n} a_k \cos(k\omega_o t) + b_k \sin(k\omega_o t)\}]^2}^{\lim n\to\infty} = \varepsilon^2 \to 0 \tag{4.8}$$

A principal modern use for the Fourier series is to determine the minimum bandwidth required to transmit and condition periodic signals. For example, the ECG waveform recorded at various sites on the body surface.

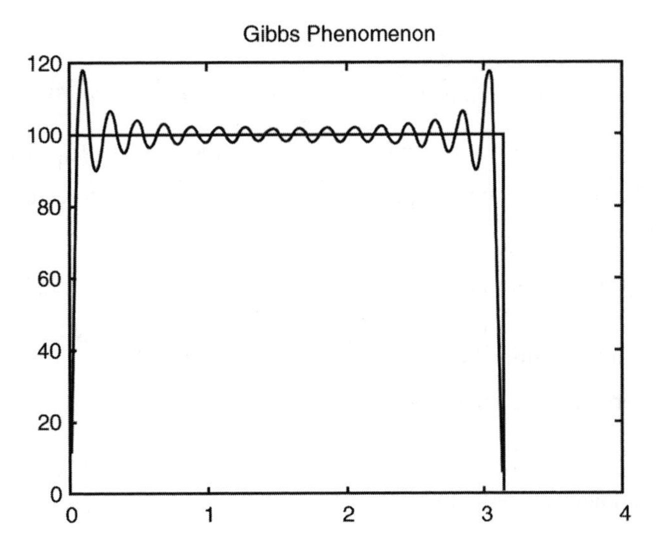

FIGURE 4.1
Illustration of the Gibbs effect ripple at the edges of one half-cycle of a square wave, $f(t)$. 16 terms were used in the Fourier series approximating $f(t)$. Note that the ripple persists the entire width of the half-cycle of $f(t)$.

4.2 Properties of the Fourier Series

Calculation of Fourier series coefficients is made easier if we note that most continuous, periodic functions, $f(t)$, can be written as either *even* or *odd functions.* If even, $f(-t) = f(t)$; if odd, $f(-t) = -f(t)$. If $f(t)$ is even, it can be shown that all the b_n coefficients $= 0$ (only $\cos(^*)$ terms are nonzero in the Fourier series). Similarly, if $f(t)$ is odd, all the a_n coefficients $= 0$ (only $\sin(^*)$ terms are nonzero in the Fourier series).

For a periodic $f(t)$ to have a Fourier series, it must satisfy the three *Dirichlet conditions* [Oppenheim and Willsky, 1983]:

Condition 1: Over a period, $f(t)$ must be absolutely integrable; that is:

$$\int_T |f(t)| < \infty \tag{4.9}$$

Condition 2: Over a period, $f(t)$ has a finite number of maxima and minima.

Condition 3: Over a period, $f(t)$ must have a finite number of discontinuities, and they must be of finite amplitude.

The Dirichlet conditions are sufficient but not strictly necessary for existence of a Fourier series.

TABLE 4.1
Some Properties of Fourier Series

Periodic Signal Property	Complex Fourier Coefficient Property
$g(t) = g(t+kT)$, (k any integer)	$\mathbf{FS}\{g(t)\}$, $\{d_k\}$ exists
$f(t) = f(t+kT)$, (k any integer)	$\mathbf{FS}\{f(t)\}$, $\{c_k\}$ exists
$Af(t)+Bg(t)$ (superposition)	$A\,c_k + B\,d_k$
$f(t-t_o)$ (time shift)	$c_k \exp(-jk2\pi t_o/T)$
$\exp(jN2\pi t/T)f(t)$ (complex multiplication)	c_{k-N}
$f^*(t)$ (complex conjugate of $f(t)$)	c^*_{-k}
$\int_{-\infty}^{t} f(t)\,dt$ (finite and periodic only if $c_o = 0$)	$\frac{c_k}{(jk2\pi/T)}$ $2\pi/T = \omega_o$
$df(t)/dt$	$(jk2\pi/T)c_k$
$f(t)g(t)$	$\sum_{n=-\infty}^{\infty} c_n d_{k-n}$
$\int_T f(\mu)g(t-\mu)d\mu$	$Tc_k d_k$
IF $f(t \pm T/2) = -f(t)$	THEN **FS** contains odd harmonics only
IF $f(t \pm T/2) = f(t)$	THEN **FS** contains even harmonics only
IF $f(t) = f(-t)$ [$f(t)$ is even]	THEN all $b_n = 0$ (no $\sin(^*)$ terms)
IF $f(t) = -f(-t)$ [$f(t)$ is odd]	THEN all $a_n = 0$ (no $\cos(^*)$ terms)
$\frac{1}{T}\int_{-T/2}^{T/2} \lvert f(t)\rvert^2\,dt$ (Parseval's relation for periodic signals)	$\sum_{n=-\infty}^{\infty} \lvert c_n\rvert^2$, c_n are coefficients of complex-form FS

Other properties of the continuous Fourier series are summarized in Table 4.1.

4.3 Fourier Series Examples

Many engineering textbooks on signals and systems analysis have examples of the calculation of Fourier series for periodic analytical waveforms commonly found in electrical, mechanical, biomedical and other engineering specialties. T is the function's period, f_o is its fundamental Hz frequency, and ω_o is its fundamental radian

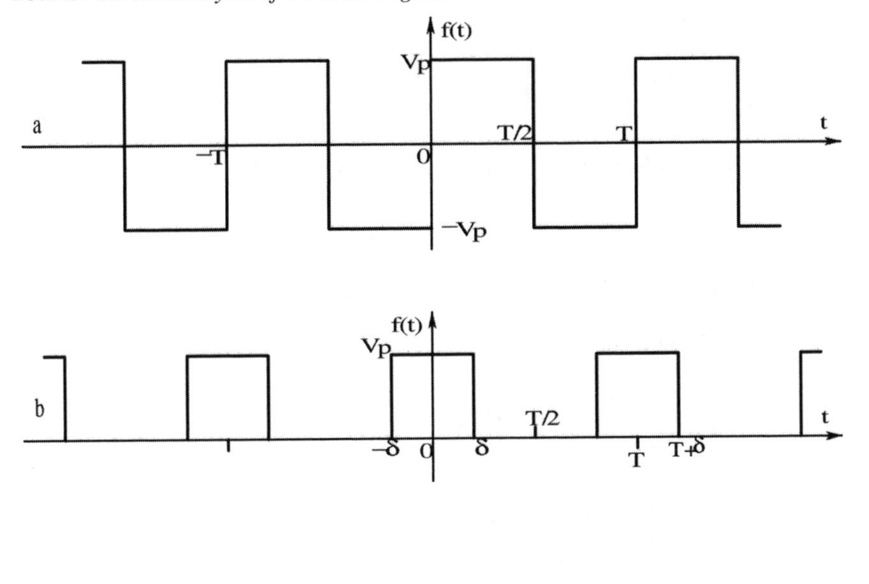

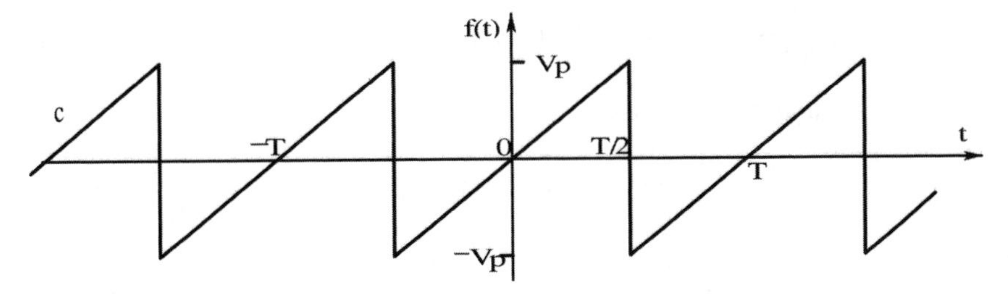

FIGURE 4.2
Three examples of periodic waves used in the text to find Fourier series: (a) An odd square wave with zero mean. (b) An even train of narrow positive pulses. (c) An odd sawtooth wave with zero average value.

frequency ($\omega_o = 2\pi/T$). Using this notation, the Fourier series can be written:

$$f(t) = a_0 + \sum_{n=1}^{\infty} [a_n \cos(n\omega_o t) + b_n \sin(n\omega_o t)] \tag{4.10}$$

Where a_0, a_n and b_n are given by Equations 4.3, 4.4 and 4.5.

As a first example of calculating a_0, a_n and b_n for a periodic $f(t)$, consider the odd ("sine") square wave shown in Figure 4.2a having peak height, V_p. Since this $f(t)$ has zero mean, $a_0 = 0$. The **FS** of the square wave also *has only odd harmonics* since it satisfies $f(t \pm T/2) = -f(t)$ in Table 4.1. Also, because *the wave is odd,* there will only be $\sin(n\omega_o t)$ terms in its **FS**. Thus we only need to evaluate the b_n coefficients for odd n:

$$b_1 = \frac{2}{T}\int_{-T/2}^{0}(-V_p)\sin(\omega_o t)\,dt + \frac{2}{T}\int_{0}^{T/2}(V_p)\sin(\omega_o t)\,dt$$

$$\downarrow$$

$$= \frac{2}{T\omega_o}\left\{-(-V_p)\cos(\omega_o t)|_{-T/2}^{0} - (V_p)\cos(\omega_o t)|_0^{T/2}\right\}$$

$$\downarrow$$

$$= \frac{2V_p}{T2\pi/T}\{1-(-1)-[(-1)-1]\} = \frac{4V_p}{\pi} \tag{4.11}$$

Now, for n = 2 (and all even values):

$$b_2 = \frac{2}{T}\int_{-T/2}^{0}(-V_p)\sin(2\omega_o t)\,dt + \frac{2}{T}\int_{0}^{T/2}(V_p)\sin(2\omega_o t)\,dt$$

$$\downarrow$$

$$= \frac{2V_p}{T2\omega_o}\left\{-(-V_p)\cos(2\omega_o t)|_{-T/2}^{0} - (V_p)\cos(2\omega_o t)|_0^{T/2}\right\}$$

$$\downarrow$$

$$= \frac{2V_p}{T2(2\pi/T)}\{1-(1)-[(1)-1]\} = 0 \tag{4.12}$$

And, in general, for all odd n values:

$$b_n = \frac{2V_p}{n\pi}\{1-(-1)-[(-1)-1]\} = \frac{4V_p}{n\pi} \tag{4.13}$$

Thus:

$$\mathbf{FS}\{f(x)\} = \sum_{\substack{n=1,\\ \text{odd}}}^{\infty} \frac{4V_p}{n\pi}\sin(n\omega_o t) = \frac{4V_p}{\pi}[\sin(\omega_o t) + (1/3)\sin(3\omega_o t) + (1/5)\sin(5\omega_o t) + \cdots] \tag{4.14}$$

As a second example, let us evaluate the *FS* for a train of positive, narrow, even (cosine) rectangular pulses, each with peak height V_p and width 2δ radians (obviously, $2\delta << 2\pi$), shown in Figure 4.2b. Because the pulse train is even, all b_n coefficients $= 0$ (there are no sin(nx) terms). a_0 is simply the average value of the waveform:

$$a_0 = \frac{1}{T}\int_{-\delta}^{\delta}(V_p)\,dt = (2\delta/T)V_p \tag{4.15}$$

and

$$a_n = \frac{2}{T}\int_{-\delta}^{\delta} V_p\cos(n\omega_o t)\,dt = \frac{2V_p}{Tn\omega_o}\sin(n\omega_o t)\Big|_{-\delta}^{\delta}$$

$$= \frac{2V_p}{Tn\omega_o}\{\sin(n\omega_o\delta) - \sin(-n\omega_o\delta)\} \tag{4.16}$$

But $\sin\theta$ is odd, so we have:

$$a_n = (4V_p\delta/T)\frac{\sin(n\omega_o\delta)}{(n\omega_o\delta)} \tag{4.17}$$

Thus,

$$\mathbf{FS}\{f(t)\} = \frac{2\delta V_p}{T} + \frac{4\delta V_p}{T}\sum_{n=1}^{\infty}\frac{\sin(n\omega_o\delta)}{(n\omega_o\delta)}\cos(n\omega_o t) \tag{4.18}$$

Note the $(\sin x/x)$ modulation of the harmonic amplitudes.

As a third example, let us calculate the **FS** of an odd, zero-mean sawtooth wave, shown in Figure 4.2c. Here, clearly, $a_0 = 0$. Because the waveform is odd, there will be no cosine terms in its **FS**. Thus, we proceed:

$$b_n = \frac{2}{T}\int_{-T/2}^{T/2}[t(V_p/T)]\sin(n\omega_o t)\,dt \tag{4.19}$$

Now from Dwight (1961), $\int \theta\sin\theta\,d\theta = \sin\theta - \theta\cos\theta$, where $\theta = n\omega_o t$. Thus, the integral can be written:

$$\begin{aligned} b_n &= \frac{2V_p}{T^2}\frac{1}{(n\omega_o)^2}\int_{-T/2}^{T/2}(n\omega_o t)\sin(n\omega_o t)\,d(n\omega_o t) \\ &= \frac{2V_p}{T^2(n\omega_o)^2}\left\{\sin(n\omega_o t)\Big|_{-T/2}^{T/2} - (n\omega_o t)\cos(n\omega_o t)\Big|_{-T/2}^{T/2}\right\} \end{aligned} \tag{4.20}$$

So we have:

$$\begin{aligned} b_n &= \frac{2V_p}{T^2(n\omega_o)^2}[\{\overset{0}{\sin(n\pi)} - \overset{0}{\sin(-n\pi)}\} - \{n\pi\overset{-1\text{ for n odd}}{\cos(n\pi)} - (-n\pi)\overset{-1}{\cos(-n\pi)}\}] \\ &= \frac{2V_p(-1)^{n+1}}{T^2(n\omega_o)^2}(2\pi n) \\ &\downarrow \end{aligned}$$

$$b_n = \frac{2V_p(2\pi n)(-1)^{n+1}}{T^2n^2(2\pi/T)^2} = \frac{V_p}{n\pi}(-1)^{n+1} \tag{4.21}$$

It is found that the second two integrals in Equation 4.21 always sum to zero for any $n = 1, 2, 3, \ldots$. Thus, the Fourier series for the positive slope sawtooth wave can be written (note the alternating signs of the b_n coefficients):

$$\mathbf{FS}\{f(t)\} = \frac{V_p}{\pi}\sin(\omega_o t) - \frac{V_p}{2\pi}\sin(2\omega_o t) + \frac{V_p}{3\pi}\sin(3\omega_o t) - \frac{V_p}{4\pi}\sin(4\omega_o t) + \cdots \tag{4.22}$$

In closed form, Equation 4.22 is:

$$f(t) = \frac{V_p}{\pi}\sum_{n=1}^{\infty}\frac{(-1)^{n+1}}{n}\sin(n\omega_o t) \tag{4.23}$$

As a fourth and final example, let us find the *complex Fourier series* of even (cosine) rectangular pulses of width 2δ and height V_p, as shown in Figure 4.2b. We first calculate the Fourier coefficient, c_n:

$$c_n = \frac{1}{T}\int_{-T/2}^{T/2} f(t)\exp(-jn\omega_o t)\,dt = \frac{1}{T}\int_{-\delta}^{\delta} V_p \exp(-jn\omega_o t)\,dt,$$
$$n = 0, \pm 1, \pm 2, \pm 3, \ldots$$

$\downarrow$

$$c_n = \frac{V_p}{T(-jn\omega_o)}[e^{-jn\omega_o\delta} - e^{+jn\omega_o\delta}] = \frac{V_p 2\delta}{T}\frac{\sin(n\omega_o\delta)}{(n\omega_o\delta)} \tag{4.24}$$

For $n = 0$, the mean value of $f(t)$ is:

$$c_0 = \frac{V_p 2\delta}{T} \tag{4.25}$$

For $n = \pm 1$, the coefficients are:

$$c_1 + c_{-1} = \frac{V_p 2\delta}{T}\left\{\frac{\sin(\omega_o\delta)}{(\omega_o\delta)}e^{j\omega_o t} + \frac{\sin(-\omega_o\delta)}{(-\omega_o\delta)}e^{-j\omega_o t}\right\} \tag{4.26}$$

Now $\sin(\theta)/(\theta)$ is even, so $\sin(\theta)/(\theta) = \sin(-\theta)/(-\theta)$ and using the Euler relation for $\cos(\phi)$, we can write:

$$c_1 + c_{-1} = \frac{4V_p\delta}{T}\frac{\sin(\omega_o\delta)}{(\omega_o\delta)}\cos(\omega_o t) \tag{4.27}$$

In general, the complex form of this Fourier series can also be written as:

$$f(t) = \frac{V_p 2\delta}{T} + \frac{4V_p\delta}{T}\sum_{n=1}^{\infty}\frac{\sin(n\omega_o\delta)}{(n\omega_o\delta)}\cos(n\omega_o t) \tag{4.28}$$

It is clear that calculating Fourier series coefficients can be tedious. Most engineering handbooks have tables of them for common waveforms found in instrumentation, communications and power supplies.

Some authors [e.g., Guillemin, 1949] give Fourier series in terms of angle argument, $x \equiv \omega_o t$ radians, instead of time. In this form,

$$f(x) = a_0 + \sum_{n=1}^{\infty} a_n\cos(nx) + b_n\sin(nx) \tag{4.29}$$

$$a_0 = \frac{1}{2\pi}\int_{-\pi}^{\pi} f(x)\,dx \tag{4.30}$$

$$a_n = \frac{1}{\pi}\int_{-\pi}^{\pi} f(x)\cos(nx)\,dx \tag{4.31}$$

$$b_n = \frac{1}{\pi}\int_{-\pi}^{\pi} f(x)\sin(nx)\,dx \tag{4.32}$$

4.4 Chapter Summary

This chapter introduced the Fourier series (FS) in both trigonometric (sine and cosine) form, as well as the equivalent complex form, as a means of approximating a periodic, time- or space-domain function. Examples of such periodic functions are square waves rectified sine waves and nondeterministic signals such as the ECG waveform.

When a FS is plotted by summing its component terms, it exhibits spike-like overshoots at discontinuities in $f(t)$. These Gibbs phenomena have been shown to be the result of using a finite number of harmonics, n, in the FS. As $n \to \infty$, the Gibbs overshoots were shown to persist in amplitude but have vanishing width, causing the mean squared error between $f(t)$ and its FS to $\to 0$. Mathematical properties of the FS were given.

Several examples of finding the FS of common periodic waveforms found in biomedical engineering were given. By examining the relative amplitudes of the component harmonics in the FS of $f(t)$, an engineer can predict how faithfully the output of a finite-width bandpass filter will reproduce a certain periodic $f(t)$ at its input. Such analysis is important in designing filters for instruments such as ECG recorders.

Problems

4.1 An even "cosine" triangle wave is shown in Figure P4.1. Note that in the interval, $-T/2 \le t \le 0$, $f(t) = V_p + 4V_p t/T$ and in the interval, $0 \le t \le T/2$ $f(t) = V_p - 4V_p t/T$. Find the Fourier series of this function in the form:

$$f(t) = a_0 + \sum_{n=1}^{\infty} \{a_n \cos(n\omega_o t) + b_n \sin(n\omega_o t)\}$$

Note that a piecewise approach to integration is required to find a_n.

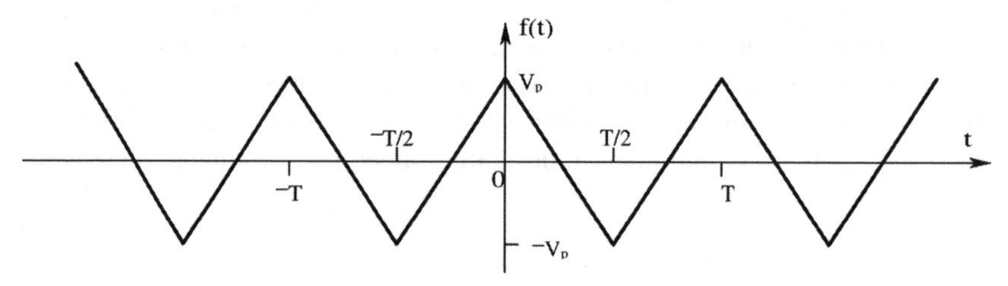

FIGURE P4.1

4.2 Narrow even triangular pulses of peak height V_p are shown in Figure P4.2. Note that, in the interval, $-\delta \le t \le 0$, $f(t) = V_p + t(V_p/\delta)$ and in the interval, $0 \le t \le \delta$, $f(t) = V_p - t(V_p/\delta)$. Find the Fourier series for $f(t)$ in the form:

$$f(t) = a_0 + \sum_{n=1}^{\infty} \{a_n \cos(n\omega_o t) + b_n \sin(n\omega_o t)\}$$

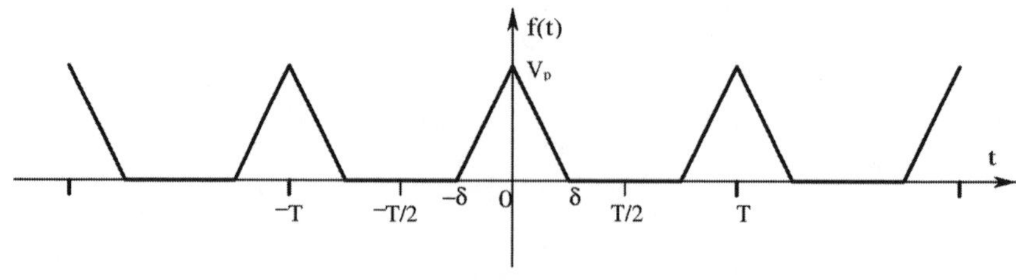

FIGURE P4.2

4.3 A nonnegative even square wave is shown in Figure P4.3. Find the Fourier series for this wave in the form:

$$f(t) = a_0 + \sum_{\substack{n=1 \\ n \text{ odd}}}^{\infty} \{a_n \cos(n\omega_o t) + b_n \sin(n\omega_o t)\}$$

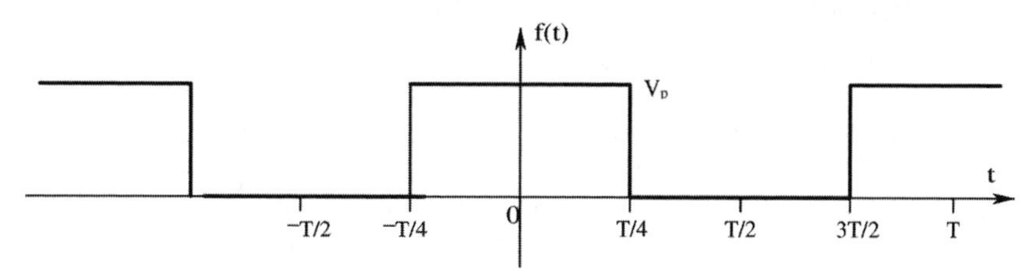

FIGURE P4.3

4.4 Consider the waveform of Figure P4.3. Find c_n for the Fourier series for this wave in the complex form:

$$f(t) = \sum_{n=-\infty}^{\infty} c_n \exp[+jn\omega_o t]$$

4.5 Consider the periodic exponential decay waveform shown in Figure **P4.5**; it is neither even nor odd, so there will be both sin and cos terms in the Fourier series. In the range of integration, $-T/2 \leq t \leq T/2$, f(t) is given by:

$$f(t) = V \exp[-a(t + T/2)]$$

Find the Fourier series for this f(t) in the form:

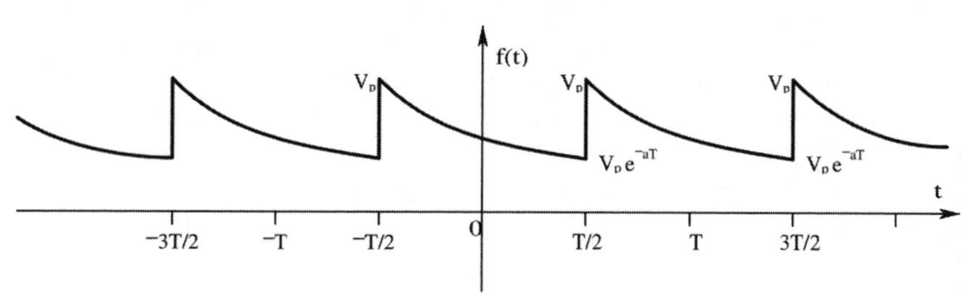

FIGURE P4.5

$$f(t) = a_0 + \sum_{n=1}^{\infty} a_n \cos(n\omega_o t) + b_n \sin(n\omega_o t)$$

Note considerable simplification results if you replace $\cos(n\pi)$ with $(-1)^n$. Also, $\sin(n\pi) = 0$, all n.

4.6 Find an expression for the Fourier series of the full-wave rectified cosine wave:

$$y(t) = |A\cos(\omega_o t)|, \quad -\infty \leq t \leq \infty, \omega_o = 2\pi/T,$$

In the form: $f(t) = a_0 + \sum_{n=0}^{\infty}\{a_n \cos(n\omega_o t) + b_n \sin(n\omega_o t)\}$.

4.7 A signal is given by:

$$y(t) = 2 + \sin(\omega_o t) + 3\cos(\omega_o t) + 5\cos(3\omega_o t + \pi/4), \quad \omega_o = 2\pi/T$$

Find the complex-form Fourier series coefficients, $\mathbf{c_k}$, for this periodic time function and write the series out. Put the $\mathbf{c_k}$ in rectangular vector form.

4.8 The positive squarewave of Figure P4.3 is delayed by δ seconds $(0 < \delta < T/2)$. Find its Fourier series in the form:

$$f(t-\delta) = a_0 + \sum_{n=1}^{\infty}\{a_n \cos(n\omega_o t + \phi_n) + b_n \sin(n\omega_o t + \theta_n)\}.$$

That is, find expressions for ω_o, a_o, a_n, b_n, ϕ_n, and θ_n.

4.9 a. Consider the periodic waveform of Figure 4.2. Find an expression for the coefficient, c_n, for the complex form of its Fourier series:

$$f(t) = \sum_{n=-\infty}^{\infty} \mathbf{c_n} \exp[+jn\omega_o t]$$

b. Now delay this waveform by some small amount, ε. Find its $\mathbf{c_n}$.

4.10 A periodic waveform, $x(t)$, with complex Fourier series, $x(t) = \sum_{n=-\infty}^{\infty} a_n \exp[+jn\omega_o t]$ is the input to a continuous LTI system with impulse response, $h(t)$. The system output is periodic $y(t)$ with a complex FS, $y(t) = \sum_{n=-\infty}^{\infty} b_n \exp[+jn\omega_o t]$. Note that, in general, by real convolution, $y(t) = \int_{-\infty}^{\infty} h(\mu)x(\mu - t)\,d\mu$ and the FS for x can be substituted into this convolution, etc. You are to derive an algebraic expression for b_n. (Note that the continuous Fourier transform of $h(t)$ is given by: $H(\omega) \equiv \int_{-\infty}^{\infty} h(t) \exp(-j\omega t)\,dt$.)

5

The Continuous Fourier Transform

5.1 Introduction

This chapter describes the derivation and reviews the mathematical properties of the *continuous Fourier transform* (CFT) from the Fourier series. Three major applications of the CFT are also treated. These include:

1. *Analog-to-digital conversion* (ADC), considered in the frequency domain, and the *sampling theorem*
2. The *analytical signal* and the Hilbert transform, and their applications in biomedical signal processing
3. The *modulation transfer function* (MTF) as a descriptor of medical imaging system performance in the spatial frequency domain.

A continuous aperiodic or transient waveform can be represented in the frequency domain by the *Fourier integral* (FI) or CFT, which can be considered to be the limiting case of the *Fourier series* for a periodic waveform, each cycle of which is the transient $f(t)$ of concern. When the waveform is periodic, we can find the complex Fourier coefficients, $\mathbf{c_n}$, using Equation 4.7. In the limit as $T \to \infty$, we can write:

$$\lim_{\substack{T\to\infty \\ \omega_o\to 0}} \mathbf{c_n} = \lim_{\substack{T\to\infty \\ \omega_o\to 0}} \int_{-\infty}^{\infty} f(t)\exp(-jn\omega_o t)\,dt, \quad \omega_o \equiv \frac{2\pi}{T}\ \text{r/sec} \tag{5.1}$$

In the limit, $n\omega_o$ approaches the continuous radian frequency variable, ω. Thus, we can finally write:

$$\lim_{T\to\infty} \mathbf{c_n} = \mathbf{F}(\omega) \equiv \int_{-\infty}^{\infty} f(t)\,e^{-j\omega t}\,dt \tag{5.2}$$

Equation 5.2 defines the continuous Fourier transform (CFT) of a transient (single) time function (note that the CFT can also be taken on a *spatial function,* $f(x)$). $\mathbf{F}(\omega)$ is, in general, a complex quantity (a 2-D vector with real and imaginary parts) and thus can be written in exponential or polar form:

$$\mathbf{F}(\omega) = |\mathbf{F}(\omega)|e^{j\varphi(\omega)} = |\mathbf{F}(\omega)|\angle\varphi(\omega) \tag{5.3}$$

The *Fourier inversion integral* allows us to recover f(t), given $\mathbf{F}(\omega)$. It can be derived from the complex form of the Fourier series given $T \to \infty$:

$$\lim_{T\to\infty} f(t) = \frac{1}{T}\frac{T}{2\pi}\sum_{n=-\infty}^{\infty} \mathbf{c_n} \exp(jn\omega_o t)\,\omega_o \equiv \frac{1}{2\pi}\int_{-\infty}^{\infty} \mathbf{F}(\omega)\, e^{j\omega t}\, d\omega \tag{5.4}$$

The continuous Fourier *inversion integral,* Equation 5.4, is sometimes written, noting that $\omega = 2\pi f$ r/s, as:

$$f(t) \equiv \int_{-\infty}^{\infty} \mathbf{F}(2\pi f)\exp(j2\pi ft)\, df, \quad f = \omega/2\pi. \tag{5.5}$$

5.2 Properties of the CFT

The CFT has many interesting properties, the more useful of which are given in Table 5.1. We consider the CFT of a *real* f(t), where t can be negative.

TABLE 5.1
Some Relations, Theorems and Transform Pairs of the Continuous Fourier Transform

	Time Domain	Frequency Domain
1.	$\int_{-\infty}^{\infty} f(t)e^{-j\omega t}\, dt$	$\mathbf{F}(\omega)$
2.	f(t) is real	*Re*$\{\mathbf{F}(\omega)\}$ is even in ω. *Im*$\{F(\omega)\}$ is odd in ω. $\lvert\mathbf{F}(\omega)\rvert$ is even in ω. $\angle\mathbf{F}(\omega)$ is odd in ω.
3.	f(t) is real and even.	$F(\omega) = 2Re\{\int_{-\infty}^{\infty} f(t)e^{j\omega t}\, dt\}$ $= 2\int_0^{\infty} f(t)\cos(\omega t)\, dt$
4.	$f(-t) = -f(t)$ (odd, real f(t))	$\mathbf{F}(\omega) = -j\int_{-\infty}^{\infty} f(t)\sin(\omega t)\, dt$ $= -2j\int_0^{\infty} f(t)\sin(\omega t)\, dt$ (even)
5.	f(at) (scale change)	$(1/\lvert a\rvert)\mathbf{F}(\omega/a)$
6.	$f(t - t_o)$ (time shift)	$\mathbf{F}(\omega)\exp(-j\omega t_o)$
7.	$\mathbf{f}(t) = \exp(j\omega_o t)$	$F(\omega) = 2\pi\delta(\omega - \omega_o)$
8.	$\mathbf{f}(t) = g(t)\exp(j\omega_o t)$	$\mathbf{G}(j\omega - j\omega_o)$
9.	F(t)	$2\pi\mathbf{f}(-\omega)$
10.	$\frac{d^n f(t)}{dt^n}$, $n = 1, 2, 3\ldots$	$(j\omega)^n\mathbf{F}(\omega)$

continued...

	Time Domain	Frequency Domain
11.	$f(t) = \cos(\omega_o t)$	$F(\omega) = \pi[\delta(\omega - \omega_o) + \delta(\omega + \omega_o)]$
12.	$f(t) = \sin(\omega_o t)$	$\mathbf{F}(\omega) = j\pi[\delta(\omega + \omega_o) - \delta(\omega - \omega_o)]$
13.	$f(t) = b(t)\cos(\omega_o t)$	$\mathbf{F}(\omega) = 1/2[\mathbf{B}(\omega + \omega_o) + \mathbf{B}(\omega - \omega_o)]$
14.	$f(t) = b(t)\sin(\omega_o t)$	$\mathbf{F}(\omega) = j1/2[\mathbf{B}(\omega + \omega_o) - \mathbf{B}(\omega - \omega_o)]$
15.	$\int_{-\infty}^{\infty} f(\sigma)g(t-\sigma)\,d\sigma$ (real convolution)	$\mathbf{F}(j\omega)\mathbf{G}(j\omega)$ (complex multiplication)
16.	$f(t)g(t)$ (real multiplication)	$\frac{1}{2\pi}\int_{-\infty}^{\infty} \mathbf{F}(\sigma)\mathbf{G}(\omega-\sigma)\,d\sigma$ (complex convolution)
17.	$\int_{-\infty}^{\infty} \lvert f(t)\rvert^2\,dt$ (Parseval's theorem)	$\frac{1}{2\pi}\int_{-\infty}^{\infty} \lvert\mathbf{F}(\omega)\rvert^2\,d\omega$
18.	$f(t) = \delta(t)$	$F(\omega) = 1, \quad -\infty \le \omega \le \infty.$
19.	$f(t) = 1(dc)$	$F(\omega) = 2\pi\delta(\omega)$
20.	$f(t) = U(t)$ (unit step)	$\mathbf{F}(j\omega) = \pi\delta(\omega) + 1/j\omega$
21.	$f(t) = \mathrm{sgn}(t)$	$2/(j\omega)$
22.	$f(t) = e^{-at}U(t)$	$\mathbf{F}(j\omega) = 1/(a + j\omega)$
23.	$f(t) = \exp(-a\lvert t\rvert)$	$F(\omega) = \dfrac{2a}{\omega^2 + a^2}$
24.	$f(t) = \exp(-at^2)$	$F(\omega) = \sqrt{(\pi/a)\exp(-\omega^2/2a)}$
25.	$f(t) = p_a(t) = 1, \quad -a \le t \le a$ $p_a(t) = 0, \quad t > a, t < -a$	$F\omega = \dfrac{2a\sin(a\omega)}{a\omega}$
26.	$\mathrm{rect}(t/T)$ $\mathrm{rect}(t/T) = 1$ for $\lvert t\rvert \le T/2$ $\mathrm{rect}(t/T) = 0$ for $\lvert t\rvert > T/2$	$F(\omega) = \dfrac{T\sin(\omega T/2)}{(\omega T/2)}$ (zeros at $\omega = k/(2\pi T), k \neq 0$)
27.	$f(t) = \left\{1 - \frac{\lvert t\rvert}{a}\right\} = \Lambda(t/a)$, $-a \le t \le a$, else 0.	$F(\omega) = \dfrac{a\sin^2(a\omega/2)}{(a\omega/2)^2}$
28.	$f(t) = t^n e^{-\alpha t}U(t), \quad \alpha > 0$	$\mathbf{F}(j\omega) = \dfrac{n!}{(j\omega + \alpha)^{n+1}}$

As in the case of the Laplace transform, if an LTI system has a weighting function $g(t)$ for $t \ge 0$ and its input $x(t)$ has a FT, $\mathbf{X}(j\omega)$, then the FT of the LTI system's output is:

$$\mathbf{Y}(j\omega) = \mathbf{X}(j\omega)\mathbf{G}(j\omega) \tag{5.6}$$

Furthermore, $\mathbf{G}(j\omega)$, is the *frequency response* of an LTI system with impulse response, $g(t)$, generally expressed as

$$AR = 20 \log_{10} |\mathbf{G}(j\omega)| \, dB \quad \text{(Bode amplitude response)} \tag{5.7A}$$

$$\varphi(\omega) = \angle \mathbf{G}(j\omega) \quad \text{(phase of frequency response)} \tag{5.7B}$$

In general, $\mathbf{G}(j\omega)$ acts on the magnitude and phase of the input, $\mathbf{X}(j\omega)$. For example, if $\mathbf{G}(j\omega)$ is a low-pass filter, it will attenuate the high frequencies in $\mathbf{X}(j\omega)$ and generally will introduce a phase lag in the attenuated terms of $\mathbf{Y}(j\omega)$. The *half-power frequency,* or *−3 dB* frequency, ω_b, of the filter is the frequency where:

$$\frac{|\mathbf{G}(j\omega_b)|}{|\mathbf{G}_{max}|} = 0.7071 \tag{5.8}$$

Another important concept in signal filtering is the *distortionless filter.* The output of a distortionless filter is of the form: $y(t) = Ax(t - t_d)$. That is, the output is the input scaled and delayed. In the frequency domain, $\mathbf{Y}(j\omega) = A\mathbf{X}(j\omega)\exp(-j\omega t_d)$. Clearly, $\mathbf{G}(j\omega) = \mathbf{Y}(j\omega)/\mathbf{X}(j\omega)$, so the filter's transfer function has the properties:

$$|\mathbf{G}(j\omega)| = A \tag{5.9A}$$

$$\angle \mathbf{G}(j\omega) = \varphi(\omega) = -\omega t_d \quad \text{radians} \tag{5.9B}$$

That is, the gain of $\mathbf{G}(j\omega)$ is constant over all ω, a property of an *all-pass filter and* the phase shift is a linear function of ω. An important descriptor of a practical, nearly distortionless filter is its *group delay,* defined as:

$$t_d \equiv -\frac{d\varphi(\omega)}{d\omega} \tag{5.10}$$

In practice, the phase shift can be made a linear function of ω (a constant t_d) only over a limited range (or *group*) of frequencies.

As a first example of the use of the theorems and identities in Table 5.1, we will derive the transform pair:

$$f(t) = p_a(t)\cos(\omega_o t) \longleftrightarrow F(\omega) = \frac{a\sin[a(\omega - \omega_o)]}{a(\omega - \omega_o)} + \frac{a\sin[a(\omega + \omega_o)]}{a(\omega - \omega_o)} \tag{5.11}$$

First, by transform # 25, $p_a(t) \longleftrightarrow \frac{2a\sin(a\omega)}{a\omega}$. We then let $p_a(t) = b(t)$ in relation # 13, $a\omega$ which is $b(t)\cos(\omega_o t) \longleftrightarrow 1/2[\mathbf{B}(\omega - \omega_o) + \mathbf{B}(\omega + \omega_o)]$, to arrive at the result above.

As a second example, we will find the CFT of $f(t) = p_a(t)[1 + \cos(\pi t/a)]$. First, we note that, by superposition, $F[g(t) + h(t)] = \mathbf{G}(\omega) + \mathbf{H}(\omega)$. Thus, $\mathbf{F}(\omega)$ can be written using the results of the previous example:

$$\mathbf{F}(\omega) = \frac{2a\sin(a\omega)}{a\omega} + \frac{a\sin[a(\omega - \pi/a)]}{a(\omega - \pi/a)} + \frac{a\sin[a(\omega + \pi/a)]}{a(\omega + \pi/a)} \tag{5.12}$$

After some algebra and noting that $\sin(\pi \pm \theta) = -, +\sin(\theta)$, we finally arrive at the not-obvious, compact form of $\mathbf{F}(\omega)$ above:

$$\mathbf{F}(\omega) = \frac{2\mathrm{a}\sin(\mathrm{a}\omega)}{\mathrm{a}\omega} \frac{1}{[1-(\mathrm{a}\omega/\pi)^2]} \tag{5.13}$$

As a third example, we will derive the time-frequency scaling theorem, # 5 in the table:

$$\mathrm{f}(\mathrm{bt}) \longleftrightarrow \frac{1}{|\mathrm{b}|}\mathbf{F}(\omega/\mathrm{b}) \tag{5.14}$$

Going to the definition of the CFT:

$$\begin{aligned}\int_{-\infty}^{\infty} \mathrm{f}(\mathrm{bt}) \exp(-\mathrm{j}\omega\mathrm{t})\, \mathrm{dt} &= \frac{1}{|\mathrm{b}|}\int_{-\infty}^{\infty} \mathrm{f}(\mathrm{x}) \underbrace{\exp(-\mathrm{j}\omega\mathrm{x}/\mathrm{a})\,\mathrm{dx}}_{\mathrm{x}\equiv\mathrm{bt}} \\ &= \frac{1}{|\mathrm{b}|}\mathbf{F}(\omega/\mathrm{b}), \quad \text{QED}\end{aligned} \tag{5.15}$$

5.3 Analog-to-Digital Conversion and the Sampling Theorem

5.3.1 Introduction

Today, we live in a world of digital signal processing (DSP). DSP is used in all areas of modern communications and instrumentation. This section examines the very important relationship between the frequency spectrum of an analog signal being sampled and digitized for DSP applications and the sampling rate at which the analog-to-digital converter operates. It will be shown that, if the sampling rate is too low, a phenomenon known as *aliasing* that effectively distorts the sampled signal will occur. In many DSP applications, the signal to be sampled is first passed through a sharp cutoff analog low-pass filter known as an *antiliasing filter* (AAF). The AAF is used to attenuate to a negligible level any high-frequency spectral energy in the signal at frequencies above one half the sampling frequency. AAFs are generally not used in digital storage oscilloscopes because, when it occurs, there is direct *visual* evidence of aliasing on the display screen. The operator can then adjust the oscilloscope controls to permit a higher sampling rate.

5.3.2 Impulse modulation and the Poisson sum form of the sampled spectrum

Let $\mathrm{y(t)}$ be a continuous, analog signal that is being converted to a number sequence periodically, every $\mathrm{T_s}$ seconds, by an ADC. $\mathrm{T_s}$ is called the *sampling period* and $\mathrm{f_s} = 1/\mathrm{T_s}$ is the *sampling frequency.* The entire sampling process can be viewed as *impulse modulation,* that is multiplication of $\mathrm{y(t)}$ by an infinite train of delta functions spaced T_s seconds apart. The output of the multiplier/modulator is a *number sequence* fed into the computer or DSP system. The number sequence will be denoted by $y^*(t)$.

$$y^*(t) = y(t) \times P_T(t) \tag{5.16}$$

The impulse train, $P_T(t)$, is periodic:

$$P_T(t) = \sum_{k=-\infty}^{\infty} \delta(t - kT_s) \tag{5.17}$$

The impulses exist only at $t = kT_s$, so at the multiplier output,

$$y^*(t) = \sum_{k=-\infty}^{\infty} y(kT_s)\delta(t - kT_s) \tag{5.18}$$

Because it is periodic, $P_T(t)$ can be written as a *Fourier series in complex form.*

$$P_T(t) = \sum_{k=-\infty}^{\infty} \delta(t - kT_s) = \sum_{k=-\infty}^{\infty} c_k \exp(+j\omega_s t), \quad \omega_s = \frac{2\pi}{T_s} \text{ r/s} \tag{5.19}$$

c_k is given by the definite integral, Equation 5.20:

$$\mathbf{c_k} = \frac{1}{T_s}\int_{-T_s/2}^{T_s/2} P_T(t)\exp(jk\omega_s t)\,dt = \frac{1}{T_s} \quad \text{(all k)} \tag{5.20}$$

Thus, the Fourier series for $P_T(t)$ is:

$$P_T(t) = \frac{1}{T_s}\sum_{k=-\infty}^{\infty} \exp(+jk\omega_s t) \tag{5.21}$$

We can rewrite $y^*(t)$ as:

$$y^*(t) = \frac{1}{T_s}\sum_{k=-\infty}^{\infty} y(t)\exp(+jk\omega_s t) \tag{5.22}$$

Now the CFT of $y^*(t)$ can be taken using the *FT theorem of complex exponentiation* on Equation 5.22. This form of the spectrum of $y^*(t)$ is called the *Poisson sum* [Ragazzini and Franklin, 1958].

$$\mathbf{F}\{y^*(t)\} = \mathbf{Y}^*(j\omega) = \frac{1}{T_s}\sum_{k=-\infty}^{\infty} \mathbf{Y}(j\omega + jk\omega_s) \tag{5.23}$$

As shown in Figure 5.1a, the Fourier spectrum of the sampled number sequence, obtained by assuming it to be a train of impulses given by Equation 5.18, is the spectrum, $(1/T_s)\mathbf{Y}(j\omega)$, repeated along the ω-axis every $k\omega_s$. That is, each spectral

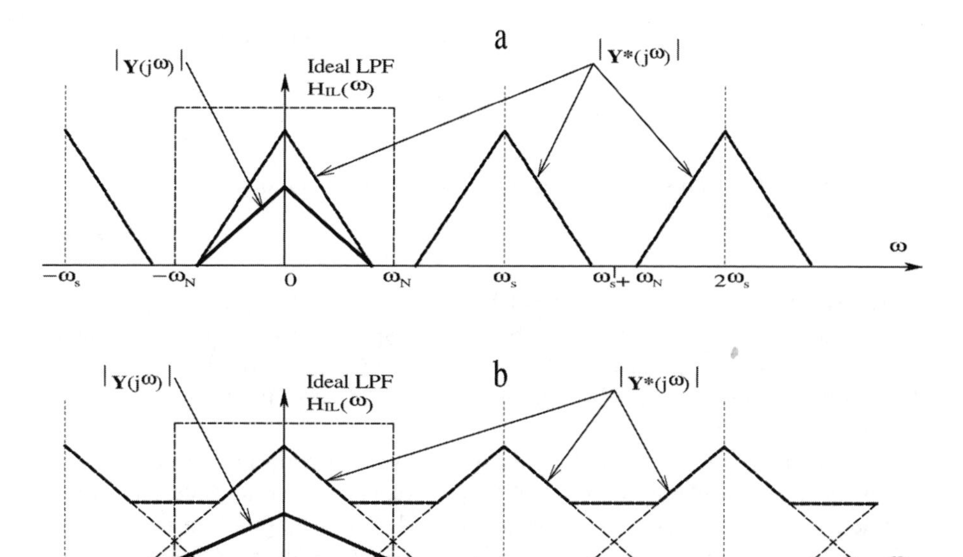

FIGURE 5.1

(a) Fourier spectrum of a periodically sampled analog signal, $y(t)$, containing no frequency components above the Nyquist frequency $f_N = \frac{1}{2T}$ Hz. Note that the magnitude of the sampled spectrum is periodic in frequency, repeating at $\pm$ integer multiples of the sampling frequency, $f_s = 1/T$. (b) Fourier spectrum of a periodically-sampled analog signal, $y(t)$, containing frequency components above the Nyquist frequency $f_N = \frac{1}{2T}$ Hz. Note the overlap of the periodic sampled spectra; this represents lost information by aliasing. $\omega_n = 2\pi f_N$.

component is centered around an integer multiple of the sampling frequency, $k\omega_s$. $\mathbf{Y}(j\omega)$ can, in theory, be recovered from $\mathbf{Y}^*(j\omega)$ by passing the $\mathbf{Y}^*(j\omega)$ spectrum through an ideal low-pass filter with unity gain spanning $\pm\omega_s/2$ (also known as the Nyquist range), *providing the high-frequency ends of the individual component sampled signal spectra do not overlap.* When the spectral components do overlap, as shown in Figure 5.1b, the condition known as *aliasing* is present and information is lost from $y^*(t)$. To ensure that aliasing cannot occur, either inherently $|\mathbf{Y}(j\omega)| \to 0$ for $\omega \geq \omega_s/2$, or $y(t)$ must be passed through an analog low-pass *antialiasing filter* to satisfy $|\mathbf{Y}(j\omega)| \to 0$ for $\omega \geq \omega_s/2$. Note that $\omega_s/2$ is called the periodically sampled signal's *Nyquist frequency,* ω_N.

5.3.3 The Sampling Theorem

The *sampling theorem* describes the analog filter required to recover an analog signal, $y(t)$, from its impulse-modulated (sampled) form, $y^*(t)$. The theorem states that if the highest frequency present in the CFT of $y(t)$ is f_{max}, then when $y(t)$ is sampled at a rate $f_s = 2f_{max}$, $y(t)$ can be exactly recovered from $y^*(t)$ by passing $y^*(t)$ through an *ideal low-pass filter,* $\mathbf{H_{IL}}(2\pi f)$.

The weighting function of $\mathbf{H_{IL}}(2\pi f)$ is [Proakis and Manolakis, 1989]:

$$h_{IL}(t) = \frac{\sin(2\pi f_{max} t)}{2\pi f_{max} t} \tag{5.24}$$

Thus, in the time domain, $y(t)$ is given by the real convolution:

$$y(t) = y^*(t) \otimes h_{IL}(t) \tag{5.25}$$

The sampling rate, $f_s = 2f_{max}$ must be at least twice the highest frequency of the signal, $y(t)$. Note that many $y(t)$s can have spectra in which their rms value approaches zero asymptotically as $f \to \infty$. In this case, the Nyquist frequency can be chosen to be the value at which the rms value of $y(t)$ is some fraction of its max value, e.g., say $1/10^3$, or -60 dB.

Note that $\mathbf{H_{IL}}(2\pi f)$ is an *ideal* LPF and is not physically realizable. In practice, the sampling rate is made three to five times f_{max} to compensate for the finite attenuation characteristics of the antialiasing low-pass filter and for any "long tail" on the spectrum of $y(t)$. Even so, some small degree of aliasing is often present in $\mathbf{Y}^*(j2\pi f)$.

5.4 The Analytical Signal and the Hilbert Transform

5.4.1 Introduction

The *analytical signal,* $\mathbf{g_a}(t)$, is defined as a *complex function of time* derived from a *real signal,* $g(t)$. When $\mathbf{g_a}(t)$ is Fourier transformed, $\mathbf{G_a}(\omega < 0)$ curiously has no negative frequency spectrum. That is, $\mathbf{G_a}(\omega < 0) \equiv 0$.

The *Hilbert transform* (HT) is used to calculate the analytic signal of a real signal, as described below. The HT and analytic signal have been found to be useful in envelope detection of amplitude and phase modulated sinusoidal signals, in the analysis of harmonic distortion produced in nonlinear systems and in wavelet-based signal processing in which a pair of wavelets form an HT pair [Selesnick, 2001]. The HT has also been applied successfully to improve images in three-dimensional differential interference contrast microscopy of chromosomes [Arnison et al., 2000]. Feldman (1997) has shown that the Hilbert transform and analytical signal approach can be used to analyze nonlinear free mechanical vibrations. Using this approach in the time domain, Feldman demonstrated that the instantaneous undamped natural frequency of the system could be extracted as well as its real, nonlinear elastic force characteristics. Feldman's approach may have utility in characterizing heart sounds.

5.4.2 The Hilbert transform and the analytical signal

This section will describe the mathematical relations between the analytical signal and the Hilbert transform. If a real signal, $g(t)$, is defined over $-\infty \le t \le \infty$ and has a CFT $\mathbf{G}(\omega)$, then the *analytical signal* of $g(t)$ is given by: $\mathbf{g_a}(t) = g(t) + \mathbf{j}\,\mathcal{h}g(t)$, where $hg(t)$ is the *Hilbert transform* of $g(t)$. Note that the analytical signal is, in general, complex. The vector $\mathbf{g_a}(t)$ can also be written in polar form:

$$\mathbf{g_a}(t) = A(t)e^{j\psi(t)} \tag{5.26}$$

Where the magnitude, $A(t) = \sqrt{g^2(t) + hg^2(t)}$ and the angle of $\mathbf{g_a}(t)$ is $\psi(t) = \tan^{-1}[hg(t)/g(t)]$. The *instantaneous energy* in the analytical signal is $E(t) \equiv A^2(t)$. If $g(t)$ is an amplitude-modulated, constant-frequency pure sinusoid, $A(t)$ is an *envelope detector*. The *instantaneous frequency* of the analytical signal is defined as:

$$f_i(t) \equiv \frac{d\psi(t)}{dt} \tag{5.27}$$

The analytical signal can also be found from the inverse Fourier transform of the positive frequency part of $\mathbf{G}(\omega)$. (Note the lower limit of integration is zero because the analytical signal has no negative frequency part. See Equations 5.28 and 5.29.)

$$\mathbf{g_a}(t) = (1/\pi)\int_0^\infty \mathbf{G}(\omega)e^{j\omega t}\,d\omega = 1/2\int_0^\infty \mathbf{G}(j2\pi f)\exp(j2\pi ft)\,df, \quad f = \omega/2\pi \tag{5.28}$$

In the frequency domain, the analytical signal can be expressed by:

$$\mathbf{G_a}(\omega) = \mathbf{G}(\omega)[1 - j\,\mathrm{sgn}(\omega)] \text{ or } \mathbf{G_a}(\omega) = 2U(\omega)\mathbf{G}(\omega) \tag{5.29}$$

Note that the analytical signal has zero spectral energy for $\omega < 0$. The name "analytical signal" comes from complex variable theory because it can be shown that the sampled $\mathbf{g_a}(t)$'s z-transform has no poles inside the unit circle on the complex z-plane. That is, $\mathbf{G_a}(z)$ is analytic in the unit circle.

The *Hilbert transform* of the real signal, $g(t)$, is defined as the imaginary part of the analytical signal. It is given by the real convolution integral:

$$hg(t) = (1/\pi)\int_{-\infty}^{\infty} \frac{g(\tau)}{(t-\tau)}\,d\tau = (1/\pi)\int_{-\infty}^{\infty} \frac{g(t-\tau)}{\tau}\,d\tau \tag{5.30}$$

and its inverse transform can be written [Guillemin, 1949]:

$$g(t) = (-1/\pi)\int_{-\infty}^{\infty} \frac{hg(\tau)}{t-\tau}\,d\tau \tag{5.31}$$

The discrete form of the HT can be written:

$$hg(n) = (1/\pi)\sum_{k=-\infty}^{\infty} \frac{g(k)}{n-k} \tag{5.32}$$

Let us examine the analytical signal in the frequency domain. The CFT of the analytical signal can be written:

$$\mathbf{G_a}(\omega) = \mathbf{G}(\omega) + j\boldsymbol{h}\mathbf{G}(\omega) = 2U(\omega)\mathbf{G}(\omega) \tag{5.33}$$

Where $\mathrm{U}(\omega)$ is the real unit step in ω; i.e., $\mathrm{U}(\omega) = 1$ for $\omega \geq 0$ and 0 for $\omega < 0$. When we solve Equation 5.33 for the CFT of $h\mathrm{g}(\mathrm{t})$, we find:

$$\boldsymbol{h}\mathbf{G}(\omega) = -\mathrm{j}\,\mathrm{sgn}(\omega)\mathbf{G}(\omega) \tag{5.34}$$

Where the signum function in ω is real and equal to $+1$ for $\omega > 0$, 0 for $\omega = 0$ and -1 for $\omega < 0$.

(Note that multiplying the vector $\mathbf{G}(\omega)$ by -1 is equivalent to subtracting a fixed π radians from its angle and multiplying it by **j** shifts the phase of $\mathbf{G}(\omega)$ by $+\pi/2$ radians. So, for $\omega < 0$, $+\pi/2$ radians is added to $\angle\mathbf{G}(\omega)$ and for $\omega > 0$, $-\pi/2$ radians is added to $\angle\mathbf{G}(\omega)$.

5.4.3 Properties of the Hilbert transform

1. The HT of a real $\mathrm{g}(\mathrm{t})$ is real.
2. The HT of an even function is an odd function and conversely, the HT of an odd $\mathrm{g}(\mathrm{t})$ is an even function.
3. The HT of an HT is the negative of the original $\mathrm{g}(\mathrm{t})$. That is: $\mathbf{HT}\{\mathbf{HT}[\mathrm{g}(\mathrm{t})]\} = -\mathrm{g}(\mathrm{t})$.
4. $\int_{-\infty}^{\infty} \mathrm{g}_1(\mathrm{t}+\tau)\mathrm{g}_2(\tau)\,\mathrm{d}\tau = \int_{-\infty}^{\infty} h\mathrm{g}_1(\mathrm{t}+\tau)h\mathrm{g}_2(\tau)\,\mathrm{d}\tau$
5. Taking the CFT of both sides of Equation 5, we have: $\mathbf{G}_1(\omega)\mathbf{G}_2(-\omega) = \boldsymbol{h}\mathbf{G}_1(\omega)\boldsymbol{h}\mathbf{G}_2(-\omega)$ [Papoulis, 1968].
6. The HT of the real convolution of two time functions is equal to the convolution of one with the HT of the other. That is: $HT\{\mathrm{f}(\mathrm{t}) \otimes \mathrm{g}(\mathrm{t})\} = \mathrm{f}(\mathrm{t}) \otimes h\mathrm{g}(\mathrm{t}) = \mathrm{g}(\mathrm{t}) \otimes h\mathrm{f}(\mathrm{t})$.
7. $\int_{-\infty}^{\infty} \mathrm{g}^2(\mathrm{t})\,\mathrm{dt} = \int_{-\infty}^{\infty} h\mathrm{g}^2(\mathrm{t})\,\mathrm{dt}$
8. If $\mathrm{g}(\mathrm{t}) \overset{\mathrm{CFT}}{\Longleftrightarrow} \mathbf{G}(\omega)$ and $h\mathrm{g}(\mathrm{t}) \overset{\mathrm{CFT}}{\Longleftrightarrow} \boldsymbol{h}\mathbf{G}(\omega)$, then $-\mathrm{sgn}(\omega)\mathbf{G}(\omega) = \boldsymbol{h}\mathbf{G}(\omega)$.
9. If $\mathrm{g}(\mathrm{t})$ is even, then $\mathrm{G}(\omega)$ is real, hence $h\mathrm{g}(\mathrm{t})$ is odd and is given by [Papoulis, 1968]: $h\mathrm{g}(\mathrm{t}) = \frac{1}{\pi}\int_0^{\infty} \mathrm{G}(\omega)\sin(\omega\mathrm{t})\,\mathrm{d}\omega$

Some HTs of common $\mathrm{g}(\mathrm{t})$s are given in Table 5.2.

Next, let us examine the use of the Hilbert definite integral in calculating HTs.

Example 1

Let us find the analytical signal for the signal, $\mathrm{g}(\mathrm{t}) = \mathrm{M}\cos(\omega_{\mathrm{o}}\mathrm{t})$. The Hilbert transform of this $\mathrm{g}(\mathrm{t})$ is:

$$h\mathrm{g}(\mathrm{t}) = (1/\pi)\int_{-\infty}^{\infty} \frac{\mathrm{M}\cos(\omega_{\mathrm{o}}\tau)}{\mathrm{t}-\tau}\,\mathrm{d}\tau \tag{5.35}$$

TABLE 5.2
Some Hilbert Transforms of Simple Signals.

Time function, g(t)	Hilbert transform, $hg(t)$
$g(t) \otimes (1/\pi t) = \int_{-\infty}^{\infty} \frac{g(\tau)}{\pi(t-\tau)} d\tau \rightarrow$	$hg(t)$
$\delta(t)$	$1/(\pi t)$
$1/t$	$-\pi\delta(t)$
$\cos(\omega t)$	$-\sin(\omega t)$
$\sin(\omega t)$	$\cos(\omega t)$
$(\omega/\pi)\frac{\sin(\omega t)}{\omega t}$	$\frac{[1-\cos(\omega t)]}{\pi t}$
$\frac{1}{1+t^2}$	$\frac{t}{1+t^2}$
rect(t) $\text{rect}(t) = 1$ for $\lvert t\rvert \leq 1/2$ $\text{rect}(t) = 0$ for $\lvert t\rvert > 1/2$	$-(1/\pi)\ln\left\lvert\frac{t-1/2}{t+1/2}\right\rvert$
$m(t)\cos(\omega t)$ (DSBSC modulation)	$m(t)\sin(\omega t)$
$m(t)\sin(\omega t)$ (DSBSC modulation)	$-m(t)\cos(\omega t)$

Now define a new variable, $u \equiv t - \tau$. Note that $d\tau = -du$ and $\tau = t + u$. Thus, we can write:

$$hg(t) = (1/\pi)\int_{-\infty}^{\infty} \frac{M\cos[\omega_o(t+u)]}{u}(-du) \tag{5.36}$$

The real integral above can be solved by using the trig identity, $\cos(\alpha+\beta) \equiv \cos\alpha\cos\beta - \sin\alpha\sin\beta$. Where $\alpha = \omega_o t$, and $\beta = \omega_o u$. Note that $\cos(\theta) = \cos(-\theta)$ (even function) and $-\sin(\theta) = \sin(-\theta)$ (odd function). Now we have:

$$hg(t) = \frac{M\cos(\omega_o t)}{\pi}\int_{-\infty}^{\infty} \frac{\cos(\omega_o u)}{u}(-du) - \frac{M\sin(\omega_o t)}{\pi} \times \int_{-\infty}^{\infty} \frac{\sin(\omega_o u)}{u}(-du) \tag{5.37}$$

The first integral is an *odd function* around u (a product of an even function times an odd function) and thus integrates to zero. The second integral is an odd function times an odd function and thus is even. Its integral is finite and is of the form,

$$\int_{0}^{\infty} \frac{\sin(ax)}{x} dx = \pi/2, \tag{5.38}$$

for $a > 0$, so considering the limits of Equation 5.37, the final HT of the cosine $g(t)$ is:

$$hg(t) = M\sin(\omega_o t) \tag{5.39}$$

Thus, using the Euler relations, the complex analytical signal for $g(t) = M\cos(\omega_o t)$ is simply:

$$\mathbf{g_a}(t) = g(t) + j\,hg(t) = M\cos(\omega_o t) + \mathbf{j}M\sin(\omega_o t) = M\frac{e^{j\omega_o t} + e^{-j\omega_o t}}{2} + Mj\frac{e^{j\omega_o t} - e^{-j\omega_o t}}{2j} = M\exp(+j\omega_o t) \quad (5.40)$$

Note that the CFT of $\mathbf{g_a}(t) = M\exp(+j\omega_o t)$ is simply $\mathbf{G_a}(\omega) = M2\pi\delta(\omega - \omega_o)$. That is, it is a single impulse in the frequency domain at $\omega = \omega_o > 0$. Also, the CFT of $g(t) = M\cos(\omega_o t)$ is

$$\mathbf{G}(\omega) = \pi M[\delta(\omega + \omega_o) + \delta(\omega - \omega_o)] \quad (5.41)$$

That is, two impulses exist at $\omega = \pm\omega_o$.

Example 2

Consider the even rectangular pulse signal, $g(t) = 1$ for $-\delta \le t \le \delta$ and 0 for $|t| > \delta$. We write its HT as:

$$hg(t) = (1/\pi)\int_{-\delta}^{\delta} \frac{1}{t - \tau}\,d\tau \quad (5.42)$$

This integral is of the form:

$$\int \frac{dx}{bx + a} = (1/b)\ln|(bx + a)| \quad (5.43)$$

where $x = \tau$, $b = -1$ and $a = t$. Thus, the definite integral Equation 5.42 can be written:

$$hg(t) = (1/\pi)[-\ln|-\delta + t| - (-\ln|-(-\delta) + t|) = (1/\pi)\ln\left|\frac{t + \delta}{t - \delta}\right|, \quad -\delta \le t \le \delta \quad (5.44)$$

Example 3

Now, consider the odd ramp function, $g(t) = (M/\delta)t$, for $-\delta \le t \le \delta$ and 0 for $|t| > \delta$. Its HT can be written:

$$hg(t) = (1/\pi)\int_{-\delta}^{\delta} \frac{(M/\delta)\tau}{t - \tau}\,d\tau \quad (5.45)$$

The integral of Equation 5.45 is of the general form:

$$\int \frac{x\,dx}{bx + a} = (1/b^2)[(a + bx) - a\ln|bx + a|] \quad (5.46)$$

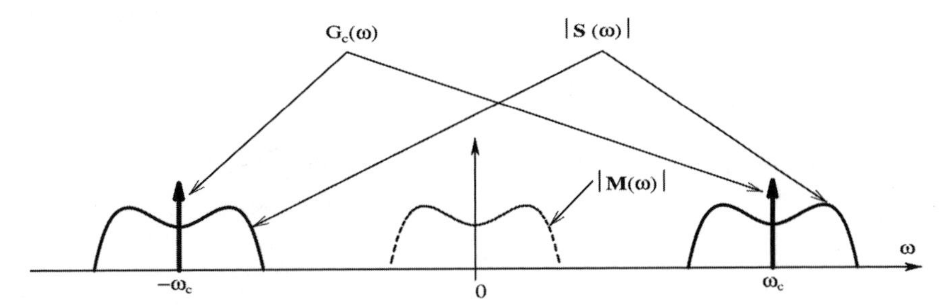

FIGURE 5.2
Plot of the spectral magnitudes of the cosine carrier, $g_c(t) = \cos(\omega_c t)$, the modulating signal, $m(t)$ and the DSBSC modulated signal, $s(t) = m(t)\cos(\omega_c t)$.

where: $x = \tau$, $a = t$, and $b = -1$. Evaluating the definite integral, Equation 5.46, we find:

$$\begin{aligned} hg(t) &= (M/\delta\pi)\{(t-\delta) - t\ln|t-\delta| - [t-(-\delta)] + t\ln|t-(-\delta)|\} \\ &= (M/\delta\pi)\left\{-2\delta + t\ln\left[\frac{t+\delta}{t-\delta}\right]\right\} \end{aligned} \tag{5.47}$$

Example 4

Let us find the analytical signal of a *double-sideband suppressed-carrier* (DSBSC) modulated signal. The DSBSC modulation scheme is widely used in instrumentation, such as in photonic systems containing light choppers, Wheatstone strain gauge bridges driven by a/c sources and in LVDT length measuring systems [Northrop, 1997]. The modulated DSBSC signal can be represented mathematically by $s(t) = m(t)\cos(\omega_c t)$. The carrier is $g_c(t) \equiv \cos(\omega_c t)$. The modulating signal is low-pass in nature; its highest frequency is $<< \omega_c$. Figure 5.2 shows the magnitude of the spectra of the cosine carrier, the modulating signal and the modulated signal, $s(t)$. The complex analytical signal corresponding to $s(t)$ is just:

$$\mathbf{s_a}(t) = s(t) + j\,hs(t) \tag{5.48}$$

The HT of the modulated DSBSC signal can be written, assuming that $\mathbf{M}(\omega)$ is low-pass [Papoulis, 1968]:

$$hs(t) = m(t)hg_c(t) = m(t)\sin(\omega_c t) \tag{5.49}$$

Papoulis shows that the relation above is valid as long as $\mathbf{M}(\omega)\mathbf{G_c}(\omega) = 0$. This condition is certainly met for $m(t) = m_o\cos(\omega_m t)$ and, in general, is approximated as long as the highest frequency in the spectrum of $m(t)$ is $<< \omega_c$. Now the CFT of $\mathbf{s_a}(t)$ can be written:

$$\begin{aligned} F\{\mathbf{s_a}(t)\} &= F\{m(t)\cos(\omega_c t) + \mathbf{j}m(t)\sin(\omega_c t)\} = 1/2[\mathbf{M}(\omega+\omega_c) + \mathbf{M}(\omega-\omega_c)] \\ &\quad + \mathbf{j}(j/2)[\mathbf{M}(\omega+\omega_c) - \mathbf{M}(\omega-\omega_c)] \end{aligned} \tag{5.50}$$

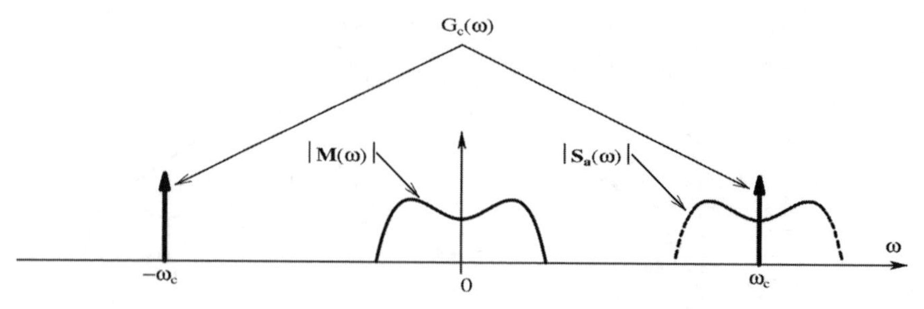

FIGURE 5.3
Plot of the spectral magnitudes of the cosine carrier, $g_c(t) = \cos(\omega_c t)$, the modulating signal, $m(t)$ and the analytical signal of $s(t)$. That is, the spectrum of $\mathbf{s_a}(t) = s(t) + j\,hs(t)$. Note that $|\mathbf{S_a}(\omega)|$ only exists for positive ω around $+\omega_c$.

$$\mathbf{S_a}(\omega) = \mathbf{M}(\omega - \omega_c)$$

$\mathbf{M}(\omega - \omega_c)$ exists only for $\omega \geq 0$, and is centered around $\omega = \omega_c$. Figure 5.3 illustrates the spectra of $\mathbf{M}(\omega)$, $\mathbf{G_c}(\omega)$ and $\mathbf{S_a}(\omega)$.

Now consider the DSBSC signal when the carrier is also angle-modulated at a low frequency (the angle modulation can be FM or PhM (see Section 1.1.5). This modulation can be expressed as:

$$s(t) = m(t)\cos[\omega_c t + \varphi(t)] \tag{5.51}$$

The complex analytical signal for this $s(t)$ can be shown to be:

$$\mathbf{s_a}(t) = m(t)\{\cos[\omega_c t + \varphi(t)] + j\sin[\omega_c t + \varphi(t)]\} \tag{5.52}$$

By the Euler relation:

$$\mathbf{s_a}(t) = m(t)\exp[j(\omega_c t + \varphi(t))] = [m(t)\exp(j\varphi(t))]\exp(j\omega_c t) \tag{5.53}$$

The factor in brackets, $\mathbf{a}(t) = [m(t)\exp(j\varphi(t))]$, is called the *complex envelope* or the *low-pass equivalent signal.* The complex analytical signal, $\mathbf{s_a}(t)$, is a bandpass signal with a one-sided spectrum. If we take the CFT of $\mathbf{s_a}(t)$, we find:

$$\mathbf{S_a}(\omega) = \mathbf{A}(\omega - \omega_c) \tag{5.54}$$

5.4.4 An Application of the Hilbert Transform

An interesting application of the Hilbert transform and analytical signal is to test the linearity of a system by the calculation of the *instantaneous energy* of the output of the system under test when its input is a pure sinusoid. The instantaneous energy of a signal is defined by [Leonhard, 2001]:

$$E^2(t) \equiv y^2(t) + [hy(t)]^2 \tag{5.55}$$

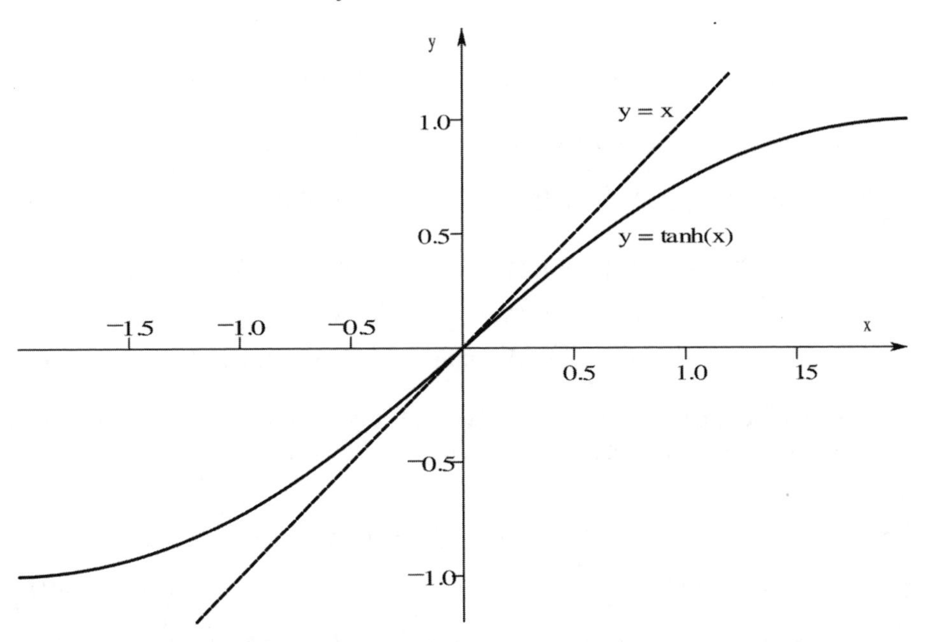

FIGURE 5.4
Plot of the odd saturating nonlinear function, $y = \tanh(x)$.

In the first example, the system is linear with no phase shift. Its input is $x(t) = A\cos(\omega_o t)$, and the output is $y(t) = KA\cos(\omega_o t)$. This system transfer function and that for the $\tan h(x)$ nonlinearity described below are shown in Figure 5.4. Thus, the instantaneous energy is:

$$E^2(t) = K^2A^2\cos^2(\omega_o t) + K^2A^2\sin^2(\omega_o t) \tag{5.56}$$

The second term is the square of the Hilbert transform of $y(t)$. Using trig identities, we find:

$$E^2(t) = (K^2A^2/2)[1 + \cos(2\omega_o t)] + (K^2A^2/2)[1 - \cos(2\omega_o t)] = K^2A^2 \tag{5.57}$$

Thus, we see that, in the case of a linear system with no distortion, the instantaneous energy of the output is a constant. Next, consider a nonlinear system with a symmetrical soft transfer function such that the output is given by $y(t) = \tanh[Kx(t)]$. Because the nonlinearity is soft, we can approximate the $\tanh(*)$ function by the first two terms of its MacLaurin's series.

$$y(t) = \tanh[Kx(t)] \cong Kx(t) - \frac{K^3x^3(t)}{3}$$
$$\downarrow$$
$$y(t) = KA\cos(\omega_o t) - \frac{K^3A^3}{3}\cos^3(\omega_o t) = KA\cos(\omega_o t) - \frac{K^3A^3}{12}[\cos(3\omega_o t) - 3\cos(\omega_o t)]$$

$$\downarrow$$
$$y(t) = KA(1 - 1/4K^2A^2)\cos(\omega_o t) - K^3A^3/(12)\cos(3\omega_o t) \quad (5.58)$$

The Hilbert transform of the distorted $y(t)$ is easily written:

$$hy(t) = KA(1 - 1/4K^2A^2)\sin(\omega_o t) - K^3A^3/(12)\sin(3\omega_o t) \quad (5.59)$$

Now the instantaneous energy in $y(t)$ is found as above in Equation 5.55:

$$\begin{aligned} E^2(t) = {} & [KA(1 - 1/4K^2A^2)\cos(\omega_o t) - K^3A^3/(12)\cos(3\omega_o t)]^2 \\ & +[KA(1 - 1/4K^2A^2)\sin(\omega_o t) - K^3A^3/(12)\sin(3\omega_o t]^2 \end{aligned} \quad (5.60)$$

Squaring the terms in Equation 5.60, then using trig functions and collecting terms, is a tedious amount of algebra. I will not terrorize my readers by repeating it here. The final result is:

$$\begin{aligned} E^2(t) = {} & [K^2A^2 - K^4A^4(1/2) + k^6A^6(1/16 + 1/144)] - (K^4A^4/6)(1 - K^2A^2/4) \\ & \times \cos(2\omega_o t) \end{aligned} \quad (5.61)$$

No fourth or sixth harmonic terms appear; they cancel out when adding the expanded $y^2(t)$ and $hy^2(t)$ terms. The presence of a nonzero second harmonic term signifies distortion is present in the output, albeit an odd-function distortion.

One way to calculate $E^2(t)$ is to excite the system under test with a pure sine wave and sample, digitize and store a steady-state record of the system's output, $y(n)$. (N samples are stored in an epoch.) $y(n)$ is squared to give $y^2(n)$, which is stored in an array. Next, $y(n)$ is windowed and its DFT is computed (generally by FFT) to give $\mathbf{Y}(k)$. Next, a point-by-point complex multiplication is performed on $\mathbf{Y}(k)$ by $\mathbf{H}(k)$. $\mathbf{H}(k) = 0 + j1$ for $0 \leq k \leq (N/2 - 1)$ and $\mathbf{H}(k) = 0 - j1$ for $N/2 \leq k \leq (N - 1)$. The complex product of $\mathbf{Y}(k)\mathbf{H}(k)$ is then inverse DFTd to finally yield the Hilbert transform of $y(n)$, $hy(n)$. $hy(n)$ is squared and its terms are added to $y^2(n)$ to give $E^2(n)$, which can then be analyzed for nondc terms, indicating nonlinearity and distortion in the output signal. This process is shown in Figure 5.5.

The conventional way of examining output harmonics produced by system distortion is to sample the steady-state output, $y(t)$, when the system is given a pure sinusoidal input. $y(n)$ is organized into M epochs, each of N samples. Each epoch of $\{y(n)\}$ is DFTd to give $\mathbf{Y_p}(k)$, then $|\mathbf{Y_p}(k)|^2$ is computed for each epoch. Then the average power spectrum is calculated:

$$\overline{|\mathbf{Y}(k)|^2} = (1/M)\sum_{p=1}^{M} |\mathbf{Y_p}(k)|^2 \quad \text{mean-squared volts/Hz} \quad (5.62)$$

In practice, N might be 2048, and $M = 32$. Often, the rms spectrum is displayed in which the square root of each value of $\overline{|\mathbf{Y}(k)|^2}$ is taken; its units are rms volts/$\sqrt{\text{Hz}}$. The advantage of presenting the spectrum or root power spectrum of the output signal is that the exact frequencies where the harmonics occur are displayed, as well as their relative magnitudes.

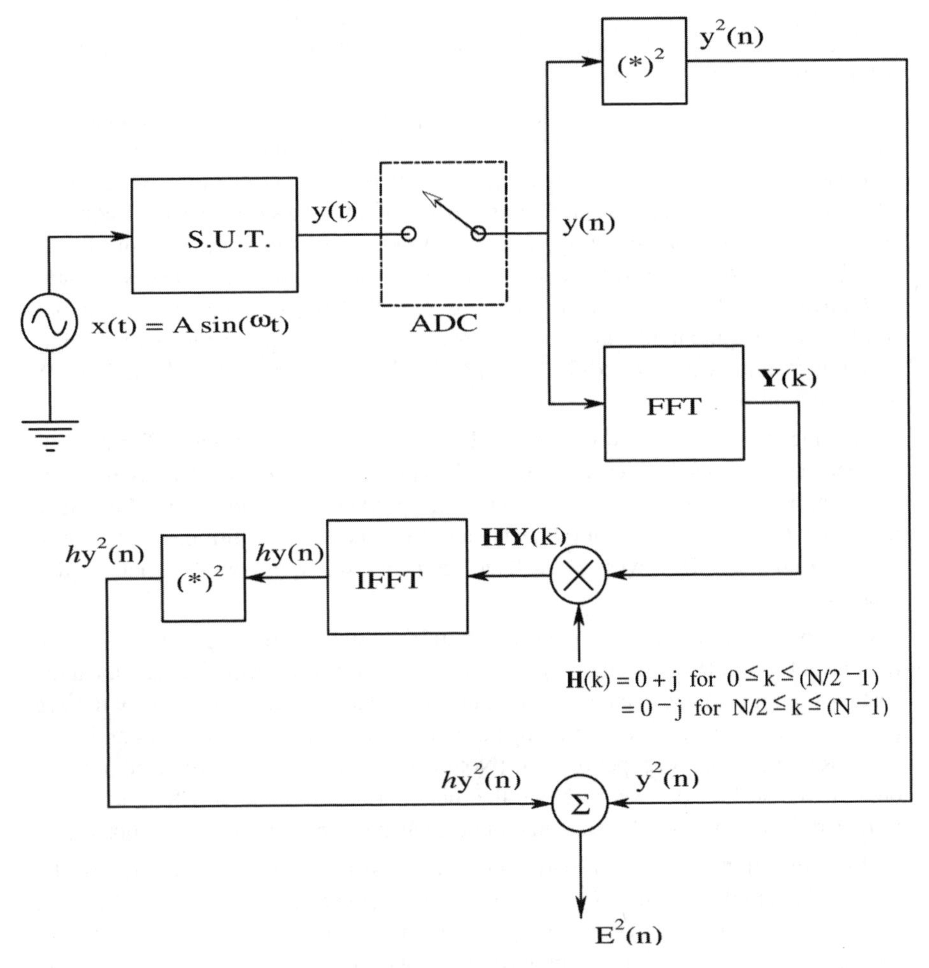

FIGURE 5.5
Block diagram of a discrete system that uses the Hilbert transform to test for nonlinearity in the output, $y(t)$, of a system given a sinusoidal input. The discrete Hilbert transform of $y(n)$ is found, squared and then added to the squared array, $y^2(n)$ to form $E^2(n)$, whose terms are analyzed. See text for description of the process.

5.5 The Modulation Transfer Function in Imaging

5.5.1 Introduction

Optical and other kinds of photon-based imaging systems (X-ray, PET, MRI, SPECT, etc.) have increasing importance in medical diagnosis and therapy. This section will examine the use of Fourier transform theory in evaluating imaging system performance, specifically their spatial resolution (i.e., their ability to resolve fine detail in the system's object).

One way to evaluate an imaging system's performance is to examine its *spatial frequency response,* where spatial frequency is an attribute of the object and image; it is measured in radians/mm, radians/degree, or cycles/mm (instead of r/sec or Hz for a temporal system). To justify further discussion of imaging system spatial frequency response, we will assume that the imaging systems under consideration are linear, i.e., they obey the properties listed in Section 2.1, which include *superposition* and *shift invariance.* In reality, imaging systems, especially those using CRT phosphors, or film, can be quite nonlinear over an expanded range of input parameters. Optical imaging systems can also exhibit nonlinearity from imperfections (aberrations) in lenses and mirrors.

Imaging systems are describable in 3-D spatial coordinate systems. Their inputs (objects) and outputs (images) can be described in terms of properties such as intensity, wavelength, polarization, etc., in rectangular, x,y planes or surfaces, or, alternately, in polar r, θ space. Images and objects can also vary in time, forming 4-D, spatio-temporal signals. However, we will not consider spatio-temporal signals in this section.

If we present a linear imaging system with a spatial impulse input, $[\mathrm{I_m}\delta(\mathrm{x})\delta(\mathrm{y})]$ (i.e., a spot of light), a spatial distribution of intensity, $\mathrm{i}(\mathrm{x},\mathrm{y})$, will be observed at the system's output (image) plane. The output image can be viewed directly by the eye (e.g., as with an endoscope, a telescope or a microscope), or can appear as an image on a CRT, or be seen on paper or film. (Note that the image can be projected in focus on a curved surface (the eye's retina, the inner surface of a curved CRT), however, film, certain sensors, and flat-screen computer displays present flat image planes.)

When the input (object) is a spatial impulse, the system's output (image) intensity, $\mathrm{h}(\mathrm{x},\mathrm{y})$, is called its *spatial impulse response* or *point spread function* [Papoulis, 1968]. An LTI imaging system's output image is given, in general, by the *2-D real convolution* of $\mathrm{h}(\mathrm{x},\mathrm{y})$ with any input (object) function.

$$\mathrm{i}(\mathrm{x},\mathrm{y}) = \mathrm{o}(\mathrm{x},\mathrm{y}) \otimes\otimes \mathrm{h}(\mathrm{x},\mathrm{y}) \tag{5.63}$$

In the spatial frequency domain, Equation 5.63 becomes:

$$\mathbf{I}(\mathrm{u},\mathrm{v}) = \mathbf{O}(\mathrm{u},\mathrm{v})\,\mathbf{H}(\mathrm{u},\mathrm{v}) \tag{5.64}$$

Where $\mathbf{I}(\mathrm{u},\mathrm{v}), \mathbf{O}(\mathrm{u},\mathrm{v})$ and $\mathbf{H}(\mathrm{u},\mathrm{v})$ are the 2-D, spatial, CFTs of $\mathrm{i}(\mathrm{x},\mathrm{y})$, $\mathrm{o}(\mathrm{x},\mathrm{y})$, and $\mathrm{h}(\mathrm{x},\mathrm{y})$, respectively. u and v are orthogonal spatial frequencies in radians/mm or radians/degree. It is often convenient to consider $\mathrm{h}(\mathrm{x},\mathrm{y})$ as even in x and y, so $\mathbf{H}(\mathrm{u},\mathrm{v})$ will be real. As a further simplification, we sometimes assume x,y isomorphism and do our Fourier analysis in the x-dimension only. (This is a weak assumption as the properties of a 2-D system with radial symmetry are not exactly the same as a 1-D system [Papoulis, 1968]).

5.5.2 The MTF

The *modulation transfer function* (MTF) is widely used as measure of imaging resolution. It is generally defined in one dimension for simplicity. To obtain the MFT experimentally, we examine the imaging system's *spatial sinusoidal frequency response,* $\mathbf{H}(u,v)$, in one dimension; that is, $\mathbf{H}(u,0)$. The object is assumed to be a 1-D, spatial intensity sine wave:

$$o(x) = (I_{om}/2)[1+\cos(u_o x)], \quad u_o \text{ in r/mm}; \quad u_o = 2\pi/\lambda \tag{5.65}$$

The dc or average component of object intensity is required because $o(x)$ is light, electromagnetic, or ionizing radiation *intensity,* and is necessarily nonnegative. λ is the period of the spatial sine wave. In the Fourier domain, the object transform is:

$$\mathbf{O}(w) = \int_{-\infty}^{\infty} o(x)\exp(-jux)\,dx = (I_{om}/2)\{2\pi\delta(u) + \pi[\delta(u-u_o) + \delta(u+u_o)]\} \tag{5.66}$$

We are interested in the x-dimension, steady-state (SS), sinusoidal response of the imaging system. The SS system output is the 1-D *image;* it can be written in general as:

$$i(x) = (\mathbf{I}_{im}/2)\{1+\cos[u_o x + \varphi(u_o)]\} \tag{5.67}$$

The linear imaging system's *SS spatial frequency response* is thus defined to be:

$$\mathbf{H}(u_o) \equiv \frac{\mathbf{I}_{im}}{\mathbf{I}_{om}}\angle\varphi(u_o) = |\mathbf{H}(u_o)|\angle\varphi(u_o), \ u_o \text{ is a specific spatial frequency.} \tag{5.68}$$

$\mathbf{H}(u_o)$ is also called the complex (vector) *optical transfer function* (OTF) evaluated at $u = u_o$ [Spring and Davidson, 2001]. Figure 5.6 illustrates a 100%-contrast 1-D spatial sinewave object; Figure 5.7 shows the image after passing through a *linear, space-invariant* (LSI) imaging system. Note the loss of contrast due to the fact that the output sine wave is attenuated by the frequency response, $\mathbf{H}(u)$, which is in general, low-pass.

The MTF of the system in the x direction is defined as the normalized *magnitude of the OTF:*

$$\text{MTF}(u) \equiv \frac{|\mathbf{H}(u,0)|}{|\mathbf{H}(0)|} \tag{5.69}$$

Most MTFs are 1 at $u = 0$ r/mm, and fall off monotonically with increasing u until they reach 0 at some u_{co}. The published MTFs of certain photographic films, e.g., Fujichrome Velvia^{TM}, are unusual in that they begin at 1 at $u/2\pi = 0$ cycles/mm, gradually rise to c. 1.25 at 10 cycles/ mm, fall to unity at c. 20 cycles/mm, then drop off sharply to be 0.06 at 200 cycles/mm, etc. The peaking of the MTF(u) for this film may be due to a thin-film (emulsion) photochemical effect during development [Koren, 2001]. If this MTF were the Bode plot of a temporal filter, we would be

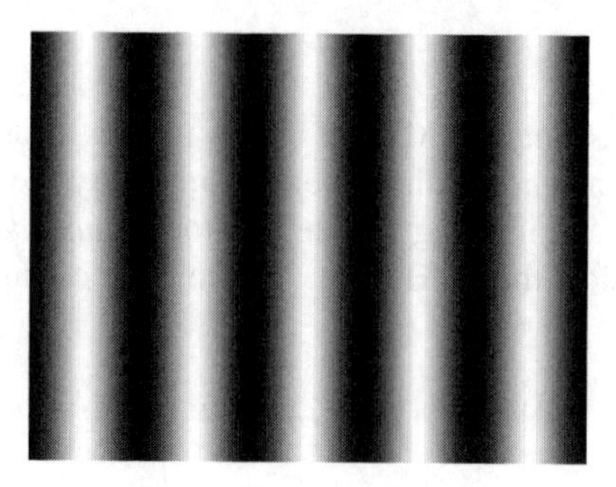

FIGURE 5.6

A 1-D, 100% contrast, spatial sine wave test object. In the x-direction, its intensity is given by: $I_o = (I_{omax}/2)[1+\sin(u_o x)]$. Note that the maximum I_o is I_{omax} and the minimum is 0, hence the object's contrast is 100%. [Northrop, 2002, CRC.]

tempted to model the response by that of a modestly under-damped, quadratic low-pass filter (one having complex conjugate poles in the s-plane with a damping factor $\xi \cong 0.5$). Optical lens MTFs, on the other hand, generally do not have a peak in their MTF(u) plots; with increasing u, they typically decrease monotonically to a cutoff point.

An alternate definition of the MTF uses the *contrast* of the input(object) and output (image). The *object contrast* or *modulation* is defined as:

$$C_o \equiv \frac{I_{omax} - I_{omin}}{I_{omax} + I_{omin}} \tag{5.70}$$

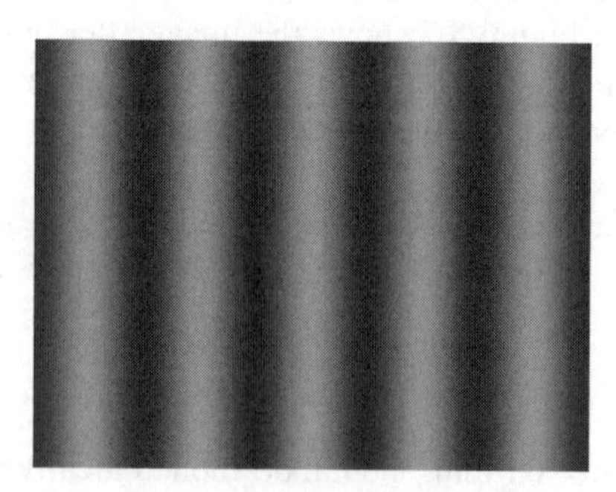

FIGURE 5.7

The imaging system's output (image), given the spatial sine wave input of Figure 5.6. The image intensity in the x-direction is given by: $I_i = (I_{omax}/2)[1+\eta\sin(u_o x)]$. The sinusoidal component of the image is attenuated by a factor of η. Note that $0 \leq \eta \leq 1$ and, in general, η decreases as the object's radian spatial frequency, u_o, increases. The sinusoidal image contrast can easily be shown to be η. (Here we have assumed that the imaging system's transfer function, H(u), is 1 at $u = u_o = 0$.) [Northrop, 2002, CRC.]

And the image contrast or modulation is:

$$C_i \equiv \frac{I_{imax} - I_{imin}}{I_{imax} + I_{imin}} \tag{5.71}$$

Where I_{omax} is the maximum intensity, and I_{omin} is the minimum intensity of the *sinusoidal object,* etc. In general, $0 \le C_o \le 1$ and $C_i \le C_o$. The MTF defined in terms of measured, sinusoidal contrasts is:

$$\mathrm{MTF(u)} \equiv C_i(u)/C_o(u) \tag{5.72}$$

In imaging systems, the spatial impulse response (image from a point source of light (or γ radiation) object) is also called the *point spread function* (PSF), $h(x, y)$. In certain optical imaging systems, the PSF can be observed as an *Airy disk diffraction pattern* [Papoulis, 1968]. The Airy disk image can be modeled in 2-D by the point spread function of Equation 5.73 which has *radial symmetry* (Here we ignore the dc component of the input, required mathematically to prevent $h(r)$ from going negative (intensity is nonnegative)):

$$h(r) = 2a^2 \frac{J_1^2(ar)}{(ar)^2}(I_{im}/2) \tag{5.73}$$

Here, $J_1(*)$ is the Bessel function of the first kind and a is a scaling constant. Papoulis uses the *Hankel transform* to find $\mathbf{H}(w)$ (w is a *radial radian spatial frequency* in r/mm). (If a 2-D function such as $h(r)$ has *circular symmetry,* then its CFT can be found from the Hankel transform.) Thus:

$$\mathbf{H}(w) = (I_{im}/2)(2/\pi)[\cos^{-1}(w/2a) - (w/2a)\sqrt{1 - w^2/(4a^2)}], \tag{5.74A}$$

$$\mathbf{H}(w) = 0 \text{ for } |w| > 2a \tag{5.74B}$$

$$\mathbf{H}(0) = (I_{im}/2) = I_0 \tag{5.74C}$$

Note that $\mathbf{H}(w)$ is real and even in w, and has circular symmetry in w, as shown in Figure 5.8.

Another model for the MTF of an aperture-lens system can be based on the approximate, 1-D x-projection of the Airy disk. This object can be modeled approximately by:

$$h(x) \cong I_{im} \frac{\sin^2(xa/2)}{(xa/2)^2} \tag{5.75}$$

The 1-D, CFT of $h(x)$ is:

$$\mathbf{H}(u) = (2\pi/a)I_{im}[1 - |u|/a], \quad \text{for } |u| \le a, \text{ else } 0. \tag{5.76}$$

This $\mathbf{H}(u)$ is a simple triangle with base width $\pm a$ and peak $I_{im}2\pi/a$. Thus the (normalized) MTF is:

$$\mathrm{MTF(u)} = \mathbf{H}(u)/(I_o 2\pi/a), \quad u \ge 0 \tag{5.77}$$

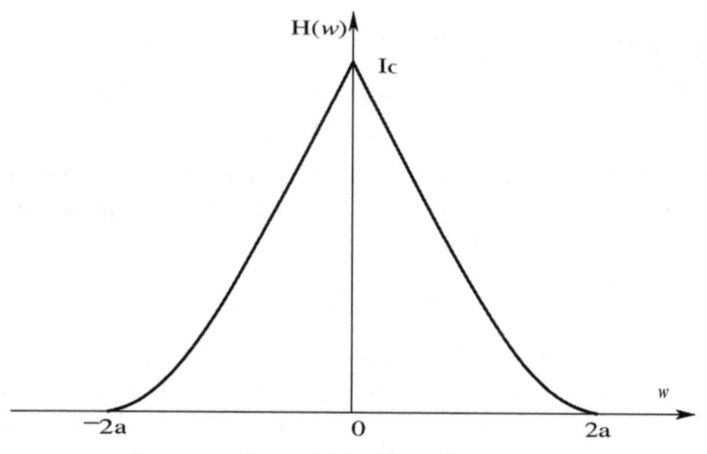

FIGURE 5.8
Plot of the Hankel transform of the image (output) of an imaging system's spatial impulse response which is an Airy disk with radial symmetry. Note that the spatial cut-off frequency for this spatial frequency response is for $|w| = 2\text{a}$. See text for mathematical description.

Note that a MTF as defined above is an even function in u. However, it is generally plotted for $\text{u} \geq 0$; that is, as a one-sided, real function. In practice, optical MTFs can have a variety of shapes; the cut-off frequency, however, is given approximately by $\text{u}_{\text{co}} = 2\ \text{NA}/\lambda$ cycles/mm, where NA is the numerical aperture of the lens and λ is the wavelength of monochromatic light. White light has a spectrum of wavelengths, hence u_{co} is poorly defined. Figure 5.6 shows a 100% contrast (input) object and Figure 5.7 shows the image. Note that the image spatial sine wave is attenuated by $|\mathbf{H}(\text{u}_\text{o})|$, thus its contrast is reduced. In the limit as $\text{u}_\text{o} \to \text{u}_{\text{co}}$, the image has zero contrast; it appears uniformly gray.

Spring and Davidson (2001) illustrate the effect on an optical microscope's MTF as the image plane is gradually defocused. The effect of *defocusing* (blur) on $\mathbf{H}(w)$ is shown in Figure 5.9. Note that, with progressive defocusing, the high spatial frequency response in the image is lost and, at extreme defocusing, $\mathbf{H}(\text{u})$ actually goes negative in a range of u, signifying an 180° phase shift. In terms of the image contrast. This means that black objects in the spatial frequency range of c. 0.25 cycles/μm will appear white and vice versa.

5.5.3 The contrast transfer function

Because of the difficulty of obtaining precision, 1-D, spatial sine wave test objects with 100% contrast, some workers seeking to characterize imaging systems resort to the more easily fabricated 1-D *spatial square wave test patterns.* With a spatial square wave object, the response of the imaging system is a low-pass-filtered square wave. The maximum contrast of a square wave (or sinusoidal) test object is a number between 0 and 1; C_o is given by Equation 5.70. C_i is the image contrast, calculated

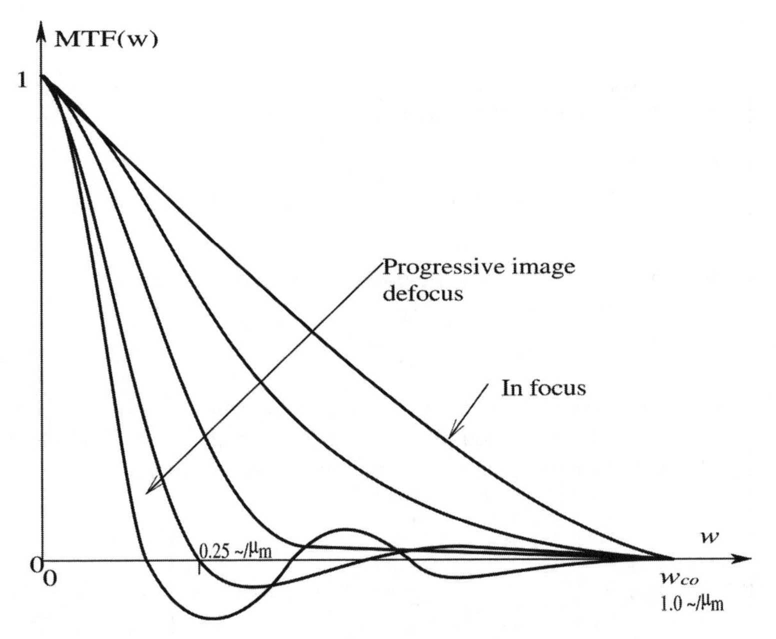

FIGURE 5.9
Plot of $\mathbf{H}(w)$ of an optical imaging system as an image is progressively defocused. There is an 180° phase shift in $\mathbf{H}(w)$ for extreme defocusing, indicating that white objects in this spatial frequency range look black and *vice versa*.

in the same way as C_o. C_o is generally made 1. The contrast transfer function for a 1-D spatial square wave is given by:

$$\mathrm{CTF(u)} \equiv \mathrm{C_i/C_0} \tag{5.78}$$

Note that, similar to the MTF, the CTF ranges $1 \geq [C_i/C_o] \geq 0$ as $0 \leq u \leq \infty$. Note that *the CTF is not the same as the MTF* (the MTF is defined for a sinusoidal input).

A spatial square wave object can be represented by its *Fourier series*. Assume a 0,1, even (cosine) spatial square wave, $o(x, \lambda)$. $o(x, \lambda)$ can be written as:

$$o(x, \lambda) = (I_{om}/2)[1 + SQ(x, \lambda)] \tag{5.79}$$

Where the average value of $o(x, \lambda)$, a_0, is $0.5I_{om}$, and $SQ(x, \lambda)$ is a zero-mean, 50% duty cycle, square wave with peak amplitude 1. Because $o(x, \lambda)$ is an even function, its *Fourier series* is even and of the general form:

$$SQ(x) = I_{om}/2 + (I_{om}/2)\sum_{n=1}^{\infty} a_n \cos(n2\pi x/\lambda) \tag{5.80}$$

Where λ is the spatial period of the square wave in mm. The Fourier series coefficient, a_n is evaluated in the usual manner for a unity peak height square wave:

$$a_n = \frac{2}{\lambda}\int_{-\lambda/2}^{\lambda/2} SQ(x)\cos(n2\pi x/\lambda)\,dx = \frac{2}{\lambda}\left\{\int_{-\lambda/2}^{-\lambda/4} -\cos(n2\pi x/\lambda)\,dx \right.$$
$$\left. + \int_{-\lambda/4}^{\lambda/4} \cos(n2\pi x/\lambda)\,dx - \int_{\lambda/4}^{\lambda/2} \cos(n2\pi x/\lambda)\,dx \right\} \tag{5.81}$$

Evaluating the definite integrals, we obtain the well known result:

$$a_n = \frac{4}{n\pi}\sin(n\pi/2)$$

Note that, for $n =$ even (2, 4, 6, 8, ...), $a_n = 0$. For $n =$ odd (1, 5, 9, ...), $\sin(n\pi/2) = +1$, and for $n =$ odd (3, 7, 1, ...), $\sin(n\pi/2) = -1$. Thus the Fourier series for the spatial cosine square wave test object can be written as:

$$SQ(x,\lambda) = (I_{om}/2)\left[1 + \sum_{\substack{n=1 \\ n\ \mathrm{odd}}}^{\infty} 2\left[\frac{\sin(n\pi/2)}{n\pi/2}\right]\cos(n2\pi x/\lambda)\right], \; u_o \equiv 2\pi/\lambda\ \mathrm{r/mm} \tag{5.82}$$

$\downarrow$

$$SQ(x,\lambda) = (I_{om}/2)[1 + \frac{4}{\pi}\cos(u_o x) - \frac{4}{3\pi}\cos(3u_o x) + \frac{4}{5\pi}\cos(5u_o x)$$
$$- \frac{4}{7\pi}\cos(7u_o x) + \frac{4}{9\pi}\cos(9u_o x) - \cdots] \tag{5.83}$$

Thus, $SQ(x,\lambda)$ is composed of a sum of sinewaves of increasing frequency. As $\lambda \to 0$, $u_o \to u_{co}$, and the square wave image can be approximated by its first harmonic; the higher-order spatial frequency harmonics of the object square wave are assumed to be attenuated to a negligible value by the low-pass action of the imaging system. Thus:

$$i(x,\lambda) \cong (I_o/2)[1 + |\mathbf{H}(u_o)|(4/\pi)\cos(u_o x)], \quad u_o = 2\pi/\lambda \tag{5.84}$$

Now by definition, $C_o = 1$ and C_i is given by:

$$C_i = \frac{I_o/2 + (2I_o/\pi)|\mathbf{H}(u_o)| - [I_o/2 - (2I_o/\pi)|\mathbf{H}(u_o)|]}{I_o/2 + (2I_o/\pi)|\mathbf{H}(u_o)| + I_o/2 - (2I_o/\pi)|\mathbf{H}(u_o)|} = \frac{(4/\pi)|\mathbf{H}(u_o)|}{1} \tag{5.85}$$

Thus, the CTF for a high spatial frequency squarewave object is:

$$CTF(u) \cong (4/\pi)|\mathbf{H}(u)| = 1.273|\mathbf{H}(u)| \tag{5.86}$$

As in the case of the MTF, —**H**(u)— is the magnitude of the OTF as a function of sinusoidal spatial frequency, u. $|\mathbf{H}(0)|$ is generally normalized to unity. In general, $\lim_{u\to\infty} |\mathbf{H}(u)| \to 0$.

5.5.4 Discussion

The ultimate goal of any medical imaging system is to be able to resolve small objects with high contrast. To do this, we need a broad, flat-topped MTF function. In practice, the MTF of most imaging systems falls off monotonically to zero at some cut-off frequency. Thus, smaller higher-spatial-frequency components in an object appear with low contrast in the image. In optical microscopes, the high-frequency portion of the optical transfer function and MTF can be enhanced by special optical techniques such as *phase contrast, differential interference contrast* and *single-sideband edge enhancement* [Spring and Davidson, 2001].

Increased high-spatial-frequency response and higher resolution of small tumors in x-ray mammography has been accomplished experimentally by x-ray *diffraction enhanced imaging* (DEI). A tightly collimated, nearly monochromatic beam of x-rays is used [Northrop, 2002]. Image features are proportional to the gradient of the x-ray refractive index in the tissue, rather than x-ray density as in conventional x-ray mammography.

5.6 Chapter Summary

This chapter has shown that the CFT can be derived from the complex form of the Fourier series by letting the period of a periodic $f(t)$ go to infinity. The CFT also results when we let $s = j\omega$ in the Laplace transform and extend the lower limit of integration to $-\infty$. In Section 5.2, we listed the mathematical properties of the CFT, including relations, theorems and certain transform pairs. For example, the CFT of a real, even $f(t)$ is a real, even $F(\omega)$.

Three important applications of the CFT were covered in this chapter: In Section 5.3, we use the Fourier series and the FT theorem of complex exponentiation to illustrate the properties of sampling in the frequency domain and to derive the sampling theorem. The analytical signal and the Hilbert transform are described in Section 5.4, including the properties of the analytical signal and the Hilbert transform. Applications and examples of the analytical signal are given in Section 5.4.4. The *modulation transfer function* (MTF) was described in Section 5.5. The MTF was shown to be the normalized spatial frequency response of an imaging system that allows quantitative prediction of the imaging system's resolution. In a linear imaging system, the CFT of the spatial impulse response (point spread function) gives the spatial frequency response of the system. The relation of the MTF to the *contrast transfer function* (CTF) was described in Section 5.5.3. The MTF and CTF were shown to be important descriptors of medical imaging system performance.

Problems

5.1 Find the CFTs of the following time functions: Note that, in our notation, $\text{rect}(t/a)$ is an even rectangular pulse of height 1.0 for $-a/2 \leq t \leq a/2$ and zero for $|t| > a/2$. $\Lambda(t/a)$ is an even triangular pulse of peak height 1.0 and width 2a. $\Lambda(t/a) = (t/a+1)$ for $-a \leq t \leq 0$, $= (1-t/a)$ for $0 \leq t \leq a$ and zero elsewhere. $U(t-a)$ is a unit step of amplitude 1.0 for $t \geq a$ and 0 for $t < a$. $p_c(t)$ is an even rectangular pulse of height 1 and width 2c; i.e., $p_c(t) = 1$ for $|t| \leq c$, and 0 elsewhere. $\otimes$ denotes the convolution operation (real or complex).

a. $\text{rect}(t/a) \otimes \text{rect}(t/a)$

b. $2\,\text{rect}[(t-2)/2]$

c. $\delta(t-1)\,\text{rect}(t/a)$

d. $\delta(t-1) \otimes \Lambda(t/a)$

e. $\cos(\omega_o t)\,\text{rect}(t/a)$

f. $\cos(\omega_o t)\,\text{rect}(t/(T/2))$

g. $\sin(\omega_o t)\,\text{rect}(t/(T/2))$

h. $2\alpha/(\alpha^2+t^2)$

i. $1/t$, for $-\infty \leq t \leq \infty$. (Note $1/t$ is odd.)

j. $\cos[(t-\pi/2)\omega_o]$

5.2 Find the inverse CFTs of the following frequency functions.

a. $b\frac{\sin(\omega b/2)}{(\omega b/2)} \otimes [\delta(\omega+b)+\delta(\omega-b)]$

b. $\frac{(a+b)+2j\omega}{[ab+j\omega(a+b)-\omega^2]}$

c. $j\pi[\delta(\omega+\omega_o)-\delta(\omega-\omega_o)] \otimes b\frac{\sin(\omega b/2)}{(\omega b/2)}$

d. $\text{rect}(\omega/a)$

e. $\pi[\delta(\omega+1/2)+\delta(\omega-1/2)]\frac{\sin(\omega/2)}{(\omega/2)}$

f. $1/\omega$

g. $j\pi[\delta(\omega+\omega_o)-\delta(\omega-\omega_o)]\exp[-j\omega\sigma]$

h. $\frac{\sin[a(\omega-\omega_o)]}{(\omega-\omega_o)} + \frac{\sin[a(\omega+\omega_o)]}{(\omega+\omega_o)}$

i. $\pi p_a(\omega)$

j. $-j\,\text{sgn}(\omega)$

5.3 A signal is $g(t) = B\sin(\omega_o t)$. Use the Hilbert transform to find the analytical signal, $\mathbf{g_a}(t)$.

5.4 An ideal *Hilbert transform filter* delays the phase of every component of a modulating signal, $m(t)$, $\pi/2$, or equivalently, has an ideal weighting function of $1/t$. Show mathematically that the system shown in Figure P5.4 generates a single sideband (SSB) signal.

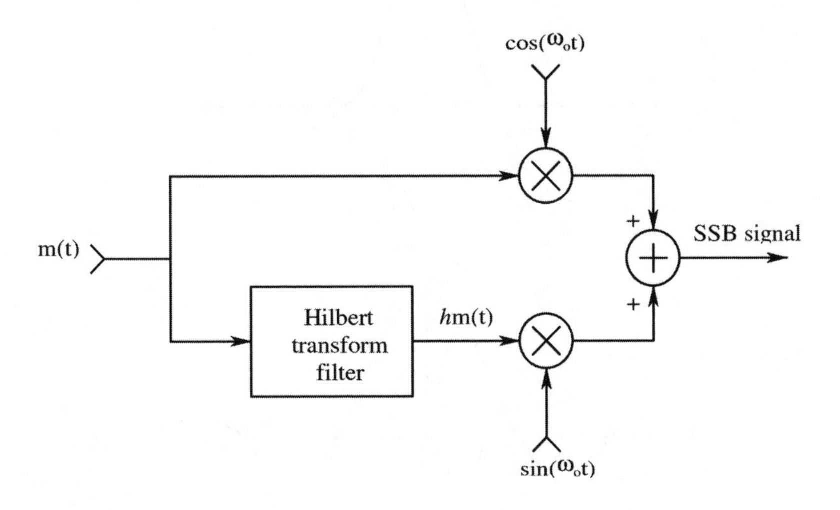

FIGURE P5.4

5.5 Find the CFT of the even time functions shown in Figure P5.5. You may use FT theorems.

5.6 The 1-D MTF of an imaging system is given by:

$$\mathrm{MTF} = [1 - |u|/a]$$

Where u is in radians/mm, $a = u_{co} = 70$ r/mm, and x is in mm.

a. Find the expression for $h(x)$, the system's point-spread function. Plot and dimension $h(x)$ for $x \geq 0$.

b. By simulation and trial and error, find the closest spacing, ε, that the impulses in an input object can have to give a 50% valley between the two peaks of the image, $I_0(x)$. The object is:

$$I_{in}(x) = I_m[\delta(x) + \delta(x - \varepsilon)].$$

5.7 The spatial impulse response of an optical imaging system is modeled by the Airy disk, which has circular symmetry. Thus r is a radial distance in mm.

$$h(r) = 2a^2 \frac{J_1^2(ar)}{(ar)^2}$$

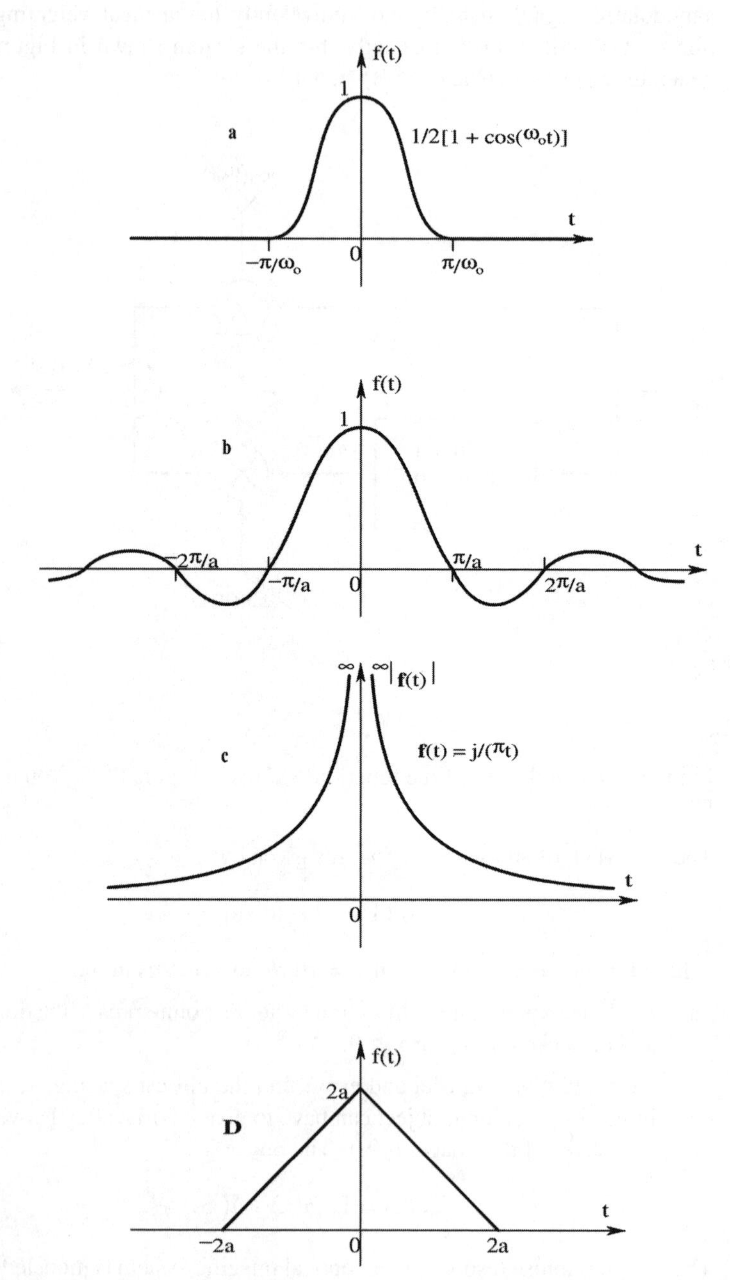

f(t)
1
a
1/2[1 + cos(ωₒt)]
t
−π/ωₒ
0
π/ωₒ
f(t)
1
b
t
−2π/a
−π/a
0
π/a
2π/a
∞
∞
|f(t)|
c
f(t) = j/(πt)
t
0
f(t)
2a
D
t
−2a
0
2a

FIGURE P5.5

To test the spatial frequency response of this system, we need a spatial sinusoidal object with circular symmetry. This can be modeled by:

$$I_{in}(r) = (I_m/2)[1 + \sin(w_o r)]$$

Where: $w_o = 2\pi/\rho_o$ radians/mm; ρ_o is the radial period of the spatial sine wave in mm, and $a \equiv 100$ r/mm.

a. Plot and dimension $I_{in}(r)$ in the polar (r, θ) plane.

b. Find the radial periods of the object sine wave, ρ_o, that will cause this system's MTF to equal 0.707, 0.5, 0.1, and 0.

5.8 The 1-D optical transfer function of an imaging system can be approximated by:

$$\mathbf{H}(u) = 2b\frac{\sin(bu)}{bu}$$

a. Find, plot and dimension this system's point spread function, $h(x)$. Note that b is in mm, u is in radians/mm.

b. Find an expression for the first zero of $\mathbf{H}$(u), u_{o1}.

c. It is observed that for visible wavelengths of light, u_{o1} is proportional to $1/\lambda$. At $\lambda = 650$ nm, $u_{o1} = 62.8$ r/mm, find b_1. Find u_{o2} and b_2 when blue (450 nm) light is used.

5.9 An imaging system has the 1-D MTF model, $\mathbf{H}(u) = \sqrt{1 - u^2/c^2}$ for $|u| \leq c$, $\mathbf{H}(u) = 0$ for $|u| > c$, and $c > 0$.

a. Plot and dimension this MTF. What practical significance has c?

b. Find the system's 1-D point spread function, $h(x)$. Plot and dimension $h(x)$.

5.10 A 1-D imaging system has a MTF modeled by:

$$\mathbf{H}(u) = \frac{a^2}{u^2 + a^2}$$

a. Find the expression for the point spread function for this system.

b. The steady-state input to the system is the 1-D sinusoidal object, $I_{in} = (I_m/2)[1 + \sin(u_o x)]$. Find the image contrast* when $u_o = a$ r/mm. * cf. Equation 5.71 in Section 5.5.

5.11 Evaluate the definite integral:

$$\int_{-\infty}^{\infty} \frac{a^2 \sin^2(at)}{(at)^2} dt$$

Use the FT pair, $\frac{a\sin(at)}{at} \longleftrightarrow \pi p_a(\omega)$, and Parseval's theorem, # 17 in Table 5.1.

6

The Discrete Fourier Transform

6.1 Introduction

The discrete Fourier transform (DFT) is the basis for modern spectral analysis of stationary signals and noise, and also is one means used to realize joint time-frequency plots used to characterize nonstationary signals (see Chapter 7). In this chapter, we examine the relation of the DFT and inverse DFT (IDFT) to the CFT and ICFT, and describe the mathematical properties of the DFT and IDFT. Also considered are *window functions* and their role in minimizing the interaction between the spectral components of a sampled signal containing two or more periodic components at different frequencies; the choice of window function is shown to affect *spectral resolution* when calculating the power density spectrogram of a signal. Finally, we introduce the fast Fourier transform (FFT), and illustrate several ways of implementing it.

The discrete Fourier transform (DFT) is used to estimate the spectral (frequency) components of sampled, deterministic signals of finite duration, as well as signals and random noise sampled over a finite *epoch.* When working with sampled random signals and noise, the DFT can be used to estimate the *auto-power density spectrum* from the *autocorrelogram* of the finite duration, sampled waveform. The DFT is also used to calculate the cross-power spectrogram from the cross-correlogram computed from two finite-duration, sampled waveforms; one typically being the input to an LTI system and the other being the system's output. The cross-power spectrogram will be shown to be useful in estimating the LTI system's weighting function, or, alternately, its frequency response. Still another use of the DFT is the calculation of the joint *time-frequency spectrograms* of nonstationary signals (see Chapter 7 of this text) using the short-time Fourier transform (STFT), and other Fourier based transforms.

We will describe *fast Fourier transform* (FFT) algorithms in Section 6.4 that offer computational efficiency in calculating DFTs, including auto- and cross-power spectrograms. Because all DFTs and FFTs are computed from finite-length data, the sampled signals can be considered to be multiplied with a finite-width rectangular *data window.* The presence of this data window alters the shape of the resultant spectrogram from what it would be if an ideal infinite-width data record were used. In Section 6.3 on data windows, you will see that there is a trade-off between the width of spectral peaks resulting from two or more coherent (e.g., sinusoidal) components in a waveform, and the amount of ripple between peaks. Many data windows (other than rectangular) have been devised that attempt to reduce ripple and still obtain high spectral resolution in the spectrogram.

6.2 The CFT, ICFT, DFT and IDFT

6.2.1 The CFT and ICFT

For purposes of review and comparison, we repeat here the continuous Fourier transform (CFT) and its inversion integral (ICFT). For conditions under which the CFT integral converges:

$$\mathbf{F}(j\omega) = \int_{-\infty}^{\infty} f(t) e^{-j\omega t} dt \tag{6.1}$$

Complex-variable theory is often used to find the inverse transform:

$$f(t) = \frac{1}{2\pi} \int_{-\infty}^{\infty} \mathbf{F}(j\omega) e^{j\omega t} d\omega \tag{6.2}$$

The properties of the CFT and ICFT were described in Section 5.2 of this text.

6.2.2 Properties of the DFT and IDFT

Sections 2.5.3 and 5.3.2 described the discretization or sampling of continuous signals. Reality dictates that a sampled function, $x^*(t) = x(nT) = x(n)$, be of finite duration, i.e., have a finite number, N, of samples taken at $t = 0, T, 2T, \ldots, nT, \ldots, (N-1)T$. The duration of the continuous signal sampled is called the *epoch length,* which is simply, $T_e = (N-1)T$, where T is the *sampling period* (time between samples). The DFT is given by the complex summation [Proakis and Manolakis, 1989]:

$$\mathbf{X}(k) \equiv \sum_{n=0}^{N-1} x(nT) \exp[-j knT 2\pi/(NT)] = \sum_{n=0}^{N-1} x(n) \exp[-j kn\Omega_0] \tag{6.3}$$

Where $k = 0, 1, 2, \ldots, N-1$, and $\Omega_o \equiv 2\pi/N$, the sample spacing in radians. Using the Euler identity, the DFT can also be expressed as:

$$\begin{aligned}\mathbf{X}(k) &\equiv \sum_{n=0}^{N-1} x(n)\exp[-jkn(2\pi/N)] \\ &= \sum_{n=0}^{N-1} x(n)\cos(kn\Omega_0) - j\sum_{n=0}^{N-1} x(n)\sin(kn\Omega_0)\end{aligned} \tag{6.4}$$

Some authors [e.g., Cunningham, 1992; Proakis and Manolakis, 1989] substitute $\Omega_o \equiv 2\pi/N$ in Equation 6.3, and drop the sampling period, T, from $x(nT)$ to write $x(n)$. Note that, in general, the DFT $\mathbf{X}(k)$ is complex, i.e., for each k value, it has a real and an imaginary part. The frequency spacing between adjacent terms of $\mathbf{X}(k)$ is given by [Northrop, 1997]:

$$\Delta f = \frac{1}{T_e} = \frac{1}{(N-1)T}\ \text{Hz} \tag{6.5}$$

Note that $\mathbf{X}(k)$ is an abbreviated form of $\mathbf{X}\left[k\frac{2\pi}{(N-1)T}\right]$, generally approximated by $\mathbf{X}[k2\pi/(NT)] = \mathbf{X}(k\Omega_o/T) = \mathbf{X}(k\Delta\omega)$. The discrete argument of $\mathbf{X}$ is in *radians/sec.,* also, the total Hz span of the spectrogram, $\mathbf{X}(k)$, is simply 0 to $1/T_s$ Hz.

Note that the $Re\{\mathbf{X}(k)\}$ is even around $k = N/2$, and $Im\{\mathbf{X}(k)\}$ is odd around $k = N/2$. Thus, the $|\mathbf{X}(k)|$ is even around $k = N/2$ and we can conclude that *one-half of an N-point, DFT spectrum of x(n) is redundant;* in other words, N samples of $x(t)$ yield only $N/2$ useful terms in $\mathbf{X}(k)$, and the useful frequency span of the half $\mathbf{X}(k)$ is 0 to f_N, the *Nyquist frequency,* which is $f_s/2$.

The *inverse DFT* is written:

$$\begin{aligned}x(n) &= \frac{1}{N}\sum_{k=0}^{N-1} \mathbf{X}(k)\exp[j(2\pi/N)kn] \\ &= \frac{1}{N}\sum_{k=0}^{N-1} \mathbf{X}(k)\exp[j\Omega_o kn],\ n = 0, 1, 2, \ldots, N-1.\end{aligned} \tag{6.6}$$

The DFT and IDFT have many of the properties of the Fourier series and the CFT and Laplace transform pairs. Table 6.1 summarizes some of the more important properties of the CFT/IDFT pair.

Now let us examine some examples of finding the DFTs of some simple time functions. *In the first example,* we will find the DFT of a truncated ramp function:

$$x(t) = tU(t) - 4U(t-4) - (t-4)U(t-4) \tag{6.7}$$

When sampled, we find: $x(0) = 0$, $x(1) = 1$, $x(2) = 2$, $x(3) = 3$, $x(4) = 0$, $x(5) = 0, \ldots$. In this example, $N = 4$. So

$$\mathbf{X}(k) = \mathbf{X}(k2\pi/N) = \mathbf{X}(k\pi/2) = \sum_{n=0}^{N-1} x(n)\exp[-j(2\pi/N)nk] \tag{6.8A}$$

TABLE 6.1
Some Properties of the Discrete Fourier Transform

Property	If	Then
1. Linearity (superposition).	$ax_1(n) + bx_2(n)$	$a\mathbf{X}_1(k) + b\mathbf{X}_2(k)$
2. Symmetry.	$x(n)$ is a *real sequence* with the DFT: $\mathbf{X}(k) = M(k)e^{j\varphi(k)}$ $M(k) = \lvert\mathbf{X}(k)\rvert$	$M(N-k) = M(k)$ $\mathbf{X}(N-k) = \mathbf{X}^*(k) = \mathbf{X}(-k)$ $\varphi(N-k) = -\varphi(k)$
3. DFT of a real signal is conjugate-symmetric.	$x(n)$ real	$\mathbf{X}(k) = \mathbf{X}^*(-k)$
4. Periodicity of an N-point DFT and N-point IDFT.	$x(n) = x(n+N)$	$\mathbf{X}(k) = \mathbf{X}(k+N)$
5. Time- and frequency shifting.	$x(n-p)$ $x(n)\exp[j(2\pi/N)nq]$	$\mathbf{X}(k)\exp[-j(2\pi/N)kp]$ $\mathbf{X}(k-q)$
6. Real convolution or filtering.	$y(n) = x(n) \otimes h(n)$	$\mathbf{Y}(k) = \mathbf{X}(k)\mathbf{H}(k)$
7. Real multiplication or modulation/demodulation.	$y(n) = x_1(n)x_2(n)$	$\mathbf{Y}(k) = \mathbf{X}_1(k) \otimes \mathbf{X}_2(k)$
8. Convergence.	$\sum_{n=-\infty}^{\infty} \lvert x(n)\rvert < \infty$ or $\sum_{n=-\infty}^{\infty} \lvert x(n)\rvert^2 < \infty$	$\mathbf{X}(k)$exists
9. Negative time.	$\mathbf{DFT}\{x(-n)\}$	$\mathbf{X}(-k) = \mathbf{X}(N-k)$
10. Real part.	—	$Re\{\mathbf{X}(k)\} = Re\{\mathbf{X}(N-k)\}$
11. Imaginary part.	—	$Im\{\mathbf{X}(k)\} = -Im\{\mathbf{X}(N-k)\}$

Now the DFT vectors are:

$$\mathbf{X}(0) = \sum_{n=0}^{3} x(n)\exp[-j(\pi/2)n0] = 0+1+2+3+0+0+\cdots = 6+j0 \quad (6.8B)$$

$$\mathbf{X}(1) = \sum_{n=0}^{3} x(n)\exp[-j(\pi/2)n1] = 0-1j+-2+3j+0+\cdots = -2+2j \quad (6.8C)$$

Thus, $|\mathbf{X}(1)| = 2\sqrt{2}$, and in polar notation, $\mathbf{X}(1) = 2\sqrt{2}\angle{-225^\circ}$.

$$\begin{aligned}\mathbf{X}(2) &= \sum_{n=0}^{3} x(n)\exp[-j(\pi/2)n2]\\ &= 0+1\angle{-180^\circ}+2\angle{-360^\circ}+3\angle{-540^\circ}+0+\cdots = -2+j0\end{aligned} \tag{6.8D}$$

$$\begin{aligned}\mathbf{X}(3) &= \sum_{n=0}^{3} x(n)\exp[-j(\pi/2)n3]\\ &= 0+1j-2-3j+0+0+\cdots = -(2+2j) = 2\sqrt{2}\angle{-135^\circ}\end{aligned} \tag{6.8E}$$

$$\mathbf{X}(4) = \sum_{n=0}^{3} x(n)\exp[-j(\pi/2)n4] = 0 \tag{6.8F}$$

By the IDFT, we can recover x(n):

$$\begin{aligned}x(0) &= \frac{1}{N}\sum_{k=0}^{3}\mathbf{X}(k)\exp[j(2\pi/N)k0] \quad (N=4)\\ &= {}^1\!/_4[6+(-2+2j)-2+(-2-2j)]\angle 0^\circ = 0\end{aligned} \tag{6.9A}$$

$$\begin{aligned}x(1) &= \frac{1}{4}\sum_{k=0}^{3}\mathbf{X}(k)\exp[j(2\pi/4)k1\\ &= {}^1\!/_4[6+(-2j-2)+2+(+2j+2)] = 1\end{aligned} \tag{6.9B}$$

$$\begin{aligned}x(2) &= \frac{1}{4}\sum_{k=0}^{3}\mathbf{X}(k)\exp[j(2\pi/4)k2]\\ &= {}^1\!/_4[6+(-2+2j)(-1)+(-2)1-(2+2j)(-1) = 2\end{aligned} \tag{6.9C}$$

$$\begin{aligned}x(3) &= \frac{1}{4}\sum_{k=0}^{3}\mathbf{X}(k)\exp[j(2\pi/4)k3]\\ &= {}^1\!/_4[6+(-2+2j)(-j)+(-2)(-1)-(2+2j)(j) = 3\end{aligned} \tag{6.9D}$$

Now, from the *periodicity property,* #4 in Table 6.1, we know that $x(4) = x(0) = 0$, and $x(5) = x(1) = 1$, etc. *In a second example* of finding $\mathbf{X}(k)$, consider the sequence, $x(n) = a, a, a, \ldots, a$ for $n = 0, 1, 2, 3, \ldots N-1$, and $x(n) = 0, 0, 0 \ldots$ for $n \geq N$ (this is a rectangular pulse of height a, with N samples). Thus, in general:

$$\mathbf{X}(k)=\sum_{n=0}^{N-1} x(n)\exp[-jn(2\pi k/N)] \tag{6.10A}$$

Now let N = 4:

$$\mathbf{X}(0)=\sum_{n=0}^{3} x(n)\exp[-j(\pi/2)n0]=[a+a+a+a]=4a+j0 \tag{6.10B}$$

$$\begin{aligned}\mathbf{X}(1) &= \sum_{n=0}^{3} x(n)\exp[-j(\pi/2)n1] \\ &= [ae^{-j0}+ae^{-j(\pi/2)}+ae^{-j(\pi)}+ae^{-j(3\pi/2)}]\end{aligned} \tag{6.10C}$$

In rectangular form, which is easier to add, $\mathbf{X}(1)=[(a+j0)+(0-ja)+(-a)+(0+ja)]=0$.

$$\begin{aligned}\mathbf{X}(2) &= \sum_{n=0}^{3} x(n)\exp[-j(\pi/2)n2] \\ &= [(a+j0)+(-a+j0)+(a+j0)+(-a+j0)]=0\end{aligned} \tag{6.10D}$$

$$\begin{aligned}\mathbf{X}(3) &= \sum_{n=0}^{3} x(n)\exp[-j(\pi/2)n3] \\ &= [(a+j0)+(0+ja)+(-a+j0)+(0-ja)]=0\end{aligned} \tag{6.10E}$$

Curiously, $\mathbf{X}(k)=\{4a,0,0,0\}, k=0,1,\ldots 3$. That is, there is only one real nonzero value in $\mathbf{X}(k)$.

As a third example, consider $x(n)=b^n$, where $0<b<1$, and $N=9$. Now the DFT is given by:

$$\begin{aligned}\mathbf{X}(k) &= \sum_{n=0}^{N-1} x(n)\exp[-j(2\pi/N)nk] \\ &= \sum_{n=0}^{N-1} b^n\exp[-j(2\pi/N)nk] \\ &= \sum_{n=0}^{N-1} (b\exp[-j(2\pi/N)k])^n\end{aligned} \tag{6.11}$$

The final summation in Equation 6.11 can be shown to have the closed form [Cunningham, 1992]:

$$\mathbf{X}(k) = \frac{1-b^N e^{-j(\Omega_o k)N}}{1-be^{-j(\Omega_o)k}}$$

$$= \frac{1-b^N[\cos(\Omega_o kN)-j\sin(\Omega_o kN)]}{1-b[\cos(\Omega_o k)-j\sin(\Omega_o k)]}$$

$$= \frac{1-b^N\cos(\Omega_o kN)+jb^N\sin(\Omega_o kN)}{1-b\cos(\Omega_o k)+jb\sin(\Omega_o k)} \tag{6.12}$$

From the last fraction term, we learn that the magnitude of $\mathbf{X}(k)$ is:

$$|\mathbf{X}(k)| = \frac{\sqrt{1-2b^N\cos(\Omega_o kN)+b^{2N}}}{\sqrt{1-2b\cos(\Omega_o k)+b^2}} \tag{6.13A}$$

And the angle of $\mathbf{X}(k)$ is:

$$\varphi(k) = \tan^{-1}\left(\frac{b^N\sin(\Omega_o kN)}{1-b^N\cos(\Omega_o kN)}\right) - \tan^{-1}\left(\frac{b\sin(\Omega_o k)}{1-b^N\cos(\Omega_o kN)}\right) \tag{6.13B}$$

Where $k=0,1,2,\ldots,N-1$.

6.2.3 Applications of the DFT and IDFT

Recall that the output of a digital filter, $h(n)$, acting on an input signal, $x(n)$, is given by the real *discrete convolution:*

$$y(n) = \sum_{p=-\infty}^{\infty} h(p)x(n-p) \tag{6.14}$$

Now $y(n)$ can also be expressed as the IDFT of the complex product, $\mathbf{H}(k)\mathbf{X}(k)$. Recall that:

$$\mathbf{X}(k) \equiv \sum_{n=0}^{N-1} x(n)\exp[-j(2\pi/N)nk] \tag{6.15}$$

Similarly, the DFT of the filter's weighting function is:

$$\mathbf{H}(k) \equiv \sum_{n=0}^{N-1} h(n)\exp[-j(2\pi/N)nk] \tag{6.16}$$

Thus, the filter's output is given by the IDFT of $\mathbf{Y}(k)=\mathbf{X}(k)\mathbf{H}(k)$:

$$y(n) = \frac{1}{N}\sum_{k=0}^{N-1} \{\mathbf{H}(k)\mathbf{X}(k)\}\exp[j(2\pi/N)kn] \tag{6.17}$$

Equation 6.17 offers an efficient means of implementing a digital filter in the frequency domain. $\{\mathbf{H}(k)\mathbf{X}(k)\}$ is an N-point vector product, that is, for each k, $\mathbf{Y}(k) = |\mathbf{H}(k)||\mathbf{X}(k)|\angle\varphi_h(k)+\varphi_x(k)$.

6.3 Data Window Functions

Every time we calculate the DFT frequency function, $\mathbf{G}(k)$, from a finite number sequence, $g(n)$, we implicitly use a *rectangular window function,* $w(n)$, of height 1 and length N which is multiplied by a $g(n)$ of infinite length. Thus, the real, windowed function, $g_w(n) = w(n)g(n)$ has N points. In the frequency domain, $\mathbf{G_w}(k)$ is calculated from a discrete, *complex convolution* of $\mathbf{W}(k)$ with $\mathbf{G}(k)$ as illustrated in Equation 6.18:

$$\begin{aligned} \mathbf{G_w}(k) &= \sum_{p=-\infty}^{\infty} \mathbf{W}(p)\mathbf{G}(k-p) \\ &= \sum_{n=0}^{N-1} \{w(n)g(n)\}\exp[-j(2\pi/N)nk], \quad k=0,1,2,\ldots N-1 \end{aligned}$$

(Discrete complex convolution) (6.18)

The *rectangular* or *natural window* is simply $w(n)=1$ for $n=0,1,2,\ldots N-1$, and zero for the other n. The rectangular window's DFT is given by

$$\mathbf{W_r}(k) = \sum_{n=0}^{N-1} \exp[-j(2\pi/N)nk], \; k=0,1,2,\ldots N-1 \quad (6.19)$$

To better appreciate what goes on in the frequency domain when a discrete $g(n)$ is windowed, we will examine the effects of windowing using *continuous time functions,* because, in my opinion, it is easier to visualize operations with CFTs. *As a first example* of how rectangular windowing affects the spectrum of the function in question, consider the function $g(t)$ to be:

$$g(t) = A\cos(\omega_o t) = A\cos[(2\pi/T)t], \quad -\infty \le t \le \infty. \quad (6.20)$$

The CFT of this $g(t)$ is well known:

$$\mathbf{G}(j\omega) = A\pi[\delta(\omega - 2\pi/T) + \delta(\omega + 2\pi/T)] \quad (6.21)$$

This $\mathbf{G}(j\omega)$ is simply a pair of delta functions; one at $\omega = 2\pi/T = \omega_o$, and the other at $\omega = -2\pi/T$ r/s. Let us choose a window that is even and centered at $t=0$, so that its CFT will be real (zero phase). A rectangular window, $w_r(t) = 1$ for $-T_w \le t \le T_w$, and zero elsewhere. The window's CFT is:

$$\mathbf{W_r}(j\omega) = \int_{-\infty}^{\infty} w_r(t)e^{-j\omega t}dt = \int_{-Tw}^{Tw} 1e^{-j\omega t}dt = \frac{\exp[-j\omega T_w] - \exp[-j\omega(-T_w)]}{-j\omega}$$

$\downarrow$

$$\mathbf{W_r}(j\omega) = (2T_w)\frac{\sin(\omega T_w)}{\omega T_w} \quad (6.22)$$

Now we can use the complex convolution relation to find the continuous spectrum of $\mathbf{G_w}(j\omega)$:

$$\mathbf{G_w}(j\omega) = \frac{1}{2\pi}\int_{-\infty}^{\infty} \mathbf{W_r}(j\omega - ju)\mathbf{G}(ju)du = \int_{-\infty}^{\infty} (2T_w)\frac{\sin[(\omega - u)T_w]}{2\pi(\omega - u)T_w} \times A\pi[\delta(u - 2\pi/T) + \delta(u + 2\pi/T)]du \tag{6.23}$$

This convolution is easy to evaluate because of the sifting property of the delta function. Thus:

$$\mathbf{G_w}(j\omega) = AT_w\left\{\frac{\sin[(\omega + 2\pi/T)T_w]}{2\pi(\omega + 2\pi/T)T_w} + \frac{\sin[(\omega - 2\pi/T)T_w]}{2\pi(\omega - 2\pi/T)T_w}\right\} \tag{6.24}$$

The even rectangular window spectrum is plotted in Figure 6.1 for $0 \le t \le 4$; note that the ideal impulse spectrum of the pure infinite cosine wave now has finite-width peaks and lots of ripple as a result of the $\sin(\theta)/\theta$ functions. As T_w increases, the frequency and amplitude of the ripple increases, as does the amplitude of the main peak at $\omega_o = 2$ r/sec; however the width of the main peak decreases with increasing window width. For trace #1, the window included exactly 20 cosine periods ($T_w = 10$), for trace #2, 16 periods ($T_w = 8$), and for trace #3, 12 periods ($T_w = 6$).

An important property of any window is *spectral resolution.* An example of spectral resolution is the ability to identify and measure the peaks of two sinusoidal

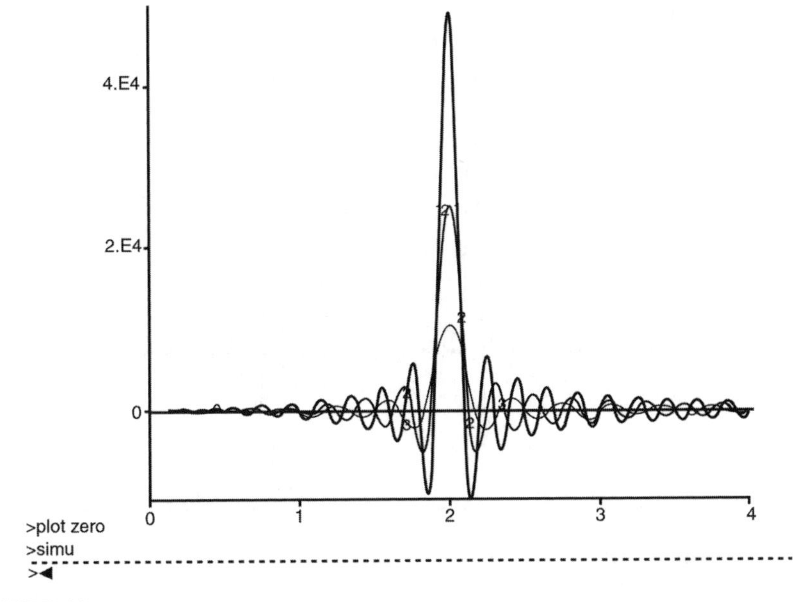

FIGURE 6.1
Plot of the spectrum of a continuous cosine wave of $\omega_o = 2$ r/sec multiplied by a rectangular, 0,1, window function of different widths. Vertical scale, relative amplitude; horizontal scale, spatial frequency.

components closely spaced in frequency. That is, to resolve the peaks of

$$g(t) = A\cos(\omega_o t) + B\cos[(\omega_o + \delta\omega)t], \quad -\infty \le t \le \infty \tag{6.25}$$

for small $(\delta\omega/\omega_o)$. Following the convolution above and recalling that convolution obeys superposition, we can write for the even rectangular window of width $2T_w$:

$$\begin{aligned} \mathbf{G_w}(j\omega) = {} & AT_w \left\{ \frac{\sin[(\omega-\omega_o)T_w]}{2\pi(\omega-\omega_o)T_w} + \frac{\sin[(\omega+\omega_o)T_w]}{2\pi(\omega+\omega_o)T_w} \right\} \\ & + BT_w \left\{ \frac{\sin[(\omega-\omega_o-\delta\omega)T_w]}{2\pi(\omega-\omega_o-\delta\omega)T_w} + \frac{\sin[(\omega+\omega_o+\delta\omega)T_w]}{2\pi(\omega+\omega_o+\delta\omega)T_w} \right\} \end{aligned} \tag{6.26}$$

We arbitrarily choose $T_w = 10T = 20\pi/\omega_o$, $A = B = 1$, and let $\omega_o = 1$ r/sec for simplicity. Note that $\mathbf{G_w}(j\omega)$ is *real*. Thus, Equation 6.26 can be written for plotting:

$$\begin{aligned} G_w(\omega) = {} & \left\{ \frac{\sin[(\omega-1)20\pi]}{2\pi(\omega-1)} + \frac{\sin[(\omega+1)20\pi]}{2\pi(\omega+1)} \right\} \\ & + \left\{ \frac{\sin[(\omega-1-\delta\omega)20\pi]}{2\pi(\omega-1-\delta\omega)} + \frac{\sin[(\omega+1+\delta\omega)20\pi]}{2\pi(\omega+1+\delta\omega)} \right\} \end{aligned} \tag{6.27}$$

A plot of Equation 6.27 is shown for $0 \le \omega \le 3$ r/sec in Figures 6.2.a, b, c and d, for $\delta\omega/\omega_o = 1, 0.125, 0.08$, and 0.07. A single peak is seen in $G(\omega)$ for $|\delta\omega/\omega_o| < 0.6$.

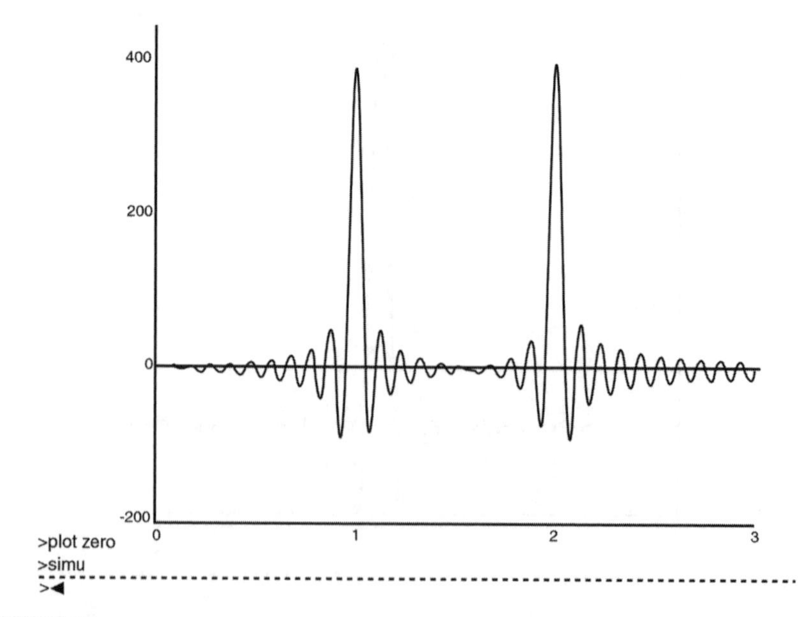

FIGURE 6.2a

Plot of the spectrums of two continuous cosine waves separated by a frequency increment, $\delta\omega/\omega_o$, multiplied by a *rectangular*, 0,1, window function of width 20T. (a) Plot for $\delta\omega/\omega_o = 1$.

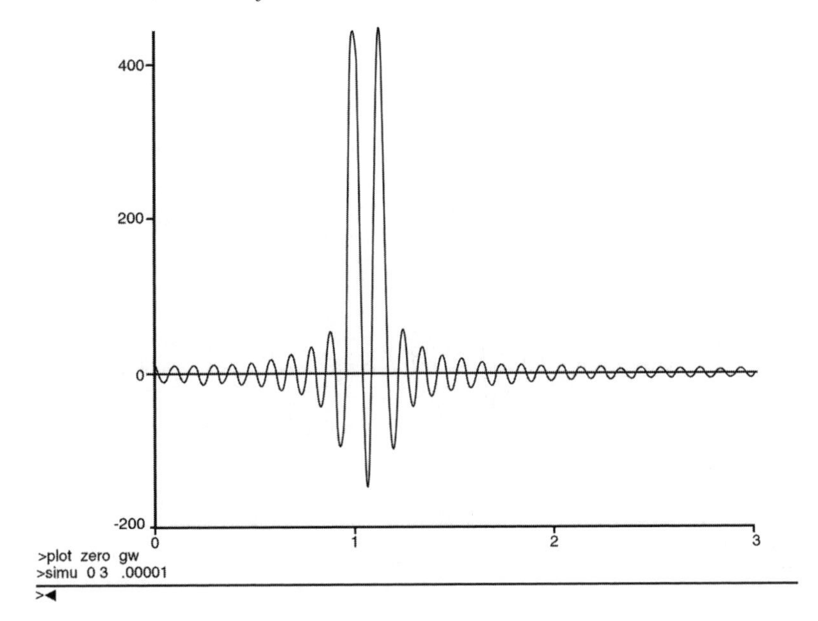

FIGURE 6.2b
(b) Plot for $\delta\omega/\omega_o = 0.125$.

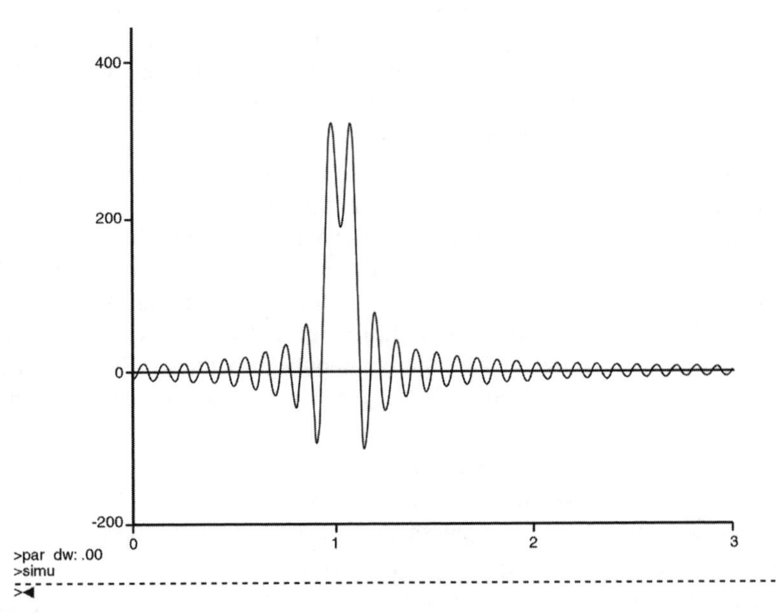

FIGURE 6.2c
(c) Plot for $\delta\omega/\omega_o = 0.08$.

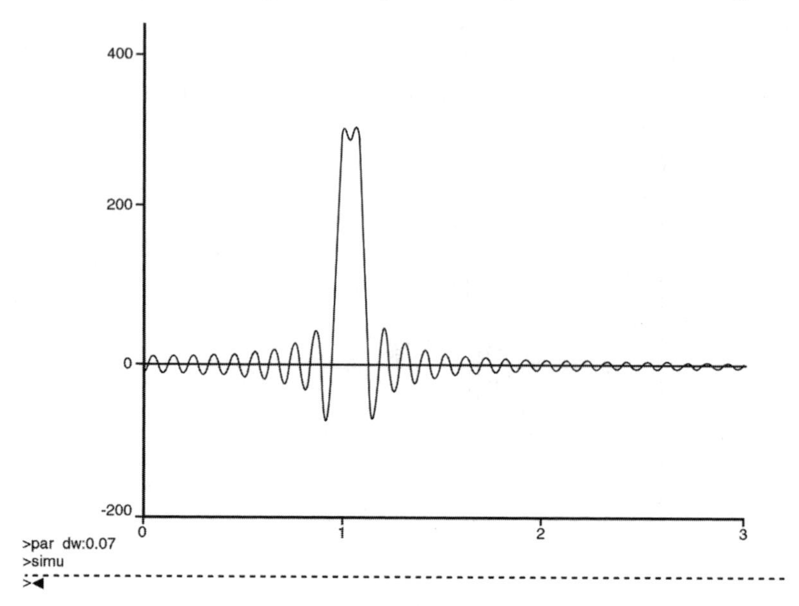

FIGURE 6.2d
(d) Plot for $\delta\omega/\omega_o$ = 0.07. Note that a small double peak is still visible in the spectrum.

Two features are evident from these plots. There is a limit to how close two frequencies can be and still be resolved in a CFT spectrum plot, and there is much ripple, even when the peaks are widely separated. Spectral resolution and ripple both improve as $T_W/T \to \infty$. However, for practical reasons, we are stuck with finite-length time data that we wish to display in the frequency domain. Thus, the windowed spectrum has ripple artifacts and limited spectral resolution.

To mitigate the effect of ripple artifact and so-called *spectral leakage,* a number of *data window functions* can be employed (other than the very ripply rectangular data window discussed above). Most data windows begin at zero at the beginning and end of the data ($n=0$ and $n=N-1$), and rise to a peak at the center of the data. Data windows are even functions around the center of the windowed data. Another general property of data windows is that the more the ripple is reduced, the wider the main lobe becomes. In the table below, we list some commonly encountered window functions, both as continuous (even) functions of time, and discrete functions of sample number, $n=0,1,2,\ldots N-1$.

Not included in Table 6.2 are the *Parzen, Blackman, Blackman-Harris* and *Lanczos* windows. In the Kaiser window, $I_o(x)$ is the zeroth order modified Bessel function. The parameter α controls the window shape, hence its ripple and spectral resolution.

Some commonly used window functions are plotted as continuous even time-domain functions from $t/T_W=-1$ to $t/T_W=+1$. In Figure 6.3 Trace #1 = Bartlett, #2 = Welch, #3 = Hann, #4 = Hamming, #5 = Blackman, #6 = Lanczos, #7 = Gaussian. Note that the Hamming and Gaussian windows do not go to zero at ± 1.

TABLE 6.2
Some Commonly Used Window Functions

Window name	As an even function of $-T_w \le t \le T_w$	As a discrete function of $n=0,1,2\ldots N-1$
Rectangular	1 for $-T_w \le t \le T_w$, else 0	1 for $0 \le n \le N-1$, else 0
Bartlett (triangular)	$(1-\lvert t\rvert/T_w)$ for $-T_w \le t \le T_w$, else 0	$w(n)=(1-\lvert 1-2n/(N-1)\rvert)$
Hann (Hanning)	$1/2[1+\cos(\pi t/T_w)]$	$w(n)=1/2[1+\cos(2n\pi/(N-1))]$ $0.5+0.5\cos(n\pi/(m+1))^*$
Hamming	$[0.54+0.46\cos(\pi t/T_w)]$	$w_n=0.54+0.46\cos(2n\pi/(N-1))$ $0.54+0.46\cos(n\pi/m)^*$
Gaussian	$2^{-(t/\sigma)^\wedge 2}$ for $-T_w \le t \le T_w$, else 0	
Kaiser	$\dfrac{I_o[\alpha\sqrt{1-(t/T_w)^2}]}{I_o(\alpha)}$	$I_o[\alpha(1-n^2/m^2)^{1/2}/I_o(\alpha)$ $^*-m \le n \le +m \quad (2m+1)$ points
Welch	$1-(t/T_w)^2$ (an inverted parabola)	

Most textbooks and authors [Williams, 1986; Cunningham, 1992; Papoulis, 1977; Theußl, 1999] that describe the properties of discrete data windows present them as functions of the sampling index, $n=0,1,2,\ldots N-1$, (N samples) as in the table above. However, the discrete window is often written as an even function of k between $k=-M$ and $+M$, giving $(2M+1)$ data points. $(2M+1)$ can be made equal to N, but is always odd. An obvious advantage of making $w(k)$ an even function is that its DFT will be real and even.

Most digital signal analysis instruments such as FFT spectrum analyzers and certain digital oscilloscopes with DSP options offer the user the choice of rectangular, Hann, Hamming, or Bartlett windows as data amplitude conditioning options. Frequency conditioning of the continuous input signal is first done by an analog antialiasing low-pass filter before it is digitized (sampled) and windowed.

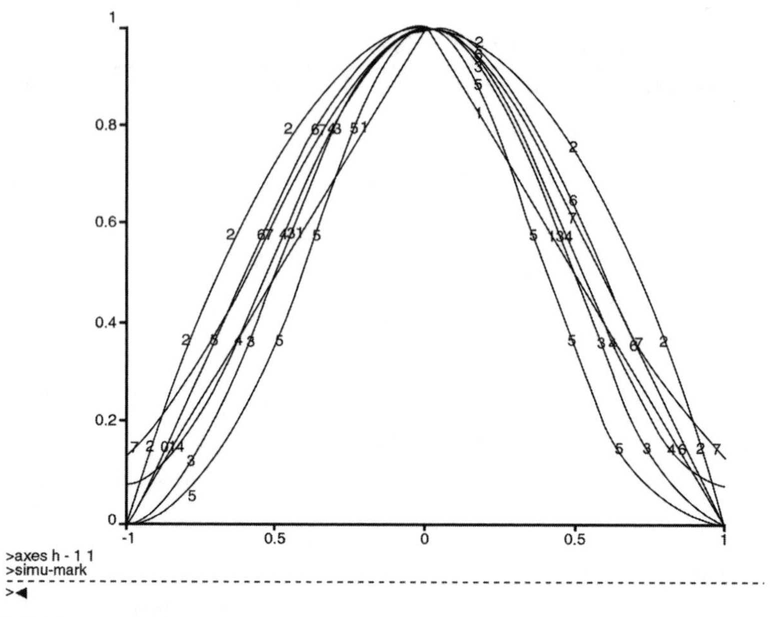

FIGURE 6.3
Normalized time-domain plots of various window functions used to suppress ripple and enhance spectral resolution. Windows are plotted as even functions from $t/T_W = -1$ to $t/T_W = +1$.

As a second example of a continuous data window applied to a signal consisting of a sum of two cosine waves closely spaced in frequency, let us examine the behavior of the *Bartlett window.* The CFT of the even Bartlett window is real and nonnegative:

$$W(\omega) = T_w \frac{\sin^2(\omega T_w/2)}{(\omega T_w/2)^2} \tag{6.28}$$

The Bartlett window is used on a cosine wave of frequency $\omega_o = 2\pi/T$ r/sec. The CFT spectrum of the windowed cosine wave of duration $2T_w$ is given by the complex convolution:

$$G_w(\omega) = \frac{1}{2\pi}\int_{-\infty}^{\infty} T_w \frac{\sin^2[(T_w/2)(\omega - u)]}{[(T_w/2)(\omega - u)]^2} A\pi[\delta(u-\omega_o) + \delta(u+\omega_o)]du$$

$$\downarrow$$

$$G_w(\omega) = \frac{AT_w}{2}\left\{\frac{\sin^2[(T_w/2)(\omega-\omega_o)]}{[(T_w/2)(\omega-\omega_o)]^2} + \frac{\sin^2[(T_w/2)(\omega+\omega_o)]}{[(T_w/2)(\omega+\omega_o)]^2}\right\} \tag{6.29}$$

Now consider the windowed signal to be the sum of two cosine waves closely spaced in frequency: $g(t) = A\cos(\omega_o t) + B\cos[(\omega + \delta\omega)t]$. As we did in the first example, let $\omega_o = 2\pi/T = 1$ r/sec, $T_w = 10\ T = 20\pi$, and $A = B = 1$. By inspection from Equation 6.29 we can write the CFT of the windowed cosine waves:

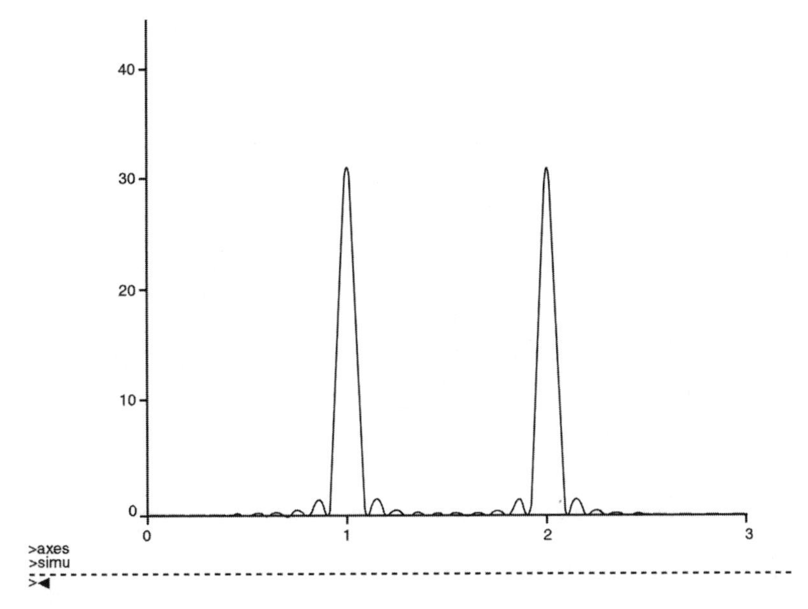

FIGURE 6.4a
Plot of the spectrums of two continuous cosine waves separated by a frequency increment, $\delta\omega/\omega_o$, multiplied by a *Bartlett window function* of total width 20T. (a) Plot for $\delta\omega/\omega_o$ = 1.

$$
\begin{aligned}
G_w(\omega) = 10\pi \bigg\{ & \frac{\sin^2[10\pi(\omega-1)]}{[10\pi(\omega-1)]^2} + \frac{\sin^2[10\pi(\omega+1)]}{[10\pi(\omega+1)]^2} \\
& + \frac{\sin^2[10\pi(\omega-1-\delta)]}{[10\pi(\omega-1-\delta)]^2} + \frac{\sin^2[10\pi(\omega+1+\delta)]}{[10\pi(\omega+1+\delta)]^2} \bigg\}
\end{aligned}
\tag{6.30}
$$

The continuous frequency response of Equation 6.30 is plotted in Figure 6.4. Note that compared with the rectangular window example, there is far lower ripple amplitude, and the ripple is positive only. The limiting frequency difference that gives two discernable peaks is $\delta\omega/\omega_o = 0.09$ for the Bartlett window, and is 0.07 for the rectangular window. This result underscores the general observation that there is a tradeoff between ripple amplitude and frequency resolution.

6.4 The FFT

6.4.1 Introduction

Fast Fourier transforms are a class of computationally efficient algorithms used to calculate the discrete Fourier transform (DFT) of a number sequence, f(n). Recall

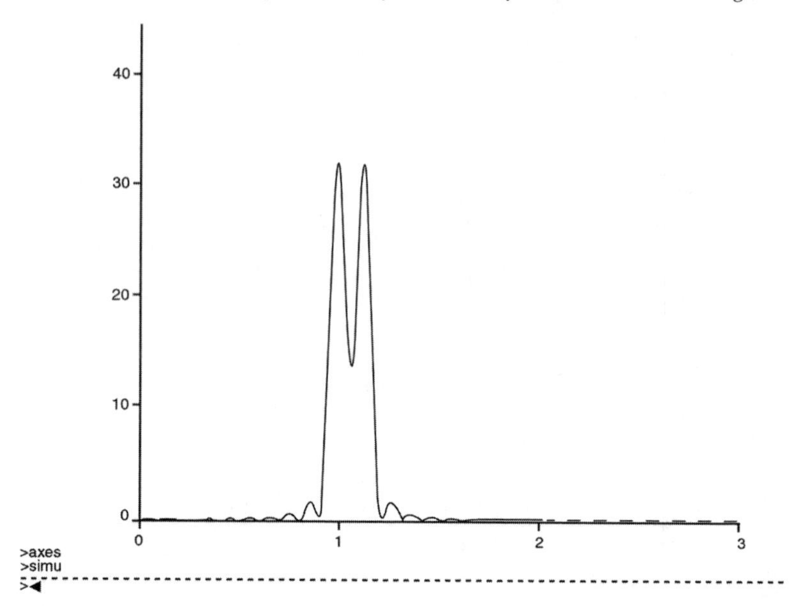

FIGURE 6.4b
(b) Plot for $\delta\omega/\omega_o = 0.125$.

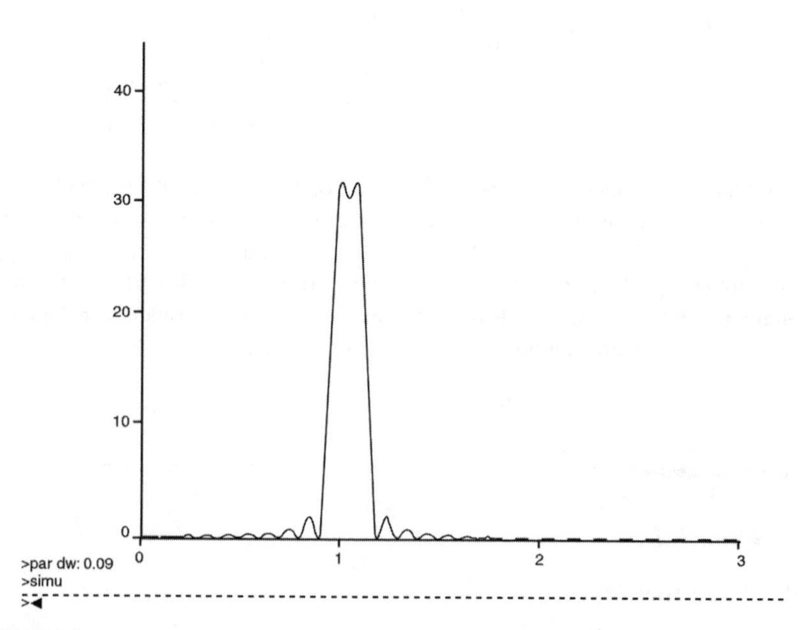

FIGURE 6.4c
(c) Plot for $\delta\omega/\omega_o = 0.08$. Note that a small double peak is still visible in the spectrum.

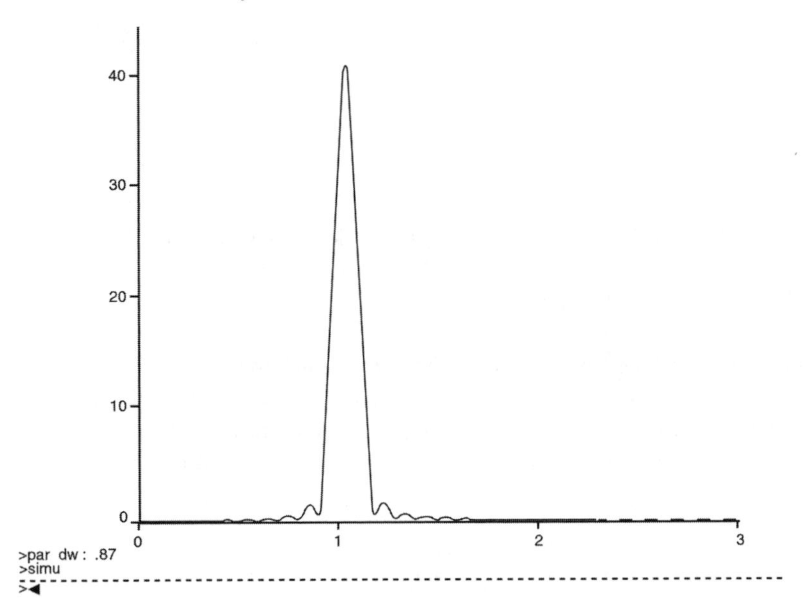

FIGURE 6.4d

(d) Plot for $\delta\omega/\omega_o$ = 0.07. Note that there is no double peak visible. Although there is less ripple surrounding the peaks, the Bartlett window has lost all resolution for $\delta\omega/\omega_o \leq 0.07$.

that the DFT can be written as:

$$\mathbf{F}(k) = \sum_{n=0}^{N-1} f(n) \exp[-jnkT2\pi/(NT)] = \mathbf{F}(k2\pi/NT), \quad \text{for } k = 0,1,\ldots N-1 \quad (6.31)$$

Note that the frequency increment for the DFTd signal is $\Delta\omega \cong 2\pi/NT$ r/sec. The total frequency span of the DFT is $2\pi/T$ r/sec. Also $f(n) = f(nT)$, where T is the sampling period, and N is the epoch length (N samples). The index, n, is usually taken from 0 to $N-1$, where N is some even number that is an integer power of 2 (e.g., $2^{10} = 1024$).

The DFT in Equation 6.31 can also be written using the complex vector **W**, defined as $\mathbf{W} \equiv \exp[-j2\pi/N]$. In polar form, $\mathbf{W} = 1\angle-(2\pi/N)$. We can write $\mathbf{W}^{nk}$ in rectangular form with the Euler relation:

$$\mathbf{W}^{nk} = \sin(2\pi nk/N) - j\cos(2\pi nk/N) \quad (6.32)$$

Thus, the DFT can be written:

$$\begin{aligned} \mathbf{F}(k) &= \sum_{n=0}^{N-1} f(n)\mathbf{W}^{nk} \\ &= \sum_{n=0}^{N-1} f(n)\sin(2\pi nk/N) - j\sum_{n=0}^{N-1} f(n)\cos(2\pi nk/N), \\ & k = 0,1,\ldots N-1 \end{aligned} \quad (6.33)$$

When $k=n=(N-1)$, $\mathbf{W}^{(N-1)(N-1)}=1\angle-[(N^2-1)2\pi/N]$. The IDFT is written::

$$f(n)=\frac{1}{N}\sum_{k=0}^{N-1}\mathbf{F}(k)\mathbf{W}^{-kn}, \quad n=0,1,\ldots N-1. \tag{6.34}$$

The FFT and IFFT are computationally efficient ways of computing the DFT and IDFT as given in Equations 6.33 and 6.34. As we remarked above, N is generally made a power of 2 to compute the FFT or IFFT. That is, $N=2^m$, where, for example, $m=10,12$, etc. If the actual data record length, D, is not a power of two, it is customary to pad the data sequence with P zeros such that $D+P=2^m=N$.

Evaluation of the DFT by ordinary means requires c. N^2 complex operations. Computation of $\mathbf{F}(k)$ by a FFT has been shown to require about $N\log_2(N)$ operations [Williams, 1986]. Thus, the fractional saving in computations can be written:

$$S=\frac{N^2-N\log_2(N)}{N^2}=1-(1/N)\log_2(N) \tag{6.35}$$

For example, if $N=1024$, $N^2=1.0486$ E6, then $S=0.99023$, or a 99% savings in computations. Actual computation of the FFT also makes use of the *angle symmetry property* of $\mathbf{W}^{nk}$.

6.4.2 The fast Fourier transform

To obtain a good approximation to the CFT of a bandwidth-limited waveform, we must calculate the DFT of the signal with a sampling rate above twice the highest frequency in the PDS of $x(t)$, and use enough samples to ensure a close spacing, Δf, between adjacent values of $\mathbf{X}(k)$. It is common to calculate spectra using Ns ranging from $256=2^8$ to $4096=2^{12}$, and higher. Use of the DFT algorithm as written above is seen to require 2N calculations (multiplications and additions) to calculate each $\mathbf{F}(k)$ coefficient's real and imaginary parts. However, there are N coefficients, so a total of N^2 multiplications and additions are required to obtain the DFT, $\{\mathbf{F}(k)\}_N$. If the magnitudes of each $\mathbf{F}(k)$ are to be displayed, then we must apply the Pythagorean theorem N times as well. It is clear that a large DFT calculated by the direct method will involve many high-precision computer operations, and will take a long time. For example, computation of an $N=4096$ point DFT involves over 33.5 million multiplications and additions. This can be time-consuming.

To overcome the computational burden of direct computation of large DFTs, Cooley and Tukey (1965) devised a fast Fourier transform (FFT) means of calculating the DFT. There are now several variations on the original Cooley-Tukey FFT. It is not our purpose here to describe in detail the steps involved in calculating an FFT. Rather, we will outline the strategy used and explain why it is efficient.

Using the complex form of the conventional DFT, direct calculation of the kth complex term can be written out as:

$$\mathbf{F}(k) = \Big\{ \overbrace{f(0)e^{-j(2\pi k0/N)}}^{\mathbf{W}^{k0}} + \overbrace{f(1)e^{-j(2\pi k1/N)}}^{\mathbf{W}^{k1}} + \cdots + \overbrace{f(n)e^{-j(2\pi kn/N)}}^{\mathbf{W}^{kn}}$$
$$+ \cdots + \overbrace{f(N-1)e^{-j[2\pi k(N-1)/N]}}^{\mathbf{W}^{k(N-1)}} \Big\} \quad k=0,1,\ldots N-1. \tag{6.36}$$

In rectangular form we have:

$$\begin{aligned} F(k) = {} & f(0)[\cos(0) - j\sin(0)] + f(1)[\cos(2\pi k/N) - j\sin(2\pi k/N)] \\ & + f(2)[\cos(4\pi k/N) - j\sin(4\pi k/N)] \\ & + \cdots f(n)[\cos(2\pi kn/N) - j\sin(2\pi kn/N)] \\ & + \cdots + f(N-1)[\cos(2\pi k(N-1)/N)] - j\sin(2\pi k(N-1)/N) \end{aligned} \tag{6.37}$$

Note that there are $N^2(kn)$ values. In rectangular form, there are $2N^2$ real multiplications.

Each of the N complex terms in Equation 6.37 has an angle, θ_{kn}, for the corresponding $\mathbf{F}(k)$. Thus, N vector summations are required in order to find the value of $\mathbf{F}(k)$ in the conventional DFT, and a total of N^2 vector summations must be done to find the entire DFT, $\{\mathbf{F}(k)\}_N$.

In computing an FFT, use is made of the fact that the exponential angle operator is periodic in kn/N. This periodicity leads to redundancy in the DFT calculations, which is taken advantage of in an FFT algorithm by rearranging the order of the calculations so that there are $\log_2 N$ columns of vector summers, each of which contains N summers, for a total of $N\log_2(N)$ complex summers in an FFT array. Each summer sums two vectors. The angles of the vectors must still be calculated when the FFT array is set up and stored as constants. Their values depend only on k, n, and N. It is not practical to try to illustrate the signal flow graph of an FFT operation for Ns over 8; it is just too complex. In Figure 6.5, we illustrate a signal flow graph representation of the computation of the N-point complex DFT, $\mathbf{F}(k)$, using one of several *decimation-in-time* (DIT) algorithms. The input signal is windowed and reordered for greater computational efficiency. Note that an eight-point FFT is shown. (SFG branches not labeled are understood to have transmissions of $+1$.)

The efficiency, η, of the FFT vs. the DFT calculated in the direct method can be calculated by assuming that computation speed is inversely proportional to the number of vector additions required in each case. So we can write

$$\eta = \frac{S_{FFT}}{S_{DFT}} = \frac{N^2}{N\log_2(N)} \tag{6.38}$$

For a 4096-point FFT, $\eta = 341.3$, for $N = 1024$, $\eta = 102.4$, etc.

In the preceding section, we saw that *windowing* the sampled function, $f(n)$, had a beneficial effect in reducing sidelobe interference in the computed $\mathbf{F}(k)$, permitting

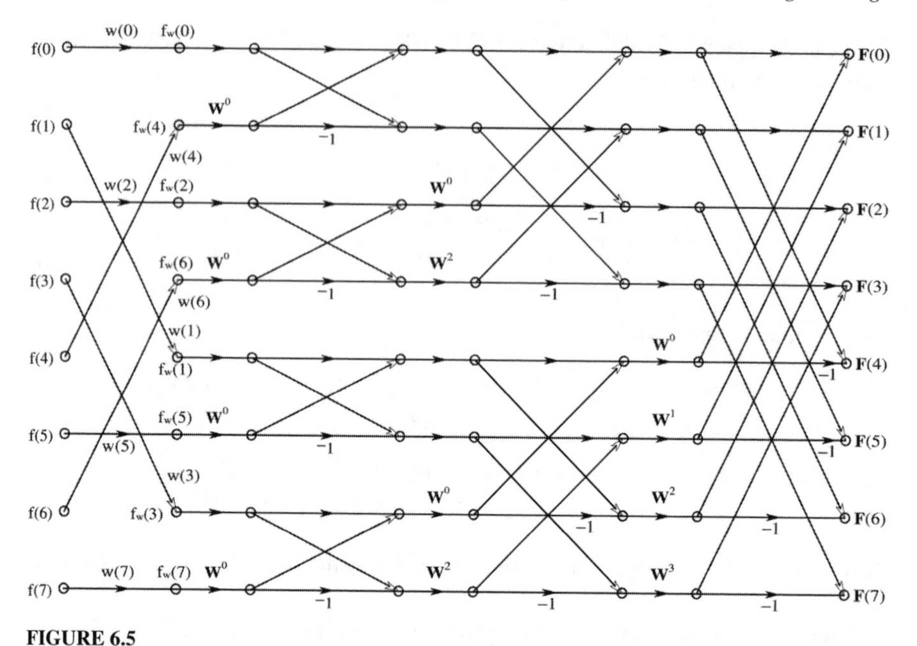

FIGURE 6.5
Signal flow graph representation of an eight-point, decimation-in-time, FFT algorithm.

resolution of closely spaced low-amplitude spectral components of $f(t)$. The windowing operation can be done as a sample-by-sample multiplication of $f(n)$ by the *windowing function,* $w(n)$. What is then FFTd is the windowed signal, $f_w(n)$. Simply put,

$$f_w(n) = f(n)w(n) \tag{6.39}$$

and the DFT is then:

$$\mathbf{F}(k) = \sum_{n=0}^{N-1} f_w(n)\mathbf{W}^{nk}, \quad k = 0, 1, 2, \ldots N-1. \tag{6.40}$$

6.4.3 Implementation of the FFT

The FFT was conceived well before 1965 and computers, going back to K.F. Gauss, and Yates in 1937 [see Rockmore, 1999]. Since its first *practical* inception by Cooley and Tukey in 1965, mathematicians, computer scientists and engineers have been devising alternate strategies to compute $\mathbf{F}(k)$ even more efficiently. Figure 6.6 shows a *decimation in time* (DIT) FFT computational strategy in which the 8 sample input array order is left sequential, however, the output array is in natural order. Note that, in this algorithm, and in all others, there are dyadic summations at each intermediary

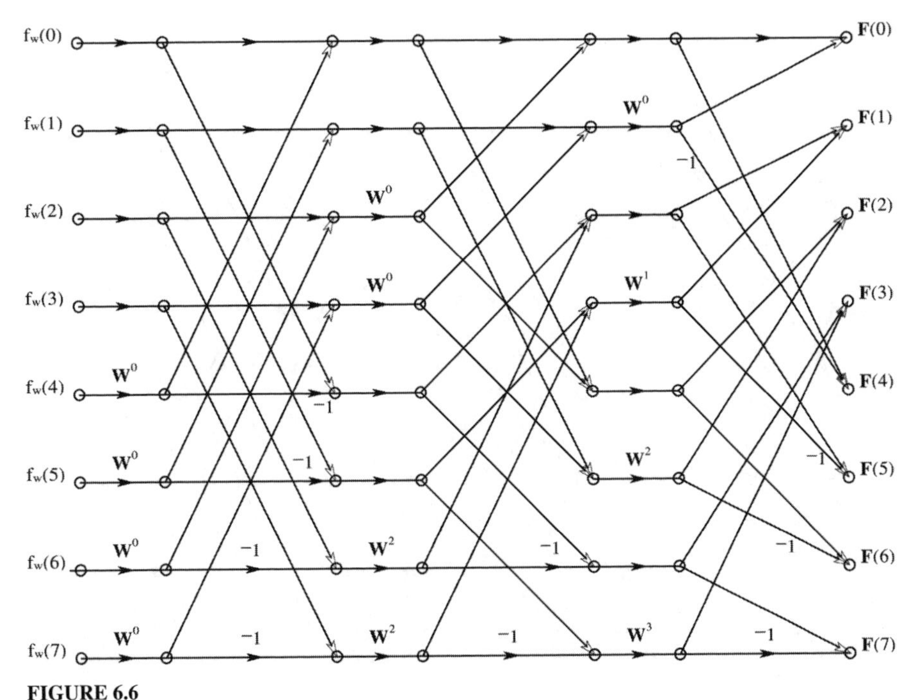

FIGURE 6.6
Another example of an eight-point, decimation in time, FFT algorithm.

SFG node. Note that $\mathbf{W}^{\mathrm{nk}} = \mathbf{W}_{\mathbf{N}}^{\mathrm{nk}}$ in some FFT notations. For $\mathrm{N}=8$, we have:

$$\mathbf{W_8}^{\mathrm{nk}} = \exp[-\mathrm{j}2\pi \mathrm{nk}/8] = \exp[-\mathrm{j\,nk}\pi/4] \tag{6.41}$$

The complex $\mathbf{W}^{\mathrm{nk}}$ factor can range from $\exp[-\mathrm{j}0\pi/4] = 1\angle 0°$ for n and/or k $= 0$. Other values of the angle argument are: $\exp[-\mathrm{j}1\pi/4] = 1\angle -45°$ for $\mathrm{n}=\mathrm{k}=1$, $\exp[-\mathrm{j}2\pi/4] = 1\angle -90°$ for $\mathrm{n}=1$, $\mathrm{k}=2$ and $\mathrm{n}=2$ and $\mathrm{k}=1$, all the way up to $\exp[-\mathrm{j}49\pi/4] = 1\angle -4365°$ for $\mathrm{n}=\mathrm{k}=7$. In fact, nk can have only the values: 0, 1, 2, 3, 4, 5, 6, 7, 8, 9, 10, 12, 14, 15, 16, 18, 20, 21, 24, 25, 28, 30, 35, 36, 42 and 49. Note that the angle of $\mathbf{W}^{\mathrm{nk}}$ repeats for certain nk values. That is, $\mathbf{W}^{\mathrm{nk}+8} = \mathbf{W}^{\mathrm{nk}}$ for $\mathrm{N}=8$. For example, when $\mathrm{nk}=1,9,$or 25, the angle of $\mathbf{W}^{\mathrm{nk}}$ is $-45°$.

An additional class of FFT algorithms is based on the *decimation in frequency* (DIF) strategy. Figure 6.7 illustrates an eight-point FFT procedure where input and output array orders are kept natural. Contrast this SFG with the Figure 6.6, where DIT is used and input and output array orders are kept natural. The creation of more efficient FFT arrays is an active area in applied mathematics. Algebraic details on the DIT and DIF approaches to the FFT, as well as windowing can be found in references such as Williams (1986), Stern (2000), Cunningham (1992), Proakis and Manolakis (1989) and Lecture notes from University of Strathclyde, U.K. (2001).

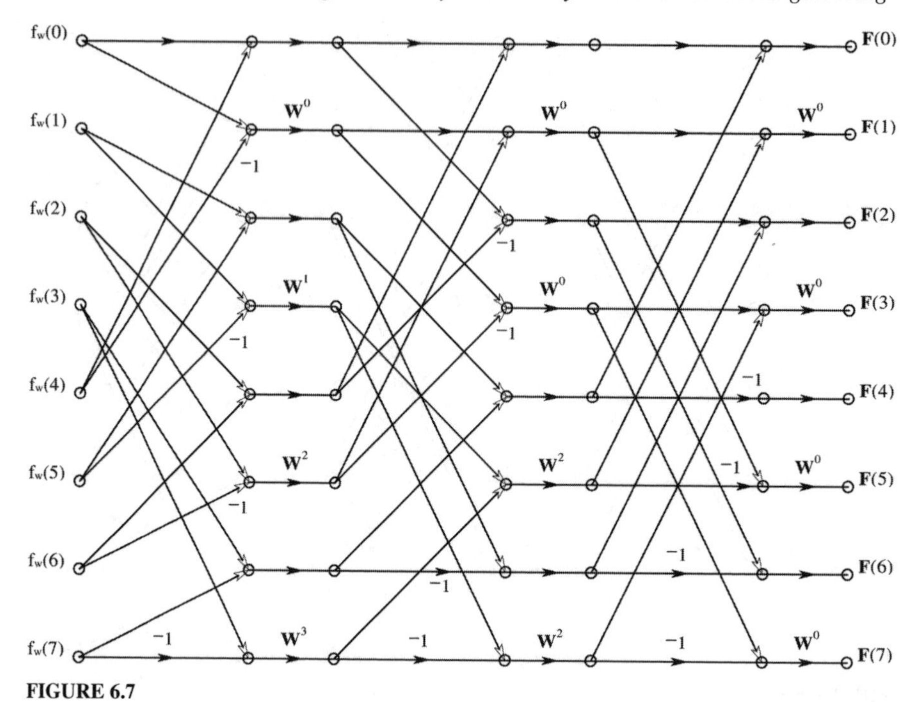

FIGURE 6.7
An example of an eight-point, decimation in frequency, FFT algorithm.

6.4.4 Discussion

There are very good odds that you, the reader, will never need to develop your own FFT routine. Many FFT software routines written in various computer languages including FORTRAN, C++, etc. are available free on the internet. Matlab™ has FFT subroutines. Also, companies offering data acquisition interface cards and software for PCs, such as National Instruments™, offer their proprietary versions of FFT routines. Thus there is little chance that a people setting up a DSP capability to examine the steady-state frequency characteristics of various biomedical signals will have to write their own FFT routine from scratch. It is important to know what is happening inside the FFT "black box," however. Note that the FFT $\{f(n)\}$ can be displayed as: $|\mathbf{F}(k)|$ and $\angle\mathbf{F}(k)$ vs. k, $Re\{\mathbf{F}(k)\}$ and $Im\{\mathbf{F}(k)\}$ vs. k, or $|\mathbf{F}(k)|^2$ vs. k. Note that $f = k/NT$ Hz. Because the $Re\{\mathbf{F}(k)\}$ is even around $k = N/2$, it is customary to only display $Re\{\mathbf{F}(k)\}$ for $0 \leq k \leq N/2$. Also, $Im\{\mathbf{F}(k)\}$ is odd around $k = N/2$, so it is customary to display $Im\{\mathbf{F}(k)\}$ for $0 \leq k \leq N/2$, as well. This means that the maximum frequency of $Re\{\mathbf{F}(k)\}$ and $Im\{\mathbf{F}(k)\}$ is $f_{max} = (N/2)/(NT) = 1/(2T) = f_N = f_s/2$, the *Nyquist frequency* of the sampled signal, $f(n)$.

When a stationary $f(n)$ is contaminated with noise, it is common practice to average M FFT spectra computed from M separate epochs cut from $f(n)$. It can be shown that the root-mean-squared noise on the averaged $|\mathbf{F}(k)|$ decreases as $1/\sqrt{M}$. Also, in displaying a large N FFT, it is customary to "connect the dots" of the discrete display by a interpolation routine, so a smooth curve appears on the CRT approximating the ideal CFT, $|\mathbf{F}(j2\pi f)|$, etc.

6.5 Chapter Summary

In this chapter we have examined the properties and applications of the DFT. Data window functions were covered in Section 6.3. The simplest window is the 0,1 rectangular window, which is inherent in taking a finite number of samples of a continuous $f(t)$ defined over all time. By considering the complex convolution of a finite-duration window function with CFT, $\mathbf{W}(\omega)$, with the signal function CFT, $\mathbf{F}(\omega)$, we were able to show how window function shape, $w(t)$, affects the sidelobes of the resultant spectrum of $\mathbf{F_W}(\omega)$, hence, the spectral resolution of closely spaced frequency components in $f(t)$.

Various schemes to calculate the fast Fourier transform were examined in Section 6.4. The FFT is implemented to efficiently calculate (in terms of computer time and memory) DFTs of sampled time functions.

Problems

6.1 A rectangular pulse time function is sampled giving $x(n) = 1,1,1,\ldots 1.$ for $n = 0,1,2\ldots,N-1$, and $x(n) = 0,0,0,\ldots$ for $n \geq N$. In closed form, the DFT, $\mathbf{X}(k)$, of this $x(n)$ this can be written as [Williams, 1986; Equation 8.10]:

$$\mathbf{X}(k) = \sum_{n=0}^{N-1} (1)\exp[-jn(2\pi k/N)] = \frac{1-\exp[-jN(2\pi k/N)]}{1-\exp[-j(2\pi k/N)]}$$

a. Show that this $\mathbf{X}(k)$ can also be written in the form:

$$\mathbf{X}(k) = N\frac{\text{sinc}(A)}{\text{sinc}(B)}\exp[-jC]$$

Note that $\text{sinc}(m) \equiv \sin(\pi m)/(\pi m)$. Find expressions for A,B and C as functions of k,N, and π.

b. Let $N = 6$. Evaluate $\mathbf{X}(k)$ for $k = 0,1,2,\ldots,5$.

6.2 Find the DFT of the sequence, $x(n) = \sin(n\pi/N)$ for $n = 0, 1,2,\ldots N-1$. *Hint:* express the sinusoid in exponential form.

6.3 A sampled $x(t)$ gives $x^*(t) = e^{-bnT}, \quad n = 0,1,2,\ldots$.

a. Find the DFT of $x^*(t)$ in closed form. Use the identity $\sum_{n=0}^{N-1} \rho^n \equiv \frac{1-\rho^n}{1-\rho}. 0 < \rho < 1$. Note that, in the limit as $N \to \infty, \sum \rho^n \equiv \frac{1}{1-\rho}$.

b. Express the DFT in *polar notation* (magnitude and angle) as a function of k:

$|\mathbf{X}^*(k)|\angle\varphi(k), \quad k = 0,1,2,\ldots,N-1.$

c. Let $T = 0.2$, $b = 1$ and $N = 8$. Plot $|\mathbf{X}^*(k)|$ and $\varphi(k)$ vs. k for $k = 0,1,2,\ldots,7$.

6.4 A continuous time function is sampled, giving:
$x(n) = e^{-bnT}U(n), 0 \leq n \leq N-1, b = 10\ \text{sec}^{-1}, T = 0.01\ \text{sec}, N = 20.$

a. Find an algebraic expression for $\mathbf{X}(k)$ in rational form.

b. Give algebraic expressions for $|\mathbf{X}(k)|$ and $\angle\mathbf{X}(k)$.

c. Plot and dimension $|\mathbf{X}(k)|$ and $\angle\mathbf{X}(k)$ for $0 \leq k \leq N$. Use parameter values given above.

6.5 Find the DFT for the even sampled time function,

$$x(n) = e^{-cT|n|}, -(N-1)/2 \leq n \leq (N-1)/2,\ N = 13,\ c = 4,\ T = 0.1$$

Use $\mathbf{X}(k) = \sum_{n=-6}^{6} e^{-cT|n|}e^{-jnk2\pi/N}$

Find and plot $\mathbf{X}(k)$ for $0 \leq k \leq 13$.

6.6 A rectangular pulse is sampled yielding: $x(n)=1$ for $0 \leq n \leq 4$, and $x(n)=0$ for $n>4$. $N=5$. The sampling period is $T=0.001$ sec. (1 ms).

a. Find an algebraic expression for $\mathbf{X}(k)$. Plot and dimension $|\mathbf{X}(k)|$ and $\angle\mathbf{X}(k)$. What is the Hz frequency spacing between $\mathbf{X}(k)$ values?

b. Now let the pulse be even (centered around $t=0$). Repeat a.

6.7 Consider a cosine wave, $x(t)=\cos(\omega_o t)$, $-\infty \leq t \leq \infty$. $\omega_o = 2\pi/\tau$, where τ is the period. $x(t)$ is sampled with a sample period $T=\tau/20$. Note that $\tau = (N-1)T$, so $N=21$. Consider the DFT of $x(n)=\cos(\omega_o nT)=\cos(n\pi/10)$ taken from $n=-(N-1)/2=-10$ to $n=(N-1)/2=10$. That is:

$$\mathbf{X}(k) = \sum_{n=-10}^{10} \cos(n\pi/10)e^{-jkn2\pi/N}$$

Find $\mathbf{X}(k)$ for this even time function.

6.8 a. Find an expression for the IDFT of $\mathbf{X}(k)=1, 1, 1, 1, 1$ for $-2 \leq k \leq 2$, and $X(k)=0$ for $|k|>2$. Note $\mathbf{X}(k)$ is real and even, and $N=5$.

b. Evaluate $x(n)$ for $n=0, 1, 2$. Note $x(n)$ is even, so you do not have to find $x(-1)$ and $x(-2)$.

6.9 a. $\mathbf{X}(k)=1, 1, 1$ for $-1 \leq k \leq 1$, and $\mathbf{X}(k)=0$ for $|k|>1$. In this problem, $N=3$. Find, plot and dimension the IDFT, $x(n)$, for $0 \leq n \leq 6$. Comment on the periodicity of $x(n)$.

b. The frequency spacing of $\mathbf{X}(k)$ is 0.1 Hz between adjacent values. Find the time spacing, T, between $x(n)$ elements.

6.10 A sampled cosine pulse on a pedestal is given by the even real function:

$x(n)=½[1+\cos(n\pi/5)]$ for $-5 \leq n \leq 5$, and $\chi(n)=0$ for $|n|>5$. $N=11$.

Find an expression for and plot and dimension the DFT of $x(n)$, $\mathbf{X}(k)$. Plot $\mathbf{X}(k)$ for $0 \leq k \leq 10$.

7

Introduction to Time-Frequency Analysis of Biomedical Signals

7.1 Introduction

This chapter will introduce an important mathematical tool for describing non-stationary (NS) biomedical signals; i.e., *joint time-frequency analysis* (JTFA). The following sections describe various transforms used to make JTF plots. These include the *short-term Fourier transform,* the *Gabor* and *adaptive Gabor* transforms, the *Wigner-Ville* and *psuedo-Wigner-Ville* transforms, *Cohen's general class* of JTF transforms, and the use of *wavelets* in JTF analysis. In addition, some applications of JTFA in biomedicine are described, and certain sources of JTFA software on the www are given.

JTFA is a mathematical process whereby a one-dimensional signal in time, such as an electroencephalogram recording (EEG), is transformed into a two-dimensional distribution revealing the signal's magnitude, intensity or power at various frequencies as a function of time. A JTF plot can be two-dimensional with time on the x-axis, frequency on the y-axis, and intensity coded by shades of gray or colors. Alternately, a JTF plot can be a 3-D contour diagram ("waterfall" plot), with intensity (or signal power) plotted in the z direction, normal to the X-Y plane. Such 3-D plots can be displayed from different viewpoints to illustrate the 3-D JTF features of the nonstationary signal. JTF analysis has also been extended to the characterization of two-dimensional (spatial) signals (e.g., images, fingerprints) in terms of intensity vs. spatial frequency vs. x and y dimensions.

We remarked in Chapter 1 that most signals in biomedicine are nonstationary (NS). These include but are not limited to the EEG, ECG, heart sounds, the instantaneous heart rate, breath sounds, joint sounds, speech, animal sounds, etc. Intuitively, we know that the information in speech is carried by its intensity, its frequency content, and how these vary in time. Historically, the first application of JTF analysis sought to describe human speech sounds by their intensity and frequency content as they occurred in time; it was called a *"voice-print" spectrogram.* The sound intensity (in Watts/m^2) at a given frequency and time was coded as gray-tone density on the *voiceprint JTF spectrogram* paper. (A spectrogram is the magnitude squared of the Fourier transform or JTF transform of a signal; a spectrogram is positive-real.) An intensity-coded JTF spectrogram of a wren's song is shown in Figure 7.1 [Birds

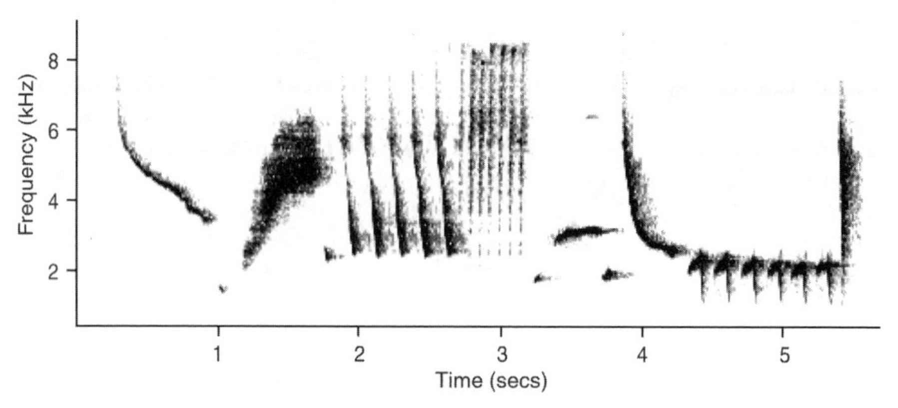

FIGURE 7.1
An intensity-coded JTF spectrogram of a wren's song. (Courtesy of Sandra Vehrencamp.)

2001]. (The blacker the marking, the higher the intensity. This type of gray scale can generally be read subjectively with 3 or 4 bit resolution.) Note the complicated time-frequency structure of the song. An example of a 3-D, *waterfall, JTF spectrogram* for gurgling breath sounds is shown in Figure 7.2. Three inhale/exhale cycles are shown. Note that the inhales are noisier and contain more high frequencies. Here the sound intensity is coded as height on the vertical axis.

The earliest speech spectrograms were made by purely analog means. A short utterance of ca. 2.5 seconds was picked up by a microphone, amplified, and recorded on an analog magnetic tape loop. The tape loop was repeatedly played back, and

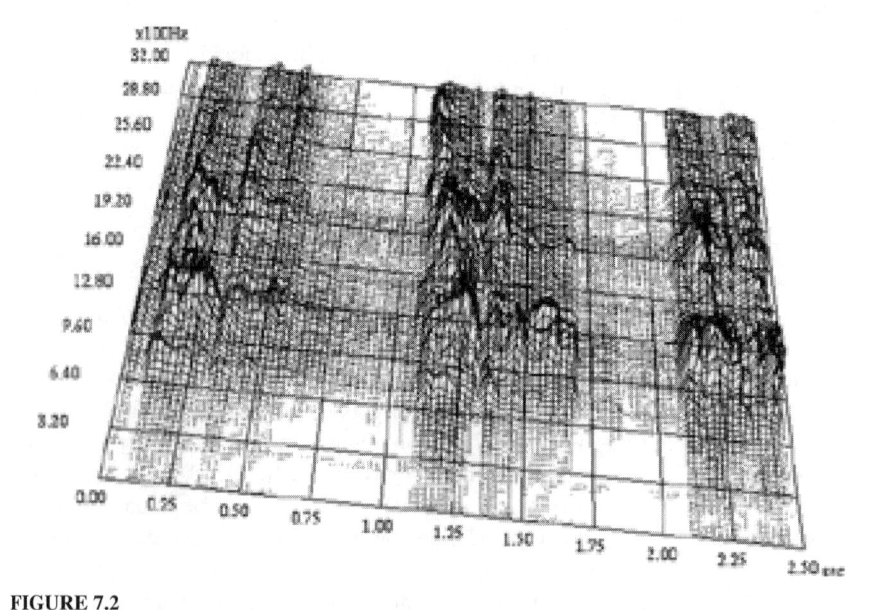

FIGURE 7.2
A 3-D waterfall-type JTF spectrogram of gurgling breath sounds. Three inhale/exhale breath cycles are shown.

the playback signal voltage was passed through an analog, narrow band-pass filter whose center frequency was proportional to the vertical height of a thermal stylus writing on a rotating drum covered with heat-sensitive paper. Drum rotation angle was synchronized with the point in time on the tape being played back, i.e., $360° =$ 2.5 seconds. Stylus temperature was proportional to the mean-squared output voltage from the tuned filter; the more speech sound intensity at a given center frequency, the higher the output voltage^2 hence stylus temperature, and the blacker the mark on the paper. Many scans had to be done to cover a wide range of filter center frequencies which were generally spaced as closely as possible in order to have minimum overlap in their bandpass characteristics.

A trade-off in the time vs. frequency resolution was seen to exist; to obtain high frequency resolution, the filters had to have high Qs (half-power bandwidths divided by center frequency). However, the transient response of a high Q filter is slower than that for a low Q filter of the same center frequency. So the higher the Q, the less certain when in time the center frequency energy burst occurred. Many playback cycles at a given filter center frequency were required when closely spaced high-Q filters were used because high-Q filters also have lower outputs because of their narrow bandwidths.

To summarize: Narrow-band filters resolve harmonics but blur temporal details such as exactly when bursts occur. On the other hand, low-Q filters enable the resolution of events in time at the cost of frequency detail. This trade-off in resolution of time vs. frequency is a demon characteristic of all types of JTF analysis algorithms, including modern JTFA systems that use numerical algorithms on sampled data to calculate the spectrogram. Stated simply, $\Delta f \Delta t = W$, where W is a constant, and Δf and Δt are the closest resolvable two frequencies and two events, respectively. Much research is being carried out to find JTFA algorithms that reduce W. We will examine some of the newer, more innovative algorithms.

JTF spectrosopy has applications in geophysical science, economics, biology, medicine, as well as in engineering and genomics. Another major use includes submarine sonar to identify targets and sense target Doppler shifts. JTFA is also used in imaging to describe an object's *spatial frequencies* vs. x and y dimensions. The Internet is full of sites showing JTF spectrograms of all sorts of animal sounds — shrimp, fish, dolphins, whales, bird songs, even insects. Visit the Cornell University Bioacoustics Research Program (BRP) web site to see (and hear) many interesting examples of JTF spectrograms. And, as mentioned above, JTFA has been applied to ECG, EMG and EEG waveforms for diagnostic purposes, and also to heart and breath sounds.

The following sections will examine some of the many transforms and algorithms currently used to find JTF spectrograms. As you will see, some algorithms are better than others for different applications. In general, JTFA algorithms can be divided into two categories: *linear* and *quadratic*. The linear JTFA algorithms include the *short-term Fourier transform* (STFT) and the *Gabor transfom* (GT) and its related forms. The quadratic JTFA forms include the *Wigner-Ville Distribution* (W-VD), the *psuedo-Wigner-Ville distribution* (pW-VD), the *Choi-Williams Transform* (C-WT), *Cohen's class* of JTFA transforms, and the *cone-shaped distribution.*

Three major considerations exist that govern one's choice of which algorithm to use:

1. Computational complexity and time
2. Trade-offs in time-frequency resolution
3. Interference between harmonics in a spectrogram leading to the display of artifacts.

As you will see, some JTFA algorithms are better suited for certain types of signals than others. Below, we first examine the widely used STFT.

7.2 The Short-Term Fourier Transform

Chapter 5 examined the properties and uses of the continuous Fourier transform (CFT) and its inversion integral. For convenience, we repeat them below:

$$\mathbf{U}(j\omega) \equiv \int_{-\infty}^{\infty} u(t)e^{-j\omega t}dt \tag{7.1}$$

$$u(t) \equiv \int_{-\infty}^{\infty} \mathbf{U}(j2\pi f)\exp(j2\pi ft)df, \quad \omega = 2\pi f \tag{7.2}$$

Use of the CFT and ICFT assumes that the signal, $u(t)$ is *stationary.* A peak in $|U(j\omega)|$ gives no information about when in time a certain frequency component occurred, or whether it was present at all times in $u(t)$. Because we are interested in describing NS time functions, we need a means of localizing in time when certain frequency components are present in an NS signal.

Section 6.3 described the effect of the data window shape on the ability of a CFT to resolve closely spaced coherent frequencies in a $u(t)$ consisting of a superposition of spectral components. It was shown that a simple rectangular window of a given width gave the sharpest resolution of signal spectral peaks but also manifested high-amplitude side lobes that affected the resolution of closely spaced low-amplitude, coherent components in $u(t)$. It was also shown that, in using other window functions of the same width, there was a trade-off between spectral resolution and side lobe interference. The side lobes produce *frequency leakage,* which causes *interference* between the different adjacent components in the windowed $u(t)$. The side lobe magnitudes are generally dependent on window shape; window width is inversely related to spectral resolution.

The *short-time* or *short-term Fourier transform* provides a means of selecting a certain section of $u(t)$ of duration $2T_w$ in which we assume that $u(t)$ is short-term-stationary and can be Fourier transformed. The continuous STFT transform of $u(t)$

is written:

$$\mathbf{U}_{\mathrm{ST}}(\omega,\tau)=\int_{-\infty}^{\infty}\mathrm{u(t)w^*(t-\tau)e^{-j\omega t}dt}=\frac{1}{2\pi}\int \mathbf{U}(\sigma)\mathbf{W}_{\tau}^{*}(\omega-\sigma)\mathrm{d}\sigma \tag{7.3}$$

(complex convolution)

Note that $\mathrm{u(t)}$ is assumed to exist for $-\infty \leq \mathrm{t} \leq \infty$, and the window, $\mathrm{w(t)}$, is generally of a finite duration, $2\mathrm{T_w}$. The w^* denotes that the complex conjugate of $\mathrm{w(t)}$ is used in the STFT integral. Except in unusual cases, $\mathrm{w(t)}$ is a real, even function, and has no conjugate. The *JTF spectrogram* is defined as the magnitude-squared of each of the STFTs $(\tau=\mathrm{n}\Delta\mathrm{T})$:

$$\mathrm{S_{uu}}(\omega,\,\tau)\equiv|\mathbf{U}_{\mathrm{ST}}(\omega,\,\tau)|^2=\mathbf{U}_{\mathrm{ST}}(\omega,\,\tau)\mathrm{U}_{\mathrm{ST}}^{*}(\omega,\,\tau) \tag{7.4}$$

The simplest $\mathrm{w(t)}$ is the even rectangular window, $\mathrm{w(t)}=1$ for $-\mathrm{T_W}\leq\mathrm{t}\leq\mathrm{T_w}$, and $\mathrm{w(t)}=0$ for $|\mathrm{t}|>\mathrm{T_w}$. For other commonly used window functions, the reader should consult Table 6.2.

In the STFT, the window is used to select subintervals of the signal under analysis (SUA), $\mathrm{u(t)}$. These subintervals of the SUA defined by the window have a finite data length. Each time the window is slid along by τ, the STFT is calculated using a new parameter $\mathrm{n}\Delta\mathrm{T}$ for every integration. The windows are commonly allowed to overlap 50% for best T-F resolution. Thus, the center of the first window is at $\tau=0$. The next STFT integral is computed for $\tau=\mathrm{T_w}$, etc. Finally, the last and Nth STFT integral is computed for $\tau=\mathrm{NT_w}$. Clearly, $\Delta\mathrm{T}=\mathrm{T_w}$. It is expedient to divide the total $\mathrm{u(t)}$ record length of interest, $\mathrm{T_e}$, into $(\mathrm{N}-1)$ segments or *epochs,* each of length $\mathrm{T_w}$, so $\mathrm{T_e}=(\mathrm{N}-1)\mathrm{T_w}$.

Intuitively, we can see that *time resolution* of the JTF spectrogram calculated with the N STFTs will *increase* as N becomes large and the window width, $\mathrm{T_w}$, becomes smaller. *At the same time that the window width is decreased, the frequency resolution in the JTF spectrogram becomes poorer.* As we remarked above, this trade off between time- and frequency resolution is a general property of all JTF spectrograms. This uncertainty was stated above in general form as $\Delta\mathrm{f}\Delta\mathrm{t}=\mathrm{W}$, where W is a constant. Gabor (1946) derived the time-frequency uncertainty relation in a more formal form as:

$$\sigma_{\mathrm{t}}\sigma_{\mathrm{f}}\geq\frac{1}{4\pi} \tag{7.5}$$

Where σ_{t} and σ_{f} are the standard deviations of the time and frequency density functions. The normalized variance of the power density spectrum of the signal is given by [Steeghs, 1997]:

$$\sigma_{\mathrm{f}}^{2}\equiv\frac{\int(\mathrm{f}-\bar{\mathrm{f}})^2\Phi_{\mathrm{uu}}(\mathrm{f})\mathrm{df}}{\int\Phi_{\mathrm{uu}}(\mathrm{f})\mathrm{df}} \tag{7.6}$$

Where: $\Phi_{\mathrm{uu}}(\mathrm{f})$ is the two-sided power density spectrum of a NS signal, $\mathrm{u(t)}$, and $\bar{\mathrm{f}}$ is the normalized mean frequency of $\Phi_{\mathrm{uu}}(\mathrm{f})$. $\Phi_{\mathrm{uu}}(\mathrm{f})$ is defined as the magnitude squared of the Fourier transform of $\mathrm{u(t)}$. That is:

$$\Phi_{uu}(f) \equiv |F\{u(t)\}|^2 \tag{7.7}$$

and

$$\bar{f} \equiv \frac{\int f\Phi_{uu}(f)df}{\int \Phi_{uu}(f)df} \tag{7.8}$$

Similarly, the variance, σ_t, is found from:

$$\sigma_t^2 = \frac{\int (t-\bar{t})^2 \Phi_{uu}(t)dt}{\int \Phi_{uu}(t)dt} \tag{7.9}$$

Where:

$$\Phi_{uu}(t) \equiv |u(t)|^2 \tag{7.10}$$

and

$$\bar{t} = \frac{\int t\Phi_{uu}(t)dt}{\int \Phi_{uu}(t)dt} \tag{7.11}$$

In practice, the STFT is computed numerically by periodically sampling $u(t)$ and using the DFT on the product $[u(n)w(n-s)]$, where s is the shift integer. Note that the inverse STFT recovers the kernel:

$$u(t)w(t-\tau) = \frac{1}{2\pi}\int_{-\infty}^{\infty} \mathbf{U}_{ST}(\omega, \tau)e^{j\omega t}d\omega \tag{7.12}$$

In an attempt to improve JTF resolution when the STFT is used, the window duration and shape can be manipulated to optimize the JTF spectrogram resolution for a particular NS signal. The signal itself, reflected and shifted in time, can be used as a window to find the JTF spectrogram by Fourier transform. This approach is called the *Wigner-Ville distribution.*

7.3 Gabor and Adaptive Gabor Transform

In the seemingly endless search for "better" algorithms for JTF spectral analysis that have both high time and frequency resolution, low cross-term artifacts and good noise immunity, we next direct our attention to the *Gabor transform,* which is a special form of the STFT, described above. The continuous representation of the GT for a simple 1-D, NS signal, $u(t)$, is:

$$\mathbf{G}(\tau, \omega) = \int_{-\infty}^{\infty} u(t)\{g(t-\tau)\exp[-j\omega(t-\tau)]\}\exp(-j\omega\tau)dt \tag{7.13}$$

Where one form of the fixed-width Gabor windowing function is the Gaussian function:

$$g(t,\tau) = \frac{1}{\sqrt{2\pi}\alpha}\exp[-(t-\tau)^2/(2\alpha^2)] \tag{7.14}$$

τ gives the center of the weighting function, with $\alpha > 0$ controlling the effective window width. $B^{\alpha}_{\tau,\omega}$ is the Gabor *basis function,* given by:

$$B^{\alpha}_{\tau,\omega}(t) = g^*(t-\tau)\exp(-j\omega t) \tag{7.15}$$

The Fourier transform of the basis function is given by the real and complex shifting relations of Fourier transforms:

$$F\{B^{\alpha}_{\tau,\omega}(t)\} = \widehat{B}^{\alpha}_{\tau,\omega}(\mu) = \exp[-j\tau(\mu-\omega)]\mathbf{G}(j\mu - j\omega) \tag{7.16}$$

Note that the GT is basically the STFT with a Gaussian-type window function centered at $t=\tau$. The 2-D GT has recently found application in the spatial frequency analysis of images in pattern recognition. Image spatial frequency is presented as a function of the image coordinates. For practical computation of the GT, one must use the discrete form, such as given in the text by Qian and Chen (1996).

In summary, one interpretation of the GT is that it is a real convolution between the nonstationary signal, $u(t)$, and a frequency-modulated $g(t)$. Note that $g(t)$ multiplied by $\exp(-j\omega t)$ in $\exp(-j\omega t) \overset{F}{\longleftrightarrow} \mathbf{G}(j\mu + j\omega)$, the time domain is equivalent to the Fourier transform pair, $g(t)$ and the GT integral can be viewed as a real convolution with t as the dummy variable. Thus, the GT integral can also be considered to be the local Fourier transform in a time interval around τ, or a bandpass-filtered version of all of $u(t)$ at a certain frequency interval.

7.4 Wigner-Ville and Pseudo-Wigner Transforms

The continuous *Wigner-Ville transform* of an NS signal, $u(t)$, is given by the integral:

$$W_{Vu}(t,\omega) \equiv \int_{-\infty}^{\infty} u(t+\tau/2)u^*(t-\tau/2)\exp[-j\omega\tau]d\tau \tag{7.17}$$

The quadratic Wigner-Ville JTF transform (W-VT) has four serious limitations:

1. Cross-term calculations may artifactually give rise to negative energy.
2. *Aliasing effects* may distort the spectrogram such that high-frequency components may cause low-frequency artifacts.
3. The W-VT deals poorly with noisy signals.

4. If more than one coherent frequency is present in $u(t)$, there will be *cross-term artifacts* in the W-V spectrogram. (This is a disadvantage when examining speech, animal sounds, certain biomedical sounds and musical instrument sounds having harmonics.)

On the plus side, the W-VT, $W_u(t,\omega)$, is *real;* it does not have imaginary components like the STFT does. It is also simple and fast to compute numerically. Some mathematical properties of the W-VT given by Bastiaans (1997) follow:

1. A point signal at $t=t_0$ can be described as $u(t)=\delta(t-t_0)$. Its W-VT transform is $W_u(t,\omega)=\delta(t-t_0)$. At one point, $t=t_0$, all frequencies are present, with no contributions at other points.
2. Let $u(t)$ be an analytic harmonic signal: $u(t)=\exp(j\omega_o t)$, described in the frequency domain as $\mathbf{U}(\omega)=2\pi\delta(\omega-\omega_o)$. A plane wave and a point source are dual to each other, i.e., the FT of one function has the same form as the other function. Due to this duality, the W-VT of a plane wave will be the same as that for the point signal, but rotated in the TF domain by $90°$. The W-VT of the plane wave is $W_u(t,\omega)=2\pi\delta(\omega-\omega_o)$. At all points in time, only one frequency $\omega=\omega_0$ appears, as expected.
3. $\int W_{Vu}(t,\omega)dt=|\boldsymbol{FT}\{u(t)\}|^2$ (Intensity of the frequency spectrum.)
4. $\frac{1}{2\pi}\int W_{Vu}(t,\omega)d\omega=|u(t)|^2$(Intensity of the signal.)
5. $\frac{1}{2\pi}\int W_{Vu}(t,\omega)dtd\omega=\int|u(t)|^2dt=\frac{1}{2\pi}\int|\boldsymbol{FT}\{u(t)\}|^2d\omega$
6. Finally, an equivalent of Schwarz's inequality can be derived for two W-VTs for two NS time signals, $u_1(t)$ and $u_2(t)$ [Bastiaans, 1997]:

$$\frac{1}{2\pi}\int\int\frac{1}{2\pi}W_{Vu1}(t,\omega)W_{Vu2}(t,\omega)dtd\omega\leq\left[\frac{1}{2\pi}\int W_{Vu1}(t,\omega)dtd\omega\right][(1/2\pi)\int W_{Vu2}(t,\omega)dtd\omega\Big]$$

Using the notation used by National Instruments (1998), the discrete form of the W-VT is given by:

$$W_{VDu}(i,k)=\sum_{m=-L/2}^{L/2}u(i+m)u^*(i-m)\exp(-j2\pi km/L) \tag{7.18}$$

The time signal, $u(t)$ and its conjugate, $u^*(t)$, are antialias (low-pass) filtered before sampling. The shifting by m and multiplication is done numerically. The discrete W-VT can also be calculated from:

$$W_{VDu}(i,k)=\sum_{m=-L/2}^{L/2}\mathbf{U}(i+m)\mathbf{U}^*(i-m)\exp(+j2\pi km/L) \tag{7.19}$$

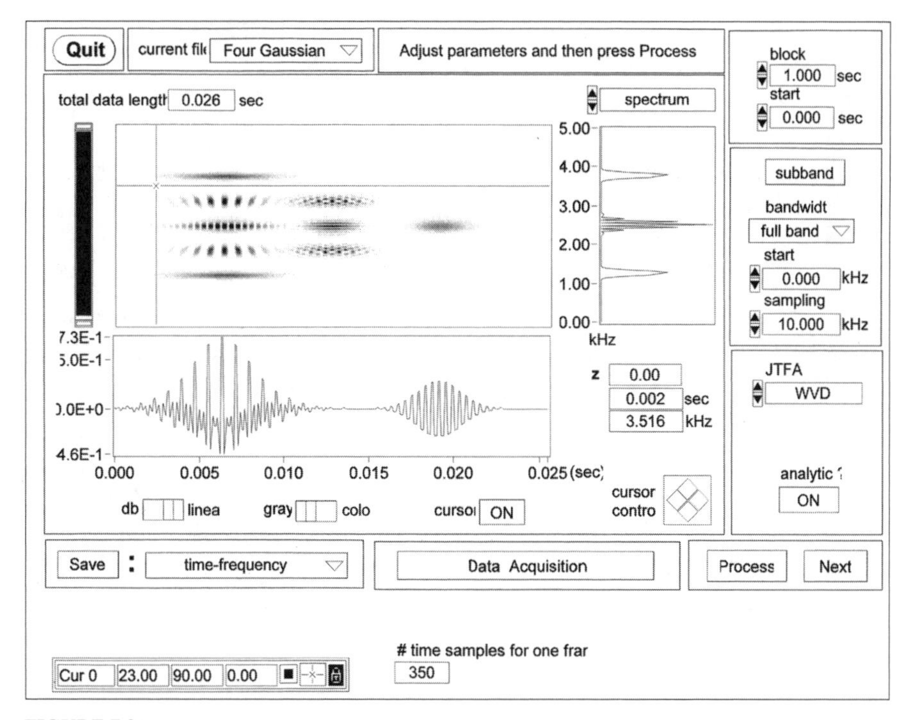

FIGURE 7.3a

(a) A Wigner-Ville JTF spectrogram of a complex signal consisting of three simultaneous Gaussian amplitude-modulated sinusoids of different frequencies, followed by a single Gaussian am burst. Note the cross-term phantoms. See the text for discussion.

Where $\mathbf{U}(\mathrm{k})$ is the STDFT of $\mathrm{u(i)}$, and the substitution, $\mathrm{k} \rightarrow (\mathrm{i+m})$ is made in $\mathbf{U}(\mathrm{k})$, etc. Note that, as in the continuous W-VT, $\mathrm{W_{VDu}(i,k)}$ is real. i is the displacement along the time axis $(\mathrm{t = iT_s})$ and k is the displacement along the frequency axis $(\mathrm{f = k\Delta f})$.

Cross term interference in the W-VD is illustrated in Figure 7.3a. Here, four signal terms consisting of Gaussian amplitude-modulated tone bursts are transformed. Three simultaneous am signals are centered at 6 msec; one at 3.75 kHz, one at 2.5 kHz and one at 1.25 kHz. A fourth Gaussian burst at 2.5 kH is centered at 19 msec. The total time span is 25 msec, and the sampling rate is 10 kHz. Note the profusion of cross-term, "phantom" artifacts that always sit halfway between the real terms in frequency or time. The two artifact spectra between the three real terms centered at 6 msec are at 3.125 and 1.875 kHz. Note also that the real 2.5 kHz term is "chopped." Three phantom terms also appear centered at 13 msec. They are at 3.125, 2.5 and 1.875 kHz. By way of contrast, examine the JTF spectrogram of the same signals done with the familiar STFT using a Hanning window 64 samples wide, shown in Figure 7.3b. It is the cross terms in the W-VT that make it unsuitable for examining NS signals with harmonics, such as heart sounds and speech in the JTF domain.

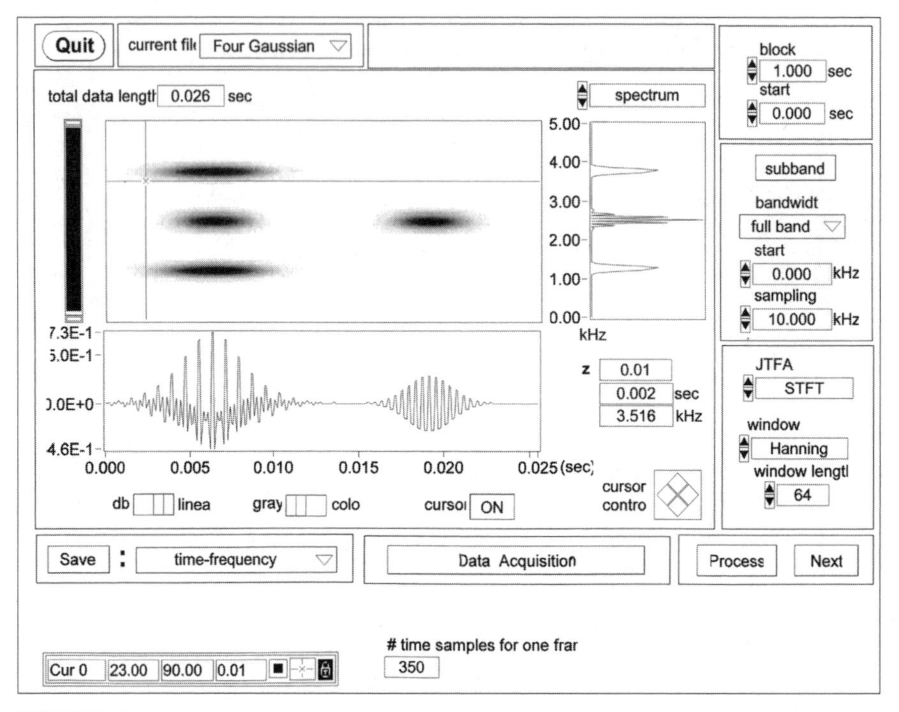

FIGURE 7.3b

(b) The JTF spectrogram of the same Gaussian signals of Figure 7.3a calculated by the short-term Fourier transform using a Hanning window 64 samples in width. Note the absence of artifacts. The data epoch in both cases was 25 msec, and the sampling period was 0.1 msec. (Joint-Time Frequency Toolkit, limited version, ©1995 National Instruments Corp. Bundled as two floppies with Qian and Chen, 1996. With permission.)

To suppress the cross-term artifacts, a window function has been introduced to form the *pseudo-Wigner-Ville transform* (pW-VT). In the time domain, this is:

$$\mathrm{pW_{VDu}(i,k)} = \sum_{\mathrm{m=-L/2}}^{\mathrm{L/2}} \mathrm{w(m)u(i+m)u^*(i-m)\exp(-j2\pi km/L)} \tag{7.20}$$

This form of the pW-VT will remove the three cross terms centered at t = 0.013 sec, shown in Figure 7.3a. However, the two cross terms centered at t = 0.006 sec are substantially unchanged. The frequency domain form of the pW-VT is:

$$\mathrm{pW_{VDu}(i,k)} = \sum_{\mathrm{m=-L/2}}^{\mathrm{L/2}} \mathbf{W}\mathrm{(m)}\mathbf{U}\mathrm{(i+m)}\mathbf{U}^*\mathrm{(i-m)\exp(+j2\pi km/L)} \tag{7.21}$$

Clearly, what is needed is a JTF spectrogram technique that removes or seriously attenuates *all* cross-term artifacts. Fortunately, several JTF transforms, such as the general JTF transform called *Cohen's class,* described below, are effective at cross-term suppression.

7.5 Cohen's General Class of JTF Distributions

In 1966, Leon Cohen described a modified DFT approach to finding the JTF spectrogram. The quadratic kernel JTF transforms that are included in *Cohen's class* are the already-considered *W-VT, pW-VT, Choi-Williams transform* and the *cone-shaped distribution transform* (CST). For a continuous signal, $u(t)$, Cohen's JTF distribution integral is given by:

$$\mathrm{CD}(t,\omega)=\frac{1}{4\pi^2}\iiint u(\sigma+\tau/2)u(\sigma-\tau/2)\varphi(\theta,\tau) \times\exp[-j(\theta t+\tau\omega+\theta\sigma)]d\sigma d\tau d\theta \tag{7.22}$$

Assume now that the signal, $u(t)$ is sampled (discrete), and can be represented by *impulse modulation* (cf. Sections 2.5 and 5.3). That is:

$$\tilde{u}(t)=\sum_n u(nT_s)\delta(t-nT_s)=u(t)P_T(t) \tag{7.23}$$

Where T_s is the sampling period. Now Cohen's distribution integral can be written:

$$\tilde{P}(t,\omega)=\frac{1}{4\pi r^2}\iiint\left[\sum_n u(nT_s)\delta(\sigma+\tau/2-nT_s)\right] \times\left[\sum_k u^*(kT_s)\delta(\sigma-\tau/2-kT_s)\right] \times\varphi(\theta,\tau)\exp[-j(\theta t+\tau\omega+\theta\sigma)]d\sigma d\tau d\theta \tag{7.24}$$

Because delta functions only exist at zero argument and there is a product of two of them in the integrand, we can set $\sigma+\tau/2-nT_s=\sigma-\tau/2-kT_s$, and solve for $\tau=(n-k)T_s$, then substitute this expression for τ into the delta function arguments. Thus:

$$\delta(\sigma+\tau/2-nT_s)=\delta(\sigma-\tau/2-kT_s)=\delta(\sigma-nT_s/2-kT_s/2) \tag{7.25}$$

We now integrate Equation 7.24 with respect to τ and obtain:

$$\tilde{P}(t,\omega)=\frac{1}{4\pi^2}\iint\sum_n\sum_k u(nT_s)u^*(kT_s)\varphi(\theta,(n-k)T_s)$$

$$\times \exp[-j(\theta t + (n-k)T_s\omega - \theta\sigma)]$$
$$\times \delta(\sigma - nT_s/2 - kT_s/2)d\sigma d\theta \tag{7.26}$$

We now let $m \equiv n+k$ in Equation 7.26, and then integrate with respect to σ, obtaining:

$$\tilde{P}(t,\omega) = \frac{1}{4\pi^2}\int \sum_n \sum_m u(nT_s)u^*((m-n)T_s)\varphi[\theta,(2n-m)T_s]$$
$$\times \exp[-j(\theta t + (2n-m)T_s\omega - \theta m T_s/2)]d\theta \tag{7.27}$$

Rearranging the orders of summation and integration we finally have:

$$\tilde{P}(t,\omega) = \sum_m \sum_n [u(nT_s)\exp(-jnT_s\omega)][u^*((m-n)T_s)\exp(j(m-n)T_s\omega)]$$
$$\times \frac{1}{4\pi^2}\int \varphi[\theta,(2n-m)T_s]\exp[-j\theta(t - mT_s/2)]d\theta \tag{7.28}$$

Equation 7.28 is a general expression for the Cohen JFT distribution [Parks, 1991]. Note that, when the kernel, $\varphi[\theta,(2n-m)T_s] = 1$, is substituted into Equation 7.22, and is integrated with respect to θ and σ, we obtain the Wigner-Ville transform (cf. Equation 7.18):

$$W-VT(t,\omega) = \frac{1}{2\pi}\int u(t+\tau/2)u^*(t-\tau/2)e^{-j\omega\tau}d\tau \tag{7.29}$$

The art in designing Cohen JTF transforms lies in the choice of the kernel to reduce cross-term interference while preserving time- and frequency resolution.

Notice that the discrete pseudo-Wigner transform, Equation 7.21, can be written as:

$$pW_{VDu}(i,k) = \sum_{m=-L/2}^{L/2}\left(\sum_n w(n)u(i-n+m)u^*(i-n-m)\right)$$
$$\times \exp(-j2\pi km/L) \tag{7.30}$$

Where $w(n)$ is the IDFT of **W**(k). Cohen wrote Equation 7.30 in a more general form:

$$C_u(i,k) = \sum_{m=-L/2}^{L/2}\sum_n \varphi(i,m)u(i-n+m)u^*(i-n-m)$$
$$\times \exp(-j2\pi km/L) \tag{7.31}$$

Where $\varphi(i,m)$ is the *discrete Cohen kernel function.*

When $\varphi_{C-W}(i,m) = \sqrt{\alpha/(4\pi m^2)}\exp[-\alpha i^2/(4m^2)]$, the result is the C-WT. The smaller α, the greater the smoothing; adjustment of α allows a tradeoff between TF resolution and cross-term interference. In an application note, National Instruments (1998) shows that the C-WT can effectively suppress the cross term caused by two auto terms with different time and frequency centers. However, the C-WT can neither completely suppress those cross terms from auto terms having the same time center and different frequencies, nor cross terms from auto terms with the same frequency and different time centers. The C-WT also is relatively slow to compute. A faster, more computationally efficient version of the C-WT is called the *Binomial Distribution* (BD) [Wood et al., 1992]. The discrete Cohen kernel in the BD is written:

$$\varphi_{\mathrm{BD}}(\mathrm{i,m}) = \left[\frac{|\mathbf{m}|}{\mathbf{i}+|\mathbf{m}/2|}\right]^{2^{-|\mathbf{m}|}} \tag{7.32}$$

Where **i** is *scale* and **m** is *shift.*

The CST of Zhao et al., (1990) uses the Cohen kernel:

$$\begin{aligned} \varphi(\mathrm{i,m}) &= \exp(-\alpha \mathrm{m}^2/\mathrm{c}) \quad \text{for } \mathrm{i}<\mathrm{m} \\ &= 0 \quad \text{otherwise.} \end{aligned} \tag{7.33}$$

The CST is ineffective in suppressing cross terms from auto terms at the same frequency but at different time centers. The CST does suppress cross-term artifacts between auto terms at different frequencies at the same time (valuable in analyzing speech, music and heart sounds), and cross terms from auto terms at different frequencies and time centers. It is quicker to compute than the C-WT, other things being equal.

Jeong and Williams (1992) modified the C-WT to further increase its resolution and decrease cross terms. They developed a new class of kernel they called the *reduced interference distribution* (RID). The Jeong-Williams RID is found from:

$$\mathrm{RID_u(t,\omega)} = \int \mathrm{R'_u(t,\tau)e^{-j\omega\tau}d\tau} \quad \text{(This is the 1-D CFT of } \mathrm{R'_u(t,\tau)}\text{.)} \tag{7.34}$$

Where:

$$\mathrm{R'_u(t,\tau)} = \int (1/|\tau|)\mathrm{h}\left(\frac{\sigma-\mathrm{t}}{\tau}\right)\mathrm{u}(\sigma+\tau/2)\mathrm{u}^*(\sigma-\tau/2)\mathrm{e}^{-\mathrm{j}\omega\tau}\mathrm{d}\sigma \tag{7.35}$$

One $\mathrm{h(t)}$ form that meets the RID criterion is the triangular function:

$$\mathrm{h(t)} = 2-4|\mathrm{t}|,\ |\mathrm{t}|<0.5, \text{ else } 0. \tag{7.36}$$

Other RID functions are given which include $\mathrm{h(t)=rect(t)}$, Hamming, a truncated Choi-Williams, and a truncated $\mathrm{h(t)} = (\alpha/2\pi)\ \sin(\alpha \mathrm{t}/2)/(\alpha \mathrm{t}/2)$. The interested reader should read the Jeong and Williams paper for details and simulation results.

Another approach to reducing the interference terms of the Wigner-Ville distribution was described by Krattenthaler and Hlawatsch (1993) in what they called the *smoothed Wigner distributions* (SWD). The SWD can be written as a discrete operation. The first summation is the real convolution of the WVD's discrete instantaneous signal product with a 2-D smoothing function, $\varphi(\mathrm{k,m})$:

$$\mathrm{c}_\varphi(\mathrm{n,m}) = \sum_{\mathrm{k}} \varphi(\mathrm{n-k,m})\mathrm{u(k+m)u^*(k-m)} \tag{7.37}$$

The SWD is the DFT of $c_\varphi(n,m)$:

$$\mathrm{SWD}_\varphi(n,q) = 2\sum_m c_\varphi(n,m)\exp(-4\pi qm) \tag{7.38}$$

The kernel $\varphi(k,m)$ is chosen so that its DFT with respect to m is real-valued and smooth.

National Instruments^{TM} (1998) offers a proprietary *adaptive spectrogram* (AS) JTFA algorithm in their JTFA toolkit. The AS performs optimally if $u(t)$ can be modeled by a sum of linear chirp-modulated Gaussian functions. The AS yields negligible cross terms, is nonnegative, and has extremely high resolution. The AS algorithm is computationally intense: computational time is slow compared to the STFT and pW-VT, for example, increasing exponentially with the length of the data record being analyzed.

7.6 Introduction to JTFA Using Wavelets

7.6.1 Introduction

A wavelet is basically an (effectively) finite-duration transient waveform, such as formed by multiplying a Gaussian envelope times a cosine wave. As you will see, there are many types of wavelets used in JTF analysis and each has its own interesting properties. A proper wavelet has some sort of damped oscillations, has zero mean and a finite norm. Some commonly used wavelet waveforms include, but are not limited to, the *Mexican hat (and other higher-order derivatives of Gaussian,* e.g., *DOG),* the *Morlet, Haar, Doubechies, Shannon, Meyer, Mallat, Paul* and *Battle-Lemarie.* No doubt others will be invented.

The wavelet approach to JTFA is long and complex: it goes back to the work of mathematician Alfred Haar in 1907. The reader interested in the evolution of wavelet analysis of NS signals should read the comprehensive review paper by Polikar (1999). The development of wavelet analysis is an active area of research today, and its applications include biomedical signal analysis, communications, geophysics, meteorology, financial analysis (stocks), vibration analysis, 2-D image processing, including fingerprints, etc.

You will see that wavelet analysis offers a very flexible and adaptable means of describing NS signals in the T-F domain. As in the case of the Fourier transform-based JTFA methods, there are a continuous wavelet transform (CWT) and a discrete wavelet transform (DWT).

Again, for pedagogical reasons, I will introduce wavelets through the CWT, and then describe the DWT and its applications. (Do not confuse the CWT with the C-WT (Choi-Williams transform.)) The CWT can be written:

$$\mathrm{CWT}(a,b) = (1/\sqrt{a})\int\!\!\int u(t)\psi^*[(t-b)/a]dt \tag{7.39}$$

(This notation follows that used by Qian and Chen (1996) and Polikar (1998).) $\psi(t)$ (with a = 1, b = 0) is called the *mother wavelet;* it can be real or complex. The * denotes its complex conjugate, used in the CWT. The time shift parameter, b, is called the *translation* of the wavelet (its units are time), and a is called the *scale* or the *dilation* of the wavelet. a is real and > 0. The scale is proportional to $1/f$ or the period of the spectral components, hence also has the dimensions of time. A scale $a > 1$ *dilates* the wavelet while $a < 1$ *compresses* it. The $(1/\sqrt{a})$ factor is for *energy normalization,* so that the transformed signal will have the same energy at every scale. Polikar (1998) compares scale to that used in maps:

"As in the case of maps, high scales correspond to a nondetailed global view (of the signal), and low scales correspond to a detailed view. Similarly, in terms of frequency, low frequencies (high scales) correspond to a detailed information of a hidden pattern in the signal (that usually lasts a relatively short time)."

The *mother wavelet* or *transforming function* was defined above as $\psi(t,\ a=1,\ b=0))$, or simply $\psi(t)$. A number of mother wavelet functions can be used; each has its pros and cons for various classes of NS signal (speech, geophysics, etc.); several will be described in the next section. Note that there is an *inverse* CWT that allows recovery of the signal, $u(t)$, from CWT(a, b).

One form of the ICWT is:

$$u(t) = \frac{1}{C_\psi a^2} \int\limits_{a>0} \int\limits_{b} CWT(a,b)\psi^*[(t-b)/a] da\, db \tag{7.40}$$

Where C_ψ is a constant that depends on $\psi(t)$.

The discrete wavelet transform given by Lin and Qu (2000) can be written as:

$$\begin{aligned} DWT(a,\ b) &= (a^{-1/2}) \sum_{k=1}^{N} u(k)\psi^*[(k-b)/a] \\ &= (a^{-1/2}) \sum_{k=1}^{N} u(k)\psi^*[(b-k)/a] \end{aligned} \tag{7.41}$$

The second summation is written in the form of a discrete real convolution under the assumption that the mother wavelet is real and even, such as the derivative of Gaussian (DOG) wavelets.

7.6.2 Computation of the continuous wavelet transform

To compute the CWT, we first select a long record (epoch) of the NS signal, $u(t)$. The wavelet is placed at the beginning of the record at $t = b = 0$, and the scale is set to a_1 = 1. The product, $[u(t)\psi(t,\ 1,\ 0)]$ is integrated over all time. Its numerical value is the functional, CWT(1, 0). The wavelet is then shifted forward by b_1, and the product $[u(t)\psi(t,\ 1,\ b_1)]$ is again integrated to find the numerical value of $CWT(1,\ b_1)$. The process is repeated for equally spaced $\{b_k\}$ until the end of the epoch is reached. The spacing of the $N\{b_k\}$ is generally chosen to cause some overlap between $\psi^*(t, 1, b_k)$ and $\psi^*(t, 1, b_{k+1})$.

Next, the scale a is incremented to $a_2 > 1$, and the integrals are again computed for $N\{b_k\}$ values. The process is repeated for a total of $M\{a_j\}$, including $a_1 = 1$, giving a total of NM CWT(a_j, b_k) values, effectively filling the 2-D, a, b space. It can be shown by example that the CWT has good time and poor frequency resolution at high signal frequencies, and poor time and good frequency resolution at low signal frequencies. In fact, one can view the wavelets as constant-Q bandpass filters where the Q is independent of the scale, a [Qian and Chen, 1996].

7.6.3 Some wavelet basis functions, $\Psi(t)$

A wavelet basis function must satisfy the *admissibility condition:*

$$\int_{-\infty}^{\infty} \Psi(t)dt = 0 \tag{7.42}$$

and its *norm* must be finite:

$$C_\Psi = \frac{1}{2\pi}\int_{-\infty}^{\infty} \frac{|\Psi(\omega)|^2}{|\omega|} d\omega < \infty \tag{7.43}$$

$\Psi(\omega)$ is the CFT of $\Psi(t)$. Note that $C_\Psi$is the constant used in the ICWT of Equation 7.40.

Several mother wavelet functions are in common use. The first described is the "Mexican hat" wavelet (MHW). The MHW belongs to the *DOG* (derivative of Gaussin) class of wavelets. Recall that the Gaussian probability density function, p(t), is given by:

$$p(t) = \frac{1}{\sigma\sqrt{2\pi}} \exp[-t^2/(2\sigma^2)] \tag{7.44}$$

The MHW is simply the negative second derivative of p(t):

$$\Psi_{mh}(t) = -\frac{d^2p(t)}{dt^2} = -\frac{1}{\sigma^3\sqrt{2\pi}}(t^2/\sigma^2 - 1)\exp[-t^2/(2\sigma^2)] \tag{7.45}$$

Note that its peak is $(1/(\sigma^3\sqrt{2\pi}))$ at $t = 0$. ($\ddot{p}(t)$ is really an *inverted* Mexican hat.)

The *Morlet wavelet* mother function [de Marchi and Craig, 1999] is given by:

$$\Psi_{mo}(t) = (\pi^{-4})\exp(-t^2/2)[\exp(jt\omega_o) - \exp(-(\omega_o t)^2/2] \tag{7.46}$$

The second term in the brackets is so the Morlet wavelet meets the admissibility criterion; it is small numerically for $\omega_o > 3$, i.e., its value is < 0.0111. Thus, in practice, we use

$$\Psi_{mo}(t) \cong (\pi^{-4})\exp(-t^2/2)[\cos(\omega_o t) + j\,\sin(\omega_o t)] \tag{7.47}$$

for the Morlet mother wavelet. It is clear that the Morlet wavelet is complex, so that its conjugate is simply:

$$\begin{aligned}\Psi_{mo}^{*}(t) &= (\pi^{-4})\exp(-t^2/2)\exp(-jt\omega_o) = (\pi^{-4})\exp(-t^2/2)\\ &\quad\times[\cos(\omega_o t) - j\sin(\omega_o t)]\end{aligned} \tag{7.48}$$

Another form of the Morlet wavelet function, used by Lin and Qu (2000), is:

$$\Psi_{mo}(t) = \exp(-\beta^2 t^2/2)\cos(\omega_o t) \tag{7.49}$$

Note that these authors drop the enigmatic (π^{-4}) factor and use only the real part of the complex exponential term. When the scaling and shifting is done, they obtained the real even Morlet wavelet form:

$$\Psi_{mo}[(t-b)/a, \beta] = \exp[-\beta^2(t-b)^2/(2a^2)]\cos[\omega_o(t-b)/a] \tag{7.50}$$

Note that the parameters a, b and β move the cosine wavelet around on the time axis and also change its shape. (Many other wavelet workers do not use the β factor or the (π^{-4}) factor.)

De Marchi and Craig (1999) argue that the CWT is, in fact, a convolution. That is:

$$\mathrm{CWT}(a, b) = \int u(t)\Psi^*[(t-b)/a]dt = \int u(\mu)\Psi^*[(b-\mu)/a]d\mu \tag{7.51}$$

The second integral is clearly a real convolution of $u(t)$ with $\Psi^*[(t-b)/a]$; it is made possible by letting $t \to \mu$, and making $\Psi^*(t)$ *even* and real so its argument can be reversed. Now, by the CFT real convolution theorem, it can be shown that the CWT of the NS signal, u(t), can be written as the ICFT of the product of the CFT of $u(t)$ and $\Psi^*[(t-b)/a]$. That is:

$$\begin{aligned}\mathrm{CWT}(a, b) &= \boldsymbol{F}^{-1}\{\mathbf{U}(j\omega)\boldsymbol{\Psi}^*(\omega, a, b)\}\\ &= \frac{1}{2\pi}\int_{-\infty}^{\infty} \mathbf{U}(j\omega)\boldsymbol{\Psi}^*(\omega, a, b)e^{j\omega t}d\omega\end{aligned} \tag{7.52}$$

De Marchi and Craig show that, for the Morlet wavelet,

$$\boldsymbol{\Psi}^*(\omega, a, b) = \sqrt{a}\exp[-1/2(a\omega - \omega_o)^2]\exp[j\omega b] \tag{7.53}$$

Thus, the CWT of $u(t)$ can be finally written as:

$$\mathrm{CWT}(a,b) = \sqrt{a/(2\pi)}\int_{-\infty}^{\infty} \mathbf{U}(j\omega)\exp[-1/2(a\omega - \omega_o)^2]\exp[j\omega(t+b)]d\omega \tag{7.54}$$

Thus, the CWT of $u(t)$ can be found by taking the FFT of $u(k)$ (the sampled $u(t)$), multiplying it by $\{\exp[-1/2(a\omega - \omega_o)^2]\exp[j\omega b]\}$, and then taking the IFFT. This process enjoys some computational efficiency, and is based on the criterion that $\Psi^*(t)$ be real and even.

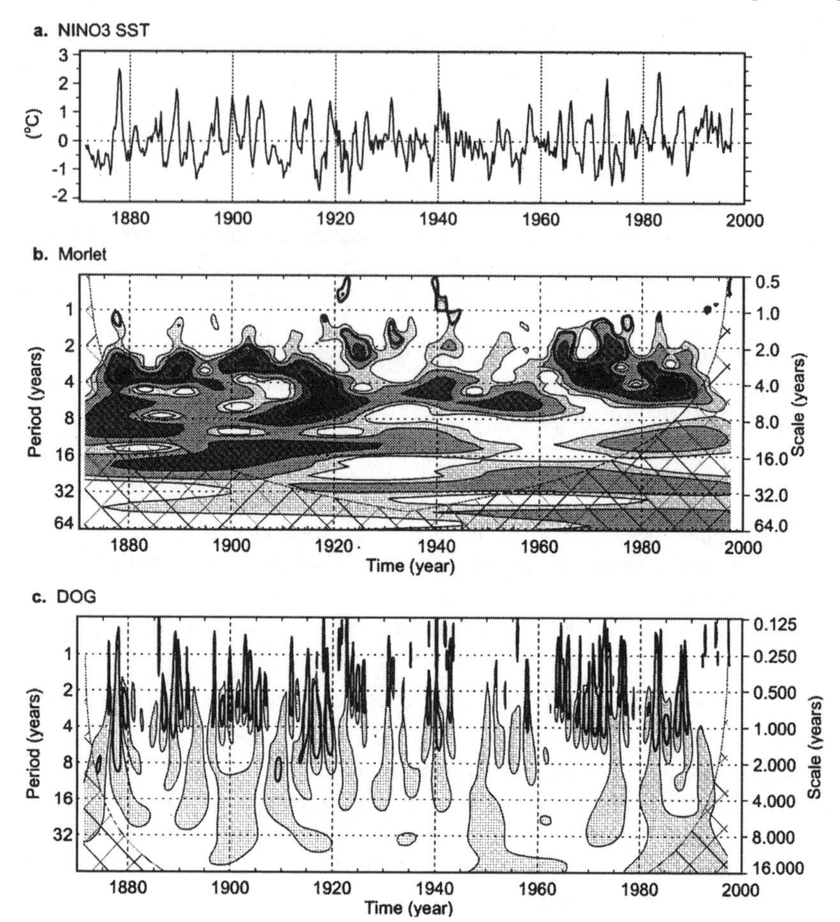

FIGURE 7.4

A geophysical example of JTFA in which the natural periodicities in ocean temperature are revealed. (a) The Niño3 sea surface temperature (SST) vs. time from 1870 to 2000. (b) JFT power spectrogram of the SST data calculated using the Morlet wavelet normalized by $1/\sigma^2$, where $\sigma^2 = 0.54\ °C^2$. (c) JTF spectrogram calculated using the second derivative of Gaussian wavelet (DOG_2); same SST data was used. Note the sharper resolution in time and poorer resolution in period than for the Morlet wavelet JTF plot. (Torrance and Compo, 1998, A practical guide to wavelet analysis. Bull. Amer. Meteorol. Soc. With permission.)

Torrence and Compo (1998) give a comparison of JTF power spectra calculated for a sea surface temperature record spanning from 1870 to 2000. An example of their raw data and two JTF spectrograms are shown in Figure 7.4. The first JTF spectrogram is calculated using the Morlet wavelet normalized by $1/\sigma^2$, where $\sigma^2 = 0.54°C^2$. The bottom spectrogram was done using the DOG_2 (Mexican hat) wavelet. Note that the Mexican hat spectrogram has much sharper resolution in time, and more uncertainty in period than the Morlet spectrogram. Torrence and Compo stated:

"This is because the Mexican hat is real valued and captures both the positive and negative oscillations of the time series as separate peaks in wavelet power. The Morlet wavelet is both complex, and [it] contains more oscillations than the Mexican hat, and hence the wavelet power combines both positive and negative peaks into a single broad peak. A plot of the real or imaginary part of $W_n(s)$ using the Morlet would produce a plot similar to Figure 1c" [Figure 7.4c].

Also note that, instead of frequency on the y axis, the spectrograms are plotted vs. decreasing period in years, which is easily converted to frequency in cycles/year. Torrence and Compo used the *continuous wavelet transform* of a discrete (sampled) time sequence, $x(n)$. They defined the CWT as the real convolution of $x(n)$ with a scaled and translated wavelet function, $\Psi^*(n)$. That is:

$$\mathrm{CWT}(a, n) = \sum_{n'=0}^{N-1} x(n')\Psi^*[(n-n')\delta t/a] \tag{7.55}$$

In the discrete real convolution above, a is the scale or dilation factor, n is the discrete shift of the wavelet and δt is the sampling period. Now, using the development that led to Equation 7.52, we can write the *inverse DFT:*

$$\mathrm{CWT}(a, n) = \sqrt{2\pi a/\delta t}\,\frac{1}{N}\sum_{k=0}^{N-1} \mathbf{X}(k)\Psi^*(a\omega_k)\exp[+j\omega_k n\delta t] \tag{7.56}$$

Where $\mathbf{X}(k)$ is the DFT of the sampled $x(t)$, $\Psi^*(a\omega_k)$ is the DFT of $\Psi^*[(n-n')\delta t/a]$, $\sqrt{2\pi a/\delta t}$ is the *energy normalization factor,* and

$$\omega_k = 2\pi k/(N\delta t) \quad \text{for } k \le N/2 \tag{7.57A}$$

$$\omega_k = -2\pi k/(N\delta t) \quad \text{for } k > N/2. \tag{7.57B}$$

We next examine the *Haar wavelets,* which were devised around 1909. The Haar wavelets found little practical application until the 1930s, when physicist Paul Levy used them to investigate Brownian motion. One property of the Haar wavelets is that they have "compact support," which means that they vanish outside of a finite interval (e.g., 0,1). Being step-like in nature, Haar wavelets are not continuously differentiable, thus they are poorly localized in frequency, which limits their applications in TFA. The Haar mother function is a simple square wave cycle, shown in Figure 7.5a. $\Psi(t) = 1$ for $0 \le t < 0.5$, $\Psi(t) = -1$ for $0.5 < t \le 1$, and zero elsewhere.

Figure 7.5b shows another member of the Haar wavelet family. Note that the wavelet height is proportional to the inverse square root of its width.

The Haar system of wavelets is orthonormal; that is:

$$\int \Psi_{\mathbf{Ha}}(t-\mu)\Psi_{\mathbf{Ha}}(t-\sigma)dt = \delta(\mu-\sigma) \tag{7.58}$$

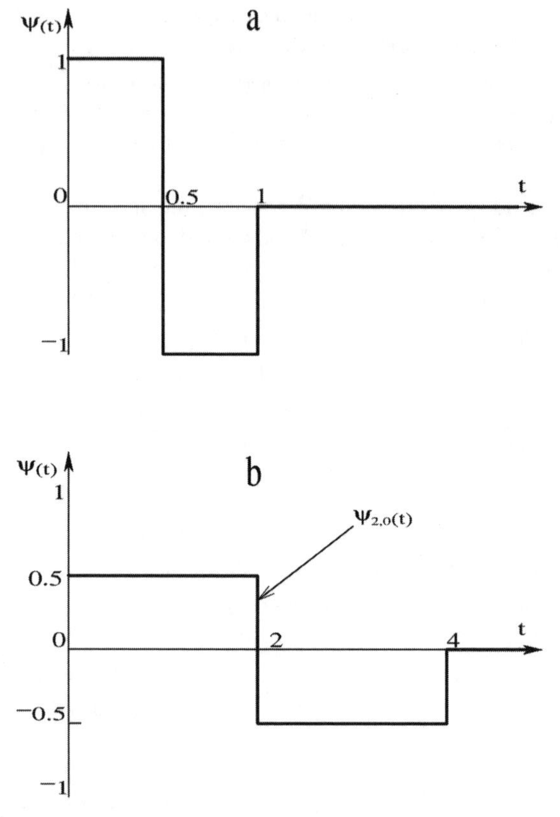

FIGURE 7.5a
(a) The Haar mother wavelet. (b) Another Haar wavelet.

The general form for the dilated and shifted Haar wavelet is derived from the mother wavelet by:

$$\Psi(\mathrm{t}, \alpha, \delta) = (\sqrt{2})^{\alpha}\Psi(2^{\alpha}\mathrm{t} - \delta) \tag{7.59}$$

Where α is the *scale* or *dilation.* Note that $\alpha = 0$ gives no scale change because $2^0 = 1$. δ is the time shift.

Although their poor frequency localization makes Haar wavelets ineffective for most for JTF analysis, Kaplan (2001) applied Haar wavelets to make JTF spectrograms of financial time series, such as the daily closing price of certain stocks or stock indices. These spectrograms were presented as 3-D contour plots. To evaluate the effectiveness of the Haar wavelet approach to this data, one needs to apply other JTFA algorithms as well, including other smooth wavelets and various RIDs, etc.

7.7 Applications of JTF Analysis to Physiological Signals

7.7.1 Introduction

This section will elaborate on applications of certain of the various forms of JTF analysis to physiological signals. First, we will examine the use of JTF analysis on heart sounds to detect valve pathologies. The EEG can also be examined by JTFA to detect incipient epilepsy, Alzheimer's disease, and other conditions. JTFA has also been applied in biomechanical studies of how vestibular disease affects the sense of balance, and to the analysis of EMG waveforms.

7.7.2 Heart sounds

It is well known that heart sounds can have great significance in the noninvasive diagnosis of heart valve pathologies [Northrop, 2002]. The sounds emitted by artificial (implanted) heart valves can also be used to detect incipient malfunction. The traditional approach to the diagnosis of bad heart valves by heart sounds is to listen to them in real time through a stethoscope (auscultation). The preliminary diagnosis is performed by the mind of the experienced listener. Diagnostic corroboration is usually done by imaging, such as by an x-ray camera imaging the beating heart while radio-opaque dye is injected into a large vein. An alternate approach to listening to the heart sounds through a stethoscope and its frequency-selective audio band-pass characteristics is to use a high-fidelity microphone with a short direct acoustic coupling to the chest surface by an *inverse horn* [Northrop, 2002]. The microphone output voltage is proportional to the sound pressure at the chest surface, without the distorting acoustic filtering characteristics of the stethoscope's bell, diaphragm and tubes. Sound from the amplified microphone output voltage can be listened to, and the voltage can also be used to make JTF spectrograms (generally synchronized to the ECG QRS spike). A number of workers have explored the diagnostic usefulness of examining heart sound JTF spectrograms [Sikiö, 1999; Bentley et al., 1998; Wood and Barry, 1995; Wood et al., 1992].

Figure 7.6a illustrates the analog sound voltage recorded from the chest of a normal subject containing heart sounds 1 and 2. Sound 1 (S_1) is generated concurrently with the contraction of the ventricles. It involves three valvular events: Mitral valve closure, tricuspid valve closure, and pulmonic and aortic valve opening. The actual closing and opening of the valve tissues is believed to be noiseless. It is believed that the sounds are generated by the interaction of the moving blood's kinetic energy with elastic tissues such as the *chordae tendonae* that snub the valve sections, and vibrations in the elastic muscle of the heart walls and aorta. Any acceleration or deceleration of a blood mass induces vibrations [Wood and Barry, 1995; Guyton, 1991]. These acoustic vibrations propagate through the pericardium and thorax to the skin, where they are sensed by a microphone with good low-frequency response. The frequency of the S_1 vibrations is believed to be determined by density and tension

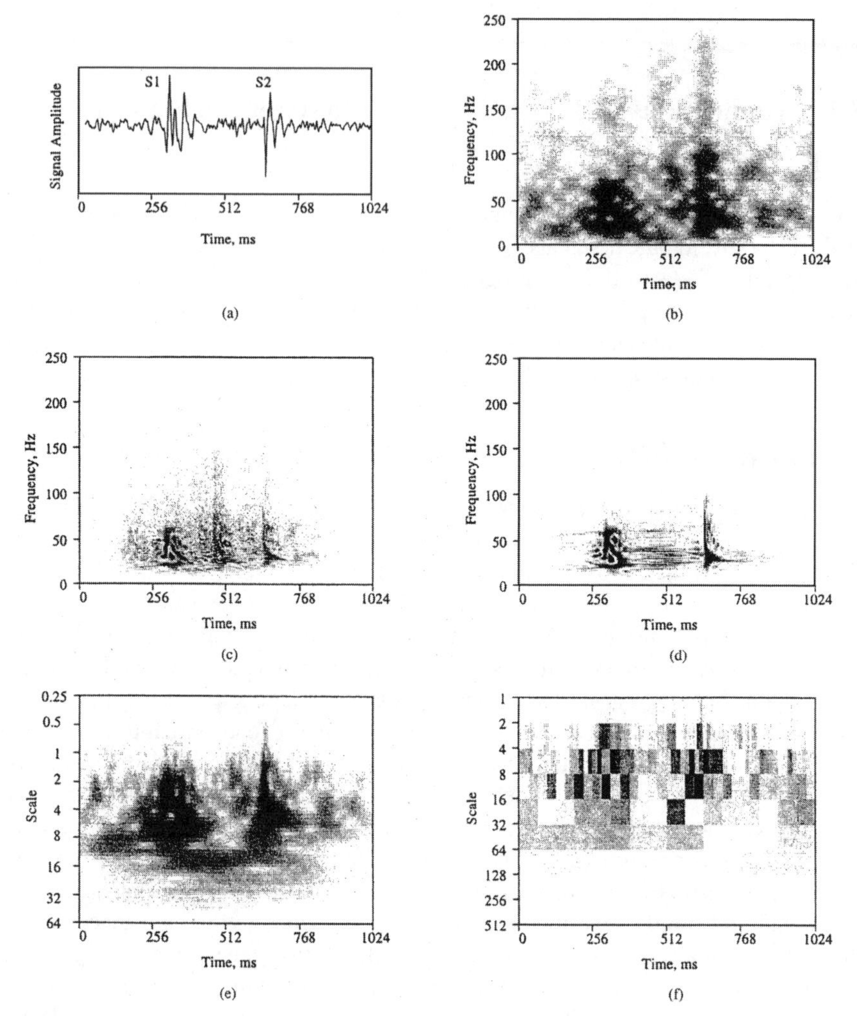

FIGURE 7.6

A study of different JTFA algorithms applied to heart sounds. (a) Heart sound waveform. (b) STFT JTF spectrogram of the heart sounds. (c) W-V transform JTF spectrogram of the heart sounds; note large artifact at $t \cong 500$ msec. (d) Choi-Williams JTF spectrogram. (e) Continuous wavelet transform JTF spectrogram using the Morlet wavelet. (f) A 20-coefficient, Daubechies wavelet JTF spectrogram. (Bentley et al. Time-Frequency and time-scale techniques for the native and bioprosthetic heart valve sounds. *Trans. Biomed. Eng.* 45(1) 1998. IEEE. With permission.)

(stiffness) of the myocardium and the shape and volume of the heart chambers, all of which change throughout the cardiac cycle. The valves themselves may vibrate in the process of closing or opening.

The second heart sound (S_2) is associated with the abrupt closure of the aortic and pulmonary (semilunar) valves, which causes them to bulge backward toward the ventricles. The kinetic energy of the decelerating blood mass causes the elastic walls of the arteries to vibrate (and perhaps the valves, as well).

Bentley et al. (1998) compare the JTF plots for five JTFA methods. In Figure 7.6b, we see the classical short-time Fourier transform of the signal with S_1 and S_2. A 128 msec (out of an epoch length of 1024 msec) window was used (window shape not given). Resolution in both time and frequency is medium, and there is much noise (including mysterious "snowflakes"). In Figure 7.6c, the authors used the Wigner-Ville distribution. Resolution is now sharper, but observe the misleading large artifactual cross term at ca. 500 msec (of course, there is no peak of energy in the signal at 500 msec). The cross term and noise are both suppressed in the Choi-Williams distribution, shown in Figure 7.6d. The Choi-Williams transform, described above, belongs to Cohen's class of JTF transforms, and may be classed as one of the reduced interference distributions (RIDs). It appears to be about the best for examining heart sounds. In Figure 7.6e, we see the result of the continuous wavelet transform (CWT) using the Morlet wavelet. In this distribution, recall that the scale (a) is proportional to the signal's period, so small a corresponds to a high signal frequency. Again, we see background phantoms and "snowflakes;" the time-frequency resolution is poor as well. The discrete wavelet transform using a 20-coefficient Daubechies wavelet is shown in Figure 7.6f. This JTF distribution is very crude and pixelated with the settings used. Evidently, the C-WT is best to represent the heart sounds in JTF space.

Wood and Barry (1995) and Wood et al. (1992) also reported on the use of different JTF transforms to characterize the first heart sound. Wood and Barry showed that the *binomial* version of the C-WT gave superior performance in suppressing noise and cross-term interference when transforming S_1. These authors cemented ultralight accelerometers directly to dog's heart walls to pick up sound vibrations, rather than the more conventional use of a microphone on the chest wall as a sound pickup. The accelerometer's frequency response was ± 3 dB from 0.1 to 400 Hz. Note that myocardial wall acceleration due to sound generated within the heart is not the same as the actual sound pressure, although the two are related.

Figure 7.7 shows a typical heart wall acceleration trace due to S_1, its Fourier power spectrum, and the bottom panel shows the binomial JTF transform of the acceleration. All noise was clipped < -40 dB from the peak intensity of the JTF transform. A dominant feature in all S_1 acceleration JTF spectra is the intense, linearly rising frequency component that begins shortly after the ECG R wave. In a second epicardial, S_1 acceleration waveform, shown in Figure 7.8, the binomial JTF transform shows a curious three-component triangular form. A rising chirp goes from about 30 Hz beginning at the R peak of the ECG to ca. 150 Hz about 49 msec later. This upward chirp is followed by a downward chirp from 150 Hz back to 30 Hz in ca. 20 msec. A constant frequency component at ca. 15 Hz begins a few msec before the R peak, and fades out gradually at the base of the downward chirp. Inside the triangle formed by the major intensity components, there are five intensity "dots" arranged on an ellipse. These may be artifacts. Finally, to demonstrate the effectiveness of the binomial JTF transform, Wood et al. compared a JTF sound spectrogram using simulated bandpass filters, a power spectrogram computed using the STFT, and finally, the result of a binomial JTF transform. These plots are shown in Figure 7.9. Clearly, the binomial distribution has the best time-frequency resolution, and the least cross-term interference of the three JTFA methods used in this study.

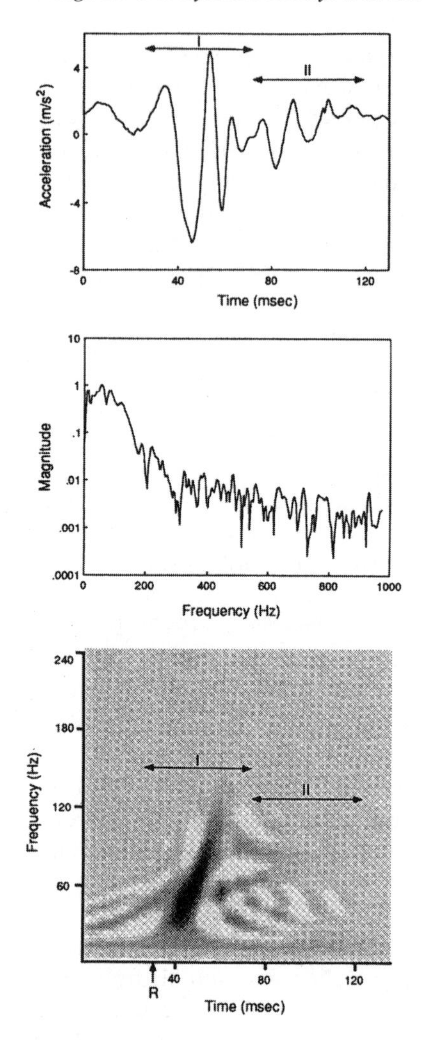

FIGURE 7.7

Beating heart wall vibrations examined by JTFA. (Top) Time record of heart wall vibrations recorded with an accelerometer. (Middle) Conventional FFT root power density spectrum of the heart vibrations. (Bottom) JTF plot of the heart vibrations done with the so-called binomial JTF transform. (Wood, J.C. et al. Time-frequency transforms: A new approach to first heart sound frequency dynamics. IEEE *Trans. Biomed. Eng.* 1992 and 1995. With permission)

7.7.3 JTF analysis of EEG signals

The EEG potentials recorded from various points on the scalp have been used for a variety of experimental and diagnostic applications [Northrop, 2002]. The EEG waveforms are typical noisy nonstationary neurophysiological waveforms. The frequency content of the EEG changes with the patient's state of consciousness (ranging

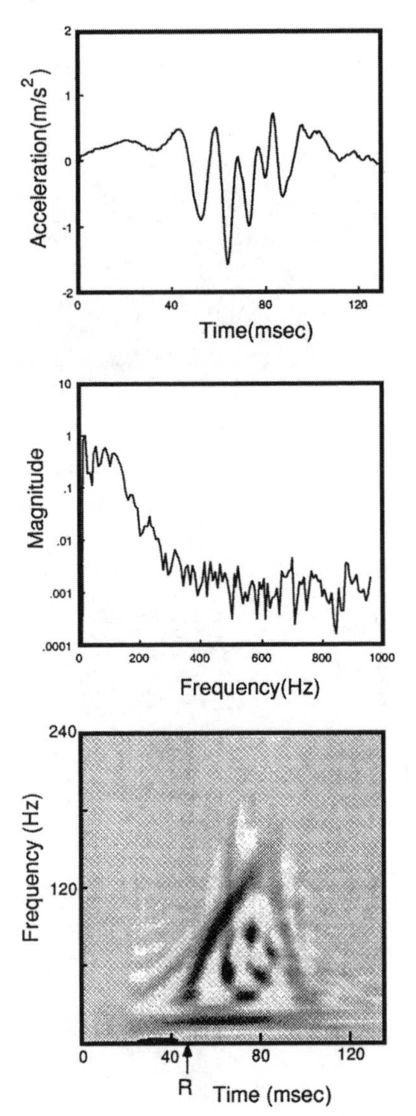

FIGURE 7.8

Figure similar to Figure 7.7. (Wood, J.C. et al. Time-frequency transforms: A new approach to first heart sound frequency dynamics. IEEE *Trans. Biomed. Eng.* 1992 and 1995. With permission.)

from deep sleep to fully awake intellectual activity). It also contains transients that accompany voluntary movements, and, in experimental studies, transients accompanying various modes of sensory stimulation. In most cases the event-related potentials (ERPs) are obscured by noise and other EEG activity, and must be recovered by signal averaging, which improves their signal-to-noise ratio [Northrop, 2002; this text, Section 8.4].

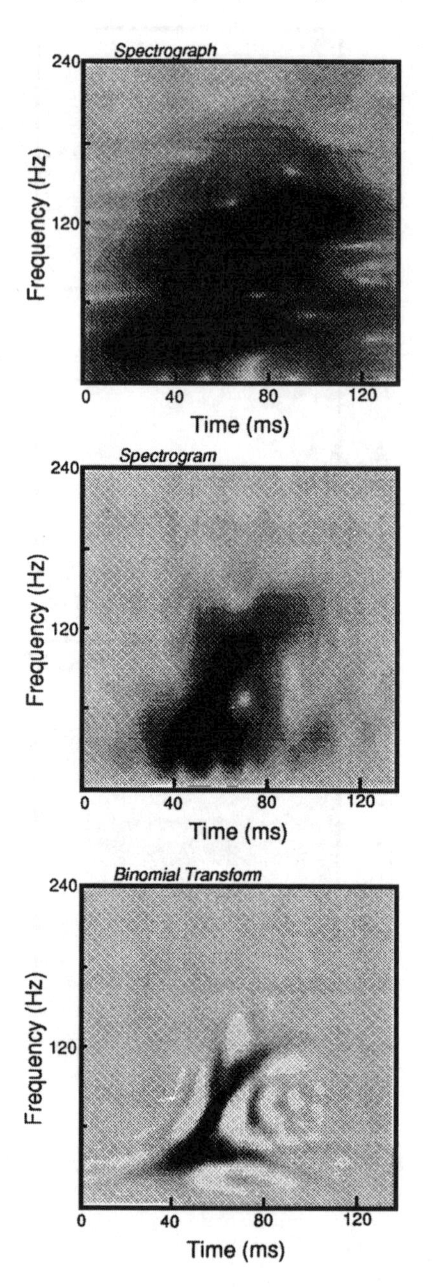

FIGURE 7.9

Comparison of three different JTF spectrograms of the heart acceleration data correlated with heart sound 1. Top plot: Result of a digital simulation of the original, McKusick spectrogram technique used with speech. Middle plot: A running window power spectrogram. Bottom plot: Result of a binomial time-frequency transform. (Wood, J.C. et al. Time-Frequency transforms: A new approach to first heart sound frequency dynamics. IEEE *Trans. Biomed. Eng.* 1992 and 1995. With permission.)

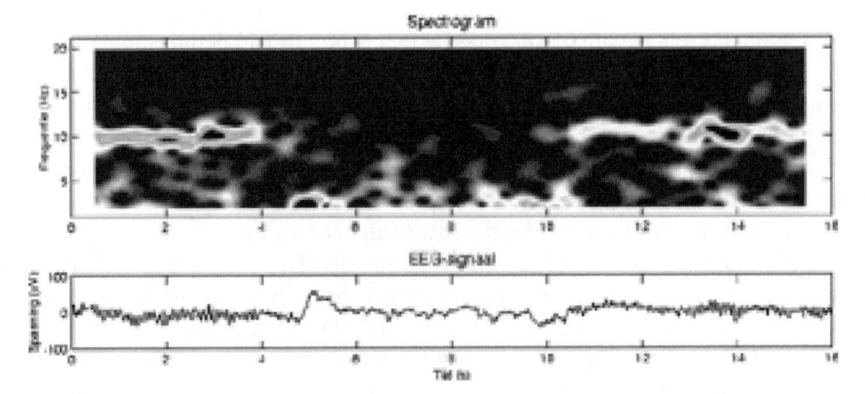

FIGURE 7.10

Top: A JTF plot of human EEG activity showing intermittent alpha wave activity. The STFT algorithm was used. Bottom: Time-domain record of the EEG. (Van Hoey, G. et al. 1997. Time-frequency analysis of EEG signals. *Proc. ProRISC Workshop on Circuits, Systems and Signal Processing.* With permission.)

One example of JTF analysis applied to an EEG waveform is shown in Figure 7.10. Here, in the time domain signal, the patient is awake and relaxed with eyes closed and is generating 10 Hz alpha rhythm. At t = 4 sec, the eyes are opened and the alpha waves vanish. When the eyes close again at 10 seconds, the alpha activity begins again after a short (c. 0.5 sec.) latency. These events are shown clearly in the JTF

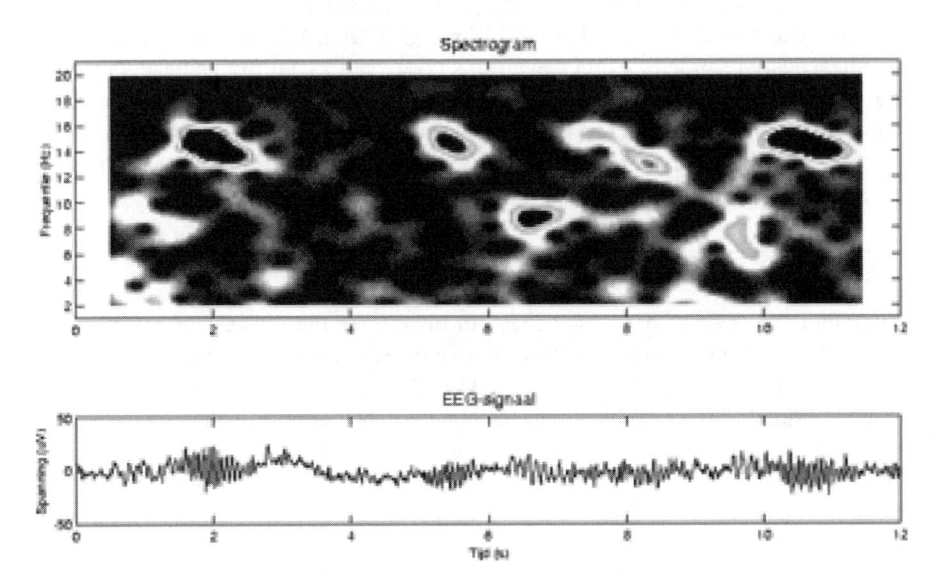

FIGURE 7.11

Another EEG JTF spectrogram showing 15 Hz beta wave spindles alternating with 9-Hz alpha bursts. The nonstationary character of this EEG waveform is made clear by the JTF plot. (Van Hoey, G. et al. 1997. Time-frequency analysis of EEG signals. *Proc. ProRISC Workshop on Circuits, Systems and Signal Processing.* With permission.)

spectrogram, presented with power coded as color. Figure 7.11 demonstrates a second EEG JTF spectrogram. In this case, large 15 Hz, beta wave "spindles" induced by tranquilizers alternate with alpha-like 9 Hz bursts. Both of these spectrograms came from the Medical Image and Signal Processing web pages of the ELIS Department of the University of Ghent, Belgium, 2001. The JTFA algorithm used was the short-term Fourier transform (STFT) [Van Hoey et al., 1997].

Williams et al., (1995) describe the use of the reduced interference distribution (RID) algorithms in forming JTF spectrograms of EEG signals in order to diagnose epilepsy. Since the EEG is an NS signal that can have coincident multiple harmonic sources, it is important to have a JTF algorithm that not only has good time and frequency resolution, but negligible cross-term artifact. Figure 7.12 a, b, c illustrates waterfall 3-D JTF plots of a test signal that has a frequency-modulated low-frequency carrier plus a coincident chirp with increasing frequency in time. In Figure 7.12a, the W-VT is shown to generate a large artifact midway in frequency between the chirp and the FM wave. The STFT spectrogram shows no artifact, but cannot faithfully reproduce the FM component in Figure 7.12b. Figure 7.12c shows the JTF spectrogram resulting from the use of the *exponential* C-WT, which uses the Cohen kernel, $\varphi(\theta,\, \tau) = \exp(-\theta^2\tau^2/\sigma)$. Note that this JTF spectrogram is crisp and has no obvious interference terms. Williams et al. go on to demonstrate the effectiveness of their exponential transform in characterizing epileptic vs. normal EEG waveforms recorded directly from the exposed cerebral cortex. We will refer to these time-domain records as electrocorticograms (ECorG), (as opposed to ECoG, the electrocochleogram [Northrop, 2001]). Williams et al. also analyzed conventionally recorded scalp EEGs. Figure 7.13 a, b, c, d from Williams et al. shows two simultaneously recorded ECorG waveforms $[x_1(t)$ and $x_2(t)]$ from adjacent recording sites during a seizure. The JTF spectrograms, displayed as contour plots, are shown in Figures 7.13b and c; Figure 7.13d shows the cross C-WT, calculated from $x_1(u+\tau/2)x_2(u-\tau/2)$. Note the virtual absence of cross terms that would render interpretation difficult if the W-VT were used.

7.7.4 Other biomedical applications of JTF spectrograms

Laughlin et al. (1996) have used JTFA to investigate the sensorimotor control of erect posture in human subjects with vestibular impairment (e.g., such as in Menière's disease). Patients and controls were asked to observe the 0.25 Hz sinusoidal motion of a three-sided wall while they try to remain upright. Figure 7.14 shows a waterfall-type 3-D JTF spectrogram for normal subjects derived from the time record output of a force plate on which the subjects were standing. Note that, as time progresses, the normal subjects sway less and less as they learn to suppress the visual input and derive stabilizing feedback from their vestibular systems. The JTF spectrogram of Figure 7.15 shows that the patients are not able to compensate for the moving visual input, suggesting that vestibular feedback for postural control is lost.

Still another application of JTFA in biomedicine was described by Duchêne et al. (1995). These authors investigated the uterine EMG activity in pregnancy using a variety of JTFA algorithms. These included: The Choi-Williams RID, the cone-shaped

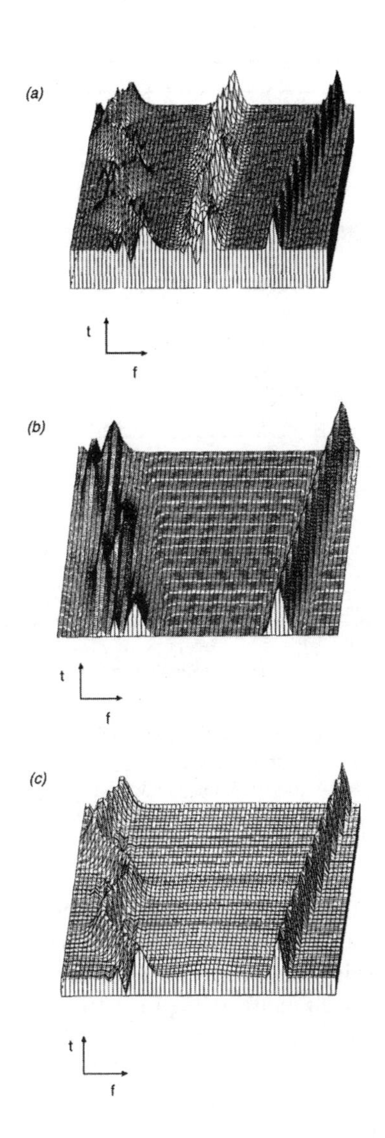

FIGURE 7.12

3-D waterfall JTF plots of a man-made signal having two components: A frequency-modulated low-frequency sinusoid plus a high-frequency chirp with linearly increasing frequency. (a) JTF plot made with the Wigner-Ville transform, showing the artifact "phantom signal" between the chirp and the FM. (b) JTF plot made with the STFT cannot faithfully reproduce the FM component. However, there is no phantom signal. (c) JTF plot made using the C-WT with the Gaussian Cohen kernel. Note that both signal components are clearly displayed with no artifact. (Williams, W.J. et. al. 1995. Time-frequency analysis of electrophysiological signals in epilepsy. *IEEE Eng. in Med. and Biol.* March/April. With permission.)

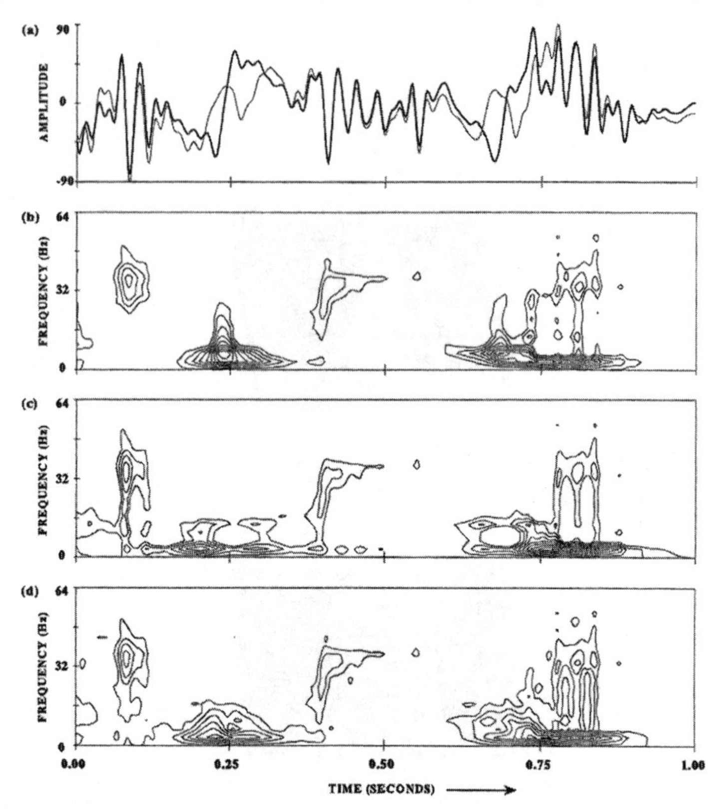

FIGURE 7.13

EEG derived from direct cortical recording. (a) Simultaneous EEG time records (x_1 and x_2) from two sites on the same brain surface. (b) JTF contour plot mae from $x_1(t)$ using the C-WT. (c) JTF contour plot made from $x_2(t)$ using the C-WT. (d) A cross-JTF magnitude plot using $x(u+\tau/2)x(u-\tau/2)$ in the C-WT. (Williams, W.J. et. al. 1995. Time-frequency analysis of electrophysiological signals in epilepsy. *IEEE Eng. in Med. and Biol.* March/April. With permission.)

kernel distribution of Zhao et al. (1990), the smoothed pseudo-Wigner-Ville distribution, and the STFT with Gaussian and Blackman windows. A typical spontaneous uterine EMG was recorded using wire electrodes embedded directly into the smooth muscle of the uterus of a pregnant monkey. Figure 7.16 shows two JTF spectra, one of a synthetic (model signal), the other from the sample EMG. The pseudo-smoothed Wigner-Ville distribution was used. These distributions and the pair done with the cone-shaped kernel of Zhao et al. appeared to me to give the highest resolution with this particular class of signals.

There is an enormous body of information on all kinds of animal sounds on the World Wide Web. These range from human speech, primate sounds, sounds from cetaceans (whales and dolphins), bat cries while hunting, reptile sounds, amphibian sounds, insect calls, etc. Actual sounds are available to listen to or download in WAV format; some sites show JTF displays. Lack of space prevents us from going into the JTF analysis of these sounds in any sort of detail. Human speech, cetacean calls

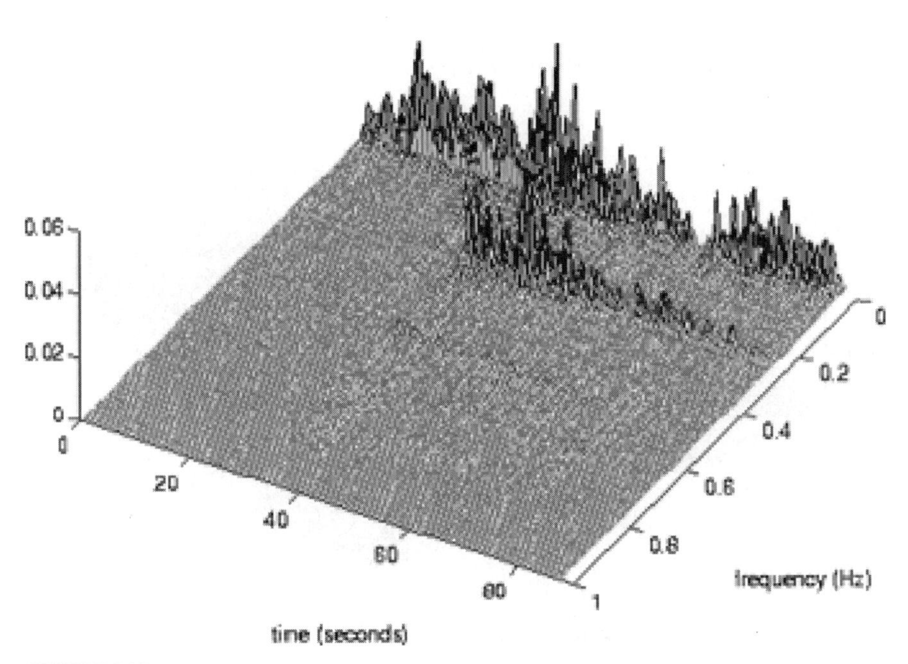

FIGURE 7.14

A 3-D waterfall-type JTF spectrogram of the force exerted on a force-plate by the feet of a human subject attempting to compensate for a disturbing visual input (see text). Note that the 0.25 Hz force component dies out for normal human subjects as they adapt to the input. (Laughlin et al. 1996. Time-varying characteristics of visually induced postural sway. *IEEE Trans. on Rehab. Eng.* 4(4). With permission.)

and bat cries have certainly been thoroughly studied. The interested reader can visit the Cornell Bioacoustics Research Programs web pages; for example, see the pages on whale communications research at URL: http://birds.cornell.edu/BRP/IUSS.html. Sound JTF spectrograms of the calls of four whale species are shown.

7.8 JTFA Software

Several sources of JTFA software modules available for those persons who wish to investigate these algorithms on biomedical (and other) signals with minimum effort. A signal processing group at the University of Nantes (France) [Auger, 2002] offers a *free* collection of c. 100 Matlab ™ m-files for various JTFA algorithms and operations. A list of the m-files is available at: ftp://ftp.univ-nantes.fr/pub/universite/iutstnazaire/tftb/newfiles/contents.m. A wide variety of JTFA algorithms and related functions is offered.

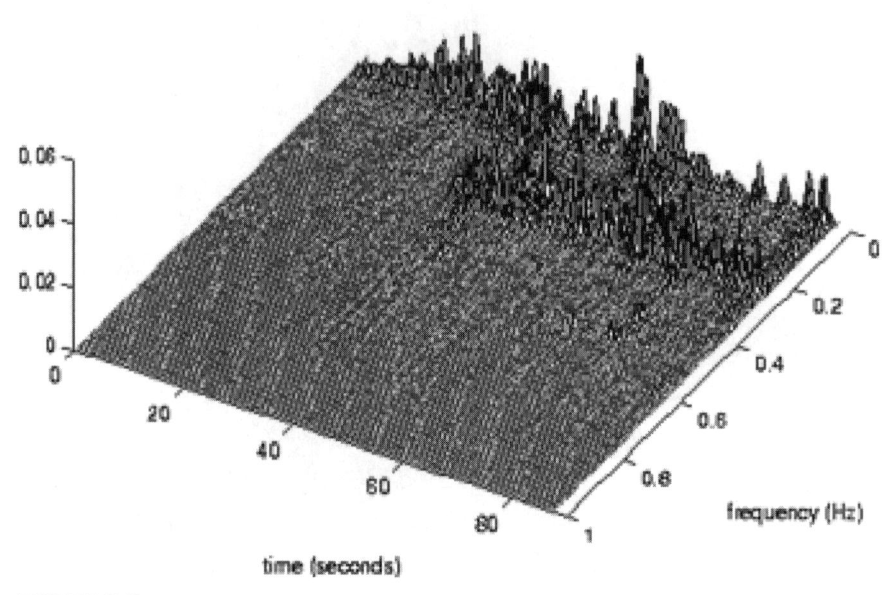

FIGURE 7.15

A 3-D waterfall-type JTF spectrogram of the force exerted on a force-plate by the feet of a human subject attempting to compensate for a disturbing visual input. Note that the 0.25 Hz force component does not dies out for human subjects with vestibular impairment because they are unable to adapt to the input. (Laughlin et al. 1996. Time-varying characteristics of visually induced postural sway. *IEEE Trans. on Rehab. Eng.* 4(4). With permission.)

The MathWorks offers a *Wavelet Toolbox* $v2.1$ that runs with Matlab and other Matlab toolboxes, such as the venerable *Signal Processing Toolbox,* $v5.1$. The Wavelet Toolbox contains a library of standard wavelet families including Daubechies wavelet filters, complex Morlet and Gaussian (DOG) wavelets, and real reverse biorthogonal and discrete Meyer wavelets. Also featured are wavelet and signal processing utilities, including a function to convert scale to frequency, the ability to add wavelet families, customized data presentation programs and interactive GUI tools for continuous and discrete wavelet analysis. Wavelet packets are implemented as Matlab objects; both 1- and 2-D transforms can be implemented. For further information, see the MathWorks web site: www.mathworks.com/products/wavelet.

A list of the URLs where some 44 wavelet software packages, most free, many developed at various universities around the world, is given on *Amara's Wavelet Page* [Graps, 2000]. (The problem with such lists is that they are ephemeral; by the time you read this, some may be "404d," and new ones may be added.)

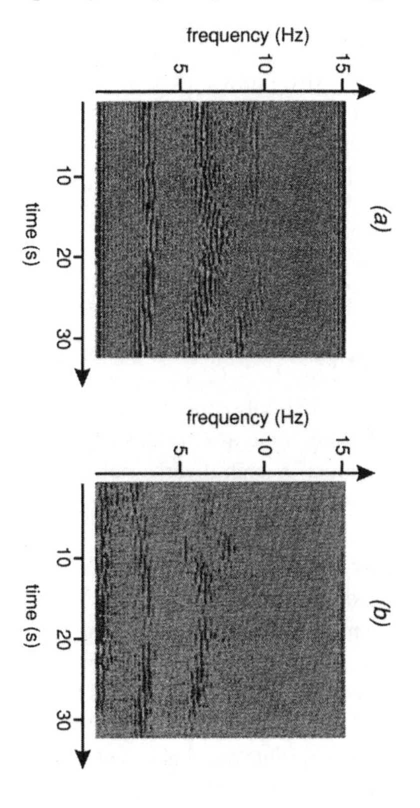

FIGURE 7.16

(a) A JTF spectrogram made with the Zhao-Atlas-Marks (cone-shaped kernel) distribution on synthetic data. (b) A JTF spectrogram made in the same manner from a spontaneous EMG signal recorded directly from the uterus of a pregnant monkey. (Duchêne, J.D. et al. 1995. Analyzing uterine EMG: Tracking instantaneous burst frequency. *IEEE Eng. in Med. and Biol.* With permission.)

National Instruments (NI) has available the LabVIEW™ Joint Time-Frequency Analysis Toolkit and the *Joint Time-Frequency Analysis Toolkit Reference Manual* (1998). National Instruments has developed their own JTFA toolkit to go with their real-time data acquisition computer card hardware and their other data acquisition software. The *Reference Manual* describes the following *linear* JTF algorithms: The STFT, the Gabor expansion, and the adaptive and inverse adaptive transform. The following *quadratic* JTF algorithms are also presented: Wigner-Ville, pseudo-Wigner-Ville, Cohen's class, including the Choi-Williams distribution, the cone-shaped distribution, the Gabor spectrogram and the NI proprietary adaptive spectrogram. NI gives the numerical (discrete) forms of the various JTF algorithms in their reference manual.

Two JTFA Toolkit demo disks by NI are bundled with the text by Qian and Chen (1996). This software runs under all the popular Windows® operating systems. It allows JTF analysis of 11 included nonstationary waveforms with each of the following JTFA algorithms: the STFT: Gabor-, C-W-, cone-shaped-, adaptive-, and

W-V distributions. The JTF diagrams are plotted as 2-D graphs, with intensity coded as color or B-and-W density. Also plotted are the classical power density spectrum of the signal, and the signal vs. time. This is a useful demo software package via which to become familiar with the idiosyncrasies of the various JFTA routines and see which one produces the fewest JTF artifacts for a given class of waveform.

7.9 Chapter Summary

Joint time-frequency analysis (or simply time-frequency analysis) is enjoying a surge of interest by workers in biomedicine as a means of describing physiological signals. It also has excited interest in such diverse fields as economics, meteorology, geophysics, image processing, biometrics (e.g., fingerprints), optics, optoelectronics, and genomics.

Because there are so many JTFA algorithms, introduction to this field will at first be confusing. However, biomedical acoustical waveforms generally contain harmonics and amplitude or frequency modulation, thus, a JTFA application with reduced cross-term interference is generally selected. The classic Wigner-Ville distribution turns out to be unsuitable for most biomedical applications. RIDs such as the Choi-Williams, have enjoyed popularity in the literature.

Many investigators also are applying various wavelet JTFA algorithms to biomedical signals. Wavelet-derived JTF spectral plots can be quite different for different mother wavelets. For example, in Figure 7.4b and c, the spectrogram using the Morlet wavelet is quite different from that computed using the DOG_2 mother. At first glance, the Morlet plot appears to have poor time resolution, while the DOG_2 plot has better time- and poorer scale (or period) resolution. With so many choices for the JTFA algorithm to be used, the windowing functions and wavelet mother functions, wavelet-based JTFA is somewhat arty and application-dependent.

8

Introduction to the Analysis of Stationary Noise and Signals Contaminated with Noise

8.1 Introduction

Nearly all physiological signals that can be recorded from the body contain significant amounts of noise that affects their resolution. In some cases, the noise can be minimized by simple linear bandpass filtering, in others, a nonlinear amplitude transformation can be effective in improving the signal-to-noise ratio. *Signal averaging* is used to extract *evoked (periodic) potentials* from noisy ERG, EEG and magneto-encephalogram (MEG) recordings, and the *lockin amplifier* can extract a low-frequency signal amplitude-modulating a coherent, constant-frequency carrier buried in noise.

The noise-contaminating physiological signals can be *random* in nature, or can be *coherent interference or both.* In recording the EEG, for example, both random noise and coherent interference are generally present, added to the EEG voltage. Coherent interference is generally man made, and can come from such sources as gasoline engine ignition noise, power line frequency electric and magnetic fields, neon and fluorescent lights, periodic inductive switching transients such as from silicon-controlled rectifier (SCR) motor speed controls, also from sparking commutators in certain electric motors, etc. It is not our purpose in this chapter to consider the actual circuits used to mitigate the effects of random noise and coherent interference, but rather to describe and examine the mathematical descriptors of noise and their uses, as well as to consider means of improving the signal-to-noise ratios of recorded signals.

In keeping with the practice used in earlier chapters, key concepts, functions and transforms using continuous real variables and integrations, rather than discrete forms and functions, will be introduced.

Section 8.2 examines the various time- and frequency domain means of characterizing noise. The use of discrete mathematics and of the DFT and the IDFT in computing power spectral measures of stationary discrete random variables (SDRVs) are treated in Section 8.3. How signal averaging of evoked transient signals improves the SNR is described mathematically in Section 8.4, as well as SNR improvement of stationary noisy signals by linear filtering. Section 8.5 introduces applications of statistics and information theory to *genomics.*

8.2 Noise Descriptors and Noise in Systems

8.2.1 Introduction

The *random noise* we will examine is assumed to have zero mean (zero average value) and also be *stationary* (or at least *short-term stationary*), and be *ergodic*. (Ergodic means that one sample record is equivalent to any other record taken from the random process.) Thus, time averages can be used in lieu of ensemble or probability averaging in calculating statistics. Noise can be characterized in terms of its amplitude and also in the frequency domain. In the developments below, we will first assume the noise is a continuous *stationary random variable* (SRV) (as opposed to discrete samples), and continuous integrals will be used to define various statistical measures.

8.2.2 Probability density functions

The *probability density function* (PDF) considers only the amplitude statistics of a noise waveform, $n(t)$, and not how $n(t)$ varies in time. The PDF of $n(t)$ is defined as:

$$p(x) = \frac{\text{Probability that } x < n \leq (x + dx)}{dx} \tag{8.1}$$

Where x is a specific value of n taken at some time t_1, and dx is a differential increment in x. The PDF is the mathematical basis for many formal derivations and proofs in probability theory and in statistics. The PDF has the properties:

$$\int_{-\infty}^{\mathbf{v}} p(x)dx = P(\mathbf{v}) = \text{Prob}[x \leq \mathbf{v}] \tag{8.2}$$

($P(\mathbf{v})$ is the *probability distribution function.*)

$$\int_{\mathbf{v}_2}^{\mathbf{v}_1} p(x)dx = \text{Prob}[\mathbf{v}_1 < x \leq \mathbf{v}_2] \tag{8.3}$$

$$\int_{-\infty}^{\infty} p(x)dx = 1 = \text{Prob}[x \leq \infty] = \text{certainty} \tag{8.4}$$

Several PDFs are widely used to describe or model the amplitude characteristics of physiological, electrical and electronic circuit continuous noise processes. These include:

$$p(x) = \left(\frac{1}{\sigma_x\sqrt{2\pi}}\right)\exp\left[-\frac{(x - <x>)^2}{2\sigma_x^2}\right] \tag{8.5}$$

Univariate Gaussian or normal PDF (8.5) $<x>$ is the mean of x, σ_x^2 is its variance; σ_x is called the standard deviation of x.

$$\begin{bmatrix} p(x) = 1/2a, & \text{for } -a < x < a, \text{ and} \\ p(x) = 0 & \text{for } x > a \end{bmatrix} \tag{8.6}$$

Rectangular PDF (8.6)

$$p(x) = \left(\frac{x}{\alpha^2}\right) \exp\left[\frac{-x^2}{2\alpha^2}\right], \quad \textit{Rayleigh PDF, } x \geq 0. \tag{8.7}$$

$$p(x) = \left(\frac{x^2}{\alpha^2}\right) \sqrt{2/\pi} \exp\left[\frac{-x^2}{2\alpha^2}\right] \quad \textit{Maxwell PDF, } x \geq 0. \tag{8.8}$$

Under most conditions, we assume that the random noise arising in electronic circuits has a *Gaussian* PDF. Many mathematical benefits follow this approximation; for example, if the input to an LTI system is Gaussian noise with variance σ_x^2, the output of the system, $y(t)$, will also be Gaussian noise with variance, σ_y^2. If Gaussian noise passes through a nonlinear system, the PDF of the output noise will, in general, not be Gaussian. Examples of the Gaussian PDF are shown by the familiar "bell-shaped curves" of Figure 8.1. The standard deviation parameter, σ, controls the relative width of the Gaussian PDF curve. The mean for the curves in this figure is $<x> = 5.0$.

The *error function* of the Gaussian PDF has been defined in several ways. We use the definition given by Papoulis (1965) because it is more intuitive.

$$\mathrm{erf}(\mathbf{x}) \equiv \frac{1}{\sqrt{2\pi}} \int_0^{\mathbf{x}} \exp[-u^2/2] du = \mathrm{Prob}\{0 < x \leq \mathbf{x}\} \tag{8.9}$$

In this form, u is the normalized GRV, $u \equiv (x - <x>)/\sigma_x$. Also, it is clear that $\mathrm{erf}(\infty) = 1/2$, and $\mathrm{erf}(-x) \equiv -\mathrm{erf}(x)$(erf(x) is odd). Indeed,

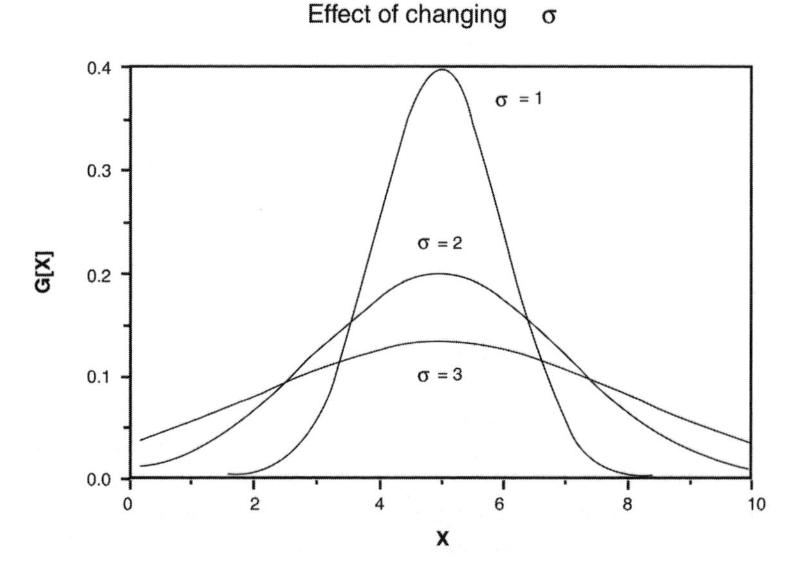

FIGURE 8.1

Examples of three Gaussian probability density functions, all with a mean of $\bar{x} = 5$. The standard deviations, σ, are 1, 2 and 3, as shown. Note that as σ decreases, the PDF becomes taller and narrower.

$$\frac{1}{\sigma_x\sqrt{2\pi}}\int_{\mathbf{x}_1}^{\mathbf{x}_2}\exp[-(x-<x>)^2/(2\sigma_x^2)]dx$$
$$=\text{erf}[(\mathbf{x}_2-<x>)/\sigma_x]-\text{erf}[(\mathbf{x}_1-<x>)/\sigma_x] \tag{8.10}$$

Where: $<x>=E\{x\}$, σ_x is the standard deviation of x, and $\mathbf{x_2}>\mathbf{x_1}$ are numerical values of the GRV, x. erf(x) is found numerically from tables; there is no closed-form algebraic solution to Equation 8.9.

The true mean of a stationary ergodic noisy voltage can be written as a time average over all time:

$$<v>=\lim_{T\to\infty}\frac{1}{T}\int_0^T v(t)dt \tag{8.11}$$

The mean of a stationary random variable (SRV), v, can also be written as an expectation, or *probability average:*

$$\mathbf{E}\{v\}=\int_{-\infty}^{\infty}vp(v)dv=<v> \tag{8.12}$$

Similarly, the mean squared v can be expressed by the expectation or probability average:

$$\mathbf{E}\{v^2\}=\int_{-\infty}^{\infty}v^2p(v)dv=<v^2> \tag{8.13}$$

The mean can be *estimated* by an average over finite time. For discrete data, this is called the *sample mean:*

$$\overline{v}=\frac{1}{T}\int_0^T v(t)dt, \quad \text{or} \quad \overline{v}=\frac{1}{N}\sum_{k=1}^{N}v_k \tag{8.14}$$

The *variance* of the random noise, v(t), is given by:

$$\begin{aligned}\sigma_v^2 \equiv <[v-<v>]^2>&=\int_{-\infty}^{\infty}[v-<v>]^2p(v)dv\\ &=\lim_{T\to\infty}\frac{1}{T}\int_0^T[v(t)-<v>]^2dt\end{aligned} \tag{8.15}$$

It is clear from Equation 8.15 that $<v^2>=\sigma_v^2+<v>^2$, or $E\{v^2\}=\sigma_v^2+E\{v\}^2$. Because the random noise we will be considering has zero mean, the mean squared noise is also its variance.

Many sources of noise accompany recorded physiological signals. An omnipresent source is the broadband random noise associated with amplifier electronics. Amplifier noise is generally modeled as an equivalent short-circuit broadband noise voltage source in series with the amplifier's input, and also a noise current source referred to the amplifier's input [Northrop, 1997].

Recording electrodes also make *thermal* or *Johnson noise;* the higher the real part of the electrode's impedance and the higher the temperature, the more noise produced. Finally, sources of random noise arise within the body itself. Unfortunately, this endogenous noise is generally nonstationary (i.e., its PDF is a $p(x,t)$), except over short time intervals, T. For example, in recording an ECG, muscle action potentials that occur when skeletal muscles contract can become superimposed on the ECG signal from the heart as broadband random noise. EMG noise can be a problem when recording an ECG while the patient is exercising (such as during a cardiac stress test). To minimize EMG noise, the standard ECG is usually recorded with the patient sitting and relaxed, or lying down. Because EMG noise is broad-band, and the ECG has a well-defined bandpass (−3 dB at 0.03 and 200 Hz), the ECG signal-to-noise ratio can be improved by sharply attenuating signal frequencies above 200 Hz. A band-reject or *notch filter* at 60 Hz can also be used to attenuate power line frequency interference on the ECG signal.

8.2.3 Autocorrelation

The *autocorrelation function* of a continuous stationary ergodic random variable can be expressed in the time domain as the average of the product, $x(t)x(t+\tau)$:

$$\varphi_{xx}(\tau) = \lim_{T\to\infty} \frac{1}{T}\int_{-T/2}^{T/2} x(t)x(t+\tau)dt = \lim_{T\to\infty} \frac{1}{T}\int_{-T/2}^{T/2} x(t-\tau)x(t)dt \quad (8.16)$$

(Some authors use $R_{xx}(\tau)$ for the ACF.) The autocorrelation function (ACF) provides an indication of the randomness or lack of correlation between samples of a stationary random variable shifted τ seconds. τ can have values $-\infty \le \tau \le \infty$. Some properties of the ACF are:

1. $\varphi_{xx}(\tau)$ is an even, real function. That is: $\varphi_{xx}(\tau) = \varphi_{xx}(-\tau)$.
2. Its value for $\tau = 0$ is the mean squared value of $x(t)$, i.e., $\varphi_{xx}(0) = E\{x^2\} = \sigma_x^2 > 0$.
3. $\varphi_{xx}(0) > |\varphi_{xx}(\tau)|$, for $\tau \neq 0$. That is, the maximum value of $\varphi_{xx}(\tau)$ is at the origin for random signals.
4. $\dot{\varphi}_{xx}(\tau) = E\{\dot{x}(t)x(t+\tau)\}$.
5. $\ddot{\varphi}_{xx}(\tau) = -E\{\dot{x}(t)\dot{x}(t+\tau)\}$.
6. The Fourier transform of $\varphi_{xx}(\tau)$ is the *two-sided auto power density spectrum* of the SRV, $x(t)$.That is, $F\{\varphi_{xx}(\tau)\} \equiv \Phi_{xx}(\omega)$ mean-squared volts/radian/second. $\Phi_{xx}(\omega)$ is positive-real and even.
7. If the SRV, $x(t)$, has nonzero mean, then $\sqrt{\varphi_{xx}(\infty)} = \langle x \rangle$.

Some interesting examples of ACFs can be found in the venerable text by Lee (1960). A few are summarized as follows:

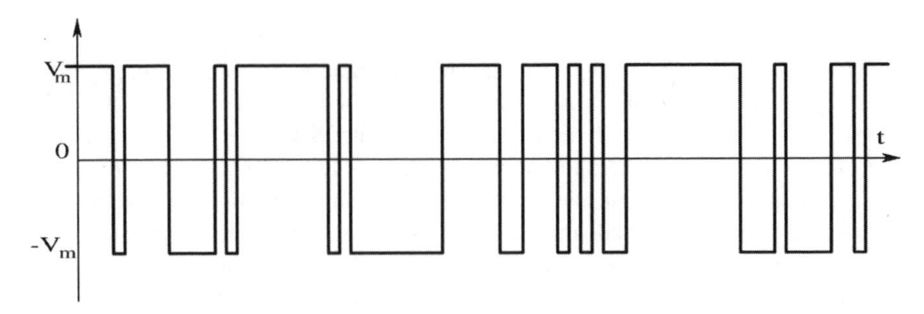

FIGURE 8.2
A random square wave with zero mean. Transition times follow Poisson statistics.

1. Let $x(t)$ be a random square wave with zero mean. The wave is shown in Figure 8.2. (Such a wave could result when the random output pulses from a Geiger counter drive a toggle flip-flop (TFF), which changes output state every time it receives an input pulse. The TFF's output must be given a negative dc offset so it will have zero mean.) The wave switches from $+V_m$ to $-V_m$ and vice versa with intervals given by the *Poisson probability function.* That is, the probability that n zeros (+ or − zero crossings) will occur in an interval, τ, is given by the *Poisson probability function* (*not* a PDF):

$$P(n,\tau) = \frac{(k\tau)^n}{n!} \exp(-k\tau) \tag{8.17}$$

Where k is the expected number of zeros per unit time. Lee shows that the ACF of this wave is: (Lee's rigorous development is rather long, so it is not repeated here.)

$$\varphi_{xx}(\tau) = V_m^2 \exp(-2k|\tau|) \tag{8.18}$$

2. Another example from Lee is the ACF of a SRV consisting of a train of randomly occurring (Poisson) positive unit impulses, as shown in Figure 8.3. Obviously, the mean value of the pulse train is k. Lee shows that the mean

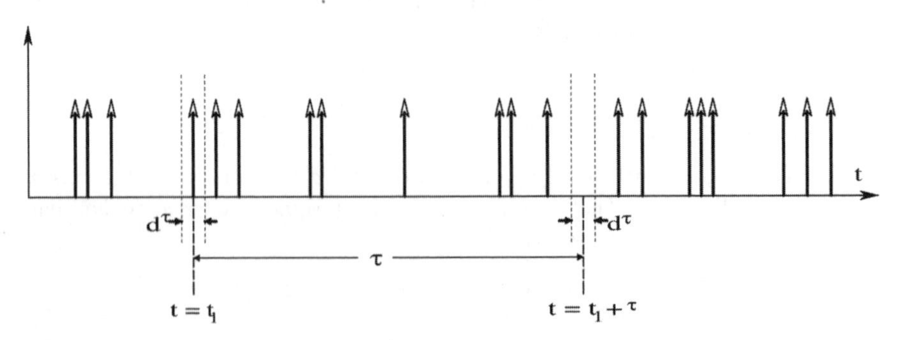

FIGURE 8.3
Randomly-occurring unit impulses. Occurrence times follow Poisson statistics.

squared value of the impulses is $\varphi_{xx}(0)=k+k^2$. The entire ACF of this SRV is shown to be:

$$\varphi_{xx}(\tau)=k\delta(\tau)+k^2 \tag{8.19}$$

3. Lee also shows that the ACF of a deterministic cosine wave of the form $x(t)=V_m\cos(\omega_o t+\theta)$ is: $\varphi_{xx}(\tau)=(V_m^2/2)\cos(\omega_o\tau)$. Note that for this deterministic waveform, $\varphi_{xx}(0)$ is not a unique maximum.
4. Very broadband (white) noise with zero mean and mean-squared value $<n^2>$ can be shown to have an ACF approximated by: $\varphi_{xx}(\tau)\cong<n^2>\delta(\tau)$. More realistically, the ACF will be of the form:

$$\varphi_{xx}(\tau)=B\exp(-\omega_c|\tau|) \tag{8.20}$$

Where ω_c is very large. It is easy to show that if the noise has a mean-squared value, $<n^2>$, then B must equal $½(\omega_c<n^2>)$ mean squared volts for the form of the ACF given in Equation 8.20.

8.2.4 Cross-Correlation

The cross-correlation function (CCF) is perhaps more useful in analyzing and describing system behavior than is the ACF. For a pair of stationary ergodic continuous random signals, the CCF is written for two stationary and ergodic random signals:

$$\varphi_{xy}(\tau)=\lim_{T\to\infty}\frac{1}{T}\int_{-T/2}^{T/2}x(t)y(t+\tau)dt=\lim_{T\to\infty}\frac{1}{T}\int_{-T/2}^{T/2}x(t-\tau)y(t)dt \tag{8.21}$$

x(t) is the input to an LTI system, and y(t) is its output. Some properties of the CCF are:

1. $\varphi_{yx}(\tau)=\varphi_{xy}(-\tau)$.
2. $\varphi_{xy}(\tau)$ is in general, neither even nor odd.
3. $\varphi_{xy}(\pm\infty)=0$.
4. $\varphi_{xy}(0)$ is not necessarily maximum.
5. $\varphi_{xy}(\tau)<½[\varphi_{xx}(0)+\varphi_{yy}(0)]$, for $-\infty\leq\tau\leq\infty$.
6. $F\{\varphi_{xy}(\tau)\}=\mathbf{\Phi_{xy}}(\omega)$, the *cross power spectral density,* which in general, will be complex. (Note that $\Phi_{xx}(\omega)$ and $\Phi_{yy}(\omega)$ are positive real.)

The cross-correlation function can also be written as an *expectation or probability average:*

$$\varphi_{xy}(\tau)=\mathbf{E}\{x(t)y(y+\tau)\} \tag{8.22}$$

The LTI system output, $y(t+\tau)$ can be given, in general, by real convolution of the system's input with the system's weighting function:

$$y(t+\tau)=\int_{-\infty}^{\infty} h(\mu)x(t+\tau-\mu)d\mu \tag{8.23}$$

Thus, we can write:

$$\varphi_{xy}(\tau)=E\{x(t)\int_{-\infty}^{\infty} h(\mu)x(t+\tau-\mu)d\mu\} \tag{8.24}$$

Since the integral in Equation 8.24 depends on μ, not t, we can bring $x(t)$ inside the integral:

$$\varphi_{xy}(\tau)=E\left\{\int_{-\infty}^{\infty} x(t)h(\mu)x(t+\tau-\mu)d\mu\right\} \tag{8.25}$$

Now we can interchange the linear operations of expectation and convolution. $h(\mu)$ is a deterministic function, not an RV, so we can write:

$$\varphi_{xy}(\tau)=\int_{-\infty}^{\infty} h(\mu)E\{x(t)x(t+\tau-\mu)\}d\mu \tag{8.26}$$

Note that the expectation is simply the definition of the autocorrelation of the SRV, $x(t)$, with time shift, $(\tau-\mu)$. Thus, the final relation is that the *CCF is equal to the real convolution of the SLS weighting function with the ACF of the input SRV,* $x(t)$*:*

$$\varphi_{xy}(\tau)=\int_{-\infty}^{\infty} h(\mu)\varphi_{xx}(\tau-\mu)d\mu=h(\tau)\otimes\varphi_{xx}(\tau) \tag{8.27}$$

Two of the many useful applications of the CCF from Lee (1960) are as follows:

1. The CCF can be used to extract a periodic signal buried in noise by cross-correlating it with a periodic train of impulses in which the impulse period is made, *a priori,* the same as the periodic signal in the noise. Stated mathematically, $x(t)=n(t)+A\sin(\omega_o t+\theta)$, and

$$y(t)=P_T(t)=\sum_{k=-\infty}^{\infty} \delta(t-k2\pi/\omega_o). \tag{8.28}$$

Thus

$$\varphi_{xy}(\tau)=\mathbf{E}\left\{\left[n(\tau)+A\sin(\omega_o\tau+\theta)\right]\left[\sum_{k=-\infty}^{\infty} \delta(t-k2\pi/\omega_o+\tau)\right]\right\} \tag{8.29}$$

Because the noise has zero mean and is uncorrelated with $\mathrm{P_T(t)}$, the first term goes to zero. By the sifting property of the delta function, the second term is:

$$\begin{aligned}\varphi_{xy}(\tau) &= \mathrm{A}\sin[\omega_o(\tau - \mathrm{k}2\pi/\omega_o)+\theta] \\ &= \mathrm{A}\sin[\omega_o\tau - \mathrm{k}2\pi+\theta] \\ &= \mathrm{A}\sin[\omega_o\tau+\theta] \end{aligned} \tag{8.30}$$

Lo and behold, the signal is recovered as a function of the cross-correlation delay variable, τ. The $\mathrm{k}2\pi$ term can be dropped because $\sin(\alpha+\mathrm{k}2\pi)=\sin(\alpha)$, i.e., the sine function is periodic. In practice, with finite data, there would be noise added to $\mathrm{A}\sin[\omega_o\tau+\theta]$, giving uncertainty to the exact A and θ parameter values. (Recall that ω_o was known, *a priori*.)

2. Another very important application of cross-correlation is the identification of the impulse response or weighting function of an LTI system, given a noise input, $\mathrm{x(t)}$. Let the system have weighting function $\mathrm{h(t)}$. As we have seen before, the system's output, $\mathrm{y(t)}$, can be put in general form using real convolution:

$$\mathrm{y(t)} = \int_{-\infty}^{\infty} \mathrm{h}(\mu)\mathrm{x}(\mathrm{t}-\mu)\mathrm{d}\mu \tag{8.31}$$

Now

$$\varphi_{xy}(\tau) \equiv \mathrm{E}\{\mathrm{x(t)y(t}+\tau)\}$$

can be written:

$$\varphi_{xy}(\tau) = \lim_{\mathrm{T}\to\infty}\frac{1}{\mathrm{T}}\int_{-\mathrm{T}/2}^{\mathrm{T}/2}\mathrm{x(t)}\overbrace{\left\{\int_{-\infty}^{\infty}\mathrm{h}(\mu)\mathrm{x}(\mathrm{t}+\tau-\mu)\mathrm{d}\mu\right\}}^{\{\mathrm{y}(\mathrm{t}+\tau)\}}\mathrm{dt} \tag{8.32}$$

By exchanging the order of integrations in Equation 8.32, we obtain:

$$\begin{aligned}\varphi_{xy}(\tau) &= \int_{-\infty}^{\infty}\mathrm{h}(\mu)\left[\lim_{\mathrm{T}\to\infty}\frac{1}{\mathrm{T}}\int_{-\mathrm{T}/2}^{\mathrm{T}/2}\mathrm{x(t)x}(\mathrm{t}+\tau-\mu)\mathrm{dt}\right]\mathrm{d}\mu \\ &= \int_{-\infty}^{\infty}\mathrm{h}(\mu)\varphi_{xx}(\tau-\mu)\mathrm{d}\mu \end{aligned} \tag{8.33}$$

In other words, CCF of SLS system input with its output can be given by the convolution of the system's weighting function with the random input's autocorrelation function. Now if the system's input is broadband Gaussian noise, its ACF can be approximated by $\varphi_{xx}(\mu) \cong \langle \mathrm{x}^2 \rangle \delta(\mu)$. When this CCF is convolved with the SLS system's weighting function, we have:

$$\varphi_{xy}(\tau) = \int_{-\infty}^{\infty}\mathrm{h}(\mu)\langle \mathrm{x}^2\rangle\delta(\tau-\mu)\mathrm{d}\mu = \langle \mathrm{x}^2\rangle \mathrm{h}(\tau) \tag{8.34}$$

Thus, the system's weighting function, $h(\tau) = \varphi_{xy}(\tau)/\langle x^2 \rangle$. As you will see below, system identification can be made in the frequency domain using the cross-power density spectrum.

8.2.5 The continuous auto- and cross-power density spectrums

Stated succinctly, the *auto-power density spectrum* (APS), $\Phi_{xx}(\omega)$, is the Fourier transform of the autocorrelation function; it has the units of mean-squared units (e.g., volts) per r/sec. Because $\varphi_{xx}(\tau)$ is real and even, $\Phi_{xx}(\omega)$ is positive-real and even (i.e., is two-sided). To reiterate:

$$\Phi_{xx}(\omega) = \int_{-\infty}^{\infty} \varphi_{xx}(\tau)\exp(-j\omega\tau)\,d\tau, \quad -\infty \leq \omega \leq \infty \tag{8.35}$$

Often, we encounter the *one-sided APS,* which is often used in describing amplifier noise, noise from resistors, etc. The one-sided spectrum is simply $S_{xx}(\omega) \equiv 2\Phi_{xx}(\omega)$ for $0 \leq \omega \leq \infty$. Often, $S_{xx}(\omega)$ in msu/r/sec is expressed as $S_{xx}(f)$ msu/Hz. Since $f = \omega/2\pi$, i.e., a radian $(57.3°)$ is smaller than a cycle $(360°)$, hence $S_{xx}(f) = 2\pi S_{xx}(\omega)$ msu/Hz. Of course, the ACF can be found from the two-sided APS by the inverse CFT. That is:

$$\varphi_{xx}(\tau) = \frac{1}{2\pi}\int_{-\infty}^{\infty} \Phi_{xx}(\omega)\exp(j\omega\tau)d\omega = \frac{1}{2\pi}\int_{-\infty}^{\infty} \Phi_{xx}(\omega)\cos(\omega\tau)d\omega \tag{8.36}$$

The second (cosine) ICFT is possible from the Euler relation because $\Phi_{xx}(\omega)$ is an even function. Note that, from Equation 8.36, we can write:

$$\varphi_{xx}(0) = E\{\mathbf{x}^2\} = \sigma_x^2 = \frac{1}{2\pi}\int_{-\infty}^{\infty} \Phi_{xx}(\omega)d\omega = \int_{-\infty}^{\infty} \Phi_{xx}(2\pi f)df \tag{8.37}$$

That is, the total area under $\Phi_{xx}(2\pi f)/2\pi$ is the mean-squared value of the SRV, $\mathbf{x}(t)$.

White noise (WN) is an ideal model for broadband noise with a flat APS over a significant span of frequency. The APS of *ideal white noise* is $\Phi_{nn}(\omega) = \eta$ msu/r/sec for $-\infty \leq \omega \leq \infty$. This definition implies that $\sigma_n^2 \to \infty$ for ideal WN, which clearly is not real-world realistic. The inverse CFT of a constant is well known:

$$\varphi_{xx}(\tau) = \frac{1}{2\pi}\int_{-\infty}^{\infty} \eta\exp(j\omega\tau)d\omega = \eta\delta(\tau) \tag{8.38}$$

That is, the autocorrelation function of white noise with zero mean is an impulse function at the origin of the time-shift axis. An APS of the form:

$$\Phi_{xx}(\omega) = \frac{2\omega_h\sigma_x^2}{\omega^2 + \omega_h^2} \tag{8.39}$$

Has the well-known autocorrelation function,

$$\varphi_{xx}(\tau) = \sigma_x^2\exp(-\omega_h|\tau|), \tag{8.40}$$

and an ideal bandwidth-limited APS of the form $\Phi_{xx}(\omega)=\pi\sigma_x^2/\omega_c$ for $|\omega|\leq\omega_c$, and $\Phi_{xx}(\omega)=0$ for $|\omega|>\omega_c$, has a corresponding ACF:

$$\varphi_{xx}(\tau)=\sigma_x^2\frac{\sin(\omega_c\tau)}{\omega_c\tau} \tag{8.41}$$

The cross-power density spectrum (CPS) is simply the CFT of the cross-correlation function (CCF):

$$\mathbf{\Phi}_{\mathbf{xy}}(\omega)\equiv\int_{-\infty}^{\infty}\varphi_{xy}(\tau)\exp(-j\omega\tau)d\tau \tag{8.42}$$

Note that the CPS is in general complex. If we substitute Equation 8.33 into Equation 8.42, we have:

$$\mathbf{\Phi}_{\mathbf{xy}}(\omega)=\int_{-\infty}^{\infty}\int_{-\infty}^{\infty}h(\mu)\varphi_{xx}(\tau-\mu)\exp(-j\omega\tau)d\mu\, d\tau \tag{8.43}$$

Now we let $\tau\equiv\xi+\mu$, so Equation 8.43 becomes:

$$\begin{aligned}\mathbf{\Phi}_{\mathbf{xy}}(\omega)&=\int_{-\infty}^{\infty}\int_{-\infty}^{\infty}h(\mu)\varphi_{xx}(\xi)\exp[-j\omega(\xi+\mu)]d\mu d\xi\\&=\int_{-\infty}^{\infty}h(\mu)\exp[-j\omega\mu]d\mu\int_{-\infty}^{\infty}\varphi_{xx}(\xi)\exp[-j\omega\xi]d\xi\end{aligned} \tag{8.44}$$

$$\downarrow$$

$$\mathbf{\Phi}_{\mathbf{xy}}(\omega)=\mathbf{H}(\omega)\Phi_{xx}(\omega)$$

Thus, from Equation 8.44, we see that the SLS frequency response function can be found by forming the vector quotient:

$$\mathbf{H}(\omega)=\frac{\mathbf{\Phi}_{\mathbf{xy}}(\omega)}{\Phi_{xx}(\omega)} \tag{8.45}$$

Clearly, the angle of $\mathbf{H}(\omega)$ is the angle of the cross-power spectrum, $\mathbf{\Phi}_{\mathbf{xy}}(\omega)$. If very broadband input noise is used (white over the bandpass region of $\mathbf{H}(\omega)$, then $\Phi_{xx}(\omega)=\eta$, and

$$\mathbf{H}(\omega)=\mathbf{\Phi}_{\mathbf{xy}}(\omega)/\eta. \tag{8.46}$$

Equations 8.45 and 8.46 illustrate classic means of LTI system characterization in the frequency domain, using a very broadband (white) Gaussian noise input.

A problem that often arises in describing noise at the inputs of LTI continuous or discrete systems is how to handle multiple independent uncorrelated noise sources. For example, the input signal can be contaminated with a noise voltage, $e_{ns}(t)$, which appears in series with the equivalent short-circuit input noise from the signal conditioning amplifier, $e_{na}(t)$. Common sense tells us that, in the time-domain, these noise voltages add at the amplifier's input to form $e_{nin}(t)=e_{ns}(t)+e_{na}(t)$. However, we generally do not treat noise in the time domain. Because we have assumed these noise sources are independent and uncorrelated, they can only be added in a mean-squared sense [Northrop, 1990]. That is, the msec $\overline{e_{nin}^2} = \overline{e_{ns}^2} + \overline{e_{na}^2}$. As a further consequence of the independence and uncorrelation assumption, we can also show that the autopower spectrum at the amplifier's input is simply the sum of the autopower spectra of $e_{ns}(t)$ and $e_{na}(t)$. That is: $\Phi_{nin}(\omega) = \Phi_{ns}(\omega) + \Phi_{na}(\omega)$. This important result has far-reaching consequences when finding the net input noise autopower spectrum from ≥ 2 independent and uncorrelated noise sources at a system's input.

In practice, finite-length records of discrete data are used to calculate auto- and cross-correlograms, and the corresponding auto- and cross-power spectrograms are found by use of the fast Fourier transform (FFT) version of the DFT. In Section 8.3, we examine some of these discrete algorithms.

8.2.6 Propagation of noise through stationary causal LTI continuous systems

It is not difficult to prove [Lee, 1960] that, when the input to a stationary analog LTI system is a stationary Gaussian random variable having a two-sided autopower spectrum, $\Phi_{xx}(\omega)$, then the output of the SLS will have an autopower spectrum given by:

$$\Phi_{yy}(\omega) = |\mathbf{H}(\omega)|^2 \Phi_{xx}(\omega) \tag{8.47}$$

Where $|\mathbf{H}(\omega)|$ is the magnitude of the (complex) frequency response function of the LTI system. As an example of this relation, let us assume the SLS is a simple low-pass filter with frequency response function given by:

$$\mathbf{H}(\omega) = \frac{K_v \omega_o}{j\omega + \omega_o} \tag{8.48}$$

The magnitude squared of $\mathbf{H}(\omega)$ is:

$$|\mathbf{H}(\omega)|^2 = \frac{K_v^2 \omega_o^2}{\omega^2 + \omega_o^2} \tag{8.49}$$

Now, if the input noise is white, with APS $\Phi_{xx}(\omega) = \eta$ msv/r/sec, the two-sided, output APS is simply:

$$\Phi_{yy}(\omega) = \frac{\eta K_v^2 \omega_o^2}{\omega^2 + \omega_o^2} \text{ msv/r/sec} \tag{8.50}$$

In other words, the SLS shapes the input APS by its frequency response magnitude squared. (This simple relation *does not hold for nonlinear systems,* or for input noise that does not have a Gaussian probability density spectrum.)

The variance of the output noise is found by taking the IFT of $\Phi_{yy}(\omega)$ with $\tau \to 0$. We use the well-known definite integral:

$$\int_0^\infty \frac{a\,dx}{a^2 + x^2} \equiv \pi/2 \tag{8.51}$$

To find:

$$\sigma_y^2 = \varphi_{yy}(0) = \frac{1}{2\pi}\int_{-\infty}^{\infty}\frac{\eta K_v^2\omega_o^2}{\omega_o^2+\omega^2}d\omega = \frac{\eta K_v^2\omega_o}{2\pi}2(\pi/2) = (\eta K_v^2\omega_o)/2 \quad (8.52)$$

8.2.7 Propagation of noise through stationary causal LTI discrete systems

Introduction to the characterization of a discrete noise sequence, $\mathbf{x}(n)$, defined at periodic sampling instants, $t = nT$, is made easier if we assume the sequence is composed of *real numbers* and is *stationary* and *ergodic*. The expected value of **x** is defined by [Papoulis, 1977, Chapter 9]:

$$E\{\mathbf{x}(n)\} \equiv \eta(n) = \eta \quad (8.53)$$

The autocorrelation of **x** is defined as:

$$E\{\mathbf{x}(n_1)\mathbf{x}(n_2)\} \equiv R_{xx}(n_1 - n_2) = R_{xx}(m) \quad (8.54)$$

Because the RV is stationary, the autocorrelation R_{xx} is a function of the *time difference,* $n_1 - n_2 = m$, between the samples in the stationary sequence, $\mathbf{x}(n)$. It can be shown that $R_{xx}(m)$ is real and even in m. If we assume that the random process generating $\mathbf{x}(n)$ is *ergodic* as well as stationary, we can write the discrete autocorrelation function as a time average:

$$R_{xx}(m) = \lim_{n\to\infty}\frac{1}{2N+1}\sum_{n=-N}^{+N} x(nT)x(nT+mT) \quad (8.55)$$

The discrete cross-correlation between two stationary random sequences is defined similarly;

$$\begin{aligned} E\{\mathbf{x}(n_1)\mathbf{y}(n_2)\} &\equiv R_{xy}(n_1 - n_2) = R_{xy}(m) \\ &= \lim_{N\to\infty}\frac{1}{2N+1}\sum_{n=-N}^{+N} x(nT)y(nT+mT) \end{aligned} \quad (8.56)$$

Figure 8.4 illustrates the process of discrete cross-correlation with two discrete deterministic, transient signals, $x(n)$ and $y(n)$. You can see for $m > 0$, the summed product of $x(n)$ and $y(n+m)$ only needs to be computed for $0 \le n \le (N - m)$; otherwise, it is zero.

We can take the two-sided z-transforms of the discrete auto- and cross-correlation functions as defined above and obtain the sampled autopower spectrum and the sampled cross-power spectrum in z, respectively. Because $R_{xx}(mT)$ is real and even, the discrete auto-power spectrum is real and even, and is given by:

$$S_{xx}(z) = \sum_{m=-\infty}^{\infty} R_{xx}(mT)z^{-m} \quad (8.57)$$

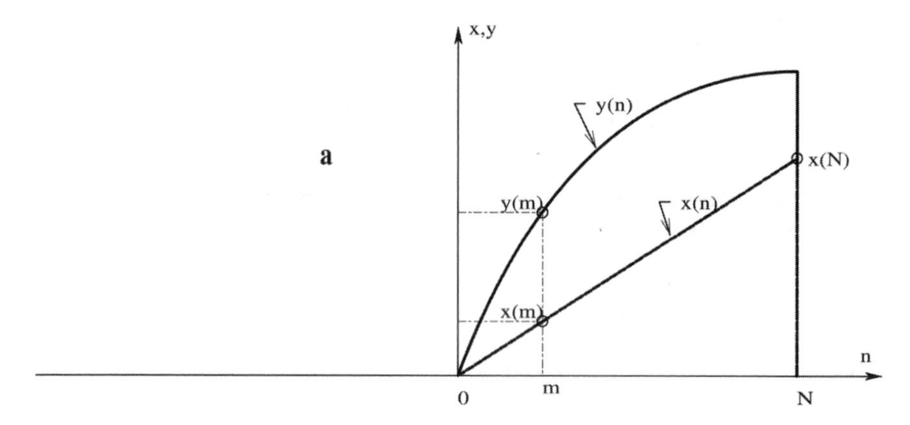

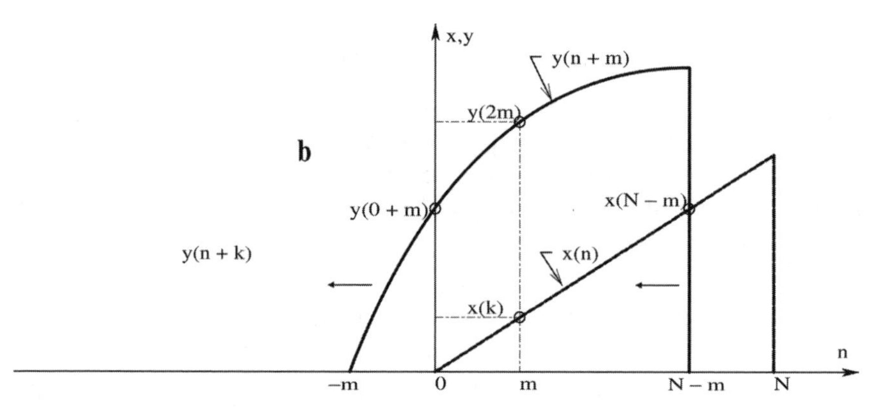

FIGURE 8.4

The process of discrete cross-correlation. $x(n)$ and $y(n)$ are shown as truncated, continuous functions for clarity. (a) Both $x(n)$ and $y(n)$ are discrete, causal signals, shown with zero time-shift. Both $x(n)$ and $y(n)$ are defined over $0 \leq n \leq N$. That is, both signals have $N+1$ samples. (b) $y(n)$ is time shifted by $t = mT$ (integer m) to form $y(n+m)$. Corresponding points in time on $x(n)$ and $y(n+m)$ are multiplied together and summed, as indicated in Equation 8.56, then divided by $N+1$.

Where it is clear that $\mathbf{z} \equiv e^{sT}$. Similarly, the cross-power spectrum is given by:

$$S_{xy}(z) = \sum_{m=-\infty}^{\infty} R_{xy}(mT) z^{-m} \tag{8.58}$$

Note that $R_{xy}(mT)$ is generally real but not even. Thus $S_{xy}(z)$ must be found with appropriate attention to regions of convergence.

It is well known that the output of a DLTI system for any input can be given by real discrete convolution. When the input is a random sequence, $\mathbf{x}(n)$, the output, $\mathbf{y}(n)$ will also be a random sequence.

$$\mathbf{y}(n)=\sum_{k=-\infty}^{\infty}\mathbf{x}(n-k)h(k) \tag{8.59}$$

From real convolution, we can write:

$$\mathbf{x}(n_1)\mathbf{y}(n_2)=\sum_{k=-\infty}^{\infty}\mathbf{x}(n_1)\mathbf{x}(n_2-k)h(k) \tag{8.60}$$

$$\mathbf{y}(n_1)\mathbf{y}(n_2)=\sum_{k=-\infty}^{\infty}\mathbf{y}(n_2)\mathbf{x}(n_1-k)h(k) \tag{8.61}$$

The cross- and autocorrelation functions are found by taking the expectations of the equations above.

$$\begin{aligned}R_{xy}(n_1-n_2)=R_{xy}(m)&=\sum_{k=-\infty}^{\infty}R_{xx}(m-k)h(k)\\&=\sum_{k=-\infty}^{\infty}R_{xx}(k)h(m-k)\end{aligned} \tag{8.62}$$

$$\begin{aligned}R_{yy}(n_1-n_2)=R_{yy}(m)&=\sum_{k=-\infty}^{\infty}R_{xy}(m-k)h(k)\\&=\sum_{k=-\infty}^{\infty}R_{xy}(k)h(m-k)\end{aligned} \tag{8.63}$$

Because the system, $h(n)$, is causal, $h(m-k)=0$ for $m-k<0$.
It can be shown [Ragazzini and Franklin, 1958; Cunningham, 1992] that the sampled crosspower spectrum in z, $S_{xy}(z)$, can be written:

$$S_{xy}(z)=S_{xx}(z)H(z) \tag{8.64}$$

And the sampled output autopower spectrum in z is given by:

$$S_{yy}(z)=S_{xx}(z)H(z)H(-z) \tag{8.65}$$

We have particular interest in the noise variance (msec noise) at the filter output, given by:

$$\sigma_y^2=\underset{m=0}{R_{yy}(0)}=\sum_{k=-\infty}^{\infty}R_{xy}(0-k)h(k)=\sum_{k=-\infty}^{\infty}R_{yx}(k)h(k) \tag{8.66}$$

To find $R_{yy}(0)$, we can also evaluate the complex inversion integral with $m=0$:

$$R_{yy}(m\to 0)=\frac{1}{2\pi j}\int_{\mathbf{C}}S_{yy}(z)z^{m-1}dz\to\frac{1}{2\pi j}\int_{\mathbf{C}}R_{yy}(z)z^{-1}dz=\sigma_y^2 \tag{8.67}$$

The contour **C** is the unit circle, —z— = 1. Now suppose the input noise is *white sampled noise with zero mean.* That is,

$$R_{xx}(m) = \sigma_x^2 \delta(m). \tag{8.68}$$

Now from Equation 8.62:

$$R_{xy}(m) = \sum_{k=-\infty}^{\infty} \sigma_x^2 \delta(m-k) h(k) = \sigma_x^2 h(m), \quad m \geq 0, \text{ else } 0. \tag{8.69}$$

The mean-squared noise output of a causal LTI digital filter with discrete weighting function, $h(n)$, is $R_{yy}(0)$. This variance can be written [Cunningham, 1992; Phillips and Nagle, 1984]:

$$\underset{m=0}{R_{yy}(0)} = \sigma_y^2 = \sigma_x^2 \sum_{k=0}^{\infty} h^2(k) \tag{8.70}$$

Note that, because $h(n) = h(nT)$ is causal, $h(n) = 0$ for $n < 0$. Thus, the square of the discrete transfer function, $h(n)$, conditions the white sampled input noise.

8.2.8 Characteristic functions of random variables

The characteristic function (CHF) of a RV, **x**, is defined as the complex expected value:

$$\boldsymbol{\Psi}(\omega) \equiv E\{e^{j\omega\mathbf{x}}\} = \int_{-\infty}^{\infty} e^{j\omega\mathbf{x}} f(x) dx \tag{8.71}$$

Where $f(x)$ is the probability density function (PDF) of the RV, **x**. It is evident that $\boldsymbol{\Psi}(\omega)$ is the Fourier transform of the PDF, $f(t)$, with $\omega \to -\omega$. That is, $\boldsymbol{\Psi}(\omega) = \mathbf{F}(-\omega)$. Note that $\mathbf{F}(-\omega)$ *is not* the conjugate of $\mathbf{F}(\omega)$.

For example, consider the Gaussian random variable with PDF:

$$f(x) = \frac{1}{\sqrt{2\pi\sigma_x^2}} \exp\left[-1/2 \frac{(x-\overline{x})^2}{\sigma_x^2} \right] \tag{8.72}$$

The CHF of the GRV, x, can be shown to be [Papoulis, 1965]:

$$\boldsymbol{\Psi}(\omega) = \exp[+j\omega\overline{x}] \exp[-{}^1\!/\!_2 \omega^2 \sigma_{x]}^2 \tag{8.73}$$

The CHF has several practical uses. One application is in finding what happens to Gaussian noise that propagates through single-valued nonlinearities. In the *first example,* consider the odd exponential nonlinearity, $y = g(x) = A[e^{bx} - e^{-bx}]$. The mean output of the nonlinearity is:

$$\overline{y} = \mathbf{E}\{y\} = \mathbf{E}\{A \exp[j(b/j)x) - A \exp[j(b/-j)x]\} \tag{8.74}$$

The exponential terms in the expectation are recognized as characteristic functions in which $\omega \rightarrow (b/j)$. Thus,

$$\bar{y} = A[\boldsymbol{\Psi}(b/j) - \boldsymbol{\Psi}(b/-j)] \tag{8.75}$$

We assumed that x was a GRV *with zero mean.* Thus, from Equation 8.73, we have:

$$\bar{y} = A\{\exp[-{}^1\!/\!_2(b/j)^2\sigma_x^2] - \exp[-{}^1\!/\!_2(b/-j)^2\sigma_x^2]\} \tag{8.76}$$

Equation 8.76 is easily shown to be:

$$\bar{y} = A\{\exp[{}^1\!/\!_2 b^2\sigma_x^2] - \exp[{}^1\!/\!_2 b^2\sigma_x^2]\} = 0 \tag{8.77}$$

This result is also intuitively obvious because $y = g(x)$ is odd and x has zero mean.

We can also use the CHF to find the autocorrelation function of the nonlinearity output, y.

$$\begin{aligned}\phi_{yy}(\tau) &= \mathbf{E}\{y(t)y(t+\tau)\} \\ &= A^2\mathbf{E}\{[\exp(bx) - \exp(-bx)][\exp(bx_\tau) - \exp(-bx_\tau)]\}\end{aligned} \tag{8.78}$$

Equation 8.78 can be expanded to a more detailed notation:

$$\begin{aligned}\phi_{yy}(\tau) = {} & A^2\mathbf{E}\{\exp[j(b/j)x(t)]\exp[j(b/j)x(t+\tau)]\} \\ & - A^2\mathbf{E}\{\exp[j(b/j)x(t)]\exp[j(b/-j)x(t+\tau)]\} \\ & - A^2\mathbf{E}\{\exp[j(b/-j)x(t)]\exp[j(b/j)x(t+\tau)]\} \\ & + A^2\mathbf{E}\{\exp[j(b/-j)x(t)]\exp[j(b/-j)x(t+\tau)]\}\end{aligned} \tag{8.79}$$

Now we must introduce the *joint CHF:*

$$\begin{aligned}\boldsymbol{\Psi}_{\mathbf{uv}}(\omega_1,\omega_2) \equiv \mathbf{E}\{\exp(j\omega_1\mathbf{u})\exp(j\omega_2\mathbf{v})\} = {} & \exp[j(\omega_1\bar{u} + \omega_2\bar{v})] \\ & \times \exp[-{}^1\!/\!_2(\omega_1^2\sigma_u^2 + \omega_2^2\sigma_v^2 + 2r\sigma_u\sigma_v\omega_1\omega_2)]\end{aligned} \tag{8.80}$$

Where

$$r\sigma_u\sigma_v = \mathbf{E}\{(\mathbf{u} - \bar{u})(\mathbf{v} - \bar{v})\} = \mathbf{E}\{\mathbf{uv}\} - \bar{u}\bar{v} \tag{8.81}$$

(Note that $v(t)$ can equal $x(t)$, $u = x(t+\tau)$, $\omega_1 = b/j$ and $\omega_2 = b/-j$) Thus:

$$\begin{aligned}\phi_{yy}(\tau) = A^2[& \boldsymbol{\Psi}_{\mathbf{xx}}(b/j, b/j) - \boldsymbol{\Psi}_{\mathbf{xx}}(b/j, b/-j) \\ & - \boldsymbol{\Psi}_{\mathbf{xx}}(b/-j, b/j) + \boldsymbol{\Psi}_{\mathbf{xx}}(b/-j, b/-j)]\end{aligned} \tag{8.82}$$

Expanding:

$$\begin{aligned}\phi_{yy}(\tau)/A^2 = {} & \exp\{-{}^1\!/\!_2[(b/j)^2\sigma_x^2 + (b/j)^2\sigma_x^2 + 2\phi_{xx}(\tau)(b/j)(b/j)]\} \\ & -\exp\{-{}^1\!/\!_2[(b/j)^2\sigma_x^2 + (b/-j)^2\sigma_x^2 + 2\phi_{xx}(\tau)(b/j)(b/-j)]\} \\ & -\exp\{-{}^1\!/\!_2[(b/-j)^2\sigma_x^2 + (b/j)^2\sigma_x^2 + 2\phi_{xx}(\tau)(b/-j)(b/j)]\} \\ & +\exp\{-{}^1\!/\!_2[(b/-j)^2\sigma_x^2 + (b/-j)^2\sigma_x^2 \\ & +2\phi_{xx}(\tau)(b/-j)(b/-j)]\}\end{aligned} \tag{8.83}$$

Note that $(j)^2 = -1$, $(-j)^2 = -1$, $(j)(-j) = 1$, so the 4 terms of Equation 8.83 become:

$$\begin{aligned}\phi_{yy}(\tau)/A^2 = &\exp[b^2\sigma_x^2 + b^2\phi_{xx}(\tau)] - \exp[b^2\sigma_x^2 - b^2\phi_{xx}(\tau)] \\ &- \exp[b^2\sigma_x^2 - b^2\phi_{xx}(\tau)] + \exp[b^2\sigma_x^2 + b^2\phi_{xx}(\tau)]\end{aligned} \tag{8.84}$$

Now note that the variance of the RV y is Var$\{\mathbf{y}\}$ = $\phi_{yy}(0) - (\overline{y})^2, \phi_{xx}(0) = \sigma_x^2$, and $\overline{x} = \overline{y} = 0$. Var$\{\mathbf{y}\}$ is a measure of the "noisiness" of y. Finally, Var$\{\mathbf{y}\}$ can be written:

$$\sigma_y^2 = 2A^2[\exp(2b^2\sigma_x^2) - 1] \tag{8.85}$$

8.2.9 Price's theorem and applications

Often stationary, Gaussian random noise is passed through a general single-valued non-linearity. The probability density of the output of the nonlinearity is, in general, no longer Gaussian. However, as we demonstrated in the special case of an exponential nonlinearity, it is possible to describe the output signal in terms of its moments and correlation functions using characteristic functions. *Price's theorem* offers a general approach to finding certain statistical properties of the output of a single-valued non-linearity, given a stationary Gaussian random input. Papoulis (1965) developed a 1-D form of Price's theorem. Let the nonlinearity be written as: $y = g(x)$; the theorem is:

$$\frac{\partial^n E\{g(x)\}}{\partial \nu^n} \equiv \frac{1}{2^n}\int_{-\infty}^{\infty} f_x(x)\frac{\partial^{2n} g(x)}{\partial x^{2n}}dx, \ \nu = \sigma_x^2 \tag{8.86}$$

The use of the 1-D Price's theorem above will be illustrated with $n = 1$, and a half-wave rectifier nonlinearity; $y = g(x) = x$ for $x \geq 0$, and 0 for $x < 0$. We will find the *mean* of the half-wave rectifier's output, y. Mathematically, the half-wave rectifier can be written:

$$y = g(x) = (x + |x|)/2 \tag{8.87}$$

The input is a Gaussian random variable, x, having zero mean. Thus, Equation 8.86 becomes:

$$\begin{aligned}&\frac{\partial E\{y\}}{\partial \nu} = \frac{1}{2}\int_{-\infty}^{\infty} f_x(x)\frac{\partial^2 g(x)}{\partial x^2}dx = \frac{1}{2}\int_{-\infty}^{\infty}\frac{1}{\sqrt{2\pi}\sigma_x}\exp[-\tfrac{1}{2}x^2/\sigma_x^2]\delta(x)dx \\ &\downarrow \\ &\frac{\partial E\{y\}}{\partial \nu} = \frac{1}{2\sqrt{2\pi}\sigma_x} \to \to \partial E\{y\}\partial\nu = \frac{d\nu}{2\sqrt{2\pi}\sqrt{\nu}}\end{aligned} \tag{8.88}$$

Integrating, we find:

$$E\{y\} = \frac{\sqrt{\nu}}{\sqrt{2\pi}} + k = \frac{\sigma_x}{\sqrt{2\pi}} + k \tag{8.89}$$

It is seen that in the limit as $\sigma_x \to 0, k \to 0$, so $k = 0$. Equation 8.89 gives the expected (average) value of y for a zero-mean Gaussian noise input to a half-wave rectifier.

Price's theorem can be extended to the bivariate case:

$$\frac{\partial^{n} E\{g(x,y)\}}{\partial \rho^{n}} \equiv \int_{-\infty}^{\infty}\int_{-\infty}^{\infty} f_{x,y}(x,y)\frac{\partial^{2n} g(x,y)}{\partial x^{n}\partial y^{n}} dxdy \tag{8.90}$$

This somewhat awesome-looking integro-differential equation is also applied here with $n=1$. $f_{xy}(x,y)$ is a joint probability density function, and ρ is the cross-covariance, which can be written:

$$\rho = \mu_{xy} = R_{xy}(\tau) - \overline{x}\overline{y} = \sigma_x \sigma_y r \tag{8.91}$$

r is the *correlation coefficient* between x and y, and $R_{xy}(\tau)$ is the cross-correlation function between x and y. Again, we assume $\overline{x}=0$, so $\rho = R_{xy}(\tau)$.

For an *example of the use of Price's theorem in the bivariate case,* consider the system illustrated in Figure 8.5. The system is a bang-bang autocorrelator. The input is a GRV, x. x is passed through a signum function that returns $w=+1$ if $x \geq 0$ and -1 if $x<0$. The signum function can be written:

$$y = g(x) = \text{sgn}(x) = \frac{x}{|x|} = [-1 + 2U(x)] \tag{8.92}$$

Applying Price's theorem:

$$\frac{\partial E\{z\}}{\partial \rho} \int_{-\infty}^{\infty}\int_{-\infty}^{\infty} f_{xy}(x,y)\frac{\partial^{2} g(x,y)}{\partial x \partial y} dxdy \tag{8.93}$$

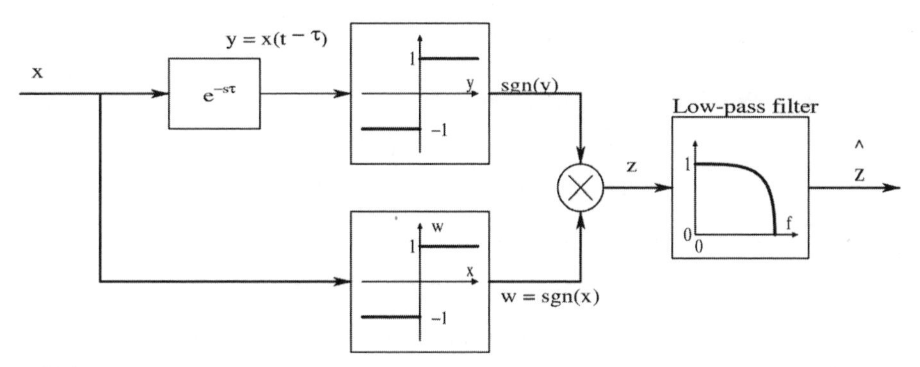

FIGURE 8.5

A continuous bang-bang (or signum) autocorrelator. The output of the analog multiplier, z, is either ± 1. Price's theorem is used to demonstrate how the system works. Note that the lowpass filtered $z(t)$ square wave can be shown to be $(2/\pi)\sin^{-1}[\phi_{xx}(\tau)/\sigma_x^2]$.

In this example, the delayed $y=x(t-\tau)$ is also a GRV. Also, $\sigma_y=\sigma_x$. First, let us calculate $\partial^2 g(x,y)/\partial x\partial y$:

$$\begin{aligned}
&\partial^2 g(x,y)/\partial x\partial y=\frac{\partial}{\partial x}\left\{\frac{\partial\{[1-2U(x)][1-2U(y)]\}}{\partial y}\right\}\\
&\downarrow\\
&\{[1-2U(x)][1-2U(y)]\}=\{1-2U(y)-2U(x)+U(x)U(y)\}\\
&\downarrow\\
&\partial\{1-2U(y)-2U(x)+4U(x)U(y)\}/\partial y=-2\delta(y)+4U(x)\delta(y)\\
&\downarrow\\
&\partial^2 g(x,y)/\partial x\partial y=\partial\{-2\delta(y)+4U(x)\delta(y)\}/\partial x=4\delta(x)\delta(y)
\end{aligned} \tag{8.94}$$

Thus, Equation 8.93 can be written:

$$\frac{\partial E\{z\}}{\partial\rho}=\int_{-\infty}^{\infty}\int_{-\infty}^{\infty} f_{xy}(x,y)[4\delta(x)\delta(y)]dxdy=4f_{xy}(0,0) \tag{8.95}$$

Now the bivariate Gaussian in RVs x and y with zero means is written:

$$\begin{aligned}
f_{xy}(x,y)=\frac{1}{2\pi\sigma_x\sigma_y\sqrt{1-r^2}}\exp\Bigg\{&-1/2\frac{1}{\sqrt{1-r^2}}[x^2/\sigma_x^2+y^2/\sigma_y^2\\
&-2rxy/(\sigma_x\sigma_y)]\Bigg\}
\end{aligned} \tag{8.96}$$

So,

$$f_{xy}(0,0)=1/[2\pi\sigma_x\sigma_y\sqrt{1-r^2}] \tag{8.97}$$

Now we let $y=x(t-\tau)$, and assume $\sigma_y=\sigma_x$ because x is a stationary RP. By definition,

$$\rho=\sigma_x\sigma_y r=\sigma_x^2 r \tag{8.98}$$

r is the *correlation coefficient* of x and y, in this case, of x and $x(t-\tau)$, hence $r=\phi_{xx}(\tau)/\sigma_x^2$.
Returning to Price's theorem, we can write:

$$\frac{\partial E\{z\}}{\partial\rho}=\frac{4}{2\pi\sigma_x\sigma_y\sqrt{1-r^2}}\rightarrow\frac{\partial E\{z\}}{\sigma_x^2 dr}=\frac{4}{2\pi\sigma_x^2\sqrt{1-r^2}} \tag{8.99}$$

Integrating both sides of Equation 8.99, we find:

$$E\{z\}=(2/\pi)\sin^{-1}(r)=(2/\pi)\sin^{-1}[\phi_{xx}(\tau)/\sigma_x^2]+k \tag{8.100}$$

By letting $\tau\rightarrow\infty$, $r\rightarrow 0$, it easy to show that the constant of integration, $k\rightarrow 0$.

To recover the desired autocorrelation function, we note that $E\{z\}$ is approximated by the output of the low-pass filter, w, in Figure 8.5. If we multiply w by $(\pi/2)$, and then pass this signal through a sin(u) nonlinearity, we recover an output proportional to the autocorrelation of the input signal, $\phi_{xx}(\tau)$.

8.2.10 Quantization Noise

In this section, we describe a little-appreciated but often important source of noise in signals that are periodically sampled and converted to numerical form by an analog-to-digital converter (ADC). The numerical samples can then be digitally filtered and then returned to analog form, $y(t)$, by a digital-to-analog converter (DAC). Such signals include modern digital audio, video and images. This noise created by converting from analog to digital form is called *quantization noise* (QN) and it is associated with the fact that when a noise-free analog signal, $x(t)$, (which has almost infinite resolution) is sampled and digitized, each $x^*(nT)$ is described by a binary number of finite length, introducing an uncertainty between the original $x(nT)$ and $x^*(nT)$. This uncertainty is the quantization noise, which can be considered to be added to either $y(t)$ or $x(t)$. (See the paper by Kollár (1986) for a comprehensive review of quantization noise. Chapter 14 in the text by Phillips and Nagle (1984) also has a rigorous mathematical treatment of QN.)

When a Nyquist band-limited analog signal is sampled and then converted by an N bit ADC to digital form, there is a statistical uncertainty in the digital signal amplitude that can be considered to be equivalent to a broadband *quantization noise* added to the analog signal input before sampling. In the quantization error-generating model of Figure 8.6, a noise-free Nyquist- limited analog signal, $x(t)$, is sampled and digitized by an *N-bit ADC of the round-off type.* The ADC's numerical output, $x^*(nT)$, is the input to an N-bit digital-to-analog converter (DAC). The *quantization error,* $e(n)$, is defined *at sampling instants* as the difference between the sampled analog input signal, $x(nT)$ and the DAC output, $y(nT)$. (Henceforth, we will use the shorter notation, $x(n)$, $y(n)$, etc.) The ADC/DAC channel has unity gain. Thus, the quantization error is simply:

$$e(n) = x(n) - y(n). \tag{8.101}$$

Figure 8.7 illustrates a nonlinear rounding quantizer function relating sampler output, $x(n)$, to the binary DAC output, $x^*(n)$. In this example, $N = 3$. (This uniform rounding quantizer has (2^N) levels and $(2^N - 1)$ steps.) When $y(n)$ is compared with the direct path, the error, $e(n)$, can range over $\pm q/2$, where q is the voltage step size of the ADC/DAC. It is easy to see that, for full dynamic range, q should be:

$$q = \frac{V_{MAX}}{(2^N - 1)} \text{ volts} \tag{8.102}$$

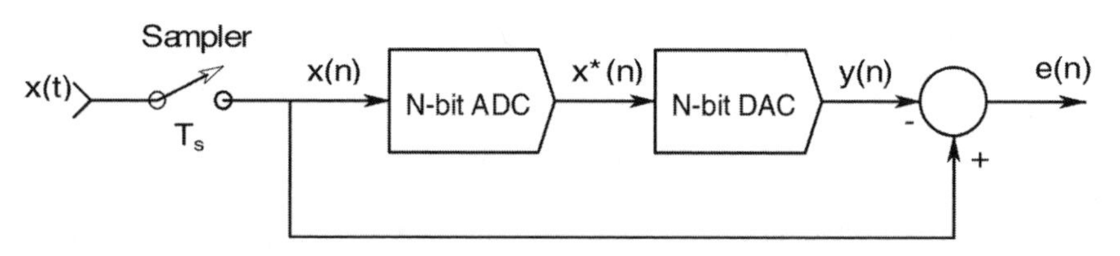

FIGURE 8.6
A quantization error generating model. See text for description.

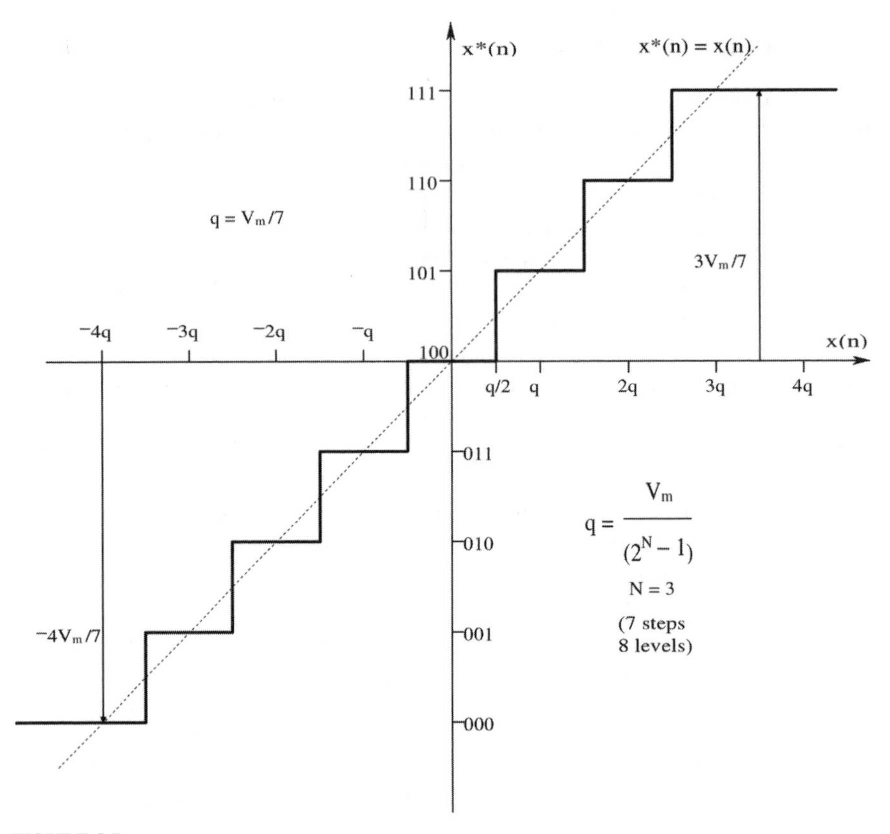

FIGURE 8.7
Transfer nonlinearity of an 8-bit rounding quantizer.

where V_{MAX} is the expected maximum (peak-to-peak) value of the input, $x(t)$, to the ADC/DAC system. For example, if a 10 bit ADC is used to convert a signal ranging from -5 to $+5$ V, then, by Equation 8.102, $q = 9.775$ mV. If $x(t)$ has *zero mean* and its probability density function (PDF) has a standard deviation $\sigma_x > q$, then it can be shown that the PDF of $e(n)$ is well modeled by a uniform (rectangular) density, $f_e(e)$ over $e = \pm q/2$. This rectangular PDF is shown in Figure 8.8; it has a peak height of $1/q$. The mean-squared error voltage is found from the expectation:

$$E\{e^2\} = \overline{e^2} = \int_{-\infty}^{\infty} e^2 f_e(e) de = \int_{-q/2}^{q/2} e^2 (1/q) de = \left.\frac{(1/q)e^3}{3}\right|_{-q/2}^{q/2}$$

$$= \frac{q^2}{12} = \sigma_q^2 \text{ msecV} \qquad (8.103)$$

Thus, it is possible to treat quantization error noise as a zero-mean broad-band noise with a standard deviation of $\sigma_q = q/\sqrt{12}$ volts, added to the ADC/DAC input signal, $x(t)$.

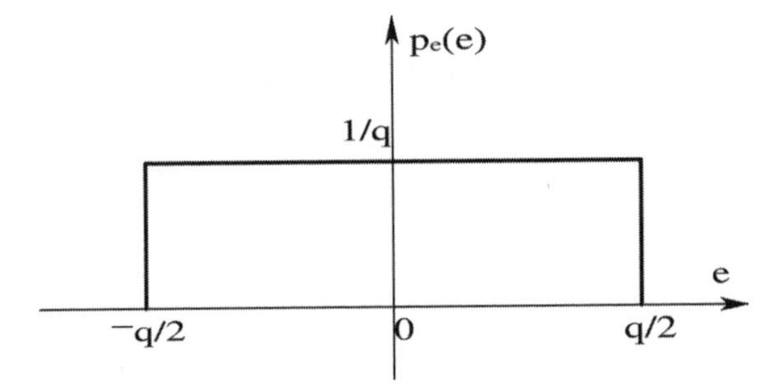

FIGURE 8.8
Rectangular probability density function of the quantization error (noise) from a rounding quantizer.

To minimize the effects of quantization noise for an N-bit ADC, it is important that the analog input signal, $x(t)$, use nearly the full dynamic range of the ADC. In the case of a zero-mean time-varying signal that is Nyquist band-limited, gains and sensitivities should be chosen so that the peak expected $x(t)$ does not exceed the maximum voltage limits of the ADC.

If $x(t)$ is a SRV and has a Gaussian PDF, the dynamic range of the ADC should be about ± 3 standard deviations of the signal. Under this condition, it is possible to derive an expression for the mean-squared signal-to-noise ratio of the ADC and its quantization noise. Let the signal have an rms value σ_x volts. From Equation 8.102, we see that the quantization step size can be written:

$$q \approx \frac{6\sigma_x}{(2^N - 1)} \text{ volts,} \tag{8.104}$$

or

$$\sigma_x = q(2^N - 1)/6 \tag{8.105}$$

From which we see that $\sigma_x > q$ for $N \geq 3$. Relation 8.104 for q can be substituted into Equation 8.103 for the variance of the quantization noise. Thus, the mean-squared output noise is:

$$N_0 = \frac{q^2}{12} = \frac{36\sigma_x^2}{12(2^N - 1)} = \frac{3\sigma_x^2}{(2^N - 1)} = \sigma_q^2 \text{ msV} \tag{8.106}$$

Hence, the mean-squared signal-to-noise ratio of the N-bit rounding quantizer is:

$$\text{SNR}_q = (2^N - 1)/3 \text{ msV/msV} \tag{8.107}$$

Note that the quantizer SNR is independent of σ_x as long as σ_x is held constant under the dynamic range constraint described above. In dB, $\text{SNR}_q = 10\log[(2^N - 1)/3]$. Table 8.2.9.1 below summarizes the SNR_q of the quantizer for different bit values. Sixteen- to 20-bit ADCs are routinely used in modern digital audio systems because

TABLE 8.2.9.1
SNR Values for an N-bit ADC Treated as a Quantizer

N	dB SNR_q
6	31.2
8	43.4
10	55.4
12	67.5
14	79.5
16	91.6

Total input range is assumed to be $6\sigma_x$ volts. Note that about 6 dB of SNR improvement occurs for every bit added to the ADC word length.

of their low quantization noise. Other classes of input signals to uniform quantizers, such as sine waves, triangle waves and narrow-band Gaussian noise are discussed by Kollár (1986).

Figure 8.9 illustrates the model whereby the equivalent QN is added to the ideal sampled signal at the input to some digital filter, H(z). Note that the quantization error sequence, $e(n)$, is assumed to be from a wide-sense stationary white-noise process, where each sample, $e(n)$, is uniformly distributed over the quantization error. The error sequence is also assumed to be uncorrelated with the corresponding input sequence, $x(n)$. Furthermore, the input sequence is assumed to be a sample sequence of a stationary random process, $\{\mathbf{x}\}$. Note that $e(n)$ is treated as *white sampled noise* (as opposed to sampled white noise). The auto-power density spectrum of $\mathbf{e}(n)$ is assumed to be flat (constant) over the Nyquist range: $-\pi/T \le \omega \le \pi/T$ r/sec. (T is the sampling period.) $\mathbf{e}(n)$ propagates through the digital filter; in the time domain this can be written as a real, discrete convolution:

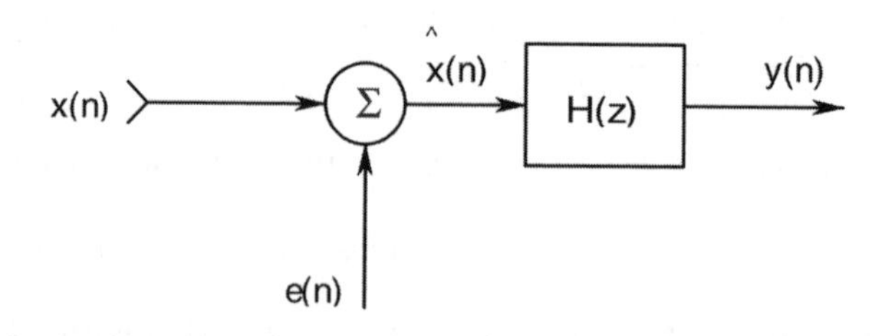

FIGURE 8.9
Block diagram showing how quantization noise, $e(n)$, is added to a noise-free digital signal, $x(n)$, which has been digitized by a sampling ADC with a rounding quantizer. The signal plus quantization noise is then filtered by an LTI discrete filter, $H(z)$.

$$\mathbf{y}(n) = \sum_{m=-\infty}^{\infty} \mathbf{e}(m)h(n-m) \quad (8.108)$$

The sampled auto-power spectrum at the output of the digital filter can be shown to be written as (letting $z \equiv e^{sT} = e^{j\omega T}$):

$$\Phi_{yy}(e^{j\omega T}) = \sigma_q^2 |\mathbf{H}(j\omega T)|^2 \quad (8.109)$$

Where σ_q^2 is the variance of the white quantization noise, and the variance of the filter's output noise can be expressed as:

$$\sigma_y^2 = R_{yy}(0) = \frac{\sigma_q^2 T^2}{2\pi} \int_{-\pi/T}^{\pi/T} |\mathbf{H}(j\omega T)|^2 d\omega, \quad \omega_N = \pi/T \quad (8.110)$$

(The integral needs to be evaluated only over the Nyquist interval because the input white QN spectrum is defined over that interval.) The integral evaluating σ_y^2 can also be written as a *contour integral* in z [Ragazzini and Franklin, 1958]:

$$\sigma_y^2 = \frac{\sigma_q^2}{2\pi j} \int_{\mathbf{C}} H(z)H(-z)z^{-1}dz \quad (8.111)$$

The CCW contour **C** encloses the poles inside the unit circle in the z-plane. As shown in Section 8.2.7, the variance of the noise output of the filter can also be written:

$$\sigma_y^2 = \sigma_q^2 \sum_{k=0}^{\infty} h^2(k) \quad (8.112)$$

8.2.11 Introduction to "data scrubbing" by nonlinear discrete filtering

Just as there are many types and designs for *linear discrete filters,* the design of *nonlinear discrete filters* (NDFs) is currently a large and evolving area of work in DSP that has a direct impact on biomedical signals. This section will introduce a class of useful easily implemented NDFs that have wide application in biomedical signal processing including medical imaging.

This section will focus (pun intended) on the design of *nonlinear filters* used to "scrub" or "clean" anomalous data outliers from one- and two-dimensional discrete signals such as telemetered EEG records and PET images, respectively. Why use a nonlinear filter instead of a linear low-pass filter? The answer is simple: the NDF permits the *impulse noise* (or *outliers*) to be selectively removed without significantly altering the normal waveform of the signal. A linear discrete low-pass filter (LPF) will attenuate the outliers but not remove them; it will also attenuate the high-frequency components of the signal. For example, the QRS complex of the ECG will be attenuated, rounded and broadened by an LPF.

We assume that, prior to sampling, the analog signal, $s(t)$, plus broadband noise, $n(t)$, is passed through an anti-aliasing LPF. The outlier noise we wish to remove can be characterized by randomly occurring *pulses* (of either polarity), $p(k)$, added to the sampled signal plus noise. The resulting 1-D sequence plus impulse noise can be written as:

$$x(k) = s(k) + n(k) + p(k), \quad 0 \le k \le N-1 \tag{8.113}$$

$p(k)$ is infrequently nonzero; its occurrence times might be governed by a Poisson process similar to radioactive decay. $|p(k)|$ is generally significantly larger than $|\overline{x_R}|$ or $|M_R|$. M_R denotes the *median* value of a set of R adjacent $x(k)$ values. R can be odd or even, although, as you will see, odd is preferred (R might be 5, 7, 9, 11, etc.). The choice of R is situation-dependent and might even be called "arty" [Pearson, 2002].

The median, $M_R(j)$ is defined as the center value of a set of R *sorted* $x(k)$ values lying in a rectangular window. For example, $M_7(j)$ is the median value of the set of $R = 7$ **x**-values: $[x(j-3), x(j-2), x(j-1), x(j), x(j+1), x(j+2), x(j+3)]$. That is, $M_7(j)$ is defined in the center of the R-window but is not necessarily the value of $x(j)$. The 7 x-values in the R-window *must be sorted for size*; we put the smallest value in the $(j-3)$ position and the largest in the $(j+3)$ position. The x-value in the center (j) position is, by definition, the median value of the set, $M_7(j)$. The R-window is then advanced one k value, and the process is repeated, etc., generating a total of N values of $M_7(j)$. Ah, you say, what happens at the ends of the x data set? If $j = k = 0$, for example, using the $R = 7$ window, we can replace the undefined $x(-3), x(-2)$ and $x(-1)$ values, each with the mean value of the four values: $x(0), x(1), x(2)$ and $x(3)$. Also, cubic splines can be used to estimate values for $x(-3), x(-2)$ and $x(-1)$, which can then be used to estimate $M_7(j)$ for $j = 0$, $j = 1$, $j = 2$ and $j = 3$, as well as $j = N-1$, $j = N-2$, $j = N-3$, and $j = N-4$ [Northrop, 1997].

Pearson (2002) describes an NDF called the *Hempel filter* for data scrubbing. This NDF uses the median value of data in a sliding window of width R to determine if a data point, $x(j)$, in the center of the window is indeed anomalous data and should be edited out. The *Hempel filter* belongs to the class of *scale-invariant filters*. This means that if we rescale the data sequence $\{x(k)\}$ to $\{mx(k) + b\}$, we do not alter the decision criterion for this filter; it still operates normally to remove any scaled outliers. The nonlinear Hempel filter does not obey superposition, however.

The Hempel filtering process can be described by the following steps:

1. Choose a moving window size, for example, let the window contain $R = 7$ samples. That is, the windowed data vector is: $\mathbf{w}(j) = [x(j-3), x(j-2), x(j-1), x(j), x(j+1), x(j+2), x(j+3)]$. (Let $j \ge k = (R-1)/2 = 3$, or let $j \le [N-(R-1)/2] = N-3$, so there will be no "end effects" to concern us in this description.)

2. Find the median value of the window vector sequence, $\mathbf{w}(j)$. This is best illustrated by an example: First, let the jth window vector have the values: $\mathbf{w}(j) = [-1.1, 0, 0.5, 2.2, 3.0, 1.2, -0.3]$. Next, order the samples to be in

ascending order: [−1.1, −0.3, 0, 0.5, 1.2, 2.2, 3.0]. By definition, the median value is in the center of the ascending ordered vector; $M_7(j)=0.5$ in this example.

3. The next step in implementing the Hempel filter is to form the *median absolute deviation* (MAD) array vector, $\mathbf{d}(j)$:

$$\begin{aligned}\mathbf{d}(j) \equiv [&|x(j-3)-M_7(j)|, |x(j-2)-M_7(j)|, |x(j-1)-M_7(j)|, \\ &|x(j)-M_7(j)|, |x(j+1)-M_7(j)|, |x(j+2)-M_7(j)|, \\ &|x(j+3)-M_7(j)|] \end{aligned} \tag{8.114}$$

Again, using our numerical example:

$$\begin{aligned}\mathbf{d}(j) = [&|-1.1-0.5|, |0-0.5|, |0.5-0.5|, \\ &|2.2-0.5|, |3.0-0.5|, |1.2-0.5|, |-0.3-0.5|] \\ &\downarrow \\ \mathbf{d}(j) = [&1.6, 0.5, 0, 1.7, 2.5, 0.7, 0.8] \end{aligned} \tag{8.115}$$

4. Now, we find the median of $\mathbf{d}(j)$ by ordering its values: $[0, 0.5, 0.7, \underline{0.8}, 1.6, 1.7, 2.5]$. The median, 0.8, is a measure of how far $x(j)$ typically lies from $M_7(j)$. The *MAD scale estimate* is defined as $Q \equiv 1.4826$ X the median of $\mathbf{d}(j)$ [Pearson, 2002].

5. To test for outliers, we compute $d_j = |x(j) - M_7(j)|$. If $d_j < \rho Q$, then we keep $x(j)$ in $\mathbf{w}(j)$. If $d_j \geq \rho Q$, then we replace the outlier $x(j)$ with $M_7(j)$. The parameters that "tune" the Hempel filter are the window width, R, and the threshold constant, ρ. If $\rho \to 0$, the Hempel filter reduces uniformly to the *median filter.*

In the *following example,* we illustrate the application of the Hempel filter. Refer to Figure 8.10, which illustrates noisy data which contains outliers we wish to scrub with a Hempel filter with $\rho=1$. The data window size is $R=7$ samples. In the first (left) window, it appears that $x(13)$ may be an outlier. We center the window on $j=k=13$ and write the samples in the window as the vector: $\mathbf{w}(13)=[16,16,16,19,17,16,15]$. The samples are next ordered to find the median: [15, 16, 16, 16, 16, 17, 19]. Clearly, $M_7(13)=16$. Next, calculate the absolute deviation vector: $\mathbf{d}(13)$ = [1, 0, 0, 0, 0, 1, 3]. We now order $\mathbf{d}(13)$, finding: [0, 0, 0, 0, 1, 1, 3]. Clearly, the median of $\mathbf{d}(13)$ is 0, so $Q=0$, and $d_{13} > 1Q$, so $x(13)$ is evidently an outlier, and we replace $x(13)=19$ with $M_7(13)=16$ to effect the smoothing.

In a *second example* of implementing a Hempel filter from Figure 8.10, we consider the center window shown centered on $k=j=26$. The windowed data vector is $\mathbf{w}(26)$ = [14, 12, 13, 12, 15, 16, 17]. Note that $x(26)=12, x(27)=15, x(28)=16$, etc. $\mathbf{w}(26)$ is next reordered to find $M_7(26): [12, 12, 13, \underline{14}, 15, 16, 17]$. Thus, $M_7(26)=14$. Next we form the absolute deviation vector: $\mathbf{d}(26)$ = [2, 2, 1, 0, 1, 2, 3]. $\mathbf{d}(26)$ is next

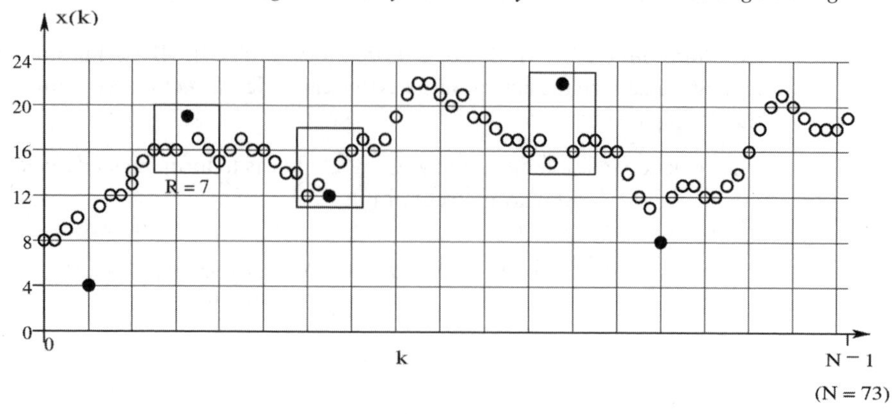

FIGURE 8.10
Example of noisy discrete data containing some outliers. The boxes delineate the surrounding data points used in the data scrubbing algorithms.

reordered to find its median: [0, 1, 1, 2, 2, 2, 3]. The Q parameter is $1.4826\times$ *median*[**d**(26)] $=1.4826\times 2=2.9652$. Now it is clear that $d_{26}=2<\rho Q=2.9652$, so we keep x(26) = 12 as a datapoint. Note that if x(26) were to equal 11, the inequality of the test would be reversed, and x(26) would be made $M_7(26)=14$ (a "seamless" smoothing).

A *second type of data scrubbing filter* is based on the *signal-dependent rank order mean* (SD-ROM) algorithm described by Chandra et al. (1998). In this NDF design, we use a sliding window of size $R=5$. The filter operates in the following steps:

1. A sample vector of size 4, *excluding the center value in the window*, x(j), is defined:

$$\mathbf{w}(j)\equiv[x(j-2),x(j-1),x(j+1),x(j+2)] \tag{8.116}$$

2. Next, the four samples in **w**(j) are sorted and arranged in ascending order:

$$\mathbf{r}(j)\equiv[r_1(j),r_2(j),r_3(j),r_4(j)],\text{ where } r_1(j)\le r_2(j)\le r_3(j)\le r_4(j) \tag{8.117}$$

3. The rank-ordered mean (ROM), $\mu(j)$ is computed from $\mathbf{r}(j)$:

$$\mu(j)\equiv[r_2(j)+r_3(j)]/2 \tag{8.118}$$

4. *The rank-ordered differences,* $d_i(j)$, are defined as:

$$d_i(j)\equiv\begin{bmatrix} r_i(j)-x(j), & \text{if } x(j)\le\mu(j) \\ x(j)-r_{4-i}(j), & \text{if } x(j)>\mu(j)\end{bmatrix} \quad i=1,2 \text{ for } R=5. \tag{8.119}$$

5. The algorithm decides that x(j) is an outlier if: $d_1(j)>\varphi_1$, *or if* $d_2(j)>\varphi_2$.

6. If an outlier is detected, x(j) (the outlier) is replaced by the ROM, $\mu(j)$, defined above. φ_1 and φ_2 are artfully chosen threshold values; Chandra et

al. (2002) used $\varphi_1 = 4, \varphi_2 = 12$ to effectively scrub an $\{x(k)\}$ characterized by 8-bit accuracy (quantization of 255 steps). These authors point out that the $R = 5$ window size gave the best output SNR (35.78 dB); $R = 7$ gave $SNR_o = 34.42$ dB and $R = 9$ gave $SNR_o = 32.77$ dB. They also point out that all data-scrubbing filters can make two types of error:

(1) An $x(j)$ that is not an outlier can be found to be one and be replaced, or

(2) an $x(j)$, which is an outlier can be treated as data and left unchanged in $\{x(k)\}$.

Let us work a numerical example of a SD-ROM filter based on the data in Figure 8.10 seen in the right-hand window centered on $k = j = 47$. The candidate flyer is $x(j) = x(47) = 22$. The w vector is: **w**(47) = [17, 15, 16, 17]. Ordering these values gives us **r**(47) = [15, 16, 17, 17]. The rank-ordered mean is thus: $\mu(47)$ = (16 + 17)/2 = 16.5. Next, we calculate the rank-ordered differences: Note that $x(47) = 22 > \mu(47) = 16.5$, so $d_1(47) = x(47) - r_3(47) = 22 - 17 = 5$, and $d_2(47) = 22 - 16 = 6$. Now $d_1(47) = 5 > \varphi_1 = 4$, and $d_2(47) = 6 < \varphi_2 = 12$. Thus because $d_1(47) > \varphi_1$, $x(47)$ is called an outlier or noise impulse, and is replaced by $\mu(47) = 16.5$.

It should be pointed out that the design of NDFs for data scrubbing is an evolving technology; we expect many designs to evolve, some using recursive methods, others having adaptive, variable thresholds based on some error or SNR criterion. Data scrubbing NDFs have been applied to cleaning 2-D, digital image data contaminated with impulse noise. The interested reader should see papers by Moore et al. (1999) for examples.

8.2.12 Discussion

Section 8.2 introduced and examined the properties of important mathematical descriptors of random noise and statistically described signals, including the meaning of the probability density function, auto- and cross-correlation functions and their CFTs and the auto- and cross-power spectral density functions. We also derived expressions describing the propagation of noise through stationary causal LTI continuous systems and also discrete systems. These expressions were found useful in identifying the LTI system's transfer function, given its random input and output.

Characteristic functions of stationary random variables were described and shown to be the CFT of the SRV's PDF with $\omega \to -\omega$. Characteristic functions were shown to be useful in describing the propagation of noise through certain types of static (algebraic) nonlinearities. Next, the uni- and bivariate forms of Price's theorem were introduced and shown to be useful in finding certain statistical descriptors of the random outputs of no-memory nonlinearities.

Section 8.2.10 introduces the concept of quantization noise (QN). QN was seen to be broadband noise ("white sampled noise") introduced into signals that undergo analog-to-digital conversion. It is the result of the rounding process inherent in converting samples of an infinite-resolution analog signal to digital words of finite word length (e.g., 10 bits).

"Data scrubbing" to remove infrequent outliers (or impulse noise) from data records was introduced in Section 8.2.11. Data scrubbing is a form of nonlinear filtering that detects the outlier data point by a statistical thresholding function applied to surrounding sample values. If the threshold is exceeded, the offending outlier is replaced by a data value calculated from adjacent data points, producing a smoothed record. Many types of biomedical signals, especially in imaging, have impulse noise amenable to scrubbing.

8.3 Calculation of Noise Descriptors with Finite Discrete Data

Once we depart from the ideal world where data records are infinite in length and integrations are carried out over infinite time and frequency, the statistical functions we calculate, such as the *sample mean,* the *sample mean-square* and the *sample variance* have a statistical uncertainty or error associated with them. The *sample mean, variance* and *mean-squared value* of the SRV, $x(t)$ are written, respectively:

$$\overline{x} = \frac{1}{N}\sum_{i=1}^{N} x_i \tag{8.120}$$

$$\widehat{\sigma}_x^2 = \frac{1}{N}\sum_{i=1}^{N} (x_i - \overline{x})^2 \tag{8.121}$$

$$\overline{x^2} = \frac{1}{N}\sum_{i=1}^{N} x_i^2 \tag{8.122}$$

The three equations above are functions of a stationary random variable, $x(t)$, and, as such, are noisy statistics. That is, there is uncertainty or noise associated with the calculation of the sample mean, $\overline{x}$, the variance, $\widehat{\sigma}_x^2$, and the mean square, $\overline{x^2}$. The variance of a statistic is a measure of its noisiness. For example, let us calculate the *variance of the sample mean;* recall that $<x>$ is the expected value (true mean) of x:

$$\begin{aligned}
\mathrm{Var}\{\overline{x}\} &= E\left\{\left[\frac{1}{N}\sum_{j=1}^{N} x_j - \langle x\rangle\right]^2\right\} = E\left\{\left[\frac{1}{N}\sum_{j=1}^{N} x_j\right]^2\right\} - \langle x\rangle^2 \\
&= E\left\{\frac{1}{N^2}\sum_{j=1}^{N}\sum_{k=1}^{N} x_j x_k\right\} - \langle x\rangle^2 \\
&= \frac{1}{N^2}\sum_{j=1}^{N}\sum_{k=1}^{N} E\{x_j x_k\} - \langle x\rangle^2
\end{aligned} \tag{8.123}$$

For the N values where $j=k$, we have, noting that the mean value of x is zero:

$$\mathrm{Var}\{\overline{x}\} = \frac{N\overline{x^2}}{N^2} = \frac{\overline{x^2}}{N} = \frac{\sigma_x^2}{N} \tag{8.124}$$

For $j \neq k$, we have $(N^2 - N)$ terms of the form: (We assume that terms with nonalike indices are uncorrelated and independent.)

$$\frac{1}{N^2}\sum_{\substack{j=1 \\ j\neq k}}^{N}\sum_{k=1}^{N} E\{x_j x_k\} - <x>^2$$

$$= \frac{1}{N^2}\sum_{\substack{j=1 \\ j\neq k}}^{N}\sum_{k=1}^{N} E\{x_j\}E\{x_k\} - <x>^2 \to 0 \tag{8.125}$$

Thus, we see that the variance of the sample mean approaches zero as $N \to \infty$.

The *autocorrelation function* of a finite number of discrete data samples can also be computed:

$$R_{xx}(m) = \frac{1}{N-m}\sum_{n=1}^{N-m} x(n)x(n+m), \quad m = 0, 1, 2, \ldots k \tag{8.126}$$

In practice, for several practical reasons, the maximum shift, m, is kept $<N/10$ [Bendat and Piersol, 1966]. For example, N might be 4096, and m could be 256. Then $R_{xx}(m)$ would have 256 data points. Note that only positive m need be considered because, ideally, $R_{xx}(m)$ is an even function.

The *cross-correlation function* for finite discrete stationary random variables can be written:

$$R_{xy}^{+}(m) = \frac{1}{N-1-m}\sum_{n=0}^{N-1-m} x(n)y(n+m), \quad m = 0, 1, 2, \ldots k \tag{8.127}$$

$$R_{yx}(m) = \frac{1}{N-m}\sum_{n=1}^{N-m} y(n)x(n+m), \quad m = 0, 1, 2, \ldots k \tag{8.128}$$

Note that $R_{yx}(m) = R_{xy}(-m)$, so the complete two-sided discrete CCF can be obtained by adding the two CCFs above. That is, $R_{xy}(m) = R_{xy}^{+}(m) + R_{yx}(|-m|)$, for discrete $-k \leq m \leq k$.

Figure 8.4 illustrates the process of discrete cross-correlation given by Equation 8.127. In practice, N samples (an epoch) of a stationary linear system's input, $x(n)$, are taken and digitized. (In the figure, for clarity, we have used deterministic transients to illustrate the cross-correlation process. In practice, the continuous input, $x(t)$, is generally a random signal, characterized by a Gaussian PDF and some APS, $\Phi_{xx}(\omega)$. An N-sample epoch of the SLS's continuous output, $y(t)$, is also taken. $x(t)$ must have been applied to the system for a long time so that the transient response of the system will have died out so $y(t)$ and $y(n)$ will be stationary random variables (SRV). In Figure 8.4a, for simplicity, I have shown transient functions for the N-sample epochs of $x(n)$ and $y(n)$. In Figure 8.4b, $x(n)$ and $y(n)$ are shown shifted to the left by m samples to form $y(n+m)$. Note that the product, $[x(n)y(n+m)]$ is defined only for the interval, $0 \leq n \leq (N-1-k)$, $m=0, 1, 2, \ldots k$. The summation of the product is computed for each m value to obtain $R_{xy}(m)$.

When the DFTs are to be taken of $R_{xx}(m)$ and $R_{xy}(m)$, we find their finite discrete autopower spectrum and cross-power spectrum, respectively, $S_{xx}(u)$ and $\mathbf{S_{xy}}(u)$. Note that the DFT, $\mathbf{S_{xy}}(u)$, is complex because, in general, $R_{yx}(m)$ lacks symmetry (is neither even nor odd in m).

8.4 Signal Averaging and Filtering for Signal-to-Noise Ratio Improvement.

8.4.1 Introduction

The *signal-to-noise ratio* (SNR) of a signal recorded with additive noise is an important figure of merit that characterizes the expected resolution of the signal. SNRs are typically given at the input to a signal conditioning system and also at its output. SNR can be expressed as a positive real number or in decibels (dB). The SNR can be calculated from the rms (or peak) signal voltage divided by the rms noise voltage, or noise standard deviation. The noise bandwidth should be specified. The SNR can also be formed from the mean-squared signal voltage divided by the mean-squared noise voltage (noise variance). If the ms SNR is computed, the $SNR_{(dB)} = 10\log_{10}$ (msSNR), otherwise it is SNR(dB) = $20\log_{10}$(rmsSNR)

Signal averaging is widely used in both experimental and clinical electrophysiology in order to extract a repetitive quasi-deterministic electrophysiological transient response buried in noise. One example of the type of signal being extracted is the evoked cortical response recorded directly from the surface of the brain (or from the scalp) by an electrode pair while the subject is given a repetitive periodic sensory stimulus, such as a tone burst or flash of light. Every time the stimulus is given, a "hard-wired", electrophysiological transient voltage, $s_j(t)$, lasting several hundred msec. is produced in the brain. When viewed directly on an oscilloscope or recorder, each individual evoked cortical response can be invisible to the eye because of the accompanying noise.

Signal averaging is generally used to extract the evoked potential, $s(t)$, from the noise accompanying it. Signal averaging is also used to extract evoked cortical magnetic field transients recorded with SQUID sensors [Northrop, 2002], and to extract *multifocal ERG signals* obtained when testing the competence of macular cones in the retina of the eye. A small spot of light illuminating only a few cones is repetitively flashed on the macular retina. ERG averaging is done over N flashes for a given spot position to extract the local ERG flash response, then the spot is moved to a new known position on the macula, and the process is repeated until the 2-D macular ERG response of one eye is mapped [Northrop, 2002].

Signal averaging is *ensemble averaging;* following each identical periodic stimulus, the response can be written for the jth stimulus:

$$x_j(t) = s_j(t) + n_j(t), \quad 0 \le j \le N \tag{8.129}$$

where $s_j(t)$ is the jth evoked transient response, and $n_j(t)$ is the jth noise following the stimulus. t is the local time origin taken as 0 when the jth stimulus is given. The noise is assumed to be, in general, non-stationary, i.e., its statistics are affected by the stimulus. We assume that the noise has zero mean, however, regardless of time following any stimulus. That is, $E\{n(t)\} = 0, 0 \le t < T_i$. T_i is the inter stimulus interval. Also, to be general, we assume that the evoked response varies from stimulus to stimulus. That is, $s_j(t)$ is not exactly the same as $s_{j+1}(t)$, etc.

We assume that each $x_j(t)$ is sampled and digitized beginning with each stimulus; the sampling period is T_s, and M samples are taken following each stimulus. Thus, there are N sets of sampled $x_j(k)$, $0 \le k \le (M-1)$, also, $(M-1)T_s = T_D < T_i$. T_D is the total length of analog $x_j(t)$ digitized following each input stimulus (epoch length).

When the jth stimulus is given, the $x(k)^{th}$ value is summed in the kth data register with the preceding x(k) values. At the end of an experimental run, we have $[x_1(k) + x_2(k) + x_3(k) + \cdots + x_N(k)]$ in the kth data register. Figure 8.11 illustrates the organization of a signal averager. Early signal averagers were stand-alone dedicated instruments. Modern signal averagers typically use a PC or laptop computer with a dual-channel A/D interface to handle the trigger event that initiates sampling and the evoked transient plus noise, $x_j(t) = s_j(t) + n_j(t)$. Modern averagers give a running display in which the main register contents are continually divided by the running j value as j goes from 1 to N.

8.4.2 Analysis of SNR improvement by averaging

The average contents of the kth register after N epochs are sampled can be written formally:

$$\overline{x(k)}_N = \frac{1}{N}\sum_{j=1}^{N} s_j(k) + \frac{1}{N}\sum_{j=1}^{N} n_j(k), \quad 0 \le k \le (M-1) \tag{8.130}$$

Where the left-hand summation is the *signal sample mean* at $t = kT_s$ after N stimuli and the right-hand summation is the *noise sample mean* at $t = kT_s$ after N stimuli. We have shown above that the *variance of the sample mean* is a statistical measure of its noisiness. In general, the larger N is, the smaller the noise variance will be. The variance of the sample mean of x(k) is written as:

$$\mathrm{Var}\{\overline{x(k)}_N\} = E\left\{\left[\frac{1}{N}\sum_{j=1}^{N} x_j(k)\right]^2\right\} - \langle x(k)\rangle^2$$

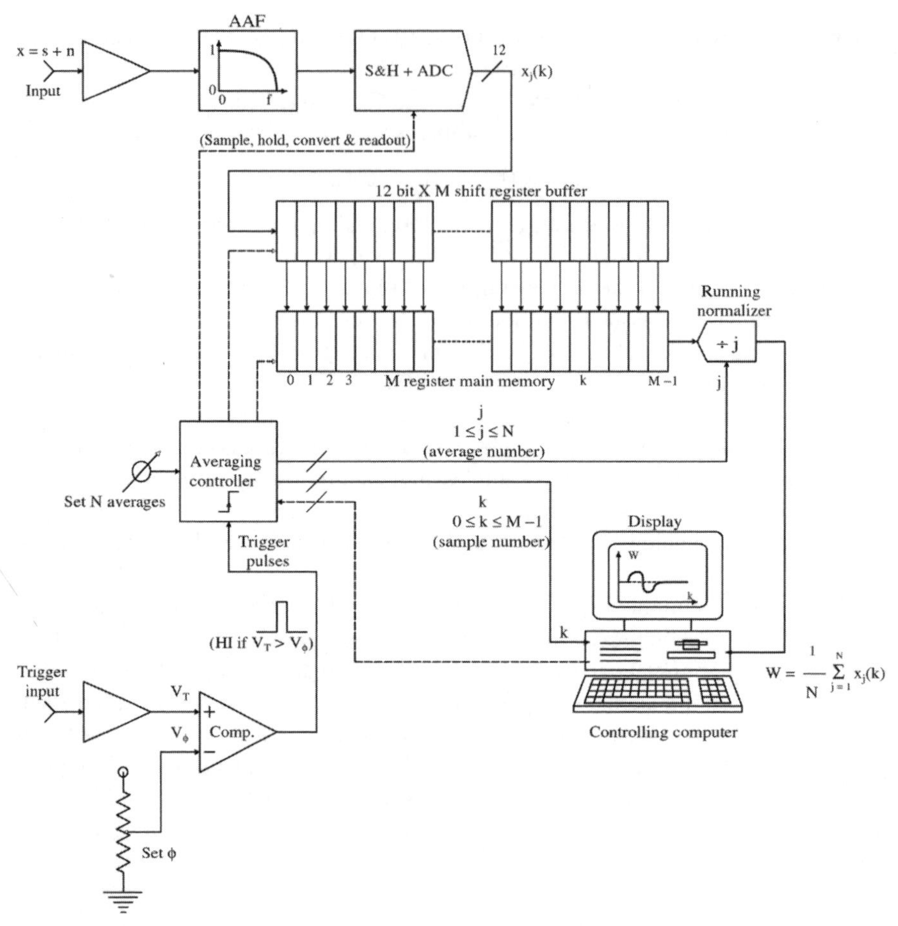

FIGURE 8.11
Block diagram of a signal averager. Note that all of the signal operations can be incorporated in a plug-in multifunction A/D–D/A card plus computer software.

$$\downarrow$$

$$\text{Var}\{\overline{x(k)}_N\} = E\left\{\left[\frac{1}{N}\sum_{j=1}^{N} x_j(k)\right]\left[\frac{1}{N}\sum_{i=1}^{N} x_i(k)\right]\right\} - <x(k)>^2$$

$$\downarrow$$

$$\text{Var}\{\overline{x(k)}_N\} = \frac{1}{N^2}\sum_{j=1}^{N}\sum_{i=1}^{N} E\{x_j(k)x_i(k)\} - <x(k)>^2$$

$$\downarrow$$

$$\text{Var}\{\overline{x(k)}_N\} = \underbrace{\frac{1}{N^2}\sum_{j=1}^{N} E\{x_j^2(k)\}}_{(N \text{ terms, } j=i)} + \underbrace{\frac{1}{N^2}\sum_{\substack{j=1 \\ j\neq 1}}^{N}\sum_{i=1}^{N} E\{x_j(k)x_i(k)\}}_{(N^2 - N \text{ terms})} - <x(k)>^2 \quad (8.131)$$

Now for the N squared terms:

$$\begin{aligned} E\{x_j^2(k)\} &= E\{[s_j(k)+n_j(k)]^2\} \\ &= E\{s_j^2(k)\}+2E\{s_j(k)\}E\{n_j(k)\}+E\{n_j^2(k)\} \\ &= \sigma_s^2(k)+<s(k)>^2+\sigma_n^2(k) \end{aligned} \tag{8.132}$$

For the (N^2-N) terms with unlike indices:

$$\begin{aligned} E\{x_j(k)x_i(k)\} &= E\{[s_j(k)+n_j(k)][s_i(k)+n_i(k)]\} \\ &= E\{s_j(k)s_i(k)\}+E\{n_j(k)n_i(k)\} \\ &\quad +E\{s_j(k)n_i(k)+s_i(k)n_j(k)\} \end{aligned} \tag{8.133}$$

Several important assumptions are generally applied to Equation 8.133: First, noise and signal are uncorrelated and statistically independent. This means that $E\{sn\} = E\{s\}E\{n\} = E\{s\}0 = 0$. Also, we assume that noise samples taken at or more than $t = T$ seconds apart will be uncorrelated; these assumptions lead to $E\{n_j(k)n_i(k)\} = E\{n_j(k)\}E\{n_i(k)\} \to 0$. So, $E\{x_j(k)x_i(k)\} = E\{s_j(k)s_i(k)\}$. We also assume that $s_j(k)$ and $s_i(k)$ taken at or more than T seconds apart are independent. So finally:

$$E\{x_j(k)x_i(k)\} = E\{[s_j(k)s_i(k)]\} = E\{s_j(k)\}E\{s_i(k)\} = \overline{s(k)}^2 \tag{8.134}$$

Now, putting all the terms together:

$$\begin{aligned} &\mathrm{Var}\{\overline{x(k)}_N\} = \frac{1}{N^2}\{N[\sigma_s^2(k)+\overline{s(k)}^2+\sigma_n^2(k)]+(N^2-N)\overline{s(k)}^2\}-\overline{s(k)}^2 \\ &\downarrow \\ &\mathrm{Var}\{\overline{x(k)}_N\} = \frac{\sigma_s^2(k)+\sigma_n^2(k)}{N} \end{aligned} \tag{8.135}$$

The variance of the sample mean for the kth sample following a stimulus is a measure of the noisiness of the averaging process. The variance of the averaged signal, x, is seen to decrease as $1/N$, where N is the total number of stimuli given and of responses averaged.

Another measure of the effectiveness of signal averaging is the *noise factor*, $F \equiv \frac{S_{in}/N_{in}}{S_O/N_O}$ where S_{in} is the *mean-squared input signal* to the averaging process, N_{in} is the *ms input noise*, S_o is the *ms output signal*, and N_o is the *ms output noise*. The noise factor is normally used as a figure of merit for amplifiers; amplifiers generally add noise to the input signal and noise, so the output signal-to-noise ratio (SNR) is less than the input SNR, so for a nonideal amplifier, $F > 1$. For an ideal, noiseless amplifier, $F = 1$. The exception to this behavior is in signal averaging, where the averaging process generally produces an output SNR > the input SNR, making $F < 1$. Note that the *noise figure* of a signal conditioning system is defined as:

$$NF \equiv 10\log_{10}(F) \text{ dB} \tag{8.136}$$

From the calculations above on the averaging process:

$$S_{in}(k) = E\{s_j^2(k)\} = \sigma_s^2(k) + \overline{s(k)}^2 \tag{8.137}$$

$$N_{in}(k) = E\{n_j^2(k)\} = \sigma_n^2(k) \tag{8.138}$$

$$S_o(k) = E\{s_o^2(k)\} = \frac{\sigma_s^2(k)}{N} + \overline{s(k)}^2 \tag{8.139}$$

$$N_o(k) = \frac{\sigma_n^2(k) + \sigma_s^2(k)}{N} \tag{8.140}$$

These terms can be put together to calculate the noise factor of the averaging process:

$$F = \frac{[\sigma_s^2(k) + \overline{s(k)}^2][1 + \sigma_s^2(k)/\sigma_n^2(k)]}{[\sigma_s^2(k) + N\overline{s(k)}^2]} \tag{8.141}$$

Note that if the evoked transient is exactly the same for each stimulus, $\sigma_s^2(k) \to 0$, and $F = 1/N$.

The reader should appreciate that this is an idealized situation; in practice, a constant level of noise, σ_a^2, is present on the output of the signal averager. This noise comes from the signal conditioning amplifiers, the quantization accompanying analog-to-digital conversion, and arithmetic round-off. The averager ms output noise can thus be written:

$$N_o = \frac{\sigma_n^2(k) + \sigma_s^2(k)}{N} + \sigma_a^2 \quad \text{mean-squared volts} \tag{8.142}$$

And as before, the ms signal is:

$$S_o(k) = \frac{\sigma_s^2(k)}{N} + \overline{s(k)}^2 \tag{8.143}$$

The averager ms output SNR is just:

$$SNR_o = \frac{\sigma_s^2(k) + N\overline{s(k)}^2}{\sigma_s^2(k) + \sigma_n^2(k) + N\sigma_a^2} \tag{8.144}$$

And if the evoked response is deterministic, $\sigma_s^2(k) \to 0$, and we have:

$$SNR_o \to \frac{N\overline{s(k)}^2}{\sigma_n^2(k) + N\sigma_a^2} \tag{8.145}$$

Note that if the number, N, of stimuli and responses averaged becomes very large, then

$$SNR_o \to \frac{\overline{s(k)}^2}{\sigma_a^2} \tag{8.146}$$

and also in the limit,

$$F \to \frac{\sigma_a^2}{\sigma_n^2(k)} \tag{8.147}$$

Signal averaging can recover a good estimate of $s(k)$ even when $\sigma_n(k)$ is 60 dB larger than $s(k)$. From Equation 8.145, we can find the N required to give a specified SNR_o, given $\sigma_n^2(k)$, σ_a^2 and $\overline{s(k)}^2$.

8.4.3 Introduction to signal-to-noise ratio improvement by linear filtering

In the previous section, we have seen how a periodically evoked (nonstationary) transient signal with a poor SNR (e.g., −40 dB) can be averaged to improve the SNR of the evoked transient. The price we pay for this SNR improvement is the time it takes to do the averaging of many experimental trials. In this section, we will introduce other means whereby the SNR of a *continuous, noisy signal* can be improved by linear filtering. The filter can be continuous (analog) or discrete (digital). Filtering the input signal plus stationary noise with an LTI bandpass filter can often give an output signal with an improved SNR when the passbands of the signal and noise do not completely coincide.

For a *first example,* consider the case where the input signal is a pure sine wave,

$$v_s(t) = V_s \sin(\omega_o t) \tag{8.148}$$

to which ideal *white* Gaussian noise is added. The white noise is characterized by a constant *two-sided* APS:

$$\Phi_{nn}(\omega) = \eta \text{ msV/r/sec} \tag{8.149}$$

In this example, signal plus noise is to be filtered by a simple analog real-pole LTI low-pass filter with the simple frequency response function, b

$$\mathbf{H}(j\omega) = \frac{b}{b + j\omega} \tag{8.150}$$

From ac circuit theory, the peak amplitude of the *output signal* sine wave is easily shown to be:

$$V_{so} = \frac{V_s b}{\sqrt{b^2 + \omega_o^2}} \tag{8.151}$$

The mean-squared output signal from the filter is one-half the peak value squared:

$$E\{v_{so}^2\} = \frac{(V_s^2/2)b^2}{b^2 + \omega_o^2} \tag{8.152}$$

It was shown above that:

$$\Phi_{no}(\omega) = \Phi_{nn}(\omega)|\mathbf{H}(j\omega)|^2 \tag{8.153}$$

The mean squared noise output from the filter is $\varphi_{no}(0) = \sigma_{no}^2$, found by taking the IFT of the two-sided noise output PDS, $\Phi_{no}(\omega)$, with $\tau \to 0$.

$$\begin{aligned}
\sigma_{no}^2 &= \frac{1}{2\pi}\int_{-\infty}^{\infty} \Phi_{nn}(\omega)|\mathbf{H}(j\omega)|^2 d\omega \\
&= \frac{2}{2\pi}\int_0^{\infty} \eta \frac{b^2}{b^2+\omega^2} d\omega \\
&= \frac{\eta b}{2\pi} 2(\pi/2) = \eta b/2 \text{ msv}
\end{aligned} \tag{8.154}$$

The ms SNR at the filter output is thus:

$$\text{SNR}_0 = \frac{\frac{(V_s^2/2)b^2}{b^2+\omega_o^2}}{\eta b/2} = \frac{V_s^2}{\eta}\frac{b}{b^2+\omega_o^2} = \frac{V_s^2}{\eta}\frac{1}{b+\omega_o^2/b} \tag{8.155}$$

Fortunately, in this case, a filter break frequency, b_{opt} r/sec, exists that will maximize SNR_o. The b that maximizes SNR_o also minimizes the denominator of the last term in Equation 8.155. This value is simply found by differentiation:

$$\frac{d[b+\omega_o^2/b]}{db} = 1 - \omega_o^2/b^2 = 0 \tag{8.156}$$

Thus, for SNR_{omax}, $b_{opt} = \omega_o$ r/sec, and

$$\text{SNR}_{omax} = \frac{V_s^2}{\eta 2\omega_o} \tag{8.157}$$

For a *second example,* we will again find the ms output SNR of an analog filter having an input of signal plus noise. Assume the input signal (or information) is an SRP describable by the two-sided PDS:

$$\Phi_{ss}(\omega) = \frac{\sigma_s^2 2\alpha}{\alpha^2+\omega^2} \text{ msV/r/sec} \tag{8.158}$$

The noise again will be white with two-sided PDS:

$$\Phi_{nn}(\omega) = \eta \text{ msV/r/sec} \tag{8.159}$$

The filter is an LTI real-pole low-pass filter with unity dc gain:

$$\mathbf{H}(j\omega) = \frac{\omega_o}{\omega_o + j\omega} \tag{8.160}$$

We will assume the signal and noise have zero means and are uncorrelated and statistically independent. Thus the input cross-power spectrum, $\Phi_{sn}(\omega) = 0$. The signal autopower spectrum at the output is:

$$\mathbf{\Phi}_{soso}(\omega) = \frac{\omega_o^2}{\omega_o^2+\omega^2}\frac{\sigma_s^2 2\alpha}{\alpha^2+\omega^2} \text{ msV/r/sec} \tag{8.161}$$

and the output noise autopower spectrum is:

$$\Phi_{\mathrm{nono}}(\omega)=\frac{\eta\omega_{\mathrm{o}}^2}{\omega_{\mathrm{o}}^2+\omega^2}\ \mathrm{msV/r/s} \tag{8.162}$$

We use the IFT to find the output mean-squared noise voltage, $R_{\mathrm{nono}}(0)=\sigma_{\mathrm{no}}^2$:

$$\sigma_{\mathrm{no}}^2=\frac{1}{2\pi}=2\int_0^\infty\frac{\eta\omega_{\mathrm{o}}\omega_{\mathrm{o}}}{\omega_{\mathrm{o}}^2+\omega^2}\mathrm{d}\omega=\frac{2\eta\omega_{\mathrm{o}}}{2\pi}(\pi/2)=\eta\omega_{\mathrm{o}}/2\ \mathrm{msV} \tag{8.163}$$

The above result comes from the fact that $\Phi_{\mathrm{nono}}(\omega)$ is even in ω; thus:

$$\int_{-\infty}^{\infty}\Phi_{\mathrm{nono}}(\omega)\mathrm{d}\omega=2\int_0^\infty\Phi_{\mathrm{nono}}(\omega)\mathrm{d}\omega, \tag{8.164}$$

and

$$\int_0^\infty\frac{\mathrm{a}}{\mathrm{a}^2+\mathrm{x}^2}\mathrm{dx}\equiv\pi/2,\quad \text{for a}>0. \tag{8.165}$$

The ms signal output is found similarly:

$$\begin{aligned}\sigma_{\mathrm{s}}^2&=\frac{2}{2\pi}\int_0^\infty\frac{\omega_{\mathrm{o}}^2}{(\omega_{\mathrm{o}}^2+\omega^2)}\frac{\sigma_{\mathrm{s}}^2 2\alpha}{(\alpha^2+\omega^2)}\mathrm{d}\omega=\frac{4\omega_{\mathrm{o}}^2\sigma_{\mathrm{s}}^2\alpha}{2\pi}\frac{\pi}{2\omega_{\mathrm{o}}\alpha(\alpha+\omega_{\mathrm{o}})}\\&=\sigma_{\mathrm{s}}^2\omega_{\mathrm{o}}/(\alpha+\omega_{\mathrm{o}})\ \mathrm{msV}\end{aligned} \tag{8.166}$$

Finally, the output ms SNR can be written:

$$\mathrm{SNR}_{\mathrm{out}}=\frac{\sigma_{\mathrm{s}}^2\omega_{\mathrm{o}}/(\alpha+\omega_{\mathrm{o}})}{\eta\omega_{\mathrm{o}}/2}=\frac{2\sigma_{\mathrm{s}}^2}{\eta(\alpha+\omega_{\mathrm{o}})} \tag{8.167}$$

As might be expected, reducing the filter's break frequency, ω_{o}, increases $\mathrm{SNR}_{\mathrm{out}}$ monotonically; however, there is no optimum break frequency in this case.

In the 1950s and '60s, much attention was given to finding the transfer function of the optimum LTI filter that minimizes the mean-squared error, $\mathrm{E}\{\mathrm{e}^2(\mathrm{t})\}$, defined by the model shown in Figure 8.12. Lee (1960) gives an exhaustive treatment of the complex derivation of the so-called *Wiener optimum filter,* found by solution of the Wiener-Hopf equation for Gaussian signals and noise described by power density spectra. We will not attempt to describe this complex derivation. The results are deceptively simple to write, however. For stationary **s**(t) and **n**(t) that are uncorrelated, Papoulis (1965) shows that the optimum filter frequency response can be written in terms of their power spectra:

$$\mathbf{H}_{\mathrm{opt}}(\mathrm{j}\omega)=\frac{\Phi_{\mathrm{ss}}(\omega)}{\Phi_{\mathrm{ss}}(\omega)+\Phi_{\mathrm{nn}}(\omega)} \tag{8.168}$$

If we let $\Phi_{\mathrm{ss}}(\omega)$ be given by Equation 8.158 and $\Phi_{\mathrm{nn}}(\omega)$ be a two-sided white noise PDS, then it is easy to show that $\mathbf{H}_{\mathrm{opt}}(\mathrm{j}\omega)$ is given by:

$$\mathbf{H}_{\mathrm{opt}}=\frac{\frac{\sigma_{\mathrm{s}}^2 2\alpha}{\alpha^2+\omega^2}}{\frac{\sigma_{\mathrm{s}}^2 2\alpha}{\alpha^2+\omega^2}+\eta}=\frac{\sigma_{\mathrm{s}}^2 2\alpha/\eta}{(\sigma_{\mathrm{s}}^2 2\alpha/\eta+\alpha^2)+\omega^2} \tag{8.169}$$

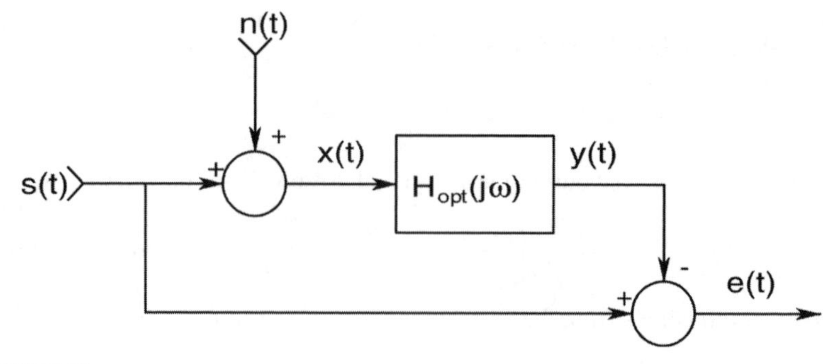

FIGURE 8.12
Error-generating model relevant to finding the filter, $\mathbf{H}_{opt}(j\omega)$, that will minimize the mean-squared error.

Inverting this CFT yields the weighting function of the optimum filter:

$$h_{opt}(t) = \frac{\alpha\sigma_s^2/\eta}{\sqrt{(\sigma_s^2 2\alpha/\eta + \alpha^2)}} \exp[-\sqrt{(\sigma_s^2 2\alpha/\eta + \alpha^2)}|t|] \tag{8.170}$$

Clearly, this optimum filter *is not causal* (its weighting function exists for negative time), a property that makes it a mathematical curiosity, rather than an engineering tool. Lee gives the following causal approximation to $\mathbf{H}_{opt}(j\omega)$ given in Equation 8.169:

$$\mathbf{H}_{opt}'(j\omega) = \frac{\alpha^2[\sqrt{(\sigma_s^2 2\alpha/\eta + \alpha^2)} - \alpha]}{j\omega + \sqrt{(\sigma_s^2 2\alpha/\eta + \alpha^2)}} \tag{8.171}$$

In general, Wiener optimum filters are algebraically difficult to find and challenging to implement with a causal approximation except for the simplest cases of $\Phi_{ss}(\omega)$ and $\Phi_{nn}(\omega)$. In addition, they are derived for statistically described signal and noise. If one (or both) of the random processes becomes nonstationary, the filter can become nonoptimal. Also, how the Wiener filter behaves for deterministic signals can be disappointing. There are better criteria for the design of filters to improve SNR_{out}.

8.4.4 Discussion

Signal averaging is widely used in biomedical research and diagnosis. A periodic stimulus (e.g., a noise, a flash, an electric shock, a pin prick, etc.) is given to a subject. The response is generally electrophysiological, i.e., an evoked cortical potential (ECP), an electrocochleogram (ECoG), or an electroretinogram (ERG), all richly contaminated with noise. By averaging, the noise is reduced (its sample mean tends to zero) as the number of averaging cycles, N, increases, while the signal remains the same. Hence, signal averaging increases the SNR in the averaged signal. However, we showed that there are practical limits to the extent of SNR improvement.

Also covered in Section 8.4 is the use of LTI filters to improve the SNR at the filter output. This SNR improvement is predicated on the requirement that the power density spectrum of the noise does not completely overlap that of the signal. Thus, by lowpass, bandpass, highpass or notch filtering the input signal plus noise, some noise power can be excluded (as well as some small amount of signal power), generally improving the SNR at the filter output, hopefully without distorting the signal excessively. The Weiner optimum filter was introduced, and shown to be generally impractical in most biomedical applications because of the nonstationarity of signal and noise.

8.5 Introduction to the Application of Statistics and Information Theory to Genomics

8.5.1 Introduction

This section assumes that the reader has some familiarity with basic cell biology and biochemistry and can describe what is meant by *amino acid, chromosome, DNA, gene, germ cells, meiosis, mitochondria, mitosis, nucleus, protein, ribosome, RNA,* etc. The section will introduce applications to *genomics* of *statistics, information theory,* and *hidden Markov models.*

Genomics is a new branch or specialization of molecular and cell biology; broadly stated, it is the detailed study of how genes transfer their stored information to proteins that are synthesized by a cell or bacterium (viruses are generally assembled by cells and bacteria). A central goal in genomics is discovering the exact genetic code contained in an animal, plant, viral or bacterial *genome.* The genome of a living organism is *all* the genetic material in its chromosomes; its size is usually specified as the total number of DNA or RNA *base pairs.* The genes contain the information that determines the sequence of amino acids in all the various proteins made by an organism's cells. The origins of many diseases can be traced to anomalous protein structures or to too little or too much of a given protein, so the ability to relate certain protein structural and regulatory defects to specific errors in genes provides medical and pharmaceutical scientists a new tool for the design of new drugs, vaccines and therapies. Rapid nucleic acid base sequencing using the new family of *gene sensors* [Northrop, 2002] promises to allow rapid direct screening of genomic DNA segments and messenger RNA (mRNA) sequences to permit the timely diagnosis or detection of certain genetic diseases and cancer. Thus, research in genomics is providing an understanding of the molecular mechanisms of disease.

Intimately associated with the discipline of Genomics is the area of *bioinformatics,* which is the art and science of creating dedicated computer databases and software applications that allow researchers to store detailed information about DNA and RNA base pairs in genes, as well as protein structures and configurations, and then compare this information statistically with new information about the structure of defective genes or proteins. Bioinformatics also allows the comparison of genes across species (e.g., man vs. chimpanzee, various strains of bacteria), and for a given species through time (evolutionary genomics) (e.g., how a given bacterial species' genome mutates over time, and develops genes for antibiotic resistance).

The following section will define certain terms used in genomics and describe the basic biochemical mechanisms whereby genes control protein synthesis. Many important *signaling substances* in the body are protein hormones (e.g., insulin, oxytocin, leptin, galanin, etc.) and defects in their structures or the structures of their *receptor proteins* located on cell membranes can cause diseases. Other important proteins serve as enzymes that catalyze biochemical reactions, including the synthesis of amino acids, other proteins, nucleic acids, steroid hormones, etc. Still other proteins are bound to and extend through cell walls, serving as ion pumps, active transport sites for amino acids, binding sites for neurotransmitters and hormones and recognition sites for certain immune system cells, etc. Life at the molecular level is very complex.

8.5.2 Review of DNA Biology

Immediately following the fertilization of a human egg, the cells produced by division of the *zygote* are diploid and normally have 23 *chromosome pairs* containing DNA derived from both egg and sperm. (At certain stages of cell development, nuclear DNA is visible with the light microscope.) At one point in embryonic development, every cell of the 8- to 16-cell *morula* stage of development apparently can grow an entire adult organism, i.e., every cell is *totipotent.* Such cells are classified as *stem cells,* and, as the embryo grows, it is their fate to differentiate and to build the specialized tissues and organs that ultimately produce a mature fetus. Understanding the control of the differentiation of stem cells has always been a central problem in embryology and now is an active area of research because of the promise of being able to grow specific tissues *in vitro* (e.g., neurons, skin, bone, pancreatic beta cells, etc.) from stem cells that can be transplanted into a host to cure disease or injury. *Pluripotent stem cells* are a second type of stem cell that is found in the inner cell layers of the *blastocyst* stage of embryonic development. Unlike totipotent stem cells, pluripotent cells cannot give rise to a fetus. They can, however, be caused to multiply as specialized tissue (e.g., skin, neurons, bone, connective tissue, blood cells, etc.) [Maienschein, 2001].

This section is not concerned with the control of stem cell differentiation, but rather how any cell transfers the information stored in its genetic code (genome) to control the synthesis of the proteins and other biochemicals needed to sustain life. The genome of nearly all organisms is carried by a molecular template or code made from sections of double-stranded *deoxyribo-nucleic acid* (DNA) that generally reside in a cell's nucleus (some DNA is also found in the extranuclear ribosomes of cells, but that is another story). (The genome of certain retroviruses (e.g., HIV) is carried in ribonucleic acid (RNA) base sequences.)

All biological macromolecules have natural complex 3-D structures in which the interatomic binding energy is minimized; DNA, RNA and proteins are no exception. Their 3-D molecular structures are generally necessary for intermolecular specificity and physiological activity. The basic organizational unit of the DNA polymer is the 2′-deoxyribose (a sugar) molecule joined to one of two *pyrimidine bases* (*cytosine*

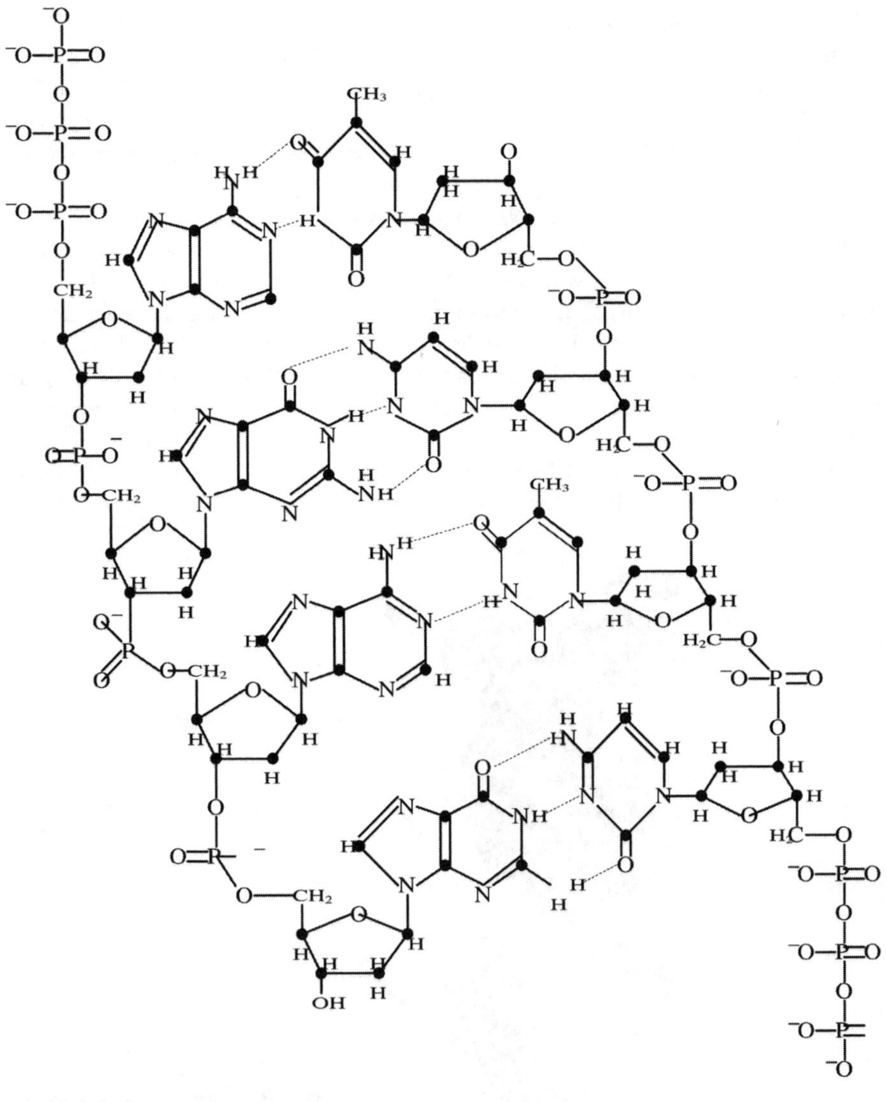

FIGURE 8.13

A 2-D schematic molecule of two-stranded DNA showing four base pairs. Base pairs are linked by hydrogen bonding.

and *thymine*), *or* one of two *purine bases* (*adenine* and *guanine*). Thus, cytosine (C), thymine (T), adenine (A), or guanine (G) can be considered to be the four *coding symbols* in a DNA molecule. The bonding between the base and the deoxyribose sugar involves the C_1' carbon of the sugar and the N_9 nitrogen of a purine base, or the N_1 nitrogen of a pyrimidine base in an N-β-glycosidic linkage.

Figure 8.13 shows a 2-D schematic view of a short section of two-stranded DNA, i.e., a DNA tetramer with four bases attached, illustrating where the covalent chemical bonds occur. A *nucleoside* subunit of DNA is one of the four bases attached to the C'_1 position of 2′-deoxy-ribose where the sugar *lacks* a phosphate group. A *nucleotide* is a nucleoside having one or two phosphate groups covalently bonded to the 3′-and/or 5′- hydroxyl group's (or groups') oxygen. A single strand of DNA thus is composed of a polymer formed from phosphodiester links between alternating nucleotide and nucleoside sugars. These links are illustrated in Figure 8.13.

In its simplest 3-D form, B-DNA contains two complementary polymer chains with the same number of bases organized as an *alpha helix.* The two DNA strands wrap around the helix axis with a right-hand spiral; the two polynucleotide chains run in opposite directions. The radius of the helix is ca. 1 nm, and the repeat length (axial period) is ca. 3.4 nm. The axial displacement between bases is ca. 0.34 nm, so about 10 base pairs are found in an axial period. Figure 8.14 illustrates the α-helix of B-DNA in a 3-D side-view. Note that, from the side, the B-DNA α-helix has a large and small groove. Most physiological DNA is of the B-form. A-DNA is a form found when DNA is dehydrated. The small groove is much smaller relative to the large groove in the A-form. (A-DNA is the "forensic form.") Z-DNA is

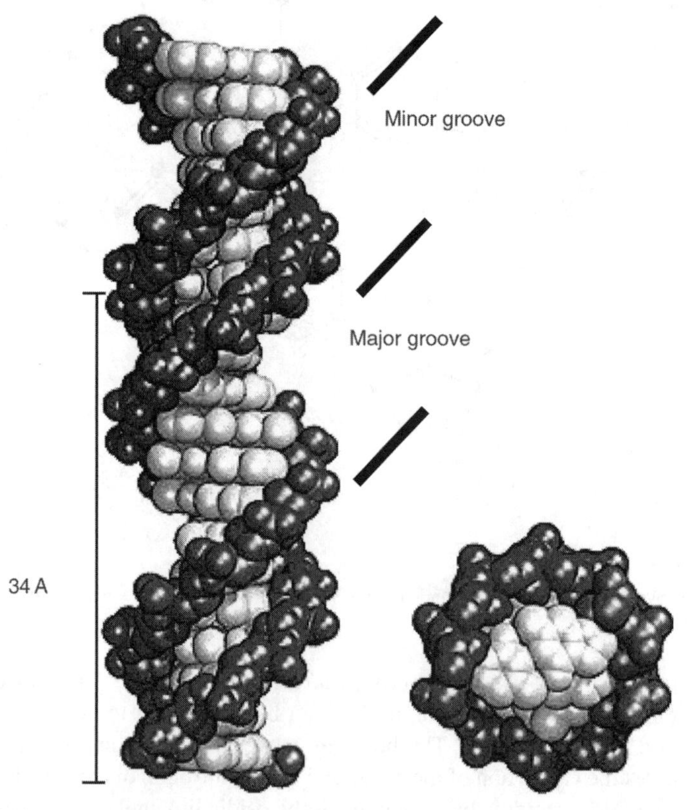

FIGURE 8.14
Left: A side view of a type B, DNA α-helix. Note the large and small grooves. Right: End view of the B-DNA molecule.

unusual in that it is a left-handed helix (A- and B-DNA have right-handed helices). Z-DNA occurs in oligonucleotides having alternating purine and pyrimidine bases, e.g., GCGCGCGC....

The sugar-phosphate links of the two DNA strands wrap around the axis like the railing of a spiral staircase, the "steps" of which are the bases in the center. The adenine on one chain *always pairs* with thymine on the opposite strand; they are held together by two weak *hydrogen bonds.* A guanine on one side *always pairs* with a cytosine on the other strand; the pair is held loosely by three *hydrogen bonds.* Figure 8.15 illustrates 2-D schematics of the purine and pyrimidine bases, and the *hydrogen bonding* between them. Approximate dimensions and angles are given. Thus, because of the complementary base structure, if we know the base sequences on one strand of the DNA helix, we know it in on the complimentary strand. This redundancy permits enzymatic repair of radiation-damaged DNA.

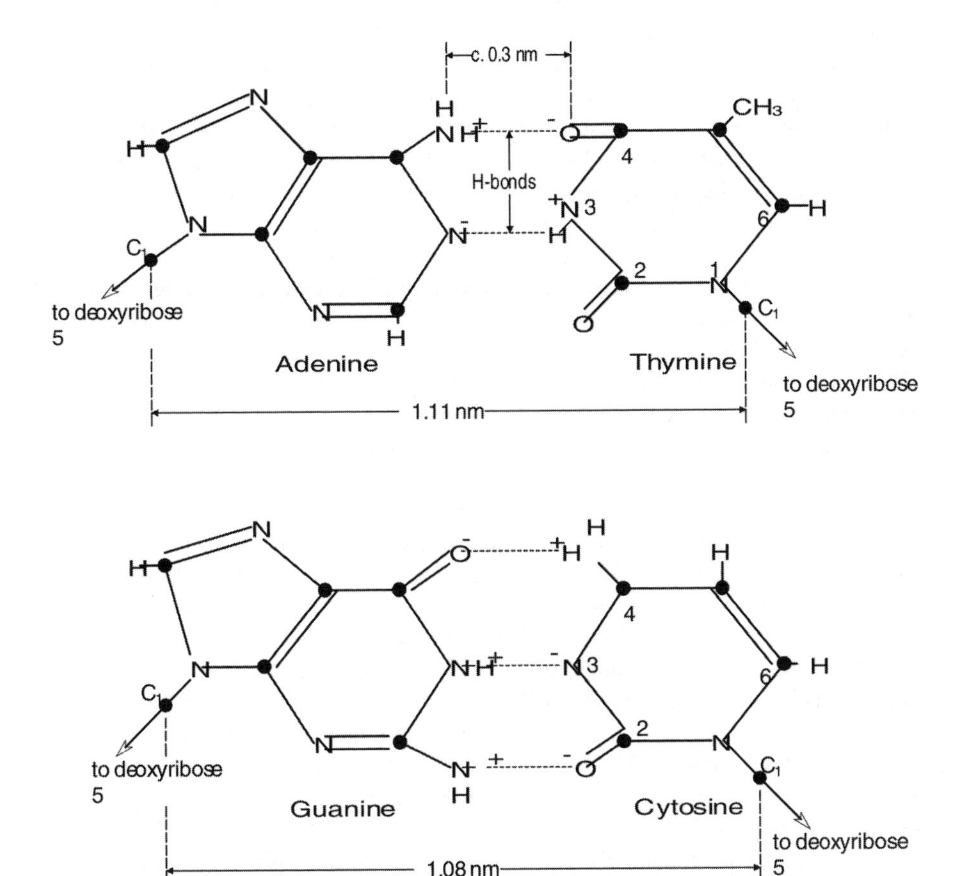

FIGURE 8.15

A detailed, 2-D view of complementary base pairing and hydrogen bonding in DNA. Black balls are carbons.

Resting DNA in the nucleus (DNA that is not being "read" for its code) is found in association with many proteins called histones. This DNA is further wrapped and folded at five different-length scales to achieve a high-density packing factor for storage in a cell's nucleus. If fully unwrapped and laid end to end, all *DNA in a human cell would be about 2 meters long* [Masum et al., 2001]. Clearly, from nuclear volume restrictions, for a gene to be read, the two DNA helix strands must be separated locally. The single-strand bases must be read sequentially and then rejoined and refolded, both in DNA replication (in mitosis) and in protein synthesis. Little is known about the *in vivo* molecular mechanisms that perform these complex 3-D molecular manipulations.

A *codon* is a sequence of *three* DNA (or RNA) bases that code for a single amino acid (AA) being incorporated into a peptide, polypeptide or protein. Since there are four possible bases in a single separated DNA strand, the total number of different codons possible is $4^3 = 64$. All 64 have been found to exist. Sixty-one have been found to code for amino acids, and three codons tell the protein synthetic mechanism to stop synthesis and release the protein. Only 20 amino acids are normally found in proteins made by human cells, so it is obvious that the genetic "code" is *degenerate,* with some amino acids being selected by more than one codon. For example, the AA leucine is coded by *six* codons: TTA, TTG, CTT, CTC, CTA and CTG. Only two AAs, methionine and tryptophan, are coded by only one codon, ATG and TGG, respectively. The complete codon matrix is shown in Table 8.5.1.

Table 8.5.2 illustrates amino acid coding from an AA point of view.

From the *Human Genome Project* a startling fact has emerged. There are some 30,000 to 40,000 different proteins (genes) in the human genome (the current estimate is 31,780 [Genomes, 2001]). The average protein contains ca. 400 AAs, so 1,200 DNA bases are required to code each protein, or a total of ca. $1{,}200 \times 40{,}000 = 48$ million bases are required. However, it is known that the entire human genome has a total of ca. 3.2 Gigabases (3.2×10^9), so it appears that only about 1.5% of the human genome is protein-coding genes; ca. 98.5% is non-coding, and has unknown or poorly understood function(s). These noncoding bases, are called *introns,* occur in packets among the coding gene base sequences, which are called *exons.* Curiously, the intron bases are transcribed into the premessenger RNA (pmRNA) for the gene, but are "edited" out of the gene sequence in the mRNA before protein synthesis occurs. The editing is done in a complex eight-step process by a set of five nuclear "caretaker" RNA molecules known collectively as a *spliceosome.* The spliceosome is composed of five subunits called *small nuclear ribonuclear proteins* (snRNP) [MCB 411, 2000]. This is a wonderful and indispensable molecular machine, because our genome is 98.5% "noise." (The details of how the spliceosome works are beyond the scope of this text; the interested reader should visit the University of Arizona MCB 411 website, Module 15.) Some workers have called intron DNA "junk" DNA. It now turns out that introns contain *cis-regulatory elements* (base sequences) that evidently determine which (and when) master control genes are activated, thus providing a clue to how embryonic development takes place. It is my opinion that it is highly unlikely that 98% of our DNA is noise or junk, just because it doesn't directly code proteins. The elaboration of the cis-regulatory DNA base sequences in introns promises to be

TABLE 8.5.1
The Human Protein Coding Codon Matrix

First	T	C	A	G	Last
T	Phe	Ser	Tyr	Cys	T
"	Phe	Ser	Tyr	Cys	C
"	Leu	Ser	Stop	Stop	A
"	Leu	Ser	Stop	Trp	G
C	Leu	Pro	His	Arg	T
"	Leu	Pro	His	Arg	C
"	Leu	Pro	Gln	Arg	A
"	Leu	Pro	Gln	Arg	G
A	Ile	Thr	Asn	Ser	T
"	Ile	Thr	Asn	Ser	C
"	Ile	Thr	Lys	Arg	A
"	Met*	Thr	Lys	Arg	G
G	Val	Ala	Asp	Gly	T
"	Val	Ala	Asp	Gly	C
"	Val	Ala	Glu	Gly	A
"	Val	Ala	Glu	Gly	G

a major challenge in genomics. Evidently, the human genome project will continue for some time.

The following section outlines the principles of protein synthesis (the "dogma"). Note that DNA carries only the information that controls synthesis — RNA, ribosomes and certain proteins carry it out.

8.5.3 RNAs and the basics of protein synthesis: transcription and translation

The transfer of the codon code for a certain gene from DNA to *messenger RNA* (mRNA) is called *transcription; translation* is the process whereby the genetic code in the mRNA is used to construct proteins. RNA is *ribonucleic acid,* a linear polymer of *ribonucleoside phosphates.* The RNA polymer is held together by covalent bonds between alternating ribose and phosphate groups. Ribose is a sugar with a five-carbon ring, as shown in Figure 8.16. Each sub unit or monomer of RNA, like DNA, also has

TABLE 8.5.2
Amino Acids Coded by DNA Codons

AA Name	Abbreviation	DNA Codons for Each AA
Tryptophan	Trp	TGG
Methionine	Met	ATG*
Aspartic acid	Asp	GAC, GAT
Glutamic acid	Glu	GAA, GAG
Cysteine	Cys	TGC, TGT
Histidine	His	CAC, CAT
Asparagine	Asp	AAC, AAT
Lysine	Lys	AAA, AAG
Phenylalanine	Phe	TTC, TTT
Glutamine	Gln	CAA, CAG
Tyrosine	Tyr	TAC, TAT
Isoleucine	Ile	ATA, ATC, ATT
Alanine	Ala	GCA, GCC, GCG, GCT
Glycine	Gly	GGA, GGC, GGG, GGT
Proline	Pro	CCA, CCC, CCG, CCT
Arginine	Arg	CGA, CGC, CGG, CGT
Threonine	Thy	ACA, ACC, ACG, AGT
Valine	Val	GTA, GTC, GTG, GTT
Leucine	Leu	TTA, TTG, CTA, CTC, CTG, CTT
Serine	Ser	TCA, TCC, TCG, TCT, AGC, AGT
Start		ATG
Stop		TAA, TAG, TGA

Note: no AA is coded by five codons.
*The DNA codon ATG codes for methionine inside a peptide sequence *or* signals the start of a sequence [UCSD, 2001].

a side chain base that is either *adenine, cytosine, guanine* or *uracil* (DNA uses thymine instead of uracil). The five common nucleic acid bases are shown in Figure 8.17.

The three major types of RNA are *mRNA, transfer RNA* (tRNA) and *ribosomal RNA* (rRNA). Other classes of small RNA molecules also exist: e.g., *small nuclear* RNA (snRNA), *small nucleolar RNA* (snoRNA) and the *4.5S signal recognition particle RNA* (srpRNA). We are concerned only with mRNA, tRNA and rRNA, because they are the species principally involved with gene expression and protein synthesis.

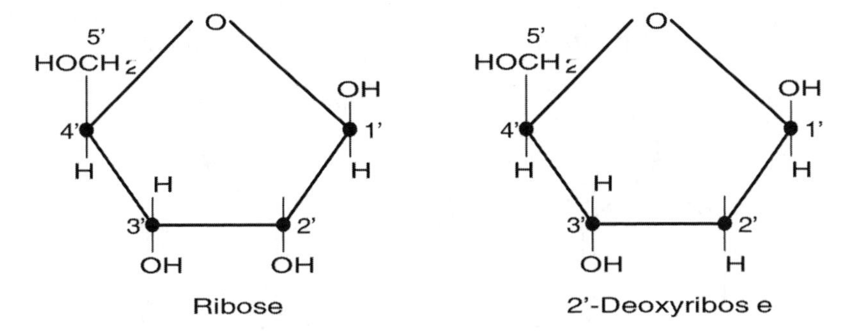

FIGURE 8.16
2-D molecular structures of the sugars ribose and $2'$-deoxyribose.

The first step in protein synthesis is the unfolding of the DNA α-helix from its storage configuration and the separation of the two complementary halves of the helix in the region of the active gene. This unraveling exposes the DNA bases so that special enzymes called *DNA-dependent RNA polymerases* (RNAP) can act to form *pre-messenger RNA* (pmRNA), which has a base structure complementary to that of the DNA template strand. Actually, there are three types of RNAP:

1. *Type I* is used to synthesize rRNA.
2. *Type II* synthesizes pmRNA.
3. *Type III* makes tRNA.

(Nothing is simple in molecular biology; enjoy the complexity.)

The uracil found in RNA pairs with adenine on the DNA strand being transcribed. Note that mRNA composes only ca. 5% of a cell's RNA (80% is rRNA, and 15% is tRNA). After the spliceosome proteins edit the intron ("noise") bases out of the pmRNA, it becomes mRNA that carries the code for the assembly of a specific protein from the gene site on the DNA, through the nuclear membrane to the ribosomes in the cytosol, where the actual protein assembly occurs.

The regulation of mRNA synthesis for a certain gene is done by *transcription factor proteins* (TFPs) that "recognize" certain DNA base sequences located upstream for the start site for RNA polymerase. When these factors bind to the DNA, the RNAP moves along the DNA, synthesizing pmRNA until it reaches a stop codon. RNAP always moves along the DNA in the same direction, from the $3'$ to $5'$ ends. The pmRNA molecule is assembled in the $5'$ to $3'$ direction. The $5'$ end of a primary transcript pmRNA has a triphosphate group. The TFPs themselves are regulated in order to turn gene expression on and off. Phosphorylation of TFPs by protein kinase enzymes (also proteins) activates them, and, no doubt, protein kinases themselves are regulated, *ad infinitum*. The codons in mRNA are read from $5'$ to $3'$, and the proteins are synthesized in the amino- to carboxyl (-COOH) direction. The process is complex, even baroque, but it works.

Purines yrimidines

NH_2
N N
H H
N N
H
Adenine

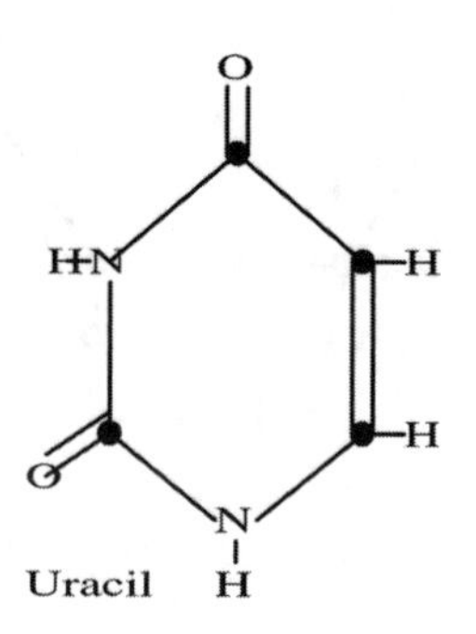

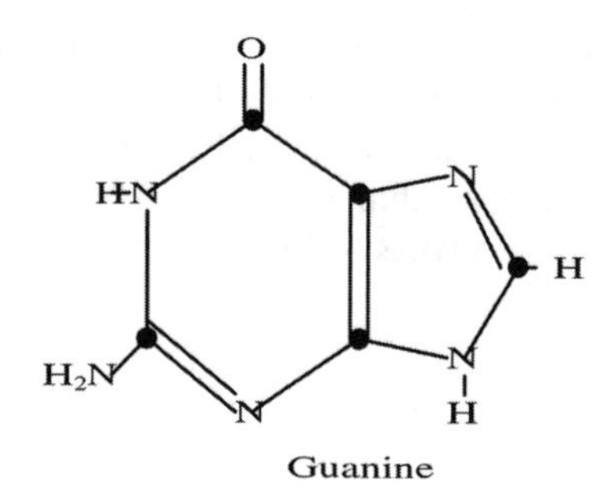

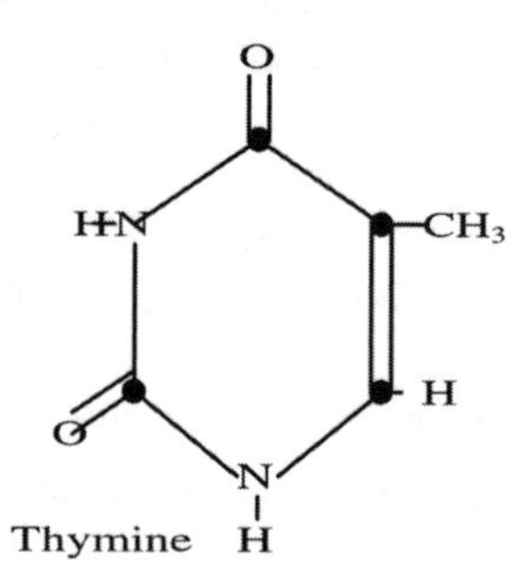

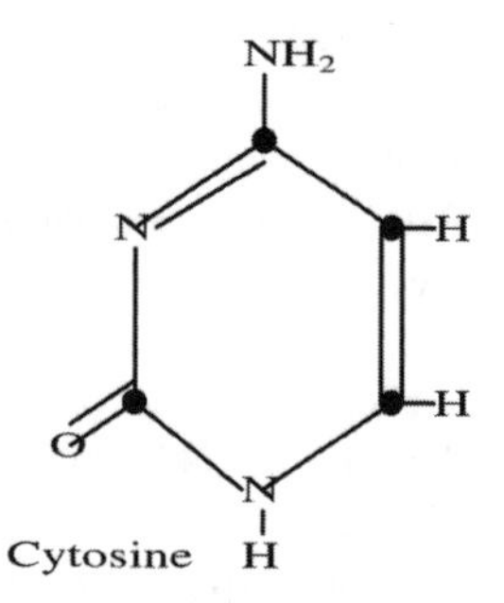

FIGURE 8.17

2-D molecular structures of the five common bases found in DNA and RNA. (The pyrimidine uracil replaces thymine in RNA.)

Transfer RNA (tRNA) molecules can have 75 to 90 nucleotide bases. Each amino acid (AA) used in human protein synthesis has one corresponding tRNA molecule that will carry the AA to a ribosome for the process of protein assembly. tRNA contains many unusual bases in addition to A, G, C and U. Some of these unusual bases are methylated or demethylated derivatives of the four normal bases. The purpose of the unusual bases may be to form a critical 3-D structure that gives tRNA its activity and specificity. The 5′ ends of all tRNAs are phosphorylated, and the terminal residue is usually pG. The base sequence at the 3′ end of all tRNAs is CCA. The activated AA to be put in the protein being assembled is attached to the free 3′-OH of the terminal adenosine (A). About half of the nucleotides in tRNA are base-paired to form short pieces of double helix. Four regions of the tRNA are not base-paired. Three bases on the anticodon loop pair with a certain codon on the mRNA molecule, i.e., they are complementary to that codon. The actual assembly of the protein from mRNA is done by another clever set of proteins and rRNA in the *ribosomes.* Figure 8.18 illustrates schematically one tRNA molecule that has the codon for the AA, phenylalanine (Phe), bound to a specific anticodon site on a mRNA molecule. Other enzyme molecules will insert the Phe AA into the protein being assembled by the ribosomal complex.

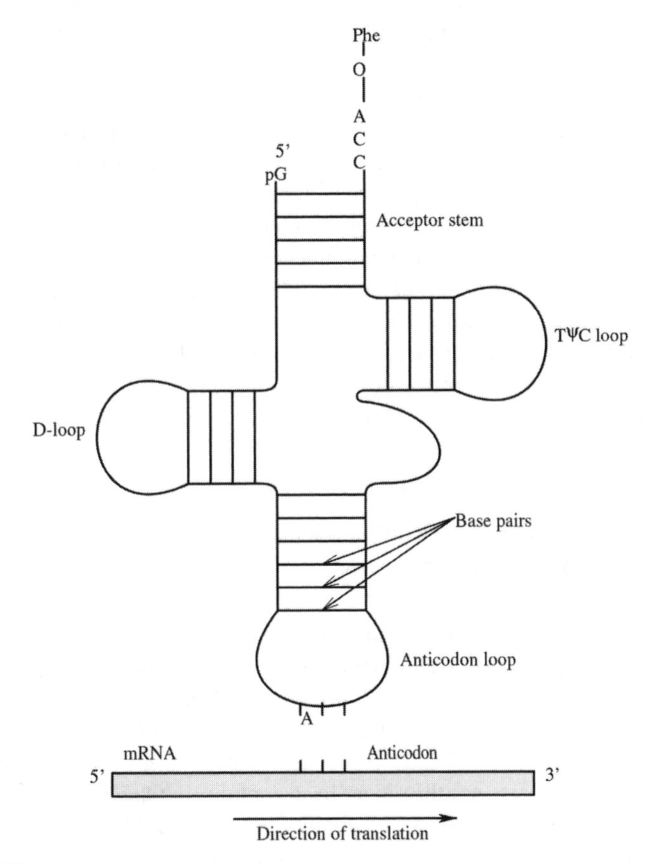

FIGURE 8.18

Highly schematic structure of a transfer RNA molecule that codes for the amino acid phenylalanine. Note that the complementary base triplet on the tRNA, AAG, is derived from the DNA triplet, TTC. The mRNA thus has the complementary anticodon, UUC.

The molecular biology of this process is very complex, and way beyond the scope of this section.

8.5.4 Introduction to statistics applied to genomics

Because there are so many genes, each one is composed of many codons, and nature has provided the genome with a huge amount of "noise" in the form of introns and random mutations, many workers use statistics to describe the molecular properties of nucleic acids when exact base sequences have not been discovered. Communications engineers have collaborated with molecular biologists in the application of *information theory* to the quantitative description of genetic coding. Such collaboration goes back to the mid-1950s, following the elaboration of DNA structure by Watson and Crick in 1953, and the formal introduction of information theory by Shannon and Weaver in 1949 [Yockey et al., 1958]. Information theory (IT) is based on finite set probabilities, so to introduce IT applications to genomics, we first must review some basic concepts from "ball-in-urn" probability and statistics.

First, let us consider the outcomes of the independent events of flipping a coin (let it be an old Indian head/buffalo nickel so the possible outcomes are truly heads or tails). If the nickel is unbiased, we know intuitively that the chance that it will come down heads is 50%. If the flips are mechanically identical each time (i.e., are done by a machine), the outcomes of the flips are no longer entirely random (physics rules), and the result is largely deterministic. However, a human coin flipper never flips exactly the same way each time, hence the randomness in the outcomes. To experimentally find the probability that the result of the flip will be a head, we toss the coin N times and count the number of times a head occurs, n_h. Then the probability of a head is approximated by the *event frequency*, $f_h = n_h/N$. The probability of a tail is estimated by $f_t = 1 - f_h$. For example, for $N = 100$ flips, $n_h = 52$, so $p_h \cong 0.52$; now if we let N = 10,000, $n_h = 4{,}980$, and $p_h \cong 0.4980$. Two things are evident:

1. As $N \to \infty$, $f_h \to p_h$, the true probability.
2. The absolute value of the difference between the number of heads and tails, $|n_h - n_t|$, grows larger as $N \to \infty$.

Now let us flip two nickels sequentially. Clearly, there are *four* possible outcomes: H_1H_2, H_1T_2, T_1H_2, T_1T_2. The outcome of the second toss is not affected by the outcome of the first toss, i.e., the *events are independent.* Thus, the probability of a given outcome is clearly $^1/_4$. The probability of one head *and* one tail in any order is $^1/_2$, and the probability of two heads *or* two tails is also $^1/_2$. Of course, in the genetic code on a DNA strand, it is not the binary heads or tails, but the quartet, A, G, C, and T. For example, if the four bases were equally frequent in DNA, then the probability of finding adenine when we pick a base at random would be $^1/_4$.

As a further example of finite-state probabilities, consider two unbiased dice. When they are rolled, we know intuitively that for either die, the probability of a number from one to six being up is 1/6 because each die has six sides with numbers from

1 to 6. Thus, the probability of rolling "snake eyes" (1 *and* 1) is the probability of rolling 1 *times* the probability of rolling 1, or 1/36. The probability of rolling a total of 11 is found by considering the ways 11 can be formed. 11 = (6 + 5) or (5 + 6). So p(11) = 1/36 + 1/36 = 1/18. The probability of rolling a 7 is found by considering the ways a total of 7 can be formed. 7 = (1 + 6) or (6 + 1) or (2 + 5) or (5 + 2) or (3 + 4) or (4 + 3). So p(7) = 6/36 = 1/6.

A general rule of determining probabilities of more than one event emerges: p(A ***and*** B) = p(A)•p(B), p(A ***or*** B) = p(*A*) + p(B). Another rule governing probability is: $p(\overline{A})$ = p(not A) = 1 −p(A). For rolling one die, the chance of getting any number, 1 to 6, is a certainty, hence p(1) + p(2) + p(3) + p(4) + p(5) + p(6) = 1. For a system with M outcomes, $\sum_{k-1}^{M} p(n_k) = 1$, i.e., there is a certainty that some outcome will occur.

Conditional probabilities are written: p(A—B). That is, the probability of A, given that we know B (i.e., B is known *a priori*). The *joint probability* of A and B can be written:

$$p(A,B) = p(A|B)p(B) \tag{8.172}$$

Bayes' theorem states:

$$p(A,B) = p(A|B)p(B) = p(B,A) = p(B|A)p(A) \tag{8.173}$$

So

$$p(A|B) = \frac{p(B|A)p(A)}{p(B)} \tag{8.174}$$

It follows from Bayes' theorem that if the two events A and B are *independent,* then:

$$p(A|B) = p(A) \text{ and } p(B|A) = p(B) \tag{8.175}$$

So it follows that

$$p(A,B) = p(A|B)p(B) = p(A)p(B) \tag{8.176}$$

Also, in dealing with probability theory and IT, it is useful to understand what is meant by *combinations* and *permutations.* In general, the *number of combinations of N things taken n at a time* is given by the well-known formula:

$$C(N,n) = \binom{N}{n} = \frac{N!}{(N-n)!n!} \tag{8.177}$$

Note that $0! \equiv 1$, and 1! = 1. When N is very large (≥20), N! can be approximated by Sterling's formula:

$$N! \cong \sqrt{2\pi N}\, N^N e^{-N} \tag{8.178}$$

Permutations give the number of ways a specific number of objects can be put in a definite order. The total number of permutations of a group of N different symbols is N!. The number of permutations of N symbols taken n at a time is given by:

$$P(N,n) = \frac{N!}{(N-n)!} \tag{8.179}$$

It is instructive to consider the total number of different codons possible given the four possible DNA bases arranged in a group of three. The first codon symbol can be one of four, the second can be one of four, and the third symbol is also one of four. Thus, a total of $4 \times 4 \times 4 = 4^3 = 64$ individual codons is possible from A, C, G and T. Of these 64 codons, three are used to stop protein coding, one is used to initiate coding or code the AA methionine, the other 60 codons are used to code the other 19 AAs used in human protein synthesis in a *degenerate code* (see the tables above). (A degenerate code is one where more than one codon can cause a given AA to be selected.)

As an example of permutations, how many different octapeptides can be made from a set of the same eight different amino acids? This is simply $8! = 40{,}320$, quite a few. Now consider how many unique octapeptides can be made from all 20 AAs *without repeating an AA in the sequence.* This is:

$$\frac{20!}{(20-8)!} = 5{,}079{,}110{,}400 \tag{8.180}$$

or more than 5 gigaoctopeptides. Mind boggling. Nucleic acids may carry the information for life, but proteins do the work.

Next, let us examine some discrete probability distributions. The *binomial distribution* gives the probability that exactly n successes will occur in N trials. The probability of one success or event's occurring is p; the probability it will not occur is $q = 1 - p$. The binomial distribution can be written:

$$P_b(N, n, p) = \frac{N!}{(N-n)!n!} p^n (1-p)^{N-n} = \binom{N}{n} p^n q^{N-n} \tag{8.181}$$

For a *first example,* consider a string of eight amino acids (an octapeptide). Calculate the probability of finding one alanine anywhere in the string. Assume $p_{ala} = 1/20 = 0.05$, and $q_{ala} = 0.95$. Then:

$$P_{b(ala)}(8, 1, 0.05) = \frac{8!}{7!1!} 0.05^1 0.95^9 = 8 \times 0.05 \times 0.6303 = 0.2521 \tag{8.182}$$

For a *second example* of application of the binomial distribution, consider a string of 12 RNA bases (an oligonucleoside). Calculate the probability of finding three uracil bases anywhere in the string. Assume $p_u = 0.25$.

$$P_b(12, 3, 0.25) = \frac{12!}{(12-3)!3!} (0.25)^3 (0.75)^9 = 0.2581 \tag{8.183}$$

And, as a *third example,* find the probability that the 12-base RNA oligonucleoside has all 12 bases uracil.

$$P_b(12, 12, 0.25) = \frac{12!}{0!12!}(0.25)^{12}(0.75)^0 = 5.9605 \times 10^{-8} \tag{8.184}$$

Another probability distribution that finds application in genomics is the *multinomial distribution.* This in an M-dimensional multivariate extension of the binomial distribution. The multinomial distribution is used to test for a certain section of DNA coding or not coding; is it an exon or intron region? Given a set of M discrete random variables: X_1, X_2, X_3, ..., X_M. The set has a probability function [Beyer, 1968]:

$$P_m(X_1 = x_1, X_2 = x_2, \ldots, X_M = x_M) = \frac{N!}{\prod_{i=1} x_i!} \prod_{i=1}^{M} p_i^{x_i} \tag{8.185}$$

Where p_i is the probability of X_i occurring, and:

$$\sum_{i=1}^{M} p_i = 1, \quad \text{and} \quad \sum_{i=1}^{M} x_i = N \tag{8.186}$$

and the mean of $X_k = \mu_k = Np_k$, the variance of X_k is $\text{Var}\{X_k\} = \sigma_k^2 = Np_k(1 - p_k)$, and the covariance of $X_j X_k$ is $-p_j p_k$.

Many other PDs are used in genomics. These include the *extreme value distribution,* the *Gaussian PDF,* the *Dirichlet-Baysian distribution,* and the *gamma distribution* used to model rates of gene evolution. Clearly, it is beyond the scope of this section to treat these distributions in detail.

8.5.5 Introduction to the application of information theory to genomics

IT was developed in the late 1940s by Claude Shannon and others. Its use in communications engineering has led to the development of efficient, error-correcting codes for data transmission in noisy channels. As early as 1958, IT was recognized as having application in genetics (and genomics) [Yockey et al., 1958]. After all, the genetic code for protein synthesis uses four symbols taken three at a time (a codon), is self-correcting in the presence of noise (see spliceosomes above), and is under tight regulation. Modern genomic research has now produced detailed quantitative material in the form of detailed DNA and mRNA base sequences that IT can be applied to and IT has led to some philosophical insight about how genes work as well as abstract details on their information content.

Some general properties of the *Shannon measure of information,* H, are:

1. $H \geq 0$.
2. H's units are bits/symbol (a binary information measure). H is continuous, not quantized or discrete.

3. If an event has an *a priori* probability of 1 (a certainty to occur), then no information is carried by that event (H = 0).

4. If two *independent* events occur (whose joint probability of occurring is the product of their individual *a priori* probabilities), the information we get from observing the joint events is the sum of the two independent Hs.

5. The function that satisfies the above properties is the *Shannon measure of average information:*

$$H \equiv -\sum_{k=1}^{M} p_k \log_2(p_k) \text{ (average bits per symbol; there are M different symbols)} \tag{8.187}$$

6. In practice, the probabilities p_k are approximated by the frequencies, $f_k = n_k/N$. n_k is the number of times event k occurs in a sequence of length N (N possible occurrences). We note that : $\lim_{N\to\infty} f_k \to p_k$.

The *Surprisal* of the kth event occurring in the sequence is defined as [Schneider, 2000]:

$$S_k \equiv -\log_2(p_k) \text{ (bits)} \tag{8.188}$$

Note that $-\log_2(p_k) = \log_2(1/p_k) \geq 0$. Convention dictates the use of logs to the base 2 because binary communications use 1s and 0s. Other log bases can be used, however, including bases 3 or 4. If the occurrence of the kth event is very infrequent, its $p_k \to \varepsilon$, and S_k will be large and positive. That is, we will be very surprised to see that symbol. Note that the Shannon measure of average information is the probability-averaged surprisal of the set of N symbols. Suppose the kth symbol appears n_k times in the set. Then it is clear that:

$$N = \sum_{k=1}^{M} n_k \quad \text{(Number of symbols in the set)} \tag{8.189}$$

There will be n_k cases where we have surprisal S_k. The average surprisal in the N symbol set is then just:

$$\overline{S} = \frac{\sum_{k=1}^{M} n_k S_k}{\sum_{k=1}^{M} n_k} \tag{8.190}$$

Substituting into Equation 8.190 from Equations 8.189 and 8.188, we obtain Equation 8.187 for the average information in the N symbol "word."

The *following example* of computing the average information in a 34-base DNA oligonucleotide (a 34-mer) is based on an example by Carter (2001). The oligonucleotide is:

AGCTTTTCATTCTGACTGCAACGGGCAATATGTC

We have no knowledge where the "spaces" are between the codons, i.e., where each codon starts, so we will calculate the average information for three codon sequences: one of 11 codons beginning with AGC (the terminal C is ignored), one of 11 codons beginning with GCT (the starting A is ignored), and a third sequence of 10 codons beginning with CTT (the beginning AG and terminal TC are ignored). We compile all the possible codons for the three cases. Those with "2" following them occurred twice in the compilation:

AAT	AAC	ACG	ACT	AGC
ATA	ATG	ATT	CAA	CAT
CGG	CTG(2)	CTT	GAC	GCA(2)
GCT	GGC	GGG	GTC	TAT
TCA	TCT	TGA	TGC	TGT
TTC(2)	TTT(2)			

The average information of the oligo is found by using Shannon's formula with codon-occurrence frequencies used to estimate codon probabilities. For example, $f_{TTT} = 2/32 = 1/16$, and $f_{TAT} = 1/32$, etc. f_{TAT} is used in lieu of p_{TAT}, etc. So the average information is:

$$\begin{aligned} H &= \sum_{k=1}^{32} f_k \log_2(1/f_k) = 5 \times 2/32 \times 4 + 22 \times (1/32) \times 5 \\ &= 4.6875 \text{ bits/codon} \end{aligned} \tag{8.191}$$

If all the codons were equally probable, i.e., all $f_k = 1/32$, then $H = \log_2(32) =$ 5 bits/codon. Note that it might be more appropriate to find H in units of trits rather than bits, since codons use three symbols, not two. This is simply achieved by using the log to the base 3 in the H formula:

$$\begin{aligned} H &= \sum_{k=1}^{32} f_k \log_3(1/f_k) = \sum_{k=1}^{32} f_k \frac{\log_{10}(1/f_k)}{\log_{10}(3)} \\ &\downarrow \\ H &= 5 \times (2/32) \times 1.20412/0.47712 + 22 \times (1/32) \times 1.50515/0.47712 \\ &= 2.9575 \text{ trits/codon} \end{aligned} \tag{8.192}$$

The bacterial, *E. coli* vs. K-12 bacteria genome has been completely mapped and has been found with certainty to contain 4,693,221 DNA base pairs coding 4401 genes encoding 116 RNAs and 4,285 proteins [Serres et al., 2001]. (Note that these numbers are constantly being revised as further work is done in the *E. coli* K-12 genome. Also *E. coli* is constantly undergoing mutations.) Some *E. coli* genes appear commonly throughout nature, while others, as might be expected, are unique to *E. coli.* The K-12 strain is not pathogenic, but some other strains of *E. coli* are toxic and have been implicated in various cases of food poisoning (e.g., strain O157:H7). The data from the K-12 genome can be compared with that from toxic strains to isolate those genes responsible for toxicity and perhaps better design drugs to fight the toxic strains or block their toxicity.

Carter (2001) gives an example of using information theory to find "interesting" sections and features of the *E. coli* genome. Carter used a sliding window to define a contiguous section of $3^8 = 6{,}561$ *base pairs* (bps) on the genome of length 4,693,221 bps. He calculated the average information for the 2187 codons in the window following the approach in the example above. The window was slid forward in steps of size $3^4 = 81$ bps, and the process repeated again and again until the window reached the end of the genome. This process generated 57,860 information data points, plotted on Figure 8.19. Notice the large downward spikes indicating analysis windows enclosing codons of low average information. Shown on the top of the figure is the result of applying the same information theory analysis to a computer-generated completely random genome of 4,693,221 bps. Note the smooth, noisy plot at nearly 6 bits/codon. A very curious phenomenon appeared when Carter took the discrete Fourier transform (DFT) of the plots of average entropy vs. window step number illustrated in Figure 8.19. Figure 8.20 illustrates the root power spectrum of the average entropy vs. window step number for the *E. coli* genome; note the periodicities that modulate the noise. (These oscillations may be an inherent property of the *E. coli* genome. They bear further investigation.) The bottom asymptote of this root power spectrum has a slope of ca. $(1/\mathrm{f})^{1.5}$. Figure 8.21 illustrates the root power spectrum of the average entropy vs. step number for the computer-generated, purely random "genome." This spectrum falls off as ca. 1/f. No periodicity is seen, so it appears that the periodicity is not a computational artifact.

Chapter 7 examined joint time-frequency analysis (JTFA) and its application to characterizing nonstationary time-domain signals. Dimitris Anasstasiou (2000) has cleverly adapted JTFA to the analysis of genetic information ("biomolecular sequences"). Instead of time, the *joint sequence frequency* (JSF) distribution is calculated using the base sequence or codon sequence position (n) going from the $5'$ toward the $3'$ end of a strand of DNA. In the case of *E. coli,* $0 \le \mathrm{n} \le (4{,}693{,}221 - 1)$. A time-domain analog signal generally has some graded value (e.g., voltage) that can be JTF transformed. A genetic sequence has the four bases, A, G, C and T. Anasstasiou converts these symbols to numbers by assigning complex numerical values to them. He uses the sliding short-term DFT to construct the JSF spectrogram and converts it to a 2-D color map to display a unique view of the genetic information. Note that JSFA can also be applied to average information plots such as shown in Figure 8.19. There is every reason to believe that genes are nonstationary random sequences and can be

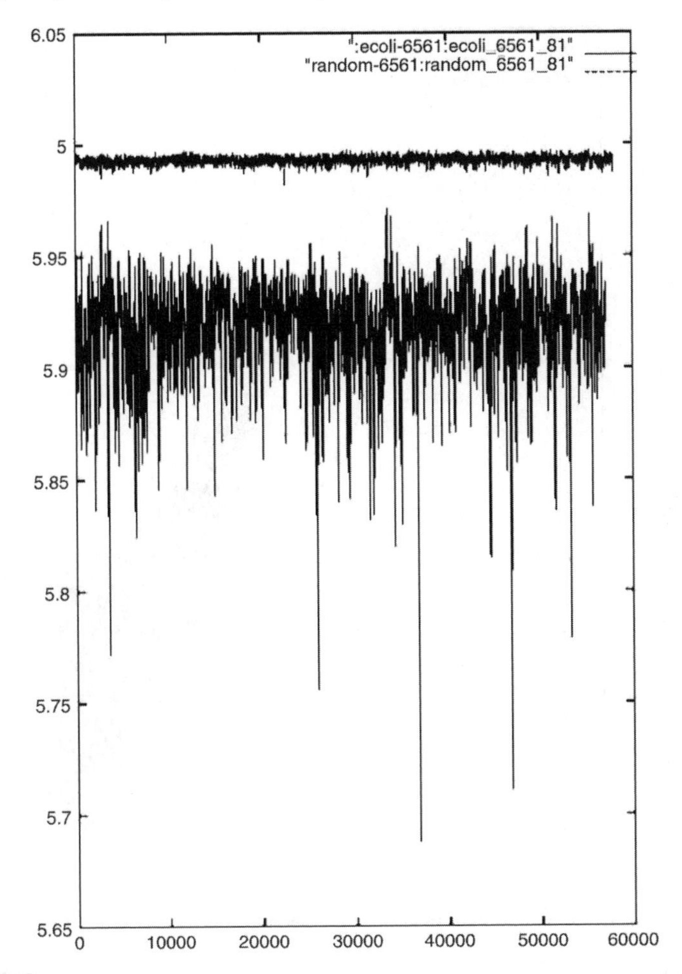

FIGURE 8.19

Plot of the average information on the *E. coli* K-12 genome of 4,693,221 base pairs (bps). A sliding window of $3^8 = 6{,}561$ bps was slid in steps of $3^4 = 81$ bps in computing the average information. Note the large spikes. The top noisy trace was obtained from an artificial, completely random genome model. Note the absence of spikes. (Carter, T. 2001. An introduction to information theory and entropy: Applications to biology. Online class notes for the Complex Systems Summer School. With permission.)

validly described by JSFA. Perhaps, once its usefulness has been demonstrated, this mode of analysis will catch on more generally in the future.

Many other applications of IT and engineering systems analysis techniques in characterizing genomes, genes and coding can be found in the literature. For example, see the many papers on this topic by Thomas D. Schneider [Schneider 2001, 2000, 1994].

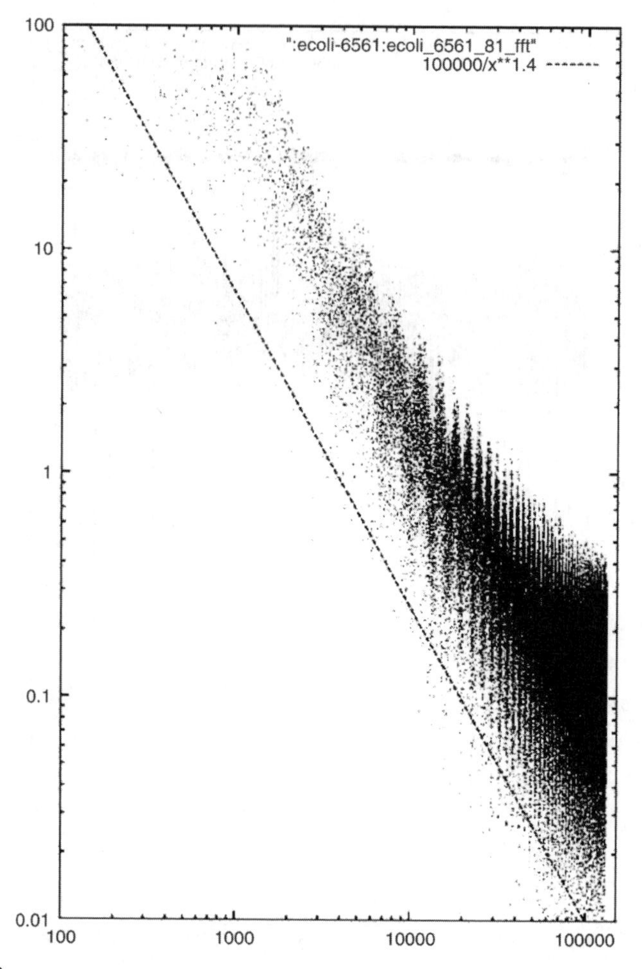

FIGURE 8.20

The information plot of Figure 8.19 was DFTd and the root power density spectrum (PDS) found. Note the curious periodicities in the root PDS. What do they mean? (Carter, T. 2001. An introduction to information theory and entropy: Applications to biology. Online class notes for the Complex Systems Summer School. With permission.)

8.5.6 Introduction to hidden Markov models in genomics

A Markov model (MM) in genomics provides a series of probabilities which tells how likely a particular *output sequence* is to have descended from a particular *ancestral sequence,* or, in reverse, given the output sequence, the MM allows the estimation of what the ancestral sequence was.

Hidden Markov models (HMMs) are a probability-based modeling method which can be used to analyze oligonucleotide base sequences, gene codon sequences and primary protein amino acid sequences. It is beyond the scope of this text to describe

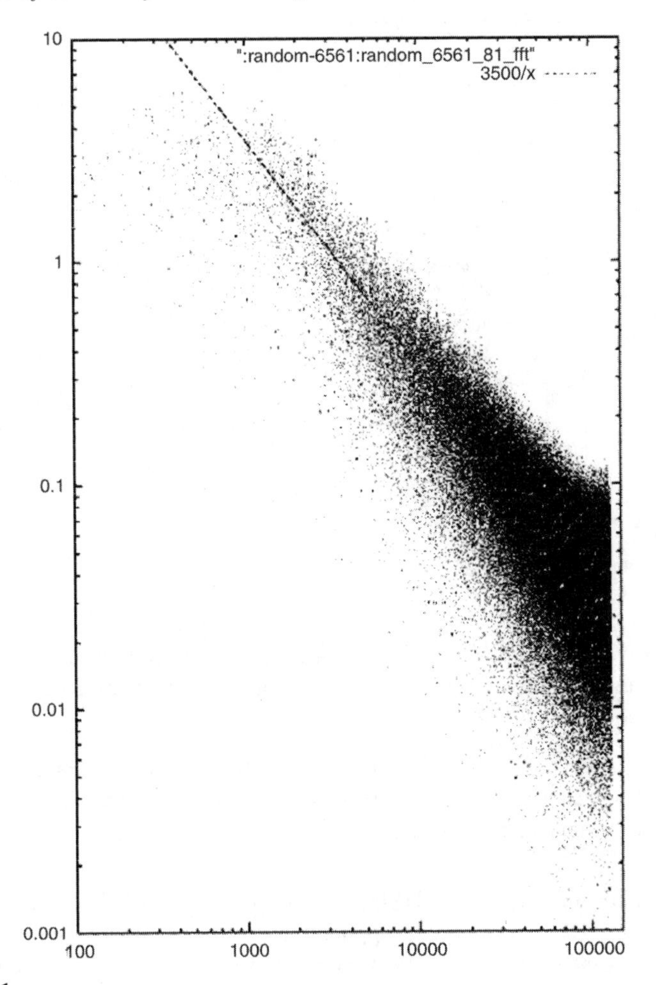

FIGURE 8.21
The root PDS of the average entropy of the computer-generated completely random "genome" shown in Figure 8.19. Note the absence of periodicities. (Carter, T. 2001. An introduction to information theory and entropy: Applications to biology. Online class notes for the Complex Systems Summer School. With permission.)

and analyze them in detail; we will examine only their salient features and discuss their applications in genomics. The reader who is interested in learning about HMMs in depth should begin by reading the tutorial papers by Rabiner and Juang (1986), and Rabiner (1989).

HMMs are suitable for solving three kinds of general problems:

1. *Evaluation:* Find with what probability a given model will generate a given sequence of observations. The *Forward Algorithm* can be used to solve this problem efficiently.

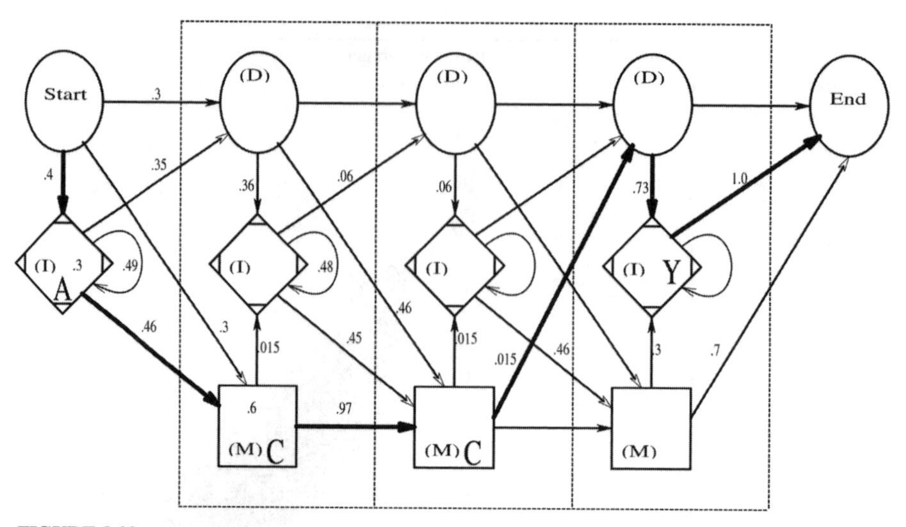

FIGURE 8.22
A three-node hidden Markov model.

2. *Decoding:* Find what sequence of hidden (underlying) states most probably generated a given sequence of observations. The *Viterbi Algorithm* is used to solve this problem.

3. *Learning:* Find what model most probably underlies a given sample of observation sequences, i.e., find the model's parameters. The *Forward-Backward Algorithm* can be used to solve this problem.

The *Hidden Markov Model* (HMM) was developed in 1989, initially for speech recognition, and has since found application in computational molecular biology (genomics, bioinformatics). HMMs have been used for protein analysis, recognition of genes in human and bacterial genomes, analysis and prediction of DNA functional sites (exons) and the compositional heterogeneity of natural DNA sequences (oligonucleotides) [Peshkin and Gelfand, 1999]. Figure 8.22 illustrates one topology for a three-node HMM. There are *Start* and *End* states; each node has a *Match State* (M), a *Delete State* (D) and an *Insert State* (I). The arrows denote position-specific *transition probabilities,* the products of which give the probabilities of transitioning into a state from a previous state. (HMMs can have up to hundreds of nodes; the number of nodes is practically limited by computational complexity and time requirements.) Transitions from state to state progress from left to right through the HMM, with the exception of the self-loops on the insertion states. The self-loops allow deletions of any length to fit the model, regardless of the length of other sequences in the family [Karchin, 1999].

An HMM is a *finite state machine* (FSM). FSMs produce some kind of output as the FSM moves from state to state or reaches a particular state. The HMM generates a protein polypeptide sequence by specifying amino acids as it progresses through a series of states. Each state has a table of AA emission probabilities, as well as a matrix of state transition probabilities such as shown in Table 8.5.3.

Consider the quadrapeptide sequence ACCY (Ala*Cys*Cys*Tyr). Referring to Figure 8.22, the probability that the first AA is Ala in position 1 is 0.3. The probability of Cys being in position 2 is 0.6. Thus, the total probability or *raw score* of ACCY along the known (dark) path shown is the product of the path and state probabilities. That is:

$$0.4^{*}0.3^{*}0.46^{*}0.6^{*}0.97^{*}0.015^{*}0.73^{*}0.01^{*}1.0 = 1.76 \times 10^{-6}$$

Calculations are simplified if the sum of the logarithms of the probabilities is used to calculate the raw score. In a real HMM, many separate paths can generate the same sequence. Thus, the correct probability of a sequence is the sum of the path probabilities in the HMM.

$$P_{seq} = \sum_{k=1}^{N} \left(\prod_{j=1}^{Mj} p_{kj} \right) \tag{8.193}$$

where there are N paths and each path has M_j probabilities. Detailed calculation of P_{seq} using Equation 8.193 is not feasible for a large number of AAs. Instead, the *forward algorithm* can be used to calculate the sum of probabilities over all possible state paths inductively. Another approach is to calculate the most probable sequence of hidden states (a path that is described by a product of probabilities) by the *Viterbi algorithm,* given the HMM and the sequence of observations. We cannot go into the details of these algorithms here. A tutorial on them can be found in the tutorial paper by Karchin (1999), and in the excellent course notes from the University of Leeds (1997), available online. Building an HMM from scratch is a nontrivial problem. The following quote is from the HMM tutorial by Karchin (1999):

"Another tricky problem is how to create an HMM in the first place, given a particular set of training sequences. It is necessary to estimate the amino acid emission distributions in each state and all state-to-state transition probabilities from a set of related training sequences.

If the state paths for all the training sequences are known, the emission and transition probabilities in the model can be calculated by computing their *expected value:* observing the number of times each transmission or emission occurs in the training set and dividing by the sum of all the transmission probabilities or all of the emission probabilities.

If the state paths are unknown, finding the best model given the training set is an optimization problem which has no closed form solution. It must be solved by iterative methods.

The algorithms used to do this are closely related to the scoring algorithms described previously. The goal is to find model parameters which maximize the probability of all sequences in the training set. In other words, the desired model is a model against which all the sequences in the training set will have the best possible scores. The parameters are reestimated after every iteration by computing a score for each training sequence against the previous set of model parameters."

Karchin goes on to discuss the applications of the *Baum-Welch* algorithm and the *viterbi* algorithm in building an HMM.

As you can conclude from the foregoing descriptions, construction and application of hidden Markov models are not for the mathematically faint of heart.

8.5.7 Discussion

Section 8.5 surveyed the application of statistics and classical information theory to the description of genomic systems. The basic molecular biology of the nucleic acids DNA and RNA was reviewed and the molecular organization of proteins described. The process of protein synthesis starting with a gene's information stored in the DNA genome through pre-messenger RNA, messenger RNA, transfer RNA, etc. was outlined. The importance of accessory proteins (enzymes) in the process of protein synthesis was underscored.

We also reviewed basic "ball-in-urn" statistics, and illustrated its application to describing nucleic acid and protein structures. Also introduced was the application of information theory to describing genes and protein structure. Hidden Markov models were introduced as yet another application of probability and statistics to the description of genomics.

8.6 Chapter Summary

This chapter has shown how we can describe noise and signals to which noise is added. Section 8.2 began by considering continuous stationary random variables (SRV) and the descriptors used to characterize them, e.g., the probability density function and its CFT, the characteristic function, the mean, the mean-squared value, the variance, the auto- and cross-correlation functions and their CFTs, the auto- and cross-power density spectra. We went on to show how the propagation of SRVs through continuous and discrete LTI systems can be described in the time and frequency domains and how the auto- and cross power density spectrum for an LTI system can be used to find its frequency response function, $\mathbf{H}(\omega)$.

Price's theorem was shown in Section 8.2.9 to offer a statistical description of how noise propagates through no-memory nonlinearities. Quantization noise associated with analog-to-digital conversion was treated on Section 8.2.10, and examples of data scrubbing were described in Section 8.2.11. Data scrubbing is a nonlinear discrete statistical filtering method that effectively removes noise pulses from discrete data records.

Section 8.3 reviewed the mathematical tools used to describe discrete noise, including discrete auto- and cross-correlation functions and their power spectra. Signal averaging, an important tool to improve the signal-to-noise ratio of evoked transient signals, was described in detail in Section 8.4. How the SNR is improved was derived mathematically. Also in this section, we introduced the application of LTI filters to improve the SNR of stationary noisy signals.

The final Section, 8.5, as described above, introduced the molecular biological concepts key to genomics, and showed how statistics, information theory and hidden Markov models can be applied to characterizing genes and protein structures.

Problems

8.1 A *signal averager* has a constant level of Gaussian output noise with zero mean whose mean-squared value, σ_a^2, is independent of s, n, the sample number k, and the number of averages, N. The evoked signal to be recovered is deterministic, so $s_i(kT_s) = s_j(kT_s)$, $j \neq i, 1 \leq j, i \leq N$. Also, $\sigma_s^2(kT_s) \rightarrow 0$ for all k, and the MS value of the noise accompanying the signal is $\sigma_n^2(kT_s) = \sigma_n^2$, $0 \leq k \leq M-1$. There are M samples spaced T_s apart taken of $(s+n)$ in each averaging cycle (experimental repetition).
Derive an expression for the number of averaging cycles, N, required to give a certain, MS SNR improvement ratio, $G(kT_sN, \sigma_a^2) = SNR_{out}/SNR_{in} > 0$.

8.2 A signal is composed of random narrow positive pulses of height P_1 added to broad band Gaussian noise with zero mean and variance σ_n^2. The mean-squared, input signal-to-noise ratio is $SNR_{in} = P_1^2/\sigma_n^2$. The Gaussian noise plus pulses are the input to an odd nonlinearity $y = g(x)$ given by:

$$y = A[e^{bx} - e^{-bx}]$$

a. Plot $y = g(x)$ vs. x for $0 \leq x \leq 3$. Let $b = 2$.

b. Find an expression for the output mean-squared signal-to-noise ratio, SNR_{out}. Assume the MS output signal is due to just the pulses and the MS output noise, σ_y^2, is due to just the input noise.

c. Let G be the MS SNR gain of the nonlinearity: $G = SNR_{out}/SNR_{in}$. In most signal conditioning systems, $G < 1$. This nonlinearity is unusual in that, under certain conditions, $G > 1$. That is, there is a signal-to-noise ratio *improvement* in going from input to output. Let $b = 2$, $P_1 = 4$, and σ_n range from 0 to 4. *Plot* $\sqrt{G}$ as a function of σ_n and demonstrate that SNR gain occurs.

8.3 Use the single variable form of *Price's theorem* to find the mean output of a *full-wave rectifier,* $y = g(x) = |x|$, given a Gaussian random input, x, with zero mean and variance σ_x^2. Note that:

$$\frac{\partial E\{y\}}{\partial \nu} = 1/2 \int_{-\infty}^{\infty} f_x(x) \frac{\partial^2 g(x)}{\partial x^2} dx, \ \nu = \sigma_x^2$$

Also, the PDF of x is: $f_x(x) = \left[1/\left(\sqrt{2\pi\sigma_x^2}\right)\right] \exp[-1/2(x^2/\sigma_x)^2]$.

8.4 Figure P8.4 illustrates a cross-correlation system. It is used to estimate the cross-correlation function between the LTI system's input, x(t), and its output, y(t). x(t) is assumed to be very broadband ("white") Gaussian noise with zero mean and with a flat power density spectrum that extends well beyond the limits of $\mathbf{H}(\omega)$. The output of the multiplier is $z = y(t)u(t-\tau)$.

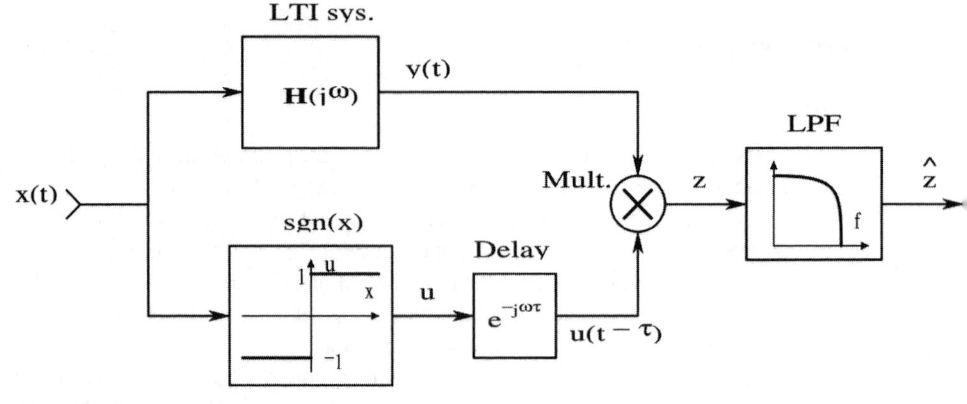

FIGURE P8.4

$u(t) = sgn(x) = [-1+2U(x)]$, and $u(t-\tau) = sgn[x(t-\tau) = \{-1+2U[x(t-\tau)]\}$. The system will be analyzed using the bivariate version of Price's theorem.

a. Find an expression for $\dfrac{\partial g(x,y)}{\partial y \partial x}$.

b. Now use text Equation 8.93 to calculate an expression for $\mathbf{E}\{z\} \cong \hat{z}$. Recall that ρ is the cross-covariance of the GRVs x and y. $\rho = \phi_{xy}(\tau) - \overline{x}\overline{y}$, but $\overline{x}$, hence $\overline{y} \equiv 0$. Also, because $\overline{x}$ and $\overline{y} = 0$, the constant of integration, $k = 0$.

c. Show how $\mathbf{E}\{z\} \cong \hat{z}$ can be used to estimate $\mathbf{H}(\omega)$ when the input noise, x, is white Gaussian noise.

8.5 Figure P8.5 illustrates a cross-correlator that uses a three-level nonlinearity, as shown. G(s) is an LTI system, x(t) is a wide-band stationary Gaussian RV.

a. Find an expression for $\partial g(x,y)/\partial y \partial x$.

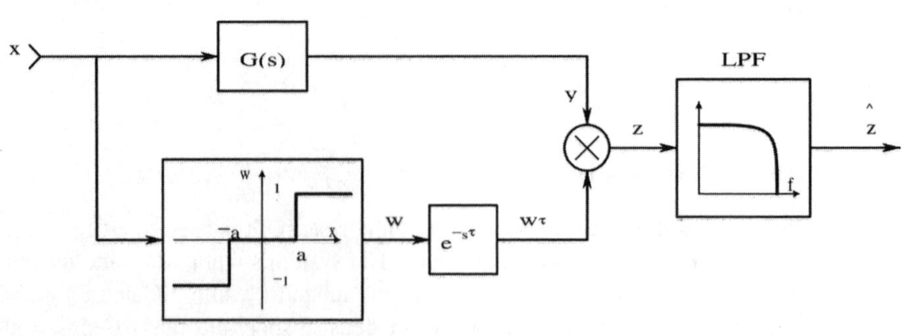

FIGURE P8.5

b. Now use text Equation 8.93 to calculate an expression for $\mathbf{E}\{z\} \cong \hat{z}$. Recall that ρ is the cross-covariance of the GRVs x and y.. $\rho = \phi_{xy}(\tau) - \overline{x}\overline{y}$, but $\overline{x}$, hence $\overline{y} \equiv 0$. Also, because $\overline{x}$ and $\overline{y} = 0$, the constant of integration, $k = 0$.

c. Show how $\mathbf{E}\{z\} \cong \hat{z}$ can be used to estimate $\mathbf{H}(\omega)$ when the input noise, x, is white Gaussian noise.

8.6 An SRV, **w**, has the probability density function shown in Figure P8.6.

a. Find a numerical value for A.

b. Find E{**w**}.

c. Find the mean-squared **w**, and the rms **w**.

d. Find Prob[0 ¡ **w** ≤rms **w**].

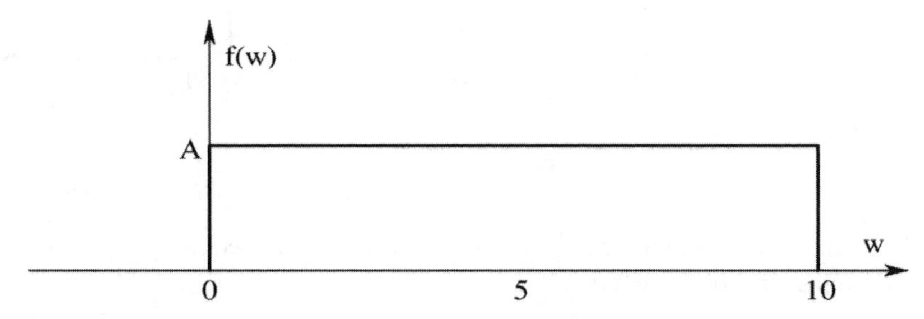

FIGURE P8.6

8.7 An SRV, **x**, is described by the Rayleigh probability density given by:

$$f(x) = kx\exp[-x^2/2\alpha^2)] \quad \text{for } x \geq 0, \text{ and}$$
$$f(x) = 0 \text{ for } x < 0.$$

a. Find an algebraic expression for k to normalize the PDF. That is, so $\int_0^\infty f(x) = 1$.

b. Find an algebraic expression for E{**x**}.

c. Find the x value where the peak of f(x) occurs; also find max f(x).

d. Find algebraic expressions for the mean-squared **x** and the rms **x** for the Rayleigh density.

e. Find the variance of **x**.

8.8 An SRV, **x**, has an exponential PDF given by $f(x) = 2e^{-2x}U(x)$.

a. Find E{**x**}.

b. Find Prob[**x** ¿ 2].

c. Find the rms **x**.

8.9 An SRV, ν, has the PDF shown in Figure P8.9.

a. Compute $E\{\nu\}$.

b. Compute var ν.

c. Show that in the limit, $\lim_{\delta\to 0} \text{var}\nu \to 1$.

d. Show that $\lim_{\delta\to 0}$ $\text{Prob}[|\nu| \geq \sigma_\nu] \to 1/4$.

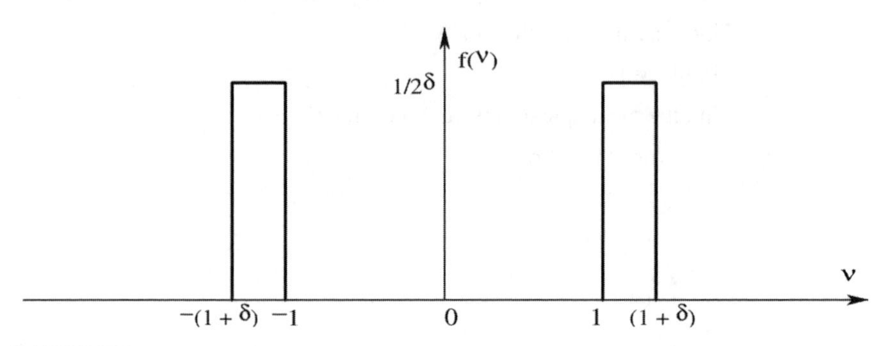

FIGURE P8.9

8.10 Find, sketch and dimension the autopower density spectra for the following autocorrelation functions:

a. $\varphi_{xx}(\tau) = \sigma_x^2 \dfrac{\sin(a\tau)}{(a\tau)}$

b. $\varphi_{xx}(\tau) = \sigma_x^2 \left(1 - \dfrac{|\tau|}{a}\right)$

c. $\varphi_{xx}(\tau) = \sigma_x^2 \exp(-{}^1\!/\!_2 \tau^2/\beta^2)$

d. $\varphi_{xx}(\tau) = \sigma_x^2 a^2/(a^2 + \tau^2)$

e. $\varphi_{xx}(\tau) = \sigma_x^2 \delta(\tau)$

f. $\varphi_{xx}(\tau) = \sigma_x^2 \dfrac{\sin^2(a\tau/2)}{(a\tau/2)^2}$

8.11 Find expressions for the output autopower spectra, given the autopower spectrum input to the LTI system frequency response function, $\mathbf{H}(j\omega)$.

a. $\Phi_{xx}(\omega) = \sigma_x^2 \sqrt{\pi/\alpha} \exp(-\omega^2/4\alpha) \to \mathbf{H}(j\omega) = \dfrac{b}{j\omega + b}$

b. $\Phi_{xx}(\omega) = \sigma_x^2 2\alpha/(\alpha^2 + \omega^2) \to \mathbf{H}(j\omega) = \dfrac{j\omega K(2\xi/\omega_n)}{[1 + (j\omega)^2/\omega_n^2] + j\omega(2\xi/\omega_n)}$

(a quadratic bandpass filter)

c. $\Phi_{xx}(\omega) = \sigma_x^2$ (white noise) $\to \mathbf{H}(j\omega) = \dfrac{K}{[1 + (j\omega)^2/\omega_n^2] + j\omega(2\xi/\omega_n)}$

(a quadratic lowpass filter)

8.12 Find the characteristic functions for the probability density functions shown in Figure P8.12.

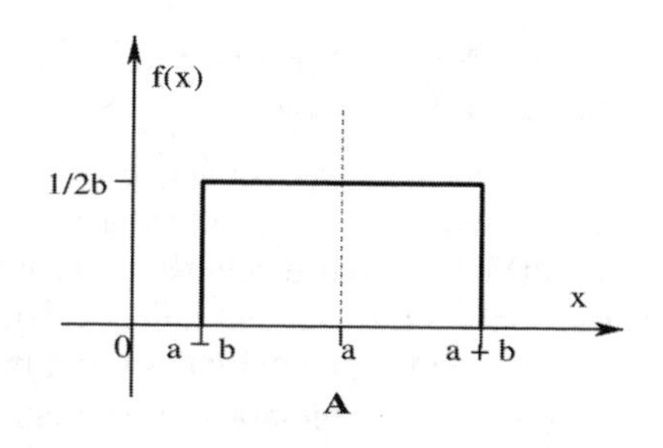

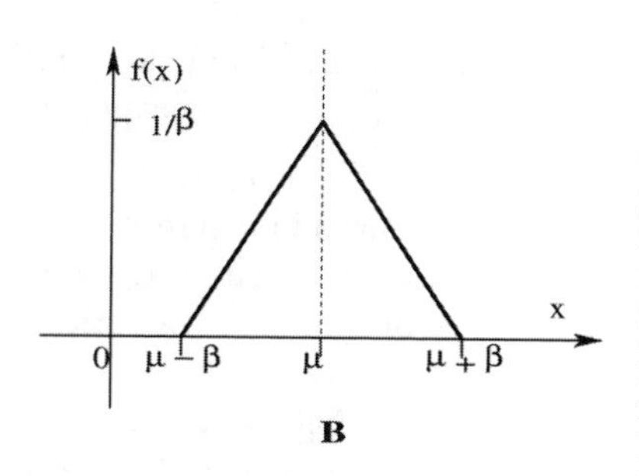

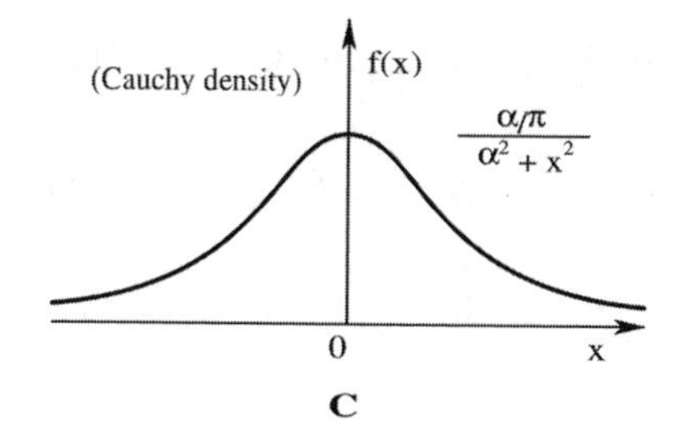

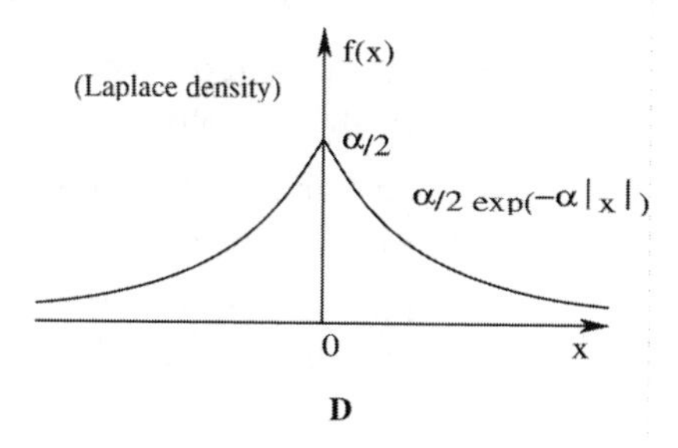

FIGURE P8.12

8.13 A 10-bit rounding A/D converter is setup to accept an input signal, $x(t)$, ranging from -1 to $+1$ volts. The output of the A/D converter is processed by a discrete LTI single-pole lowpass filter with transfer function,

$$H(z) = \frac{z}{z - e^{-aT}}$$

Let a = 500 r/sec, and the sampling period T = 1 msec.

a. Find the quantization step size, q.

b. Calculate the rms quantization noise voltage, σ_q, for this quantizer.

c. Find the rms noise at the filter output, $y(n)$. (Use the relation, $\sigma_y^2 = \sigma_q^2 \sum_{k=0}^{\infty} h^2(k)$.) $h(k)$ is the weighting function of $H(z)$.

8.14 A signal is described by the autocorrelation function, $\varphi_{ss}(\tau) = \sigma_s^2 e^{-\alpha|\tau|} \cos(\omega_o \tau)$. Added to the signal is uncorrelated white noise with the 2-sided PDS, $\Phi_{nn}(\omega) = \eta$ msV/r/sec.

a. Use the CFT modulation theorem, $f(t)\cos(\omega_o t) \Leftrightarrow \frac{1}{2}[F(\omega + \omega_o) + F(\omega - \omega_o)]$, to find an expression for the signal APS, $\Phi_{ss}(\omega)$.

b. The signal plus noise is filtered by an ideal bandpass filter, $F_i(\omega)$, as shown in Figure P8.14. Note that $0 < \alpha << \omega_o$, and that the bandpass filter frequency response and the PDSs are even functions. Because of symmetry we need to integrate only the signal and noise spectra between $\omega = \omega_o$ and $(\omega_o + B/2)$ r/sec, and then multiply this result by 4 to find the ms output signal and noise. This integration is made easier when we note that we get approximately the same results when we integrate $\Phi_{nn}(\omega)$ and $\Phi_{ss}(\omega)$ with $\omega_o = 0$ between $\omega = 0$ and $B/2$ r/sec, and again multiply by 4. Find an algebraic expression for the ms SNR at the output of the ideal bandpass filter.

c. Find an approximate expression for the ms SNR_{out} for the Hi-Q filter condition where $B/2 << \alpha$.

d. Find an approximate expression for the ms SNR_{out} for the condition where $B/2 = \alpha$.

e. Find an approximate expression for the ms SNR_{out} for the Lo-Q filter condition where $B/2 >> \alpha$.

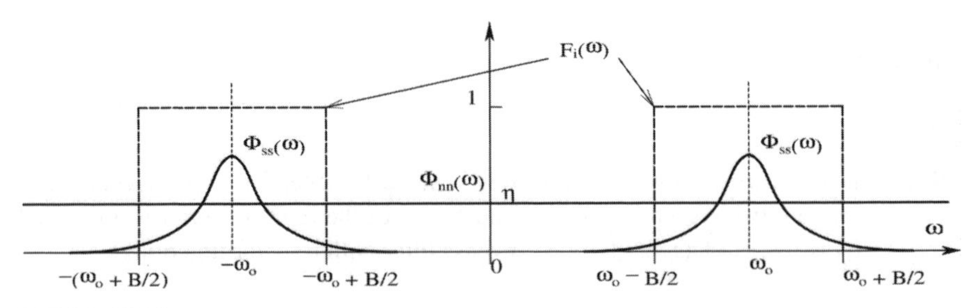

FIGURE P8.14

8.15 Calculate the average information, H, in trits/codon for the 34-base RNA fragment (oligonucletide): UCGAAAAGUAAGACUGACGUUGCCCGUUAUACAG

8.16 Apply the Hempel filtering algorithm to scrub the seven data points defined by the 7-point, x(47) window shown in Figure 8.10.

8.17 Apply the SD-ROM algorithm to scrub the five data points centered on x(56) in text Figure 8.10. Use $\varphi_1 = 4$, $\varphi_2 = 12$ for the thresholds.

8.18 A stationary, narrow-band, random signal is modeled by the APS shown in Figure P8.18. Calculate and plot to scale the signal's two-sided autocorrelation function, $\varphi_{xx}(\tau)$.

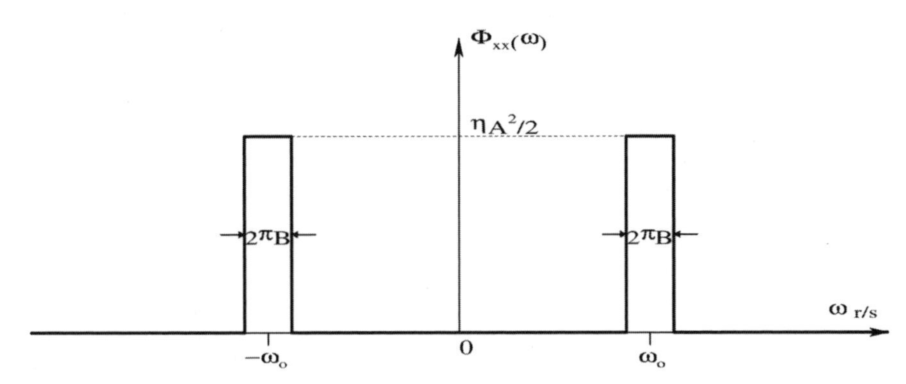

FIGURE P8.18

9

Basic Mathematical Tools Used in the Characterization of Physiological Systems

9.1 Introduction

The engineering side of biomedical engineering has traditionally attempted to describe the dynamic properties physiological systems with the tools of engineering systems analysis. The rationale for such characterization includes the need to understand the physiology and biochemistry of such systems. Such understanding can lead to better diagnosis and treatment of diseases. In some cases, the systems engineering approach has been successful in leading to better therapies (e.g., in the glucoregulatory system), in other cases, the "black box" approach has not shed light on the physiology of system components, but has provided information on the overall properties of the system.

This chapter will examine the general properties of physiological systems and, in particular, some properties of nonlinear systems. How underlying physical and chemical processes contribute to the behavior of physiological systems will be described, including diffusion and chemical mass action. We then examine some of the means used to characterize nonlinear physiological systems.

9.2 Some General Properties of Physiological Systems

This section will describe some general properties of physiological systems (PSs). These are bulk properties, i.e., they apply to entire multicomponent systems as follows:

1. Nearly all PSs are *closed-loop systems employing one or more causal feedback loops.* Feedback is generally negative. Loop gains tend to be low. Feedback can be implemented by various modalities: neural signals, *hormones, cytokines, autacoids,* etc. It is by negative feedback that living organisms maintain the steady-state conditions necessary for life. Such maintenance of dynamic equilibrium has been called *homeostasis* [Guyton, 1991].

2. *Most closed-loop physiological systems (CLPSs) generally have real-pole loop gains.* (An exception is found in the horizontal tracking control system for the eyes. Here, a CNS controller time constant is sufficiently long to allow what is in essence an integrator (a pole at the origin), creating a *type 1 closed-loop system* [Stark, 1968; Ogata, 1970]. Also, in the eye movement control system, the plant (the eyeball rotation) generally has complex-conjugate poles because of its moment of inertia coupled to the damped elasticity of the extraocular muscles.) Other neuromuscular control systems may also have complex-conjugate poles because of the mass or moment of inertia of a moving object, such as a limb, restrained by viscoelastic skeletal muscles. CLPSs based on biochemical reactions and diffusion tend to have real poles.

3. As a consequence of their real-pole loop gains, CLPSs are generally type 0 systems that have some steady-state error in response to a constant set point input [Northrop, 2000].

4. *CLPSs are usually multiple-input, multiple output (MIMO) systems. They generally have cross-coupling and interactions with related CLPSs.* Cross-coupling can arise from shared nervous system pathways, shared effector organs such as the kidneys, or a hormone affecting more than one class of target cells (pleiotropy).

5. *CLPSs generally use parametric control.* A parametric controller (PC) is one in which the difference between the set point or desired output and a function of the output is used to manipulate one or more system gains, rate constants, or parameters in order to force the output toward the desired value. By contrast, in a conventional SISO control system or regulator, the control (input to the plant), u, is varied as a function of the difference between the plant's input and output. In a PC, system output variables, especially in "wet" systems, are regulated by the alteration of diffusion and chemical reaction rate constants and loss rates by hormones and *autacoids* [Gilman, Goodman et al., 1985]. Hormones also affect the active "pumping" of certain ions and molecules across cell membranes. Hormone release rates, hence concentrations, can be a function of a controlled variable. Neurotransmitters alter specific ion permeabilities or conductances.

6. *Many CLPSs have transport lags (dead time) in their loop gains.* Such lags can arise from the time it takes an autacoid or hormone to activate a multistep, nuclear biosynthetic pathway, or from the finite time it takes nerve impulses to propagate down an axon and reach the target organ (muscle, gland, etc.). Transport lags create stability problems in high-gain closed-loop systems, however, CLPSs seldom have stability problems because their loop gains are generally low.

7. *CLPSs are generally stable, or, in certain cases, may exhibit bounded, limit cycle oscillations.* Such oscillations are seen under certain conditions in

the lens accommodation control system [Stark, 1968] and in the canine and human fasting glucoregulatory systems [Kragen and Lazarus, 1973; Yates et al., 1973].

8. *CLPSs are massively parallel systems.* Every organ is composed of thousands of cells that have similar functions, and each cell or functional groups of cells may receive inputs in parallel, e.g., from nerve fibers serving a common purpose, or a hormone that affects all the cells simultaneously. Such redundant parallel architecture insures robust behavior under conditions of injury or disease.

9. *Some "wet" CLPSs are push-pull* in the sense that two regulatory hormones having opposing effects are coupled into the system to regulate a common parameter. An example of this physiological control strategy is in the regulation of blood glucose. The pancreatic hormone *insulin* causes glucose in the blood to decrease by its being taken up by the liver for storage as glycogen, and by it diffusing into insulin-sensitive cells. The pancreatic hormone *glucagon* causes blood glucose to rise, mostly by causing glycogen stored in the liver to be broken down and released into the blood as glucose.

10. *Physiological regulators generally have no uniquely identifiable summing point* where error is generated between the set point and controlled variable. (Again, an exception is in eye movement control, where the angular position of a retinal image relative to the fovea can be considered error.) CLPSs involving hormones have what is considered to be *implicit summing points* [Jones, 1973]. Figure 9.1(a) illustrates a hypothetical linear hormonal regulatory feedback system operating in the steady-state. Block 1 contains an endocrine gland whose hormonal secretion rate is a linear, decreasing function of the concentration of the controlled variable. The hormone secretion rate in the steady state is assumed to linearly affect the controlled variable. Mathematically, we have:

$$\dot{Q}_H = \dot{Q}_{Ho} - K_G Y = K_G Y_o - K_G Y = K_G (Y_o - Y) \tag{9.1}$$

$$Y = K_R \dot{Q}_H \tag{9.2}$$

Thus, an implicit summing point is created where Y_o is the effective set point. Figure 9.1(b) illustrates the conventional feedback system block diagram with the implicit summing point. By inspection, the steady-state level of the controlled variable is:

$$Y = Y_o \frac{K_G K_R}{1 + K_G K_R} \tag{9.3}$$

Jones (1973) shows that the same strategy works to find the implicit summing point when the gland and regulated variable relations are nonlinear, as shown in Figure 9.2(a). Straight-line tangent approximations to $\dot{Q}_H = f(Y)$ and $Y = g(\dot{Q}_H)$ are drawn where the two curves intersect, and the procedure shown above is to the two resulting linear equations. See Figure 9.2(b). The linearized gain is:

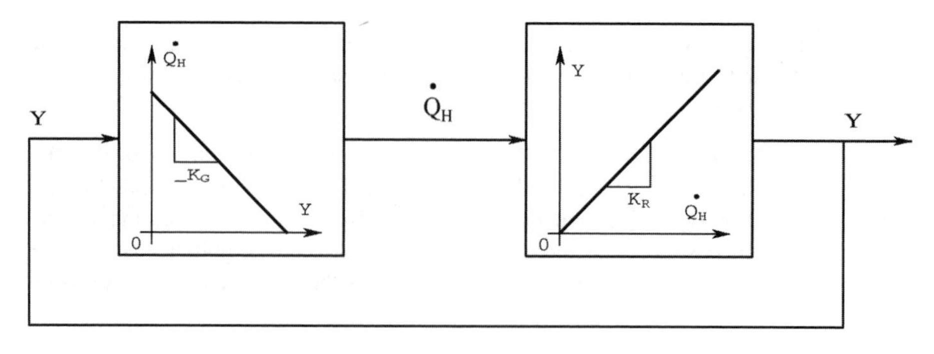

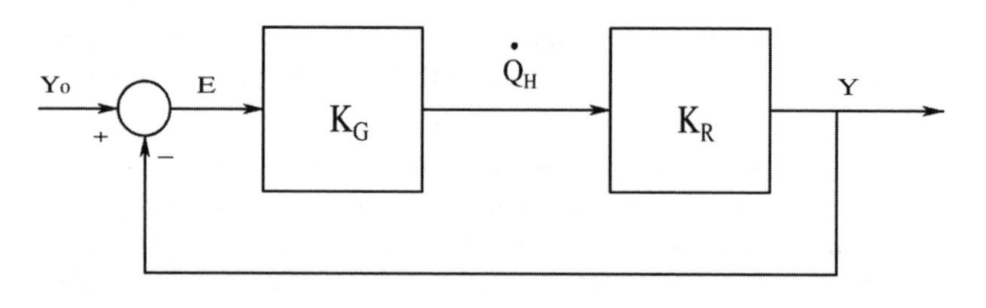

FIGURE 9.1
(a) A hypothetical, linear, static, single feedback-loop, hormonal regulatory system. (b) The hormone regulator configured as a SISO control system. Y_o is the equivalent setpoint. (Northrop, R.B. 2000. *Endogenous and Exogenous Regulation and Control of Physiological Systems.* CRC Press, Boca Raton. With permission.)

$$Y = (Y_o - Y_i)\frac{K_G K_R}{1 + K_G K_R} \tag{9.4}$$

(Linearization around an *operating point* is an established technique in engineering analysis, used for mathematical expediency.)

Twenty years ago, the fact that all CLPSs are nonlinear was a major setback for physiologists and engineers who wished to model them and predict their behavior. Systems had to be linearized for computational expediency. Linearization generated oversimplification and robbed the models of interesting behaviors that were the result of their inherent nonlinearity and complexity. Now, with the aid of modern engineering software and PCs, it is possible to model complex high-order nonlinear PSs and gain an increased understanding about how the systems work and interact and to model the dynamics of certain diseases and possible therapies.

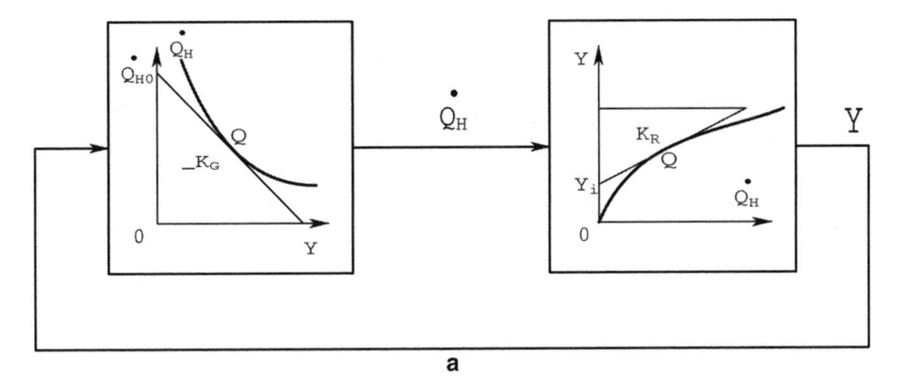

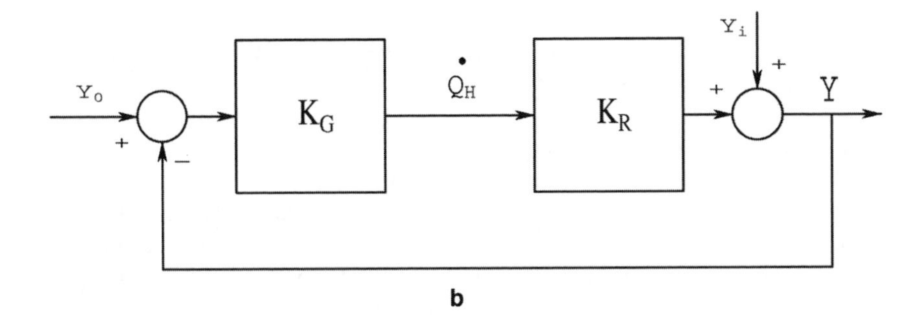

FIGURE 9.2

(a) A hypothetical, nonlinear, static, single feedback-loop, hormonal regulatory system. (b) The hormone regulator is linearized around its operating points and is configured as a linear, SISO control system. Y_o is the equivalent setpoint. (Northrop, R.B. 2000. *Endogenous and Exogenous Regulation and Control of Physiological Systems.* CRC Press, Boca Raton. With permission.)

9.3 Some Properties of Nonlinear Systems

Section 2.1 described the properties of LTI systems. In this section, we examine the attributes of *nonlinear systems,* with special attention to physiological and biochemical systems.

If a steady-state (SS) sinusoidal input is given to a dynamic LTI system, then the output is a sinusoid of the same frequency but with (in general) different phase and amplitude. The SS sinusoidal frequency response is a reliable and robust descriptor of a LTI system. When a NLTI system is given an SS sinusoidal input, the output will generally be periodic, but generally not sinusoidal. Hence, a Bode plot is generally not a valid descriptor for an NLS. However, the SS periodic output of a NLTIS can be written as a Fourier series, showing the existence of the fundamental frequency and higher-order harmonics. The amplitude distribution of the harmonics will, in general, depend on the nonlinearity and the amplitude and frequency of the sinusoidal input signal.

A nonlinear system can also generate *intermodulation distortion* terms at its output, given an input $x(t)$ which is the sum of two or more sinusoids of different frequencies. The intermodulation process can be illustrated by assuming the NLTI system to be characterized by a third-order power law *static nonlinearity:*

$$y = g(x) = a_0 + a_1 x^1 + a_2 x^2 + a_3 x^3 \tag{9.5}$$

If we let $x(t) = [b_1 \sin(\omega_1 t) + b_2 \sin(\omega_2 t)]$, then the output can be written:

$$\begin{aligned} y(t) = a_0 &+ a_1 [b_1 \sin(\omega_1 t) + b_2 \sin(\omega_2 t)] \\ &+ a_2 [b_1^2 \sin^2(\omega_1 t) + 2 b_1 b_2 \sin(\omega_1 t) \sin(\omega_2 t) + b_2^2 \sin^2(\omega_2 t)] \\ &+ a_3 [b_1^3 \sin^3(\omega_1 t) + b_2^3 \sin^3(\omega_2 t) + 3 b_1^2 b_2 \sin^2(\omega_1 t) \sin(\omega_2 t) \\ &+ 3 b_1 b_2^2 \sin(\omega_1 t) \sin^2(\omega_2 t)] \end{aligned} \tag{9.6}$$

From trig identities, we see that $y(t)$ not only contains terms at the input frequencies, but also dc terms, plus terms with frequencies of: $(\omega_1 - \omega_2)$, $(\omega_1 + \omega_2)$, $2\omega_1$, $2\omega_2$, $3\omega_1$, $3\omega_2$, $(2\omega_1 - \omega_2)$, $(2\omega_1 + \omega_2)$, $(2\omega_2 - \omega_1)$, and $(2\omega_2 + \omega_1)$. (The situation becomes even more complex if an x^4 term is present.)

Certain kinds of NLS given a SS sinusoidal input are seen to generate exact *subharmonics* at their outputs. (See Northrop (2000) for an example of a subharmonic dynamic, NLS.) The output behavior of nonlinear systems is generally dependent on the initial conditions and the input amplitude and frequency. Other types of nonlinear systems can exhibit input-dependent or initial condition-dependent *output limit cycles* that are bounded periodic oscillations of the output. An NLS can also exhibit input amplitude-dependent damping, where the system's output in response to an input step shows progressively less damping as the input amplitude is increased. In some cases, the damping can go to zero or have a negative value, causing an unbounded (unstable) output. Initial conditions can also determine whether an NLS's response is stable, oscillatory or unbounded for a given input. The complexity of NLSs is fascinating because their behavior can be counter-intuitive. For example, experimentally increasing the concentration of a certain hormone can cause a system output to increase, rather than to decrease as expected. In such cases, it is clear that our model of the system must be revised.

The nonlinearity in an NLS can often be modeled by a functional nonlinearity in series with otherwise linear dynamics. The functional nonlinearity can be half-wave rectification, otherwise known as nonnegativity, common to all physiological concentrations, or it can be a soft, odd, saturating nonlinearity such as $y = A\tanh(bx) = A(1 - e^{-2bx})/(1 + e^{-2bx}) \cong A[(bx) - (bx)^3/3 + (2/15)(bx)^5 - (17/315)(bx)^7 + \cdots]$. Many physiological systems exhibit rate saturation. For example, the steady-state secretion rate of a gland in response to a hormone concentration, [H], can be written as the (hyperbolic) *Hill function:*

$$\dot{Q}_G = \frac{[H]\, Q_{GMAX}\, K}{(1 + [H]K)}, \text{ for } [H] > 0. \tag{9.7}$$

For $K[H] >> 1$, $\dot{Q}_G \to \dot{Q}_{GMAX}$.

To be nonlinear, a NLS need not have a specific functional nonlinearity. The nonlinear behavior can be due to a set of nonlinear ODEs. This is generally the case in modeling physiological systems involving chemical kinetics. Such state equations can contain terms that have products of states and states raised to integral powers. These ODEs can be mathematically "stiff," which means that certain terms can $\rightarrow 0$ while other terms are very large. There are often problems in the numerical solutions of sets of stiff ODEs; special integration routines must be used to prevent numerical over- and underflows [Hultquist, 1988].

In conclusion, we wish to stress that nature gives us nonlinear, noisy and time-variable closed-loop physiological systems. Modeling such systems used to require linearization and severe order reduction. Now, computer simulations allow us to tackle reasonable complexity (high system order), nonlinearity, noise and time-varying coefficients directly, preserving the interesting and often unexpected counterintuitive behavior of complex nonlinear systems.

9.4 Physical Factors Determining the Dynamic Behavior of Physiological Systems

9.4.1 Diffusion dynamics

On a microscopic scale, all physiological systems contain cells, and molecules and ions suspended or dissolved in physiological fluids (in the cytosol and extracellular fluid). The molecules and ions are in constant random motion as the thermodynamic result of being above 0 Kelvin. In general, the higher the temperature, the more rapid and chaotic their movement, and the higher the pressure the particles can exert on the walls of their containers by elastic collisions. The molecules and ions, through their random movements, can also collide with like or different molecules and ions. In such collisions, chemical reactions can occur, or a transfer of momentum can occur in which electrostatic and internuclear forces play a role.

In physiological systems, Fick's Laws for *diffusion* describe the *average* or *bulk movement* of ions or molecules in response to concentration gradients set up by chemical reactions producing source or sink conditions for the ions or molecules in a volume. Physiological diffusion generally occurs through cell membranes. The ions or molecules generally pass through the membrane at discrete sites, through protein receptors or, "pores," that may have specificity for a particular species of ion or molecule. If the protein pores combine either physically or chemically with the ion or molecule diffusing through the membrane, the process is called *facilitated-* or *carrier-mediated diffusion* [Guyton, 1991]. If we plot the rate of diffusion, **J**, (ng/min/μ m^2) of a molecule or ion vs. the concentration difference across the membrane, we see that **J** saturates above a critical concentration difference. This saturation is a nonlinear behavior, and may be due to: (a) The finite number of diffusion sites or areas on the membrane or (b) The molecular processes whereby an ion or molecule binds to the receptor molecule(s) causing a configurational change that transports the ion or molecule across the membrane slowly, i.e., the actual transport process is rate-limiting [Guyton, 1991, p42].

In some cases, a *second* molecule or ion, a *messenger,* if present, can modulate the permeability of the pore, producing *ligand gated diffusion.* For example, the hormone insulin increases the diffusion for glucose molecules at glucose pore sites. In the presence of insulin, the bulk permeability for glucose (in insulin-sensitive cells) rises, increasing the rate of diffusion of glucose into those cells. In this case, insulin acts as a *parametric control* substance. The glucose diffuses from a higher extracellular concentration to a lower intracellular concentration. Other types of pores can be opened by a change in the transmembrane potential difference, producing *voltage-gated diffusion.* Voltage-gated diffusion figures largely in the generation of nerve impulses, or in their inhibition and in the triggering of muscle contraction.

In deriving a quantitative description of simple diffusion, we consider the one-dimensional model shown in Figure 9.3. The tube has cross-sectional area A. The concentration of a molecule S at x_1 is C_1; at x_2 it is C_2. Let $C_1 > C_2$. We assume that the probability of a molecule of S jumping in either $-x$ or $+x$ direction is equal.

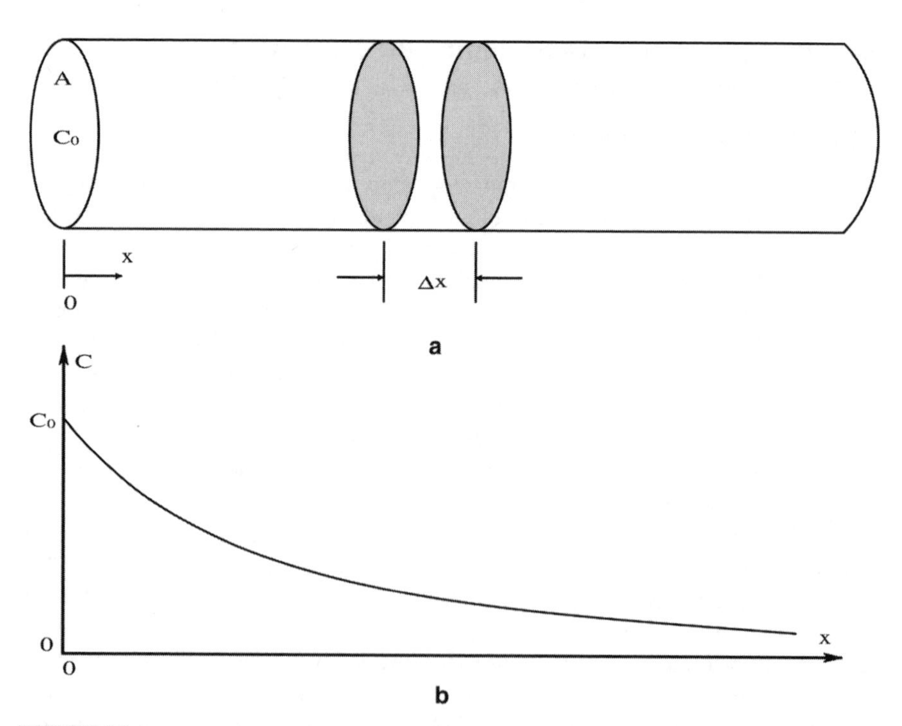

FIGURE 9.3

Geometrical model relevant to the derivation of 1-D diffusion using Fick's law. (Northrop, R.B. 2000. *Endogenous and Exogenous Regulation and Control of Physiological Systems.* CRC Press, Boca Raton. With permission.)

Furthermore, the mass/time of S going from plane 1 to plane 2 is proportional to C_1 @ x_1. Likewise, the mass/time going from plane 2 to 1 is proportional to C_2 @ x_2. The mass rates are also proportional to A. Thus, we can write:

$$\frac{\Delta m}{\Delta t} = \beta A(C_1 - C_2) = -\beta A \Delta C \text{ mg/min.} \tag{9.8}$$

β is approximated by $k/(x_2 - x_1) = k/\Delta x$. $\Delta C \equiv (C_2 - C_1) < 0$.
Substituting this relation into Equation 9.8 and letting the Δs approach 0, we can write:

$$\frac{\partial m}{\partial t} = -kA\frac{\partial C}{\partial x} \tag{9.9}$$

In the above one-dimensional diffusion equation, m is the mass diffusing, k is Fick's constant with dimensions L^2T^{-1}, and $\partial C/\partial x$ is the concentration gradient in the $-x$ direction. When a thin membrane separates C_1 and C_2, the diffusion equation can be simplified to:

$$\dot{m} = -kA\Delta C = kA(C_1 - C_2) \text{ mg/min.} \tag{9.10}$$

Because cells individually have small intracellular volumes compared with the total extracellular volume, the prolonged influx of m will raise C_2, lowering the concentration difference across the membrane, hence reducing the diffusion rate, dm/dt. If nothing happens to m once it diffuses into the cell, eventually, $C_2 = C_1$ in the steady-state, and dm/dt = 0.

The diffusion equation can be put in a general, 3-D form [Ackerman, 1962]:

$$\frac{\partial c}{\partial t} = k\left[\frac{\partial^2 c}{\partial x^2} + \frac{\partial^2 c}{\partial y^2} + \frac{\partial^2 c}{\partial z^2}\right] \tag{9.11}$$

Here c is the volume distribution of concentration at time $t, c = c(x,y,z,t)$. In vector notation, Equation 9.11 becomes:

$$\frac{\partial c}{\partial t} = k\nabla^2 c \tag{9.12}$$

The mass current density is defined as:

$$\mathbf{J} \equiv \left(\frac{1}{A}\frac{\partial m}{\partial t}\right)\mathbf{n} = k\nabla c \text{ (kg/sec)/m}^2 \tag{9.13}$$

Where **n** is a unit vector normal to the surface A. If the molecule diffusing is being manufactured in a region in x,y,z space at some rate per unit volume, we can write the *inhomogeneous diffusion equation:*

$$\frac{\partial c}{\partial t} = k\nabla^2 c + q(x,y,z) \tag{9.14}$$

Note that some diffusion equations are written in terms of mass/time and others in terms of concentration/time; concentration is simply mass/volume. In most descriptions of diffusion in physiological modeling, we try to use the simple approach as shown in Equation 9.10.

9.4.2 Biochemical systems and mass-action kinetics

Biochemical reactions, such as the regulated synthesis of hormones and proteins, underlie nearly all physiological regulatory and control processes. All chemical reactions proceed at rates governed by the concentrations of the reactants, the presence of a catalyst or enzyme, the temperature of the reaction and by the number of molecules of reactants required to produce a molecule of product. One underlying assumption in formulating *mass-action* descriptions of chemical kinetics is that the reactants are uniformly distributed (in a compartment) and are free to move around and collide with a probability that is proportional to their concentration(s). Another assumption is that mass-action formulations are based on large numbers of molecules interacting; mass action is therefore a bulk formulation of chemical behavior [Maron and Prutton, 1958]. In reality, some biochemical reactions occur between a finite number of molecules fixed in space, such as receptor proteins bound to a cell membrane, and large molecules in solution, such as hormones.

It will be seen that modeling the behavior of chemical mass action systems generally involves solutions of nonlinear ODEs. Thus, dynamic solutions are best done by computer simulation. We will give some simple examples here that illustrate the procedures to be used and also some typical biochemical reaction architectures.

9.4.2.1 Examples of mass action kinetics

1. First, let us consider a bimolecular reaction in which one molecule of A combines irreversibly with one molecule of B to form one molecule of product, C. That is, in chemical notation: $A+B \xrightarrow{k_1} C$. In the first kinetic formulation, we start at $t=0$ with a Moles of A, b Moles of B, and 0 C. $x=$ moles of C are made at time t. Using the theory of *mass action* we can write the nonlinear ODE:

$$\dot{x}=k_1(a-x)(b-x)=k_1[ab-x(a+b)+x^2] \tag{9.15}$$

   k_1 is a reaction rate constant, generally a function of Kelvin temperature, and enzyme concentration.

2. A second example of mass action kinetics is given for the *reversible oxidation* of nitrogen oxide: The chemistry is:

$$2NO+O_2 \underset{k_2}{\overset{k_1}{\rightleftharpoons}} 2NO_2 \tag{9.16}$$

$$\begin{aligned} \text{Let}: k_1 &= \text{forward rate constant.} \\ k_2 &= \text{reverse rate constant.} \\ a &= \text{initial concentration NO.} \\ b &= \text{initial concentration } O_2. \\ x &= \text{amount of } O_2 \text{ reacted at t.} \end{aligned}$$

The forward reaction rate is: $\dot{x}_f = k_1(a-2x)^2(b-x)$ (9.17A)

The reverse reaction rate is: $\dot{x}_r = k_2(2x)^2$ (9.17B)

The net reaction rate is the difference: $\dot{x}_{net} = \dot{x}_f - \dot{x}_r = k_1(a-2x)^2(b-x) - k_2(2x)^2$ (9.17C)

(Note that, when two molecules react, the concentration is squared; when three molecules react, it is cubed. The ODE above is very nonlinear.)

3. For a third example, we consider the physiologically important formation and decomposition of carbonic acid:

$$H_2CO_3 \underset{k_R}{\overset{k_F}{\Leftarrow\!\Rightarrow}} H_2O + CO_2 \quad (9.18)$$

Let x = concentration of carbonic acid, w = concentration of water, g = concentration of dissolved CO_2. Thus, we can write for the rate of appearance of carbonic acid:

$$\dot{x} = -k_F x + k_R(wg) \quad (9.19)$$

The rate of appearance of CO_2 is simply:

$$\dot{g} = +k_F x - k_R(wg) = -\dot{x} \quad (9.20)$$

If water is present in excess, then the w factor can be eliminated from the ODEs above and its effect incorporated in k_R.

4. In a fourth example, we examine a typical biochemical "two-step" reaction in which two reactants combine reversibly to form a *complex,* and then the complex is rapidly converted to the end-product, with the release of the E-reactant unchanged. (The E-reactant can be an enzyme.) The product P decays at rate k_4P. This reaction form follows the well-known *Michaelis-Menten* architecture [Godfrey, 1983; Mathews and van Holde, 1990].

$$X + E \underset{k_2}{\overset{k_1}{\Leftarrow\!\Rightarrow}} E*X \xrightarrow{k_3} E + P \xrightarrow{k_4} * \quad (9.21)$$

Where: x_1 = running concentration of substrate X; u = running concentration of free enzyme, E; x_2 = running concentration of complex, E*X; x_3 = running concentration of product P; k_1, k_2, k_3 = reaction rate constants. The reaction is assumed to take place in a closed vessel, so enzyme will be conserved. That is, $u_o = u + x_2$ or $u = u_o - x_2$. The nonlinear mass-action ODEs can be written:

$$\dot{x}_1 = -k_1(u_o - x_2)x_1 + k_2 x_2 \quad (9.22A)$$

$$\dot{x}_2 = k_1(u_o - x_2)x_1 - (k_2 + k_3)x_2 \quad (9.22B)$$

$$\dot{x}_3 = k_3 x_2 - k_4 x_3 \quad (9.22C)$$

From enzyme conservation, we see that $x_2 = -\dot{u}$. If we assume steady-state conditions, $\dot{x}_1 = \dot{x}_2 = \dot{x}_3 = 0$, and we have:

$$x_{2SS} = \frac{k_1 x_1 u_o}{(k_2 + k_3) + k_1 x_1} = \frac{x_1 u_o}{x_1 + K_M} \tag{9.23}$$

Where $K_M \equiv (k_2 + k_3)/k_1$ is the well-known (to biochemists) *Michaelis constant.*

If we set $x_1 \equiv x_{10}$ (constant) and $u \equiv u_o$ (constant) and again assume steady-state conditions where all derivative terms $\to 0$, the equilibrium concentration of P is easily shown to be:

$$x_{3ss} = \frac{k_3 x_2}{k_4} = \frac{k_3}{k_4} \frac{k_1 u_o x_{10}}{(k_2 + k_3)} = \frac{k_3 u_o x_{10}}{k_4 K_M} \tag{9.24}$$

It is clear that dynamic solutions of the three Michaelis-Menton ODEs (two are nonlinear) are best done by computer simulation.

5. As a fifth example, consider a compartment surrounded by a diffusion membrane. (Perhaps this is a cell.) In the compartment is an enzyme in excess concentration that catalyzes the reversible transformation of A into B. Furthermore, A must diffuse into the compartment, and B diffuses out. The concentration of A outside the membrane is a_o; inside the compartment it is a. Likewise, the concentration of B outside the compartment is b_o, and it is b inside (refer to Figure 9.4). The rate of increase of A and B inside the

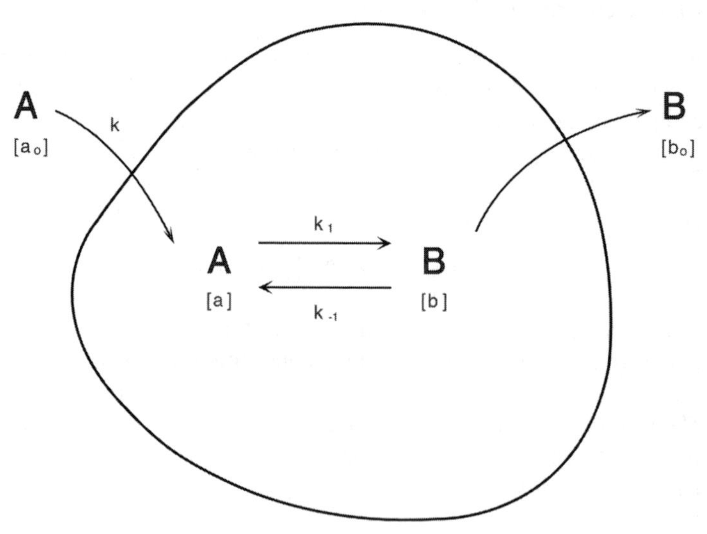

FIGURE 9.4

Linear diffusion/mass-action system of the fifth mass-action example in the text. (Northrop, R.B. 2000. *Endogenous and Exogenous Regulation and Control of Physiological Systems.* CRC Press, Boca Raton. With permission.)

compartment is thus governed by both mass action and diffusion. The ODEs are:

$$\dot{a} = K_{da}(a_o - a) + k_{-1}b - k_1 a \qquad \text{kg/sec} \tag{9.25A}$$

$$\dot{b} = -K_{db}(b - b_o) + k_1 a - k_{-1}b \qquad \text{kg/sec} \tag{9.25B}$$

K_{da} and K_{db} are diffusion rate constants. The k_1 and k_{-1} terms relate to simple mass-action. Note that, in this special case, *the system is linear,* and can be solved for its states, a and b, using conventional linear algebraic methods and Laplace transforms, or signal flow graphs.

Diffusion and mass-action dynamics are often necessarily used together to describe intracellular biochemical events, such as the synthesis of a hormone in response to a signal from a control hormone. The control hormone must enter the cell, and the synthesized hormone must diffuse out through the cell's membrane to enter the bloodstream in order to reach its intended remote target cells. In addition, reaction substrates, such as glucose and oxygen, must diffuse into the cell. The mass-action dynamics governing the hormone's synthesis are generally nonlinear and high-order; no simple Laplace solution is possible, as in example 5 above.

6. In a sixth example, consider the hypothetical situation where there is a finite number, N, of cell membrane receptors per unit volume. At any instant, there is a density F of free receptors which can bind with molecules of an input hormone, H_1, to form a complex. Once bound, the complex initiates the biosynthesis and release of a *second messenger hormone,* H_2. The complex is broken down enzymatically to release an inactivated input hormone molecule, $\overline{H_1}$, and a free membrane receptor. Intuitively, we see that this system will saturate for high concentration of H_1. That is, there can be no further increase in the rate at which H_2 is produced because nearly all of the free receptors are complexed at any time. These processes can be represented by the reactions:

$$H_1 + F \underset{k_2}{\overset{k_1}{\Leftarrow\!\Rightarrow}} H_1^*F \xrightarrow{k_3} \overline{H_1} + F \tag{9.26A}$$

$$H_1^*F \xrightarrow{k_4} H_2 \xrightarrow{k_5} * \tag{9.26B}$$

The total number of receptors $N = f + b$. f is the number of free receptors; b is the number of receptors complexed with H_1. The system's mass-action equations are:

$$\dot{b} = -(k_2 + k_3)b + k_1 h_1 f = -(k_2 + k_3)b + k_1 h_1 (N - b) \tag{9.27A}$$

$$\dot{h}_2 = -k_5 h_2 + k_4 b \tag{9.27B}$$

In the steady state, we see from Equation 9.27A above that for $h_1 >> K_M$.:

$$b_{SS} = N h_1/(h_1 + K_M) \longrightarrow N \tag{9.28}$$

As before, K_M is the Michaelis constant for the system. Also:

$$h_{2SS} = k_4 b_{SS}/k_5 \quad (9.29)$$

So the concentration of H_2 exhibits saturation as a function of H_1, as well. Remember that use of mass action kinetics depends on the assumptions that large numbers of molecules of a given species are uniformly distributed in a volume (e.g., test tube, flask) where the reaction is taking place. As we remarked above, many biochemical reactions take place on fixed cell membrane surfaces or in organelles such as mitochondria, where concentration gradients of reactants and products can exist. Such gradients invoke diffusion dynamics in addition to mass action ODEs. This latter situation is generally neglected in modeling because of the inhomogeneity of tissues surrounding the cell membranes in question.

9.5 Means of Characterizing Physiological Systems

9.5.1 Introduction

Ideally, we would like to represent a physiological system's dynamics by a detailed linear model which contains many ODEs and states. In practice, we often have access to only the system's output, and input. An important goal is to be able to deduce using I/O information as much about the internal physical, biochemical, biomechanical, and physiological mechanisms of the system as we can.

A central problem in the analysis (and modeling) of nonlinear physiological systems is what model structure to assume. That is, can the system be modeled by an LTI system, or an LTI system followed by a static no-memory nonlinearity, such as a soft [tanh(x)] saturation, or does the nonlinearity precede the LTI part? Also, what is the order of the system (i.e., how many states)? Another architecture for an open-loop NLS was described by Marmarelis and Marmarelis (1978), who placed a no-memory power law nonlinearity *between* two LTI blocks.

Stark (1968) used both transient and sinusoidal inputs to study the closed-loop and open-loop behavior of the human pupil regulator for retinal light flux, and the human lens accommodation control system. In the latter, Stark noted discrepancies in the closed-loop system's response delay to transient (step) inputs, and the phase lag in the response to sinusoidal inputs. He reported a 360 msec delay to the step changes in target radial position, but the accommodation phase lag when keeping a sinusoidally moving target in focus was found to require only a 100 msec time lag. Stark explained this discrepancy by postulating the presence of a CNS *predictor block* that operated when a periodic input was present. Such a predictor at first consideration appears to not be physically realizable (it is noncausal). However, for a stationary periodic input of fixed frequency, we note that a realizeable 270° delay is equivalent to a 90° predictor. (Effective predictors are also found in the lateral gaze control system, and in visual-motor control tasks such as manual target tracking). Stark used *describing function analysis* to approximate an odd saturation-type nonlinearity that preceded an LTI low-pass element in the closed-loop model.

9.5.2 The Nyquist stability criterion

This section describes the application and limitations of the venerable *Nyquist test* for the stability of single-loop LTI SISO feedback systems. The Nyquist test is based on the steady-state sinusoidal frequency response of the system's loop gain function, and is well suited for analysis based on experimental frequency response data. The Nyquist test is also directly related to the use of *describing functions* in the analysis and design of certain nonlinear control systems in which an algebraic odd nonlinear function is separable from linear low-pass dynamics in the control system's loop gain [Ogata, 1970].

To introduce the Nyquist test for closed-loop system stability, we call attention to the conventional SISO LTI feedback system shown in Figure 9.5. In this system, no minus sign assumption is made at the summing point. The closed-loop system transfer function is simply:

$$\frac{Y}{X}(s) = \frac{G(s)}{[1 - A_L(s)]} \tag{9.30}$$

In this negative feedback system, the loop gain, $A_L(s) = -G(s)H(s)$, so we have finally:

$$\frac{Y}{X}(s) = \frac{G(s)}{[1 + G(s)H(s)]} \tag{9.31}$$

The denominator of the closed-loop transfer function is called the *return difference,* $F(s) = [1 + G(s)H(s)]$. If $F(s)$ is a rational polynomial, then clearly *its zeros are the poles of the closed-loop system function.* The Nyquist test effectively examines the zeros of $F(s)$ to see if any lie in the right-half s plane. Know that one or more poles of the closed-loop system in the right-half s-plane produces unstable behavior. In

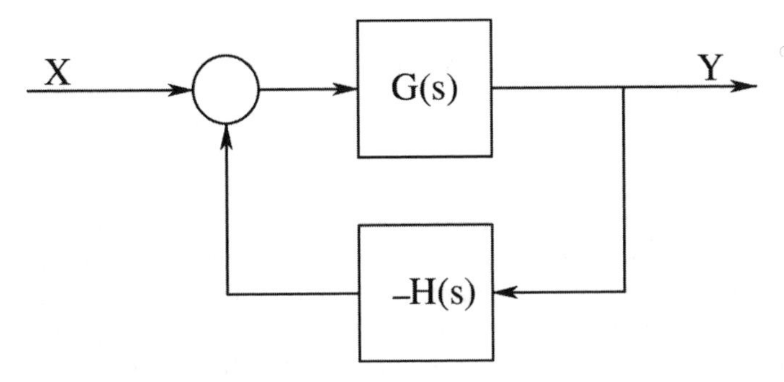

FIGURE 9.5
A simple SISO LTI feedback system.

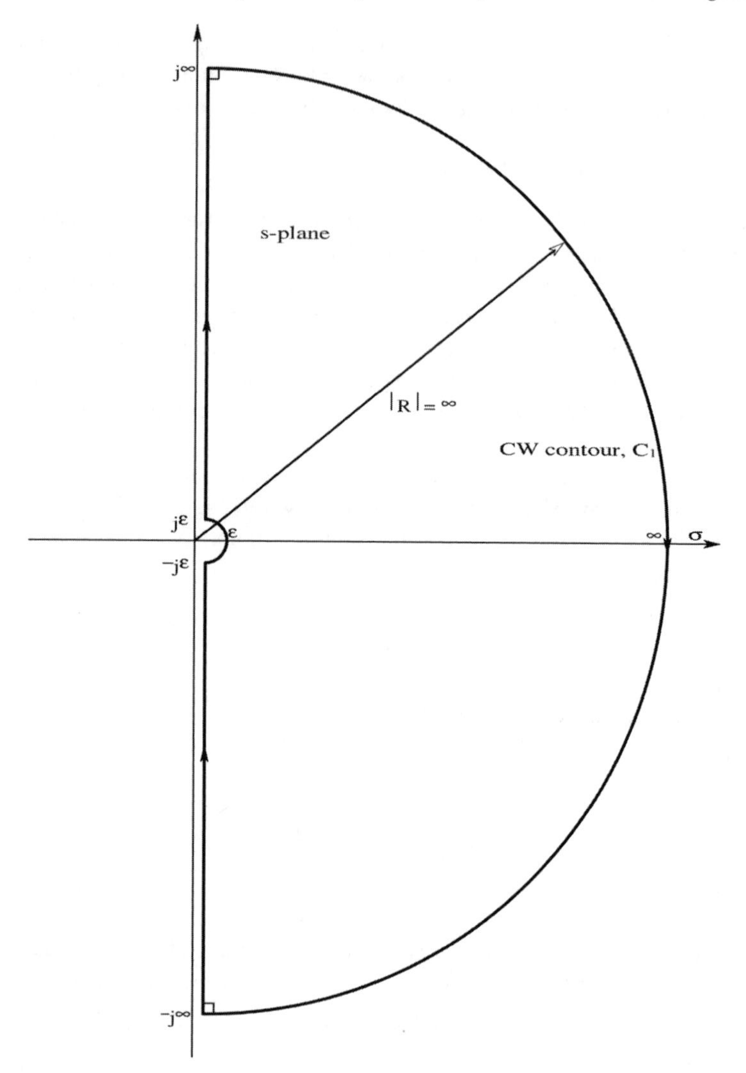

FIGURE 9.6
The clockwise contour C_1 in the **s**-plane used to define the complex s vector used in conformal mapping the vector, $\mathbf{A_L(s)}$, into the polar plane.

practice, it is more convenient to work with $A_L(s) = 1 - F(s)$, and see if there are (vector) **s** values that make $\mathbf{A_L(s)} \to 1\angle 0°$. The Nyquist test uses a process known as *conformal mapping* to examine the poles and zeros of $A_L(s)$, hence the zeros of $F(s)$. In the conformal mapping process used in the Nyquist test, the vector **s** lies on the contour shown in Figure 9.6. This contour encloses the entire right-half s-plane in a clockwise encirclement. The infinitesimal semicircle to the left of the origin is to avoid any poles of $A_L(s)$ at the origin. Because the test is a vector test, $A_L(s)$ is written in *vector difference form. For example:*

$$A_L(s) = \underset{\textit{Factored Laplace form}}{\frac{K(s+a)}{(s+b)(s+c)}} \longrightarrow \mathbf{A_L(s)} = \underset{\textit{Vector difference form}}{\frac{-K(s-s_1)}{(s-s_2)(s-s_3)}} = \underset{\textit{Vector polar form}}{\frac{K|\mathbf{A}|}{|\mathbf{B}|\,|\mathbf{C}|}\angle\theta_a - \theta_b - \theta_c - \pi} \tag{9.32}$$

The convention used in this text places a (net) minus sign in the numerator of the loop gain when the feedback system uses negative feedback. In this example, the vectors $\mathbf{s_1} = -a$, $\mathbf{s_2} = -b$ and $\mathbf{s_3} = -c$ are negative real numbers. In practice, **s** has values lying on the contour shown in Figure 9.6. The vector differences $(\mathbf{s} - \mathbf{s_1}) = \mathbf{A}, (\mathbf{s} - \mathbf{s_2}) = \mathbf{B}$ and $(\mathbf{s} - \mathbf{s_3}) = \mathbf{C}$ are shown for $\mathbf{s} = j\omega_1$ in Figure 9.7. For each **s** value on the contour C_1, there is a corresponding vector value, $\mathbf{A_L(s)}$. A fundamental theorem in conformal mapping says that if the vector **s** assumes values on the closed contour, C_1, then the $\mathbf{A_L(s)}$ vector will also generate a closed contour, the nature of which depends on its poles and zeros.

Before continuing with the treatment of the vector loop gain, let us go back to the vector return difference, $\mathbf{F(s)} = \mathbf{1} - \mathbf{A_L(s)}$, and examine the Nyquist test done on the $F(s)$ of an *unstable* system. Assume:

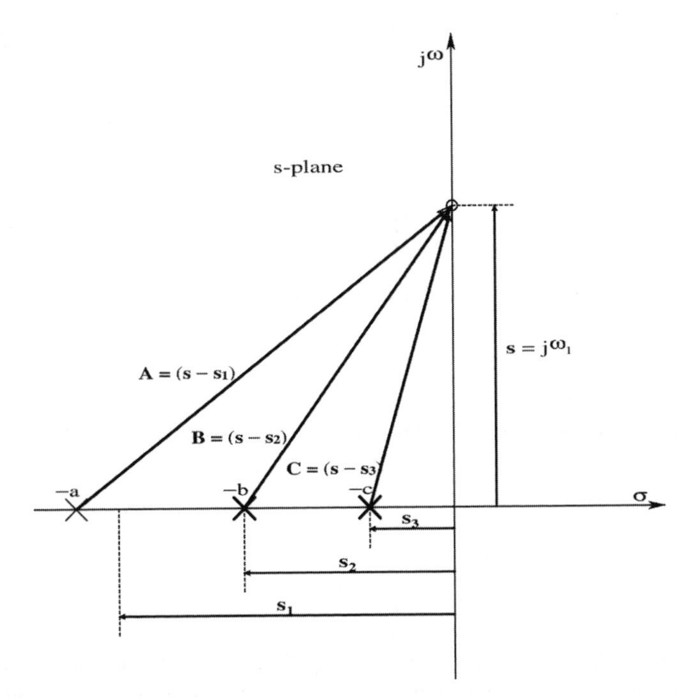

FIGURE 9.7

Vector differences in the s-plane used to calculate $A_L(s)$. In this case, $s = j\omega_1$ on the contour C_1. The infinitesimal semicircle around $s = 0$ is to avoid any singularity of $\mathbf{A_L(s)}$ at the origin. (Northrop, R.B. 2000. *Endogenous and Exogenous Regulation and Control of Physiological Systems.* CRC Press, Boca Raton. With permission.)

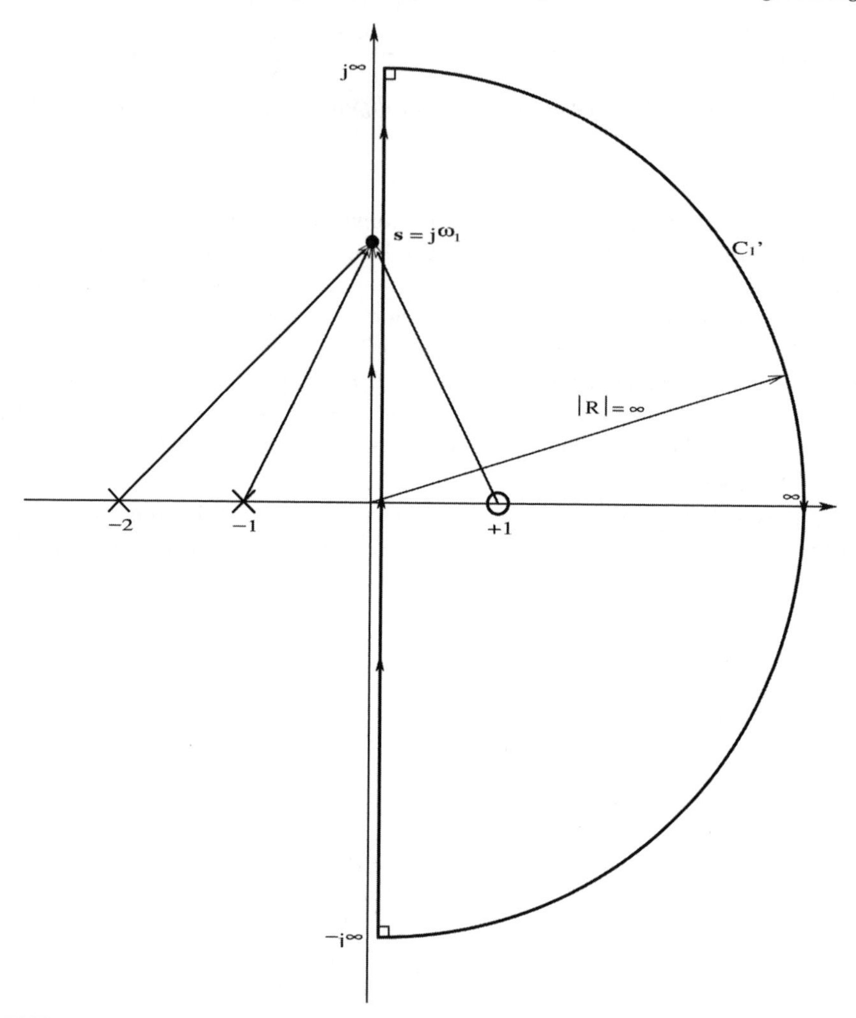

FIGURE 9.8
The vector differences $(\mathbf{s}-\mathbf{s_1})$, $(\mathbf{s}-\mathbf{s_2})$ and $(\mathbf{s}-\mathbf{s_3})$ used in Equation 9.33 for **F(s)**. Note the right-half s-plane zero.

$$\mathrm{F(s)} = \frac{\mathrm{K(s-1)}}{\mathrm{(s+2)(s+1)}} \rightarrow \mathbf{F(s)} = \frac{\mathrm{K}(\mathbf{s}-\mathbf{s_1})}{(\mathbf{s}-\mathbf{s_2})(\mathbf{s}-\mathbf{s_3})} \tag{9.33}$$

Recall that a right-half s-plane zero of F(s) is a right-half (unstable) pole of the closed-loop system. **s** assumes values on the contour C_1' in Figure 9.8. Note that C_1' does not need the infinitesimal semicircle around the origin of the s-plane because F(s) has no poles or zeros at the origin. Note that, as **s** goes from $\mathbf{s} = j0+$ to $\mathbf{s} = +j\infty$, the angle of $\mathbf{F(s)}$ goes from $+180°$ to $-90°$, and $|\mathbf{F(s)}$ goes from K/2 to 0. When $|\mathrm{s}| = \infty$, $|\mathbf{F(s)}| = 0$ and its angle goes from $-90°$ to $+90°$ at $\mathrm{s} = -j\infty$. The **F(s)**

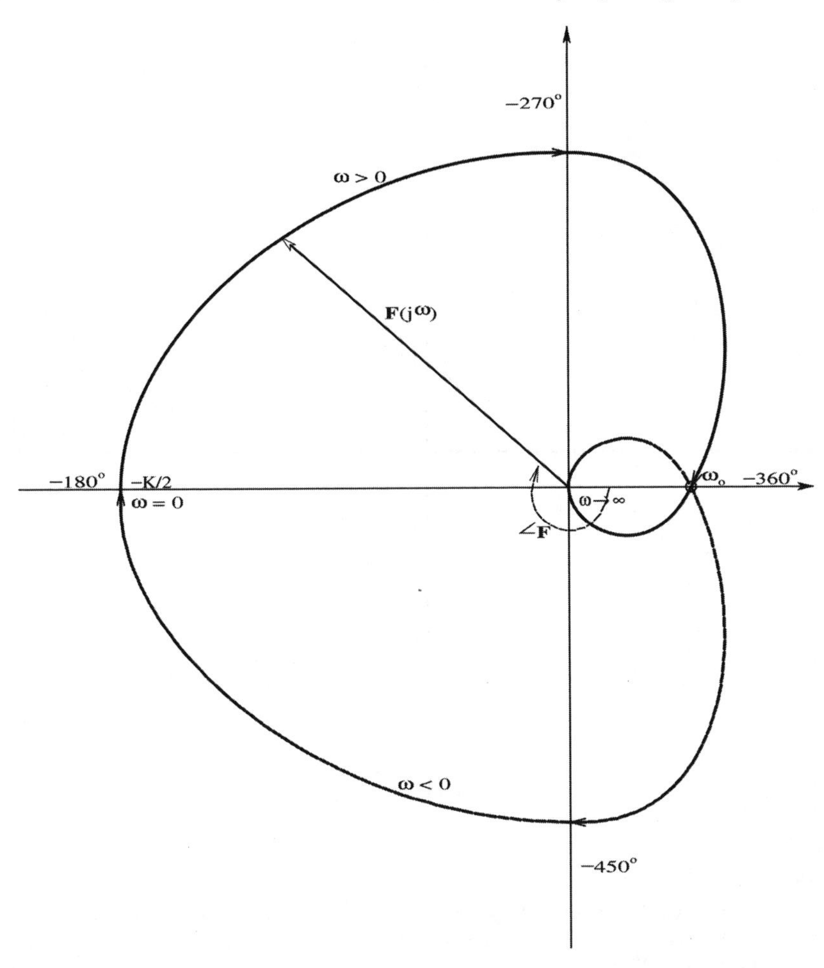

FIGURE 9.9
Polar vector plot of $\mathbf{F}(\mathbf{s})$ as the vector **s** assumes values around the contour C_1' shown in Figure 9.8.

vector contour in the $\mathbf{F}(\mathbf{s})$ plane is shown in Figure 9.9. Note that the vector contour for $\mathbf{s} = -j\omega$ values is the mirror image of the contour for $\mathbf{s} = +j\omega$ values. We also see in this case that the complete $\mathbf{F}(\mathbf{s})$ contour (for all **s** values on C_1' traversed in a *clockwise* direction in the s-plane) makes one net *clockwise* encirclement of the origin in the **F(s)** plane. This encirclement is the result of the contour C_1' having enclosed the right-half s-plane zero of $F(s)$. The encirclement is the basis for the Nyquist test relation for the return difference:

$$Z = N_{CW} + P \tag{9.34}$$

Here Z is the number of right-half s-plane zeros of $F(s)$ *or* right-half s-plane poles of the closed-loop system's transfer function. Obviously, Z is desired to be zero. N_{CW} is the observed total number of clockwise encirclements of the *origin* by the **F(s)** contour. P is the *known* number of right-half s-plane poles of $F(s)$ (usually zero).

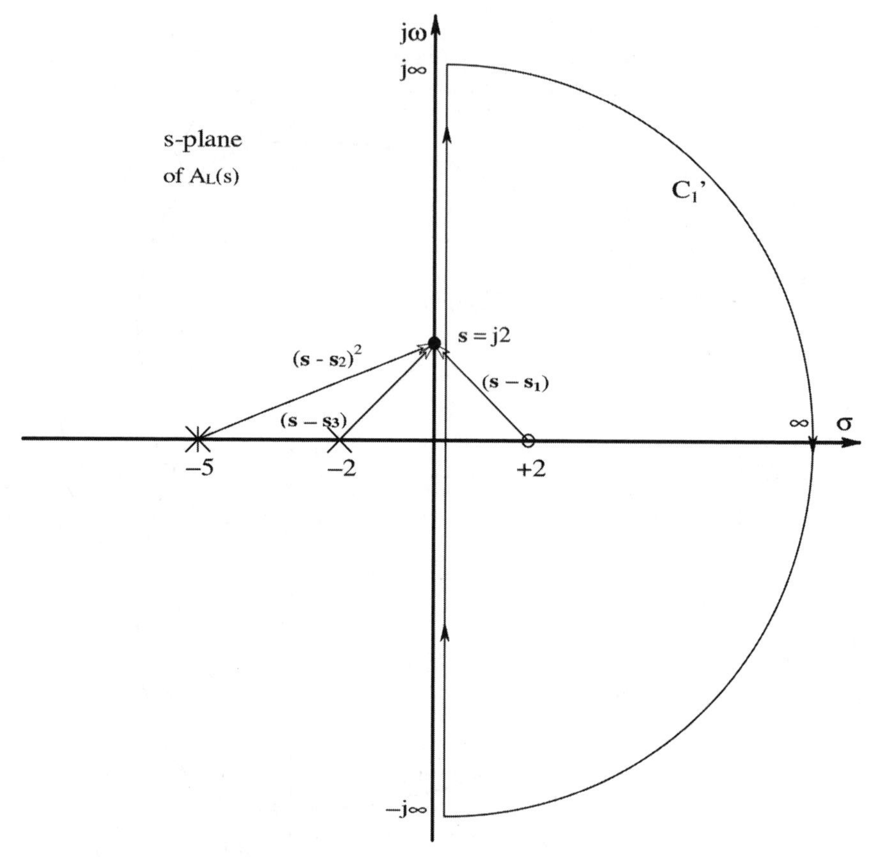

FIGURE 9.10
The vector differences in the s-plane for $\mathbf{A_L}(\mathbf{s})$ given by Equation 9.35. **s** has values defined by the contour, C_1'. (Northrop, R.B. 2000. *Endogenous and Exogenous Regulation and Control of Physiological Systems.* CRC Press, Boca Raton. With permission.)

Now we return to the consideration of the more useful loop gain transfer function, $A_L(s)$. Recall that, when $\mathbf{F(s)} = 0$, $\mathbf{A_L(s)} = +1$. For the *first example,* we take:

$$A_L(s) = \frac{-K(s-2)}{(s+5)^2(s+2)} \longrightarrow \mathbf{A_L(s)} = \frac{-K(\mathbf{s}-\mathbf{s_1})}{(\mathbf{s}-\mathbf{s_2})^2(\mathbf{s}-\mathbf{s_3})} \tag{9.35}$$

Figure 9.10 shows the s-plane with the poles and zeros of $A_L(s)$, the contour C_1', and the vector differences used in calculating $\mathbf{A_L(s)}$ as **s** traverses C_1' clockwise. Table 9.5.1 gives values of $|\mathbf{A_L(s)}|$ and $\angle \mathbf{A_L(s)}$ for **s** values on C_1'.

The polar plot of $\mathbf{A_L(s)}$ is shown in Figure 9.11. Since we are using $\mathbf{A_L(s)}$ instead of $\mathbf{F(s)}$, the point $\mathbf{A_L(s)} = +1$ is critical for encirclements, rather than the origin. The positive, real point of intersection occurs for **s** = j0. It is easily seen that if $K > 25$, there will be one net CW encirclement of the $+1$ point. We can modify the Nyquist conformal equation to:

TABLE 9.5.1
Values of $A_L(s)$ as s Traverses Contour C_1' Clockwise in the s-Plane

s	—$A_L(s)$—	$\angle A_L(s)$
$\pm j0$	$+K/25$	$0°$
$j2$	$K/29$	$-133.6°$
$j5$	$K/50$	$-226.4°$
$j\infty$	0	$-360°$
$+\infty$	0	$-180°$
$-j\infty$	0	$+360°$
$-j2$	$K/29$	$+133.6°$
$-j5$	$K/50$	$+226.4°$
$-j\infty$	0	$+360°$

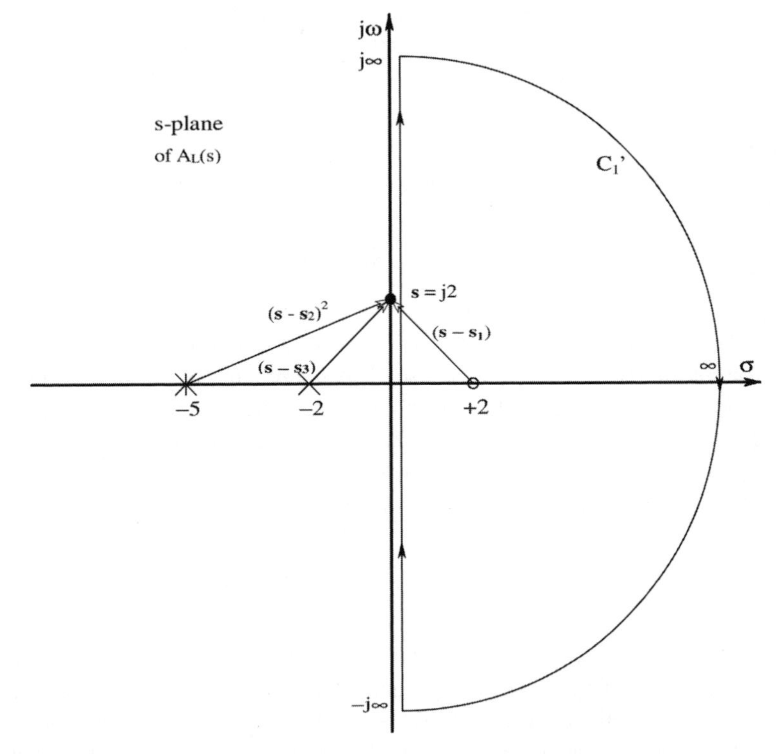

FIGURE 9.11
Polar vector plot of $A_L(s)$ as s assumes values around the contour C_1' shown in Figure 9.10. Note that the critical point $s = +1$ is encircled once clockwise if K ¿ 25 in Equation 9.35.

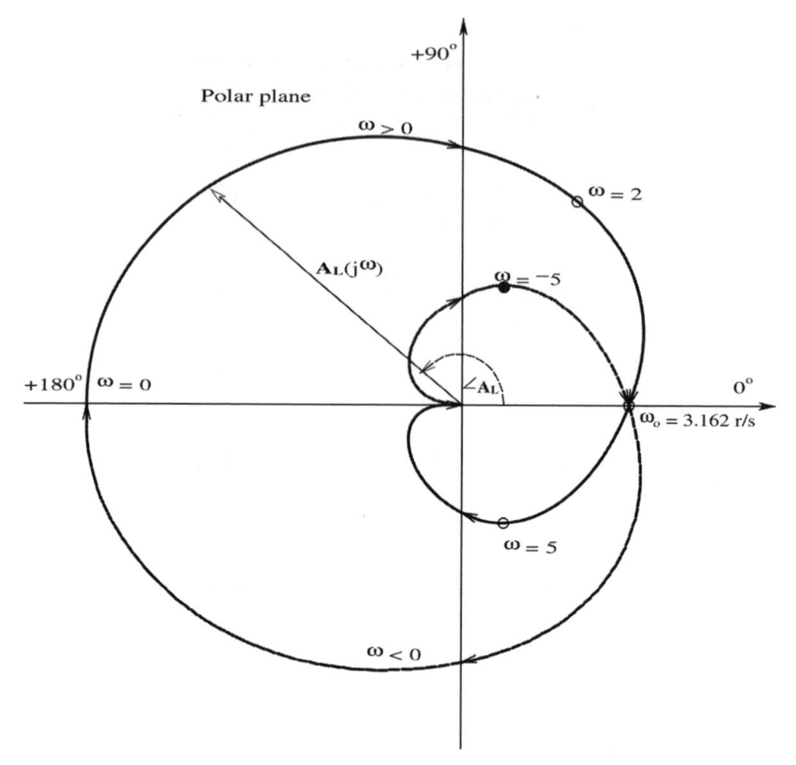

FIGURE 9.12
Polar vector plot of $\mathbf{A}_\mathrm{L}(\mathbf{s})$ for the second example.

$$\mathrm{P_{CL}} = \mathrm{N_{CW}} + \mathrm{P} \tag{9.36}$$

$\mathrm{P_{CL}}$ is the number of closed-loop system poles in the right-half s-plane (desired to be zero). $\mathrm{N_{CW}}$ is the total number of *clockwise* encirclements of $+1$ in the $\mathbf{A}_\mathrm{L}(\mathbf{s})$ plane as **s** traverses the contour C_1' clockwise. P is the number of poles of $\mathrm{A_L(s)}$ known *a priori* to be in the right-half s-plane. Thus, for the system of the first example, $\mathrm{P}=0$, and $\mathrm{N_{CW}}=1$ only if $\mathrm{K}>25$. The closed-loop system is seen to be unstable with one pole in the right-half s-plane when $\mathrm{K}>25$.

In the *second example,* we give the system of example 1 *positive feedback.* Thus:

$$\mathrm{A_L(s)} = \frac{+\mathrm{K(s-2)}}{\mathrm{(s+5)^2(s+2)}} \tag{9.37}$$

Figure 9.12 shows the polar plot of the positive feedback system's $\mathbf{A}_\mathrm{L}(\mathbf{s})$ as **s** traverses the contour C_1'. Now, we see that, if K exceeds a critical value, there will be *two* clockwise encirclements of $+1$, hence two closed-loop system poles will be in the right-half s-plane. Under these conditions, the instability will be a sinusoidal oscillation with an exponentially growing amplitude. To find the critical value of K for instability, it is convenient to first find the $\mathrm{s}=\mathrm{j}\omega_\mathrm{o}$ value at which the system will oscillate by examining the phase of $\mathbf{A_L}(j\omega_o)$ where $\mathbf{A_L}$ crosses the positive real axis:

$$-2\tan^{-1}(\omega_o/5) - \tan^{-1}(\omega_o/2) + [180° - \tan^{-1}(\omega_o/2)] = 0° \quad (9.38A)$$

$$-2\tan^{-1}(\omega_o/5) - 2\tan^{-1}(\omega_o/2) = -180° \quad (9.38B)$$

$$\tan^{-1}(\omega_o/5) + \tan^{-1}(\omega_o/2) = 90° \quad (9.38C)$$

Trial and error solution of Equation 9.38C yields $\omega_o = 3.162$ r/sec. Substitution of this ω_o value into $|\mathbf{A_L}(j\omega_o)| = +1$, and solving for K we get $K = 35.00$. Therefore, if $K > 35$, the closed-loop positive feedback system is unstable, having two net CW encirclements of $+1$ and thus a complex-conjugate pole pair in the right-half s-plane. Furthermore, the frequency of oscillation at the threshold of instability is $\omega_o = 3.162$ r/sec.

As a *third example* of the Nyquist stability criterion, we examine the Nyquist plot of a third-order negative feedback system with loop gain:

$$A_L(s) = \frac{-K\beta}{s(s+5)(s+2)} \quad (9.39)$$

This system has a pole at the origin, so in examining $\mathbf{A_L}(\mathbf{s})$, $\mathbf{s}$ must follow the contour C_1 having the infinitesimal semicircle of radius ε avoiding the origin. We will start at $\mathbf{s} = j\varepsilon$ and go to $\mathbf{s} = j\infty$. At $\mathbf{s} = j\varepsilon$, $|\mathbf{A}|_L(\mathbf{s})| \to \infty$, and $\angle \mathbf{A}_L = -270°$. As $\mathbf{s} \to j\infty$, $|\mathbf{A_L}(\mathbf{s})| \to 0$ and $\angle \mathbf{A}_L \to -450°$. Now when $\mathbf{s}$ traverses the ∞ radius semicircle on C_1, $|\mathbf{A_L}(\mathbf{s})| = 0$ and the phase goes through $0°$, thence to $+90°$, all with $|\mathbf{A_L}(\mathbf{s})| = 0$. Now as $\mathbf{s}$ goes from $-j\infty$ to $-j\varepsilon$, $|\mathbf{A_L}(\mathbf{s})|$ grows larger, and its phase goes from $+90°$ to $-90°$(or $+270°$). As $\mathbf{s}$ traverses the small semicircle part of C_1, $|\mathbf{A_L}(\mathbf{s})| \to \infty$, and the phase goes from $-90°$ to $-180°$ at $\mathbf{s} = \varepsilon$, thence to $-270°$ at $\mathbf{s} = j\varepsilon$. The complete contour, $\mathbf{A_L}(\mathbf{s})$, is shown in Figure 9.13. Note that, if $K\beta$ is large enough, there are two CW encirclements of $+1$ by the $\mathbf{A_L}(\mathbf{s})$ locus, signifying that there are two closed-loop system poles in the right-hand s-plane, hence oscillatory instability. Because $\mathbf{A_L}(j\omega_o)$ is real, we can set the imaginary terms in the denominator of $\mathbf{A_L}(j\omega_o) = 0$, and solve for ω_o. Thus:

$$j\omega_o(j\omega_o + 5)(j\omega_o + 2) = -j\omega_o^3 - 7\omega_o^2 + 10j\omega_o \textit{ must be Real} \quad (9.40)$$

Thus: $(-j\omega_o^3 + 10j\omega_o) = 0$, or $\omega_o = 3.162$ r/sec, and $K\beta > 7\omega_o^2 = 70$ for instability.

As a *fourth and final example* of application of the Nyquist test, consider the simple realpole plant with a transport lag δ in its feedback path, shown in Figure 9.14. The loop gain function is:

$$A_L(s) = \frac{-(K_1K_2/\tau_1)e^{-s\delta}}{(s + 1/\tau_1)} \quad (9.41)$$

The simple contour C_1', in the s-plane is used to define $\mathbf{s}$ values used in evaluating the $\mathbf{A_L}(\mathbf{s})$ contour. Figure 9.15 illustrates the $\mathbf{A_L}(\mathbf{s})$ contour. It begins at $\mathbf{A_L}(j0)$ = $-K_1K_2$, and spirals CW into the origin as $s = j\omega \to j\infty$. When $\mathbf{s}$ traverses the ∞ semicircle in the s-plane, the magnitude of $\mathbf{A_L}(\mathbf{s})$ = 0. Then, as $\mathbf{s}$ goes from $-j\infty$

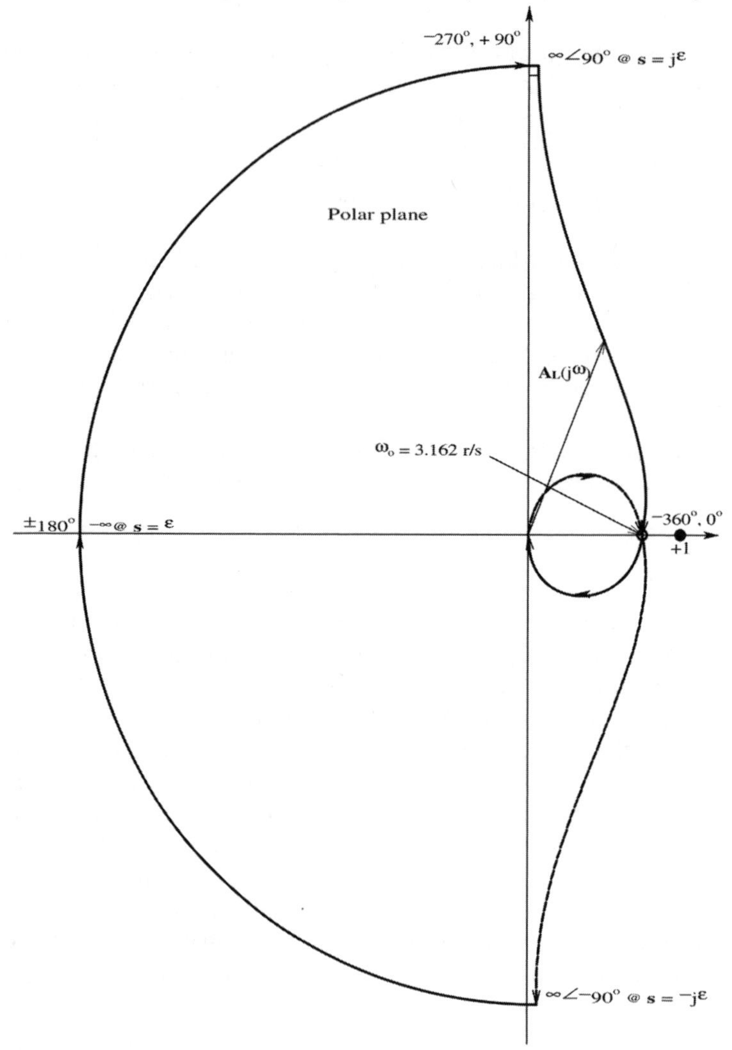

FIGURE 9.13

Polar vector plot of $A_L(s)$ for the third example. The contour C_1 is used because this loop gain function has a pole at the origin (See Equation 9.39).

to $-j0$, $\mathbf{A_L(s)}$ traces the mirror image of the vector locus for positive $j\omega$. Clearly, if the gain K_1K_2 is large enough, there can be 2,4,6,... CW encirclements of the $+1$ point, implying 2, 4, 6 ... closed-loop poles in the right-half s-plane. If there were no transport lag ($\delta = 0$), the phase would approach $-270°$, and there could be *no* encirclement of +1 for any positive gain. Hence the system would be stable. However, with $\delta > 0$, the phase of $\mathbf{A_L(s)}$ becomes:

$$\phi = -180° - \tan^{-1}(\omega\tau) - \omega\delta R \tag{9.42}$$

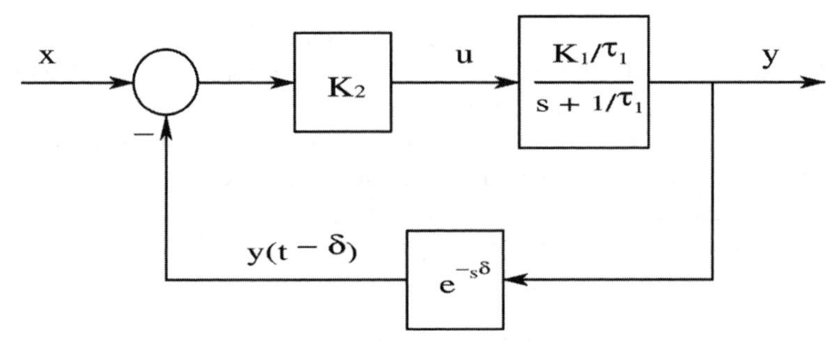

FIGURE 9.14
Linear SISO feedback system with a transport lag (signal delay) in its feedback path. $A_L(s)$ is given by Equation 9.41 in this fourth example.

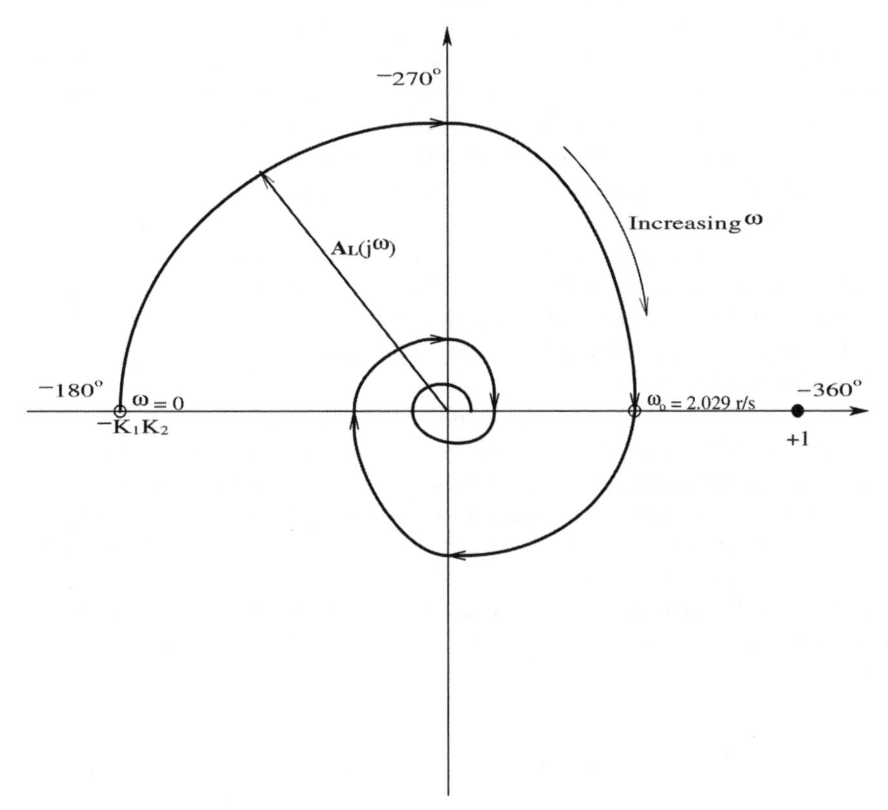

FIGURE 9.15
Polar vector plot of the vector locus of $\mathbf{A_L(s)}$ for the fourth example. Only $j0 \leq \mathbf{s} \leq +j\infty$ is considered. See text for description of stability.

$R = 57.3$ degrees/radian. Let $\delta = 1$ sec, $\tau = 1$ sec. The phase equation can be solved for the ω_o at which $\phi = -360°$. This turns out to be $\omega_o = 2.029$ r/sec. By setting $|\mathbf{A_L}(j\omega_o)| = 1$, we find that the system is unstable (two poles in the RH s-plane) if $K_1 K_2 > 2.262$. At some higher gain, there will be *four* CW encirclements of $+1$, implying that there are *two* pairs of complex-conjugate poles of the closed-loop system in the right-half s-plane. One might argue that this is quadruple instability. The critical gain, however, is that which produces one complex-conjugate pole pair in the right-half s-plane, i.e., 2.262.

9.5.3 Describing functions and the stability of closed-loop nonlinear systems

Describing functions are used in conjunction with the Nyquist stability criterion to predict the behavior of SISO closed-loop nonlinear systems, i.e., determine whether they will be stable, oscillate in a finite-amplitude limit cycle, or will be frankly unstable. The describing function (DF) method is based on a knowledge of the sinusoidal frequency response of the linear portion of the system's loop gain. DF analysis has been used to characterize certain closed-loop physiological control systems such as the pupil area regulator, and eye lateral tracking [Stark, 1968]. Instead of examining stability *per se,* the describing function method can also be used to find the approximate odd nonlinearity in a nonlinear feedback system.

The DF is the equivalent vector gain (or attenuation) of an *odd nonlinearity* in a closed-loop system's feedback loop, usually associated with the controller or effector block. That is, for the purpose of computational ease, we can replace the nonlinearity with an equivalent vector gain. A describing function's vector gain is generally a function of the amplitude and frequency of the input to the nonlinearity. The use of DFs is justified and valid under certain conditions described below [Ogata, 1970; Tompkins and Webster, 1981].

The nonlinearity which we replace with a DF has input $e(t)$ and output $u(t)$, and *must be* an odd nonlinearity, $u(e) = -u(-e)$. Often, a nonlinearity can be made odd for DF analysis by adding constant values to the input or the output. In calculating the describing function for an odd nonlinearity, *we assume that the input is a sine wave with zero mean.* That is, $e(t) = E(\sin\omega t)$. In general, the output of the nonlinearity will be nonsinusoidal, but have the same period as the input, $T = 2\pi/\omega$. Thus $u(t) = u(t+T)$, and may be represented by a *Fourier series.* We have seen in Chapter 4 that there are several formats for writing the Fourier series of a periodic function. One is:

$$\begin{aligned} u(t) &= A_o + \sum_{n=1}^{\infty} [A_n \cos(n\omega t) + B_n \sin(n\omega t)] \\ &= A_o + \sum_{n=1}^{\infty} C_n \sin(n\omega t + \phi_n) \end{aligned} \tag{9.43}$$

Where $C_n = \sqrt{A_n^2 + B_n^2}$, $\phi_n = \tan^{-1}(A_n/B_n)$, and $\omega = 2\pi/T$. A_o is the dc (average) output, here taken to be zero. If the input to the nonlinearity is an odd function of time, and $u = f(e)$ is odd, then $u(t)$ will be odd and the even (A_n) terms in the Fourier series can be shown to be zero. The harmonic amplitude coefficients are given by:

$$A_o = (1/T)\int_0^T u(t)dt = \frac{1}{2\pi}\int_0^{2\pi} u(\omega t)d\omega t \tag{9.44A}$$

$$\underset{n\geq 1}{A_n} = (2/T)\int_0^T u(t)\cos(n\omega_o t)dt = (1/\pi)\int_0^{2\pi} u(\omega t)\cos(n\omega t)d\omega t \tag{9.44B}$$

$$\underset{n\geq 1}{B_n} = (2/T)\int_0^T u(t)\sin(n\omega_o t)dt = (1/\pi)\int_0^{2\pi} u(\omega t)\sin(n\omega t)d\omega t \tag{9.44C}$$

The describing function is defined as $\mathbf{N}(E) \equiv (C_1/E)\ \angle\phi_1$. The DF has a nonzero angle if the output of the odd nonlinearity is phase-shifted with respect to the input sinusoid, $e(t)$.

Single-valued nonlinearities give rise to zero phase describing functions, which are positive real functions. The hysteresis function, encountered in certain temperature controllers, and in mechanical systems with gear backlash is called a *memory nonlinearity;* it gives rise to a complex DF.

We now examine the calculation of the describing functions of some commonly found nonlinearities. In the *first example,* we assume an algebraic, odd, nonlinear function:

$$u(t) = De^3(t) \tag{9.45}$$

For the sinusoidal input, $u(t) = DE^3\sin^3(\omega t)$. By trig. identity, this becomes:

$$u(t) = DE^3\frac{1}{4}[3\sin(\omega t) - \sin(3\omega t)] \tag{9.46}$$

Thus, by the definition, $\mathbf{N}(E) = DE^2\frac{3}{4}\angle 0°$. In this case, $\mathbf{N}(E)$ is a positive real *increasing function of E.*

In a *second example,* we examine the hard saturation nonlinearity, $u(t) = D\,\text{sgn}(e)$. Here $u = +D$ for $e(t) \geq 0$, and $u = -D$ for $e(t) < 0$. Thus, an input sine wave of any finite E generates a square wave with peak height D and the same frequency and phase. It is well-known that a square wave has a Fourier series containing odd harmonics; it is given by:

$$\begin{aligned} u(t) &= \frac{4D}{\pi}\sum_{n=1}^{\infty}\frac{1}{2n-1}\sin[(2n-1)\omega t] \\ &= \frac{4D}{\pi}[\sin(\omega t) + \frac{1}{3}\sin(3\omega t) + \frac{1}{5}\sin(5\omega t)\ldots] \end{aligned} \tag{9.47}$$

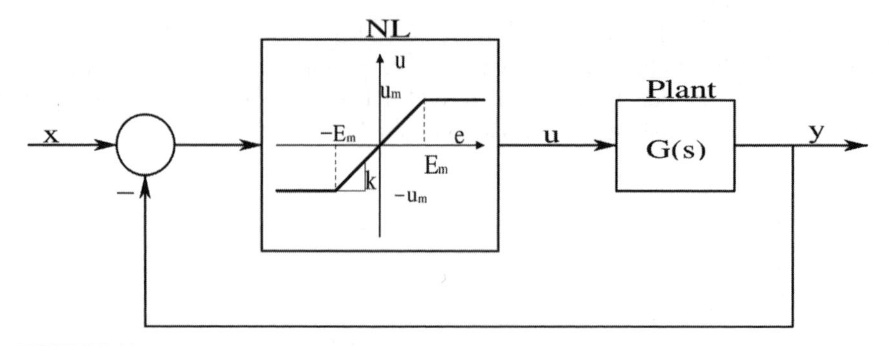

FIGURE 9.16
Block diagram of a SISO feedback system with a saturating controller.

So, the DF for the saturation nonlinearity is $\mathbf{N}(E) = \frac{4D}{\pi E}\angle 0°$. Unlike that for the cubic nonlinearity, this DF is a *decreasing real function of the input amplitude,* E.

A linear controller with output saturation nonlinearity, shown in Figure 9.16, is considered in the *third example.* In the linear region, the nonlinearity has gain $k = u_m/E_m$. Thus, if $E < E_m$, $u(\omega t) = kE\sin(\omega t)$, and $\mathbf{N}(E) = k$. When $E > E_m$, the tops and bottoms of the output sine wave are clipped to $\pm u_m$. This distorted sine wave has a Fourier series in which the (even) A_n coefficients are zero because $u(t)$ is odd in ωt. Thus, to find the DF for this nonlinearity, we only have to evaluate B_1 for $E > E_m$. $u(\omega t)$ saturates in the regions $\beta \le \omega t \le (\pi - \beta)$, and $(\pi + \beta) \le \omega t \le (2\pi - \beta)$. From simple trigonometry, $\beta = \sin^{-1}(E_m/E)$, $E > E_m$. We calculate the first harmonic peak amplitude, B_1:

$$\begin{aligned} B_1 = (1/\pi)[&\int_0^{\beta} kE\sin(\omega t)\sin(\omega t)d\omega t + \int_{\beta}^{\pi-\beta} U_m \sin(\omega t)d\omega t \\ &+ \int_{\pi-\beta}^{\pi+\beta} kE\sin(\omega t)\sin(\omega t)d\omega t - \int_{\pi+\beta}^{2\pi-\beta} U_m \sin(\omega t)d\omega t \\ &+ \int_{2\pi-\beta}^{2\pi} kE\sin(\omega t)\sin(\omega t)d\omega t] \end{aligned} \tag{9.48}$$

Calculation of the five definite integrals above is tedious, and will not be done here. Division of B_1 by E yields the DF for the saturation nonlinearity:

$$\begin{aligned} \mathbf{N}(E) = \frac{2k}{\pi}&[\sin^{-1}(E_m/E) + (E_m/E)\sqrt{1 - (E_m/E)^2}], \\ &\text{for } E > E_m \\ &\text{(Note that } \sin^{-1}(E_m/E) \text{ must be in radians.)} \end{aligned} \tag{9.49}$$

This DF is plotted in Figure 9.17.

Table 9.5.2 illustrates some common nonlinearities and their DFs. Note that one (hysteresis) has nonzero phase, and one (dead-zone with saturation, not shown) is double-valued in E [Ogata, 1970].

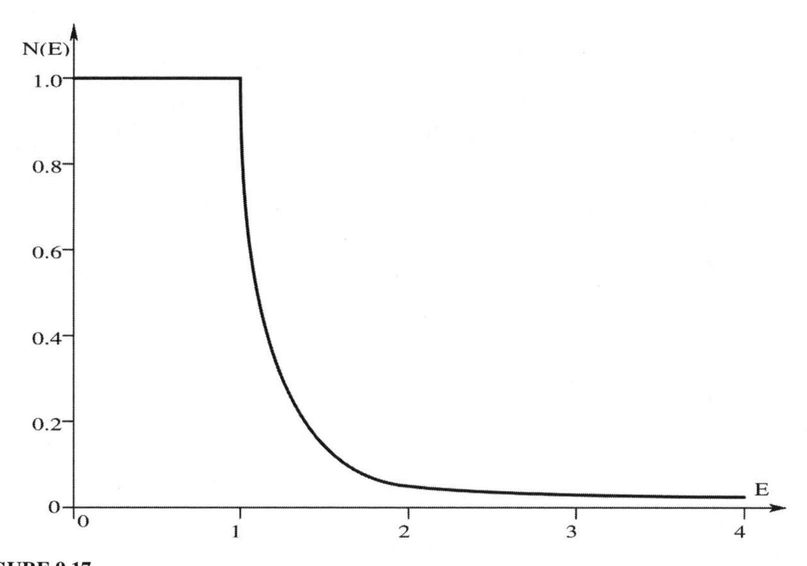

FIGURE 9.17
Plot of the describing function, N(E), of a saturation nonlinearity having unity slope and saturation level. [This figure and Figures 9.18, 9.19, 9.20, 9.21 and 9.22 from Northrop 2000. ©2000 Chapman and Hall/CRC. Used with permission.]

In the application of DFs to the analysis and design of closed-loop, nonlinear systems, we assume that the input to the odd nonlinearity at the *design center* is a zero-mean sine wave. For example, this input can be system error, defined as $e = r - y$. The set-point r at the design center is R_o. The closed-loop system (plant) output, $y(t)$, is assumed to have a dc level, $Y_o = R_o$, and a sinusoidal ripple component, $y(t) = -e(t)$. The plant input, however, is $u(t)$, the output of the nonlinearity. The higher order harmonics from $u(t)$ are assumed to be attenuated by the low-pass characteristics of the plant to a negligible level so that the sinusoidal output component of the plant can be considered to be just due to the fundamental frequency in $u(t)$. This attenuation requires that the plant be low-pass in nature when DF analysis is used.

As a *fourth example* of application of the DF method to the analysis of a closed-loop control system, consider the ON/OFF drug infusion control system shown in Figure 9.18a. The plant is a third-order low-pass system with three real poles and no zeros. An ON/OFF controller is to be designed that has specified peak error due to steady-state limit cycling.

First, we must find the U_{max} required. Let us assume that the desired average steady-state drug concentration is SP = $\overline{y} = 20\mu$g/liter. We also assume a 50% steady-state duty cycle in the controller when it is limit-cycling around the design set-point. Thus, the controller output in the steady state, $u(t)$, is a 50% duty cycle square wave with minimum value 0 and maximum U_{max}. This means that the average (dc) input to the plant is $\overline{u} = U_{max}/2$. The dc average SS plant output is then $(U_{max}/2)(20/6) = 20$, so clearly, $U_{max} = 12\mu$g/hr.

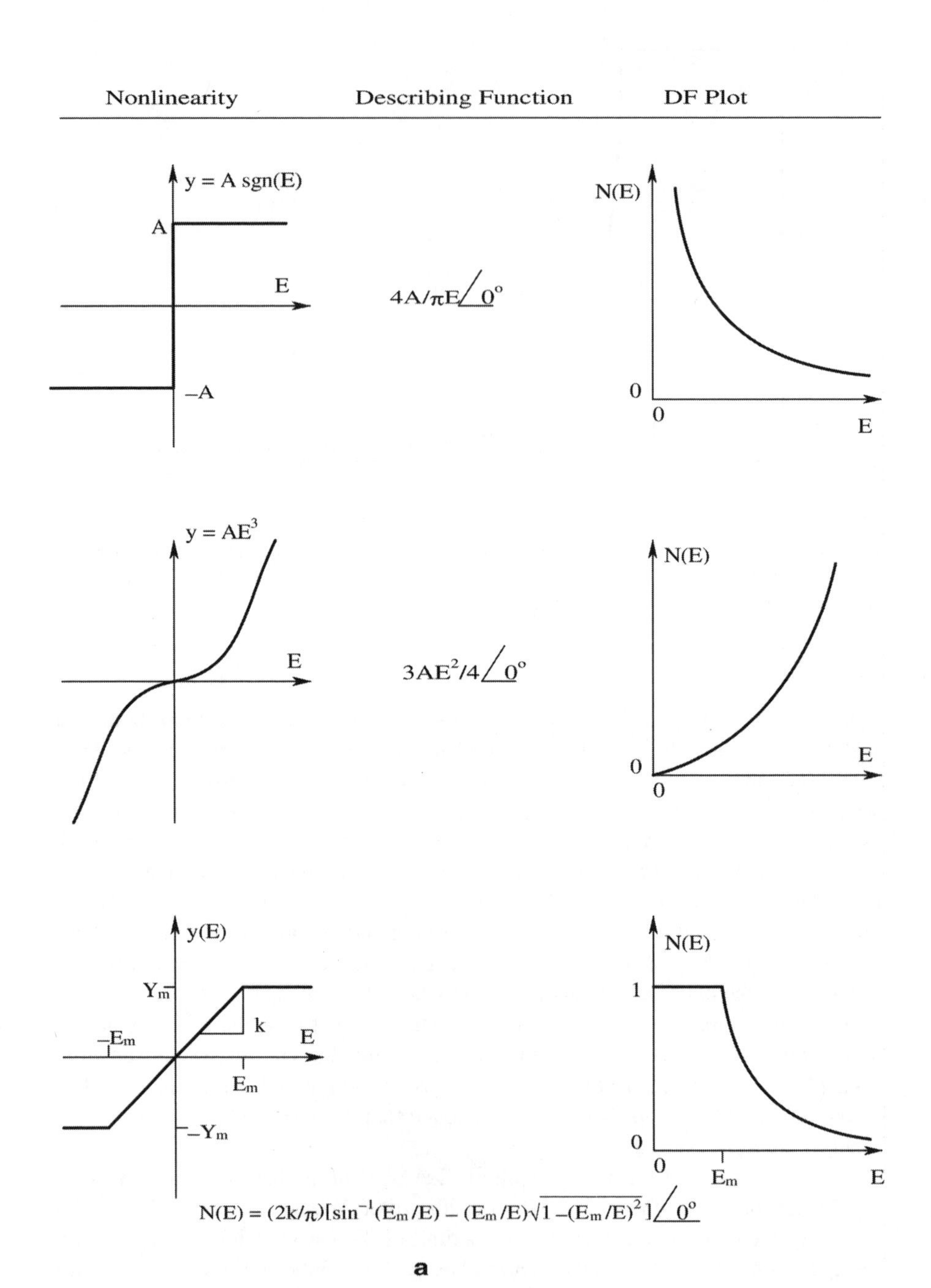
Nonlinearity
Describing Function
DF Plot
y = A sgn(E)
A
E
–A
4A/πE∠0°
N(E)
0
0
E
y = AE³
E
3AE²/4∠0°
N(E)
0
E
0
y(E)
Yₘ
k
–Eₘ
E
Eₘ
–Yₘ
N(E)
1
0
0
Eₘ
E
N(E) = (2k/π)[sin⁻¹(Eₘ/E) – (Eₘ/E)√(1 –(Eₘ/E)²)]∠0°
a

TABLE 9.5.2a

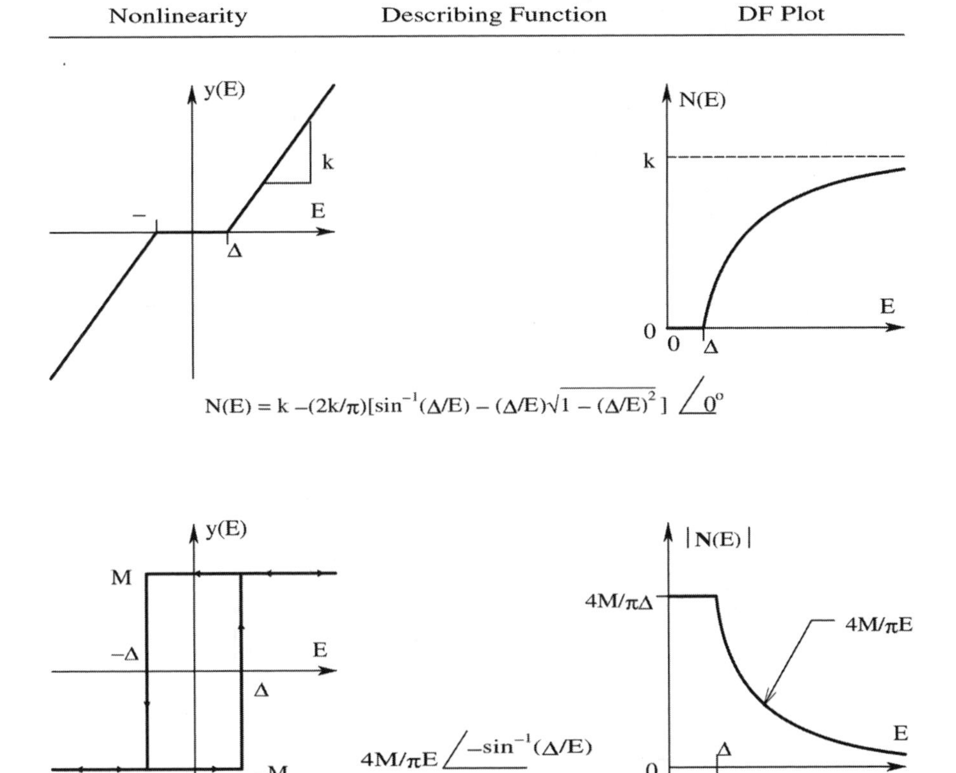

TABLE 9.5.2b

To use the describing function method, the 0, U_{max} nonlinearity must be made odd, switching between $\pm U_{max}/2$. To do this, we have assumed that, in the steady-state, the error is sinusoidal with zero mean $[e(t) = E_o \sin(\omega_o t)]$ and consequently, the $u(t)$ square wave will have a 50% duty cycle. Figure 9.18(b) illustrates the reconfigured system, which takes into account $\overline{u}$. The DF $\mathbf{N}(E) = (2U_{max})/(\pi E)$ for the symmetrical nonlinearity. However, we plot $\mathbf{N}^{-1}(E)$ in the polar plane along with $-K_F \mathbf{G}_p(j\omega)$, which is:

$$\frac{-K_F 20}{(j\omega+1)(j\omega+2)(j\omega+3)} = \frac{-K_F 20}{j\omega(11-\omega^2)+(6-6\omega^2)} \tag{9.50}$$

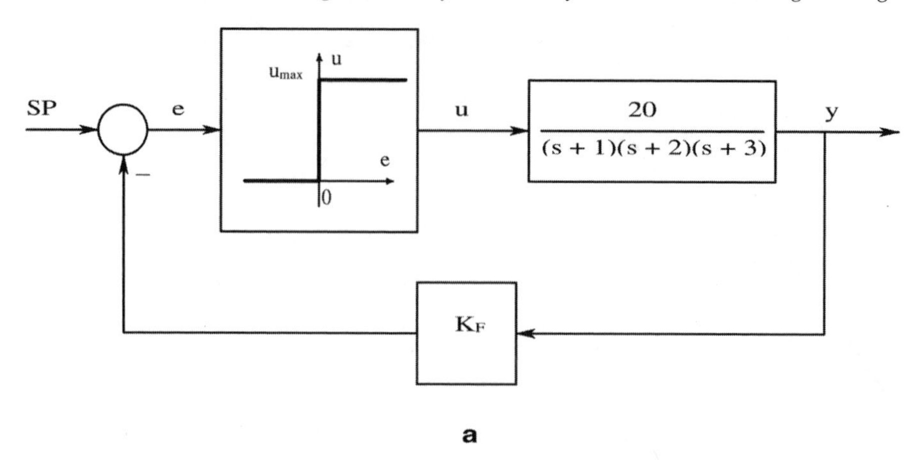

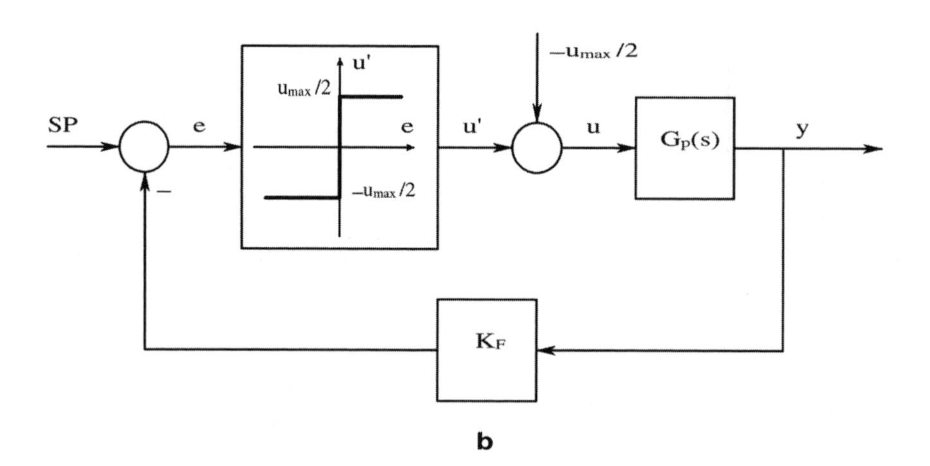

FIGURE 9.18

(a) Block diagram of a SISO feedback drug infusion system with an on-off (bang-bang) controller. The linear plant is cubic, i.e., it has three real poles. (b) The same system with the controller nonlinearity made an odd function having a defined describing function. (Northrop, R.B. 2000. *Endogenous and Exogenous Regulation and Control of Physiological Systems.* CRC Press, Boca Raton. With permission.)

Now all of $\mathbf{N}^{-1}(\mathrm{E})$ lies on the positive real axis, so where the locus of $-\mathrm{K_F}\mathbf{G}_\mathrm{p}(\mathrm{j}\omega)$ intersects $\mathbf{N}^{-1}(\mathrm{E})$, it is real. This means that the imaginary term in the denominator of Equation 9.50 must equal zero: $\mathrm{j}\omega_\mathrm{o}(11-\omega_\mathrm{o}^2)=0$, so $\omega_\mathrm{o}=\sqrt{11}$ r/hr. We now consider the magnitudes of the $\mathbf{A}_\mathrm{L}(\mathrm{j}\omega)$ and $\mathbf{N}^{-1}(\mathrm{E})$ vectors at ω_o. See Figure 9.19.

$$\frac{-\mathrm{K_F}20}{(6-6\mathrm{X}11)}=\frac{\mathrm{K_F}20}{60}=-\mathrm{K_F}/3=\frac{\pi\mathrm{E}}{2\mathrm{U}_{\mathrm{max}}} \tag{9.51}$$

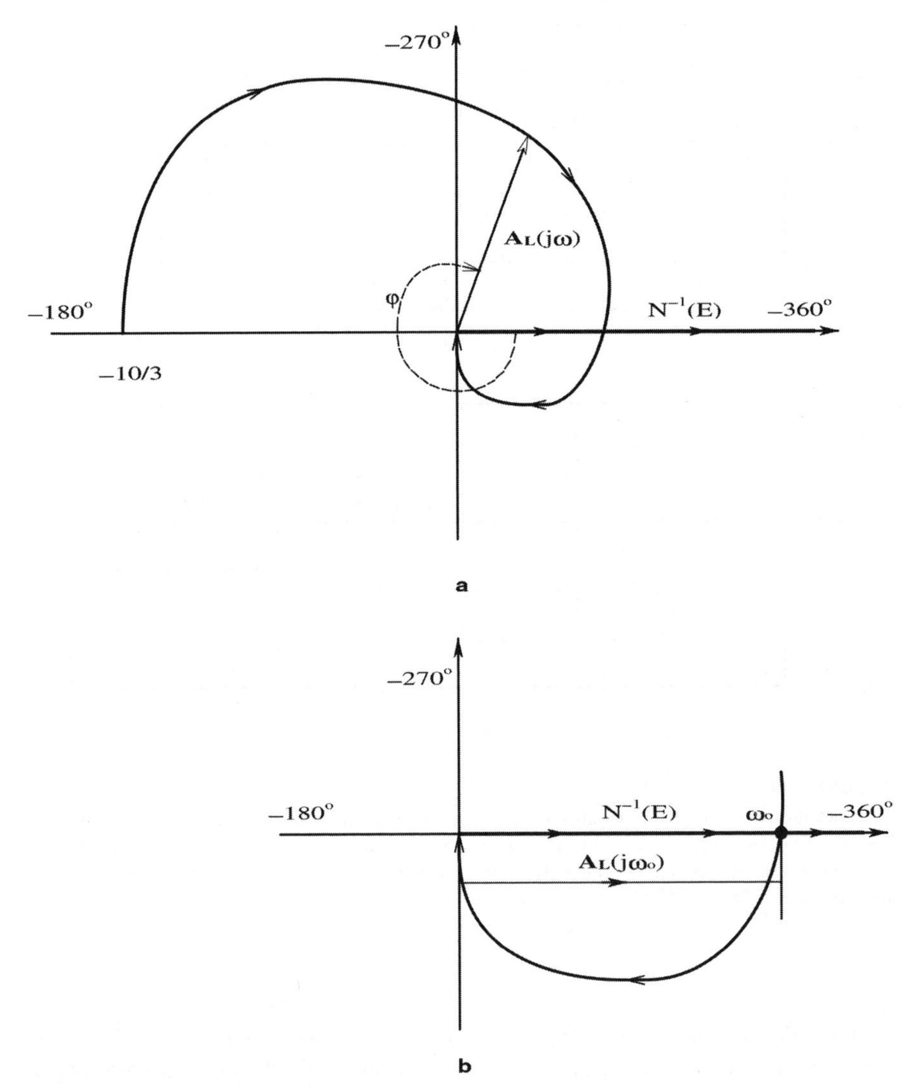

FIGURE 9.19
(a) Polar plot of $\mathbf{A_L}(\mathbf{s})$ for $j0 \leq \mathbf{s} \leq +j\infty$ and $\mathbf{N}^{-1}(E)$ for the system of Figure 9.18b. (b) Enlarged view of the polar plane in the region where the vector $\mathbf{A_L}(j\omega)$ crosses the real axis and the vector, $\mathbf{N}^{-1}(E)$. At the crossing, $\omega = \omega_o$, and $A_L(j\omega_o)$ is real and positive. (Northrop, R.B. 2000. *Endogenous and Exogenous Regulation and Control of Physiological Systems.* CRC Press, Boca Raton. With permission.)

We require that E be 5% of the set point, or 1 μg/l. Substitution of the values of U_{max} and E in Equation 9.51 yields the required value of $K_F = \pi/8$ to meet the 5% error specification. While this simple example was easily solved algebraically, the describing function method is not always so algebraically obliging, and it often is more expedient to do a graphical solution from the polar plot of $\mathbf{N}^{-1}$ and $-\mathbf{G}_p(j\omega)$, or use a simulation.

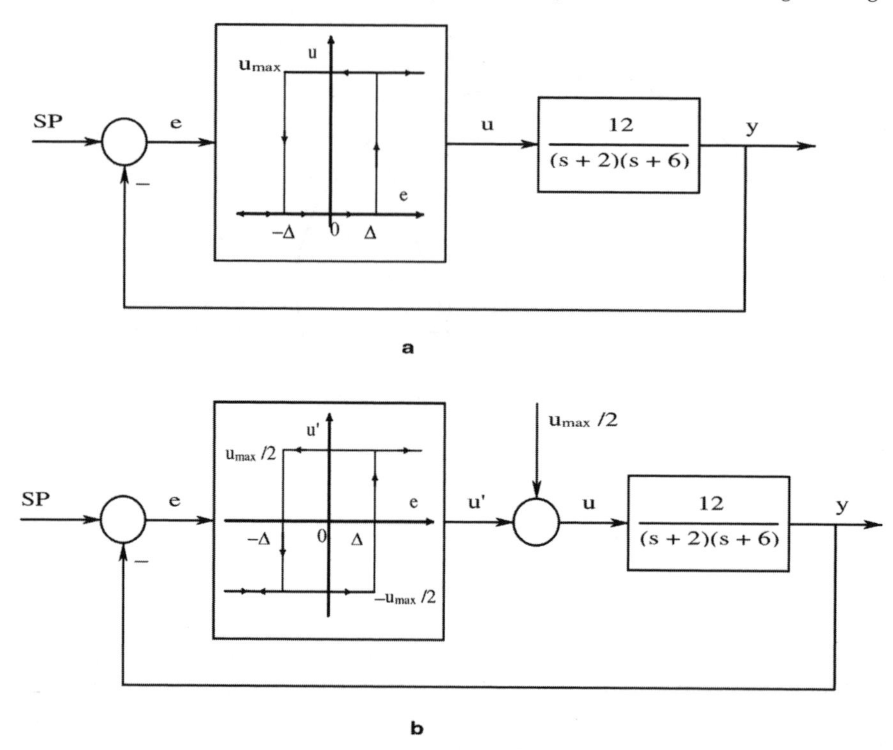

FIGURE 9.20

(a) Block diagram of a SISO drug infusion system having an on-off controller with hysterisis. The plant has two real poles. (b) Same system as in (a), but the nonlinearity has been made an odd function that has a defined describing function. (Northrop, R.B. 2000. *Endogenous and Exogenous Regulation and Control of Physiological Systems.* CRC Press, Boca Raton. With permission.)

In a *fifth example,* we examine how a graphic implementation of the DF method can be used to predict and characterize a nonlinear feedback system's stability and inherent limit cycles. The system shown in Figure 9.20 is a *drug infusion control system* designed to maintain a nearly constant concentration of a drug in a patient's blood. The pharmacokinetic dynamics are described by a second-order LTI plant. An *ON/OFF controller with hysteresis* is used. (Hysteresis controllers are widely used in ON/OFF type temperature regulators, such as home heating systems.) To use the DF method, we must convert the nonlinearity to a symmetrical (odd) form by adding the dc average controller output to the output of the symmetrical hysteresis controller. This modification is shown in Figure 9.20(b). Let us assume that the steady-state error is sinusoidal, has zero mean and 50% duty cycle. Thus, the dc steady-state input to the plant is $\overline{u} = u_{max}/2$.

The average plant output is desired to be equal to the set-point, SP. Thus we can find the required u_{max} from:

$$\mathrm{SP} = \frac{\mathrm{u_{max}}}{2}\mathbf{G}_\mathrm{p}(0) = \frac{\mathrm{u_{max}}}{2}\frac{\mathrm{K_p}}{\mathrm{ab}} \tag{9.52}$$

$\mathbf{G}_\mathrm{p}(0)$ is the dc gain of the plant. Thus $\mathrm{u_{max}} = \mathrm{SP}(2\mathrm{ab}/\mathrm{K_p})$.

We next consider the describing function of the hysteresis nonlinearity. If $\mathrm{E} > \Delta$, the hysteresis dead zone, u' will be a $\pm\mathrm{u_{max}}/2$ square wave with zero mean. There will also be an amplitude-dependent phase shift between the Fourier series terms of $\mathrm{u}'(\mathrm{t})$ and $\mathrm{e}(\mathrm{t})$. For the fundamental frequency term in $\mathrm{u}'(\mathrm{t})$, this phase lag can be shown to be: $\angle\mathbf{N} = -\sin^{-1}(\Delta/\mathrm{E})$. Thus, the complete DF for the hysteresis nonlinearity can be shown to be:

$$\mathbf{N}(\mathrm{E}) = \frac{4(\mathrm{u_{max}}/2)}{\pi\mathrm{E}}\angle - \sin^{-1}(\Delta/\mathrm{E}) \tag{9.53}$$

and its reciprocal is:

$$\mathbf{N}^{-1}(\mathrm{E}) = \frac{\pi\mathrm{E}}{2\mathrm{u_{max}}}\angle + \sin^{-1}(\Delta/\mathrm{E}) \tag{9.54}$$

Figure 9.21 shows that $\mathbf{N^{-1}}(\mathrm{E})$ for the hysteresis nonlinearity plots as a straight line parallel to the 0° axis in the first quadrant of the polar graph. $\mathbf{N^{-1}}(\mathrm{E})$ intersects the polar −270° axis at a radial distance of $\pi\Delta/2\mathrm{U_{max}}$ for $\mathrm{E} = \Delta$, and extends to

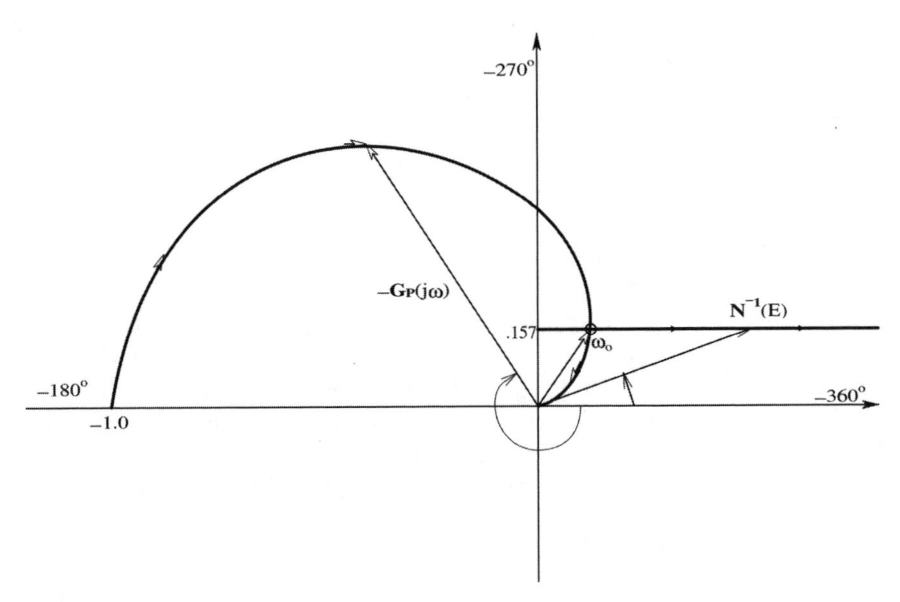

FIGURE 9.21

Polar plot of the vectors, $-\mathbf{G_P}(\mathrm{j}\omega)$ and $\mathrm{N}^{-1}(\mathrm{E})$ for $0 \leq \omega \leq \infty$, and $0 \leq \mathrm{E} \leq \infty$. Note that $-\mathbf{G_P}(\mathrm{j}\omega) = \mathbf{A_L}(\mathrm{j}\omega)$. (Northrop, R.B. 2000. *Endogenous and Exogenous Regulation and Control of Physiological Systems.* CRC Press, Boca Raton. With permission.)

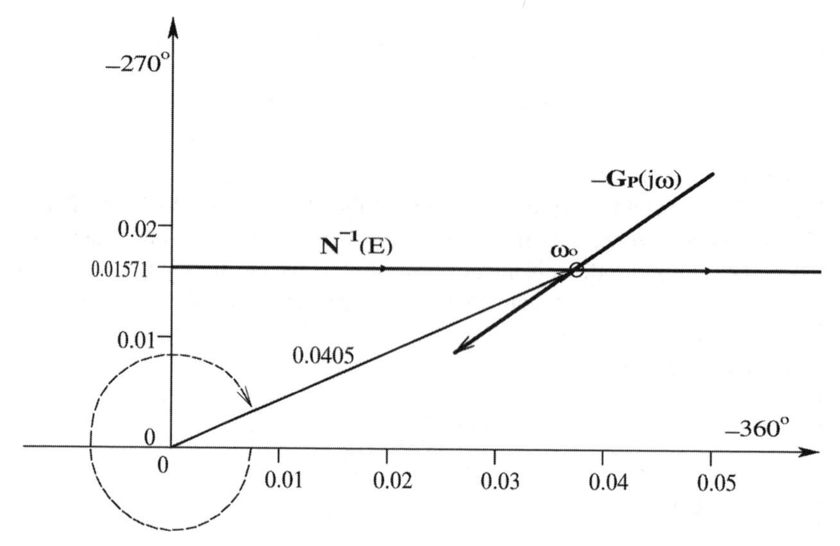

FIGURE 9.22

Enlarged view of the vector intersection of $-\mathbf{G_P}(j\omega)$ and $\mathbf{N}^{-1}(E)$ at $\omega = \omega_o$ and $E = E_o$. ω_o gives the frequency for limit cycle oscillations, and E_0 their amplitude. See text for details. (Northrop, R.B. 2000. *Endogenous and Exogenous Regulation and Control of Physiological Systems.* CRC Press, Boca Raton. With permission.)

the right with increasing E. For the system to produce stable limit cycle oscillations, the vector $-\mathbf{G}_p(j\omega)$ must intersect $\mathbf{N^{-1}}(E)$ at $\omega = \omega_o$, and $E = E_o$. We can design for the intersection within bounds by adjusting Δ and K_F.

To demonstrate the efficacy of a *graphic solution,* let us define numerical values for the system parameters: SP = 10 μg/l, $E_o \leq 5\mu$g/l, $K_p = 12$, $a = 2, b = 6$ r/hr, $\Delta = 0.2\mu$g/l. E_o, U_{max} and ω_o are to be determined: $U_{max} = (2SPab)/K_p = 2 \times 10 \times 2 \times 6/12 = 20\mu$g/hr. The intersection of $\mathbf{N}^{-1}(E)$ with the $-270°$ axis is at $R = \pi\Delta/2U_{max} = 6.283/40 = 1.571E-2$. The angle of $-\mathbf{G_p}(j\omega)$ is given by: $\varphi = -180° - \tan^{-1}(\omega/2) - \tan^{-1}(\omega/6)$. The magnitude of $-\mathbf{G_p}(j\omega)$ is $K_p/[(\sqrt{\omega^2+2^2})(\sqrt{\omega^2+6^2})]$. In order to limit-cycle, the magnitude of $-\mathbf{G_p}(j\omega)$ must exceed $1.571E-2$ at $\varphi = -270°$ so there will be an intersection of $-\mathbf{G_p}(j\omega)$ and $\mathbf{N^{-1}}(E)$. By adjusting Δ, we can affect the limit cycle frequency, ω_o, and E_o. Figure 9.22 illustrates the graphical solution for ω_o, and E_o, given the parameters above. We see that the intersection of $\mathbf{N^{-1}}(E)$ and $-\mathbf{G_p}(j\omega)$ occurs at $\omega_o \cong 16.7$ r/hr. Also, $|\mathbf{N^{-1}}(E_o)| \cong 0.0405$, so $E_o = 40 \times 0.0405/\pi = 0.516\mu$g/l peak. This represents a 5.2% peak error for the steady-state limit cycling system. Such error is acceptable in this type of controller.

9.5.4 The use of Gaussian noise-based techniques to characterize physiological systems

We saw in Sections 8.2.5 and 8.2.6 that calculation of the cross-correlation and the cross-power spectrum between the random input and the output of an LTI system can be used to find the system's weighting function, $h(t)$, and its frequency response function, $\mathbf{H}(\omega)$, respectively. To reiterate, the cross-correlation between system input and output can be written as the real convolution:

$$\varphi_{xy}(\tau) = \int_{-\infty}^{\infty} h(\mu)\varphi_{xx}(\tau - \mu)d\mu = h(\tau) \otimes \varphi_{xx}(\tau) \tag{9.55}$$

When $x(t)$ is broadband Gaussian noise, its ACF can be approximated by $\varphi_{xx}(\mu) \cong < x^2 > \delta(\mu)$. When this $\varphi_{xx}(\mu)$ is convolved with the SLS system's weighting function, we have:

$$\varphi_{xy}(\tau) = \int_{-\infty}^{\infty} h(\mu) < x^2 > \delta(\tau - \mu)d\mu = < x^2 > h(\tau) \tag{9.56}$$

Thus, the LTI system's WF is:

$$h(\tau) \cong \varphi_{xy}(\tau) / < x^2 > \tag{9.57}$$

And it was shown that in the frequency domain:

$$\mathbf{H}(\omega) = \frac{\mathbf{\Phi_{xy}}(\omega)}{\Phi_{xx}(\omega)} \cong \mathbf{\Phi_{xy}}(\omega)/\eta \quad \text{(for broadband, “white” noise)} \tag{9.58}$$

The *coherence function* of the system, $\gamma^2(\omega)$, is used as a test of the use of the input autopower spectrum and the input/output cross-power spectrum to find $\mathbf{H}(\omega)$. $\gamma^2(\omega)$ is a set of real numbers between 0 and 1, given by [Bendat and Piersol, 1966]:

$$\gamma_{xy}^2(\omega) \equiv \frac{|\mathbf{\Phi_{xy}}(\omega)|^2}{\Phi_{xx}(\omega)\Phi_{yy}(\omega)} \tag{9.59}$$

Ideally, $\gamma(\omega) \to 1$. In practice, $\gamma^2(\omega) < 1$ for several reasons:

1. The system is nonlinear.
2. Extraneous noise is present in $x(t)$ and/or $y(t)$.
3. Other (hidden) inputs besides $x(t)$ are present.
4. The signals $x(t)$ and/or $y(t)$ are aliased.

If $\gamma^2(\omega)$ is considered too small and 2, 3 and 4 above are not applicable, then the system is probably nonlinear enough to require a testing mode designed specifically for NLSs.

A noise-based method of nonlinear system characterization is the *white noise method* developed by Marmarelis (1972) and Marmarelis and Marmarelis (1978). In this method, the system input is again broadband Gaussian noise. The input modality can be sound, light, electric field, etc., depending on the physiological system under investigation. The white noise process yields one- two-, three- to n-dimensional weighting functions or *kernels* that are determined by the system's nonlinearity. (If the system were linear, the kernels of order two and higher would be zero.) It is purely a “black-box” approach; little insight is gained into the mechanism of the nonlinearity or where it occurs in the system. Also, it is conceptually difficult to visualize the third- and higher-order weighting functions and to interpret their significance

[Northrop, 2001, Section 8.3]. The white noise method has been used to characterize retinal neurons in the goldfish eye, and motoneurons. Figure 9.23 illustrates the steps required to calculate the NLS's first-order (linear) weighting function, $h_1(\tau)$, and the second-order weighting function, $h_2(\tau_1,\tau_2)$. The same white noise analysis can be carried out in the frequency domain, shown in Figure 9.24. Here the process outputs are the linear system's frequency response, $\mathbf{H}_1(\omega)$, and its second-order frequency response, $\mathbf{H}_2(\omega_1,\omega_2)$.

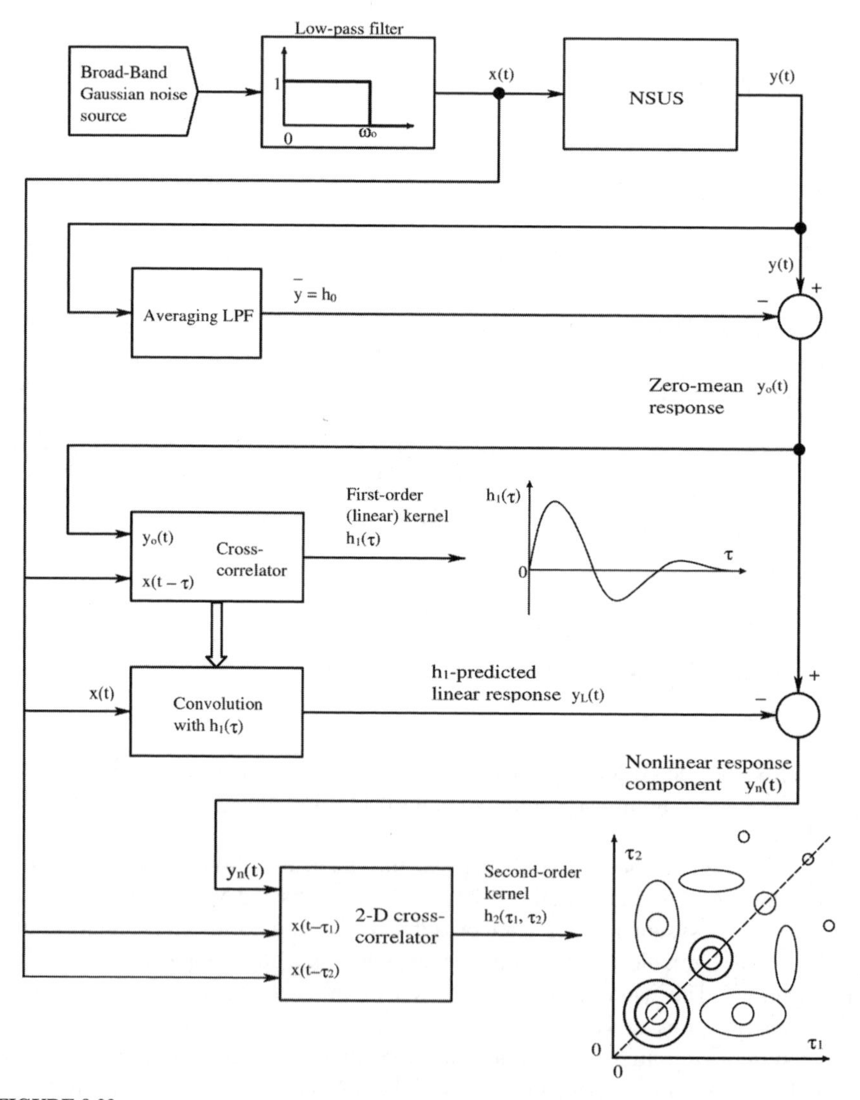

FIGURE 9.23

Block diagram illustrating the mathematical steps required to calculate the first- and second-order (time-domain) Wiener kernels for a nonlinear system excited with broadband Gaussian noise.

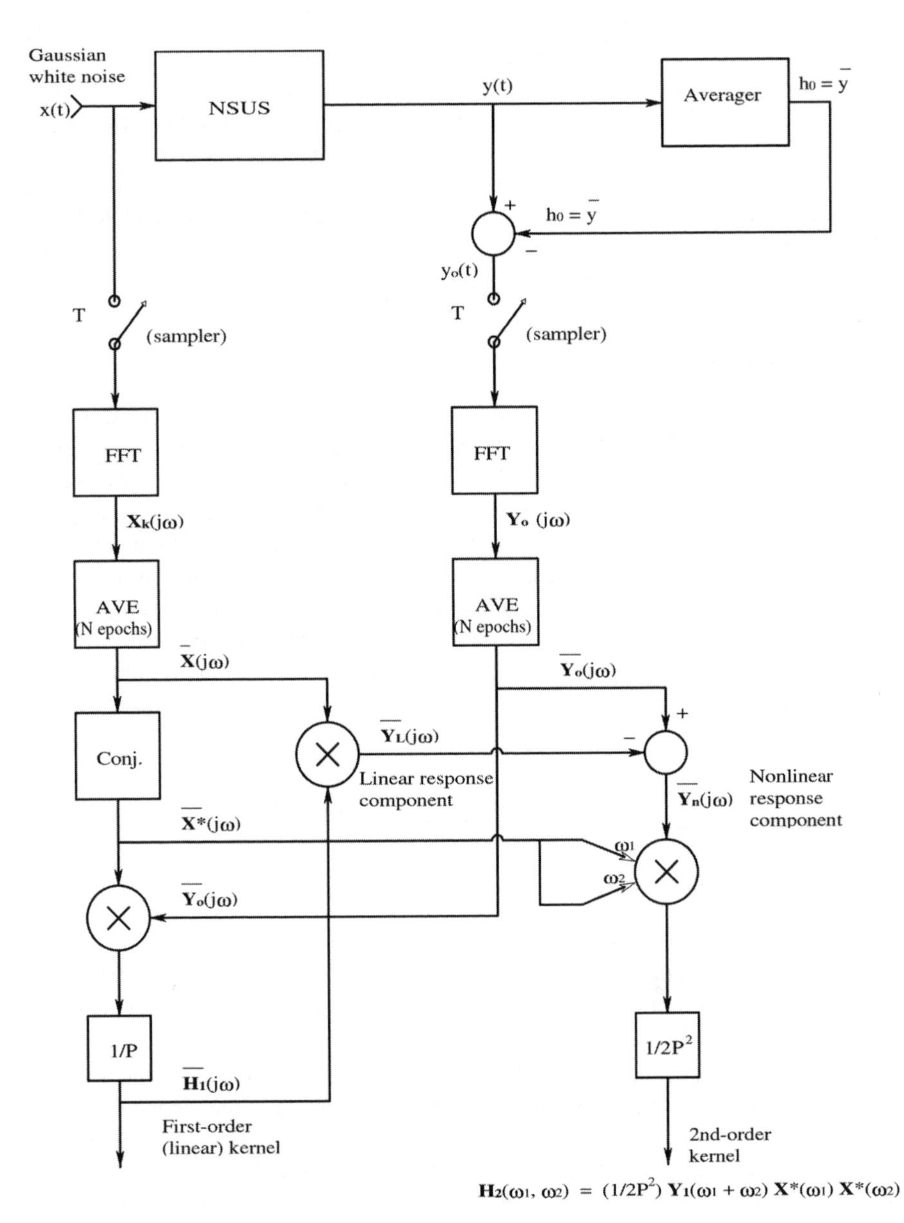

$$\mathbf{H}_2(\omega_1, \omega_2) = (1/2P^2)\,\mathbf{Y}_1(\omega_1 + \omega_2)\,\mathbf{X}^*(\omega_1)\,\mathbf{X}^*(\omega_2)$$

FIGURE 9.24
Block diagram illustrating the mathematical steps required to calculate the first- and second-order frequency-domain Wiener kernels for a nonlinear system excited with broadband Gaussian noise. These kernels are the DFTs of the time-domain kernels.

Another complex but interesting approach to the characterization of *neurosensory systems* is called *triggered correlation* (TC) [Northrop, 2001]. In TC, a neurosensory system is excited with a broadband Gaussian noise stimulus, and the system's output is the firing of a sensory (afferent) nerve fiber. The firing process is modeled as a nonlinear threshold system having conditions on its input amplitude and derivative. The input to the output spike generator is the output of the LTI system that we wish to characterize. Conditional averaging of the input noise is used to extract the weighting function of the *equivalent LTI transfer function* of the neurosensory system [Northrop, 2001, Section 8.2]. TC has been used to estimate the band-pass frequency selectivity of eigth nerve fibers in vertebrate hearing.

9.5.5 Discussion

With LTI systems, we can use the SS frequency response or the impulse or step response to characterize the system. On the other hand, characterization of nonlinear systems has always been a challenge because the output of an NLS is dependent on initial conditions, forcing input amplitude and frequency, and, in some physiological systems, the previous history of the system's states and output. A wide variety of approaches must be used to adequately characterize a frankly nonlinear system. Linearization of an NLS around some operating point may be expedient for engineering analysis and design, but, when a physiological system is considered, linearization to expedite analysis avoids the central problem of understanding why the system behaves the way it does.

9.6 Chapter Summary

We have seen that there are many powerful mathematical tools for the time- and frequency-domain analysis of LTI continuous and discrete systems. Chapter 9 focused on the attributes of *nonlinear* physiological systems and the physical and chemical processes that underlie their nonlinearity.

Unfortunately, few analytical techniques are specifically suited for the analysis of nonlinear systems. In a few cases, enough is known about the mechanisms and dynamics of a physiological system (e.g., the human glucoregulatory system) to allow a computer model to be created to enable simulations that will verify and predict the system's behavior, validating the model's architecture and parameters. In other cases, although little may be known about the details of a system's organization, we do have experimental access to an input and an output. The challenge here is to deduce as much as possible about the system's input/output characteristics by examining the output, given various classes of inputs — for example, various transient inputs, sinusoidal inputs, and random inputs. The Nyquist stability criterion, introduced in Section 9.4.2, allows one to predict the stability of a closed-loop LTI system, given the steady-state, sinusoidal frequency response of the system's loop gain function. In Section 9.4.3 the Nyquist stability test is extended to the stability analysis of closed-loop systems having an amplitude nonlinearity in their loop gain. The describing function method allows the prediction of bounded limit cycle oscillations which can occur in some closed-loop physiological regulators.

A more black-box approach to the characterization of nonlinear systems was introduced in Section 9.4.4. The use of Wiener functionals as described by Marmarelis and Marmarelis (1978) is described is used to characterize NLTI systems that contain an unknown nonlinearity. One-, two- and higher-order kernels (system weighting functions) are calculated using a broadband Gaussian noise input and the system output. Unfortunately, kernels of order 3 and higher require more than 3-D space to visualize and thus, are not practical. The kernels can be Fourier transformed, giving system frequency responses. If the system is completely linear (unlikely in a physiological system), only the first-order kernel is nonzero; its FT is the system's frequency response function.

Problems

9.1 Figure P9.1 illustrates a simple LTI system that involves simple diffusion across a cell membrane, as well as a simple one-step chemical reaction in the cell where biochemical **A** is transformed to **B**. **A** diffuses into the cell, and **B** diffuses out. For simplicity, the external concentration of **A** is a constant a_o, and the external concentration of **B** is a constant b_o. The internal (running) concentration of **A** is a, and the internal concentration of **B** is b. Assume the system is started at $t=0$ with zero initial conditions on a and b.

a. Write the two first-order linear ODEs that describe the *rate of increase* of a and b.

b. Make a signal flow graph based on the two ODEs.

c. Since the system starts at $t=0$ with zero ICs, you can treat the external concentrations like steps, $a_oU(t)$ and $b_oU(t)$. From the SFG, find expressions for $a(s)$ and $b(s)$.

d. Find algebraic expressions for the steady-state $a(t)$ and $b(t)$, a_{ss} and b_{ss}. You can use either the Laplace final value theorem on $a(s)$ and $b(s)$, or the ODEs with $\dot{a}$ and $\dot{b}$ set to zero.

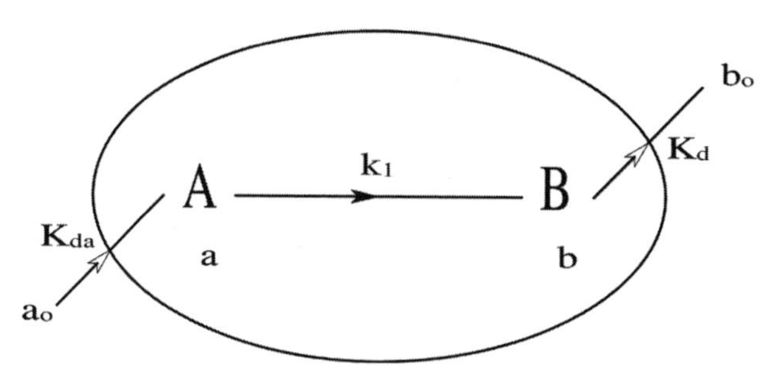

FIGURE P9.1

9.2 See Figure P9.2. A hormone is infused into the blood stream at a constant rate of $Q_{in}\mu$ g/min. The circulating blood constitutes a single pharmacokinetic compartment with volume = 5 liters. In the steady state, the blood concentration of the hormone, C_H, is 10 μg/liter. When the infusion stops, the concentration falls exponentially such that it is 5 μg/liter at $t = 2.7$ hours.

a. Write the ODE describing the system dynamics.

b. Make a signal flow graph for the linear system. Give its transfer function,. $\frac{C_H}{Q_{in}}(s)$.

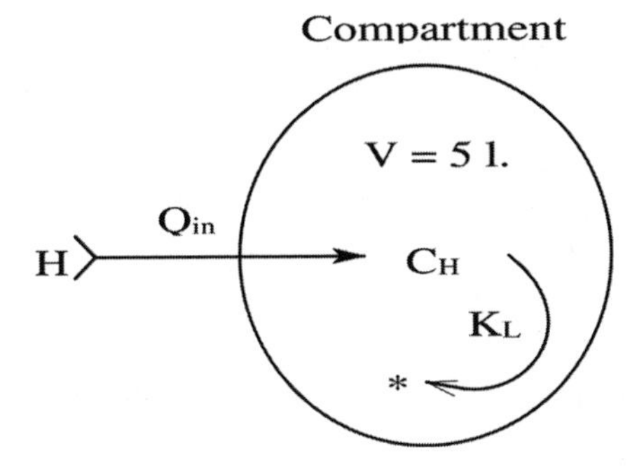

FIGURE P9.2

c. Find the steady-state input infusion rate, Q_{in}.

d. Give a numerical value for the hormone's loss rate constant, K_L.

9.3 See Figure P9.3. A concentration of hormone, H, in extracellular space controls the diffusion of a molecule, M, into a cell. The extracellular concentration of the molecule is m_e, its intracellular concentration is m_i pg/μl. The hormone is removed from the cell with first-order kinetics.

a. Write the state equation for m_i.

b. Draw a signal flow graph for the system.

c. Find an expression for the steady-state m_i vs. H. Assume $K_L >> K_{do}$.

d. Plot and dimension the system's natural frequency, ω_o, as a function of H.

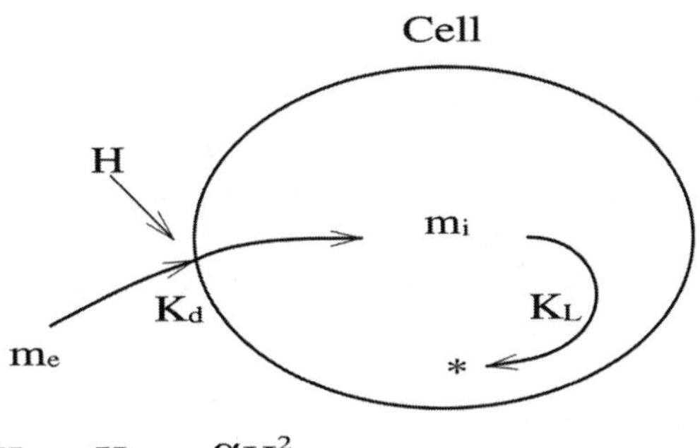

FIGURE P9.3

9.4 A Michaelis-type chemical reaction in which parametric control is present is shown below. In this reaction, the end-product concentration, p, affects the forward rate constant according to the law, $k_1 \cong \beta/p$. The enzyme E is assumed to be conserved, i.e., no new enzyme is made. Thus: $e+c=e_o$. R*E is a complex between a reactant molecule, R, and a free enzyme molecule, E.

$$\underset{r}{\mathbf{R}}+\underset{e}{\mathbf{E}} \overset{k_2\ k_1}{\Leftarrow\Rightarrow} \underset{c}{\mathbf{R^*E}} \xrightarrow{k_3} \underset{e}{\mathbf{E}}+\underset{p}{\mathbf{P}} \xrightarrow{k_4} *$$

a. Write the mass-action ODEs governing the nonlinear system's dynamics.

b. Assume r is constant $(r=r_o)$. Find an expression for the steady-state concentration of P, p_{ss}. Show that p_{ss} is independent of r. (Note: this answer is arrived at by solving a quadratic equation in p_{ss}. Use the approximation: $\sqrt{1+\varepsilon} \cong 1+\varepsilon/2, \varepsilon << 1$.)

9.5 This problem examines a hypothetical biochemical oscillator model for a "biological clock." It is based on a model suggested by Spangler and Snell (1961) that involves *cross-competitive inhibition* (CCI). The four cross-coupled biochemical reactions are written below:

$$(A_1) \xrightarrow{J_{a1}} A_1 + E_1 \underset{k_{11r}}{\overset{k_{11}}{\Leftarrow\Rightarrow}} B_1 + \xrightarrow{k_{21}} E_1 + P_1 \xrightarrow{k_{31}} *$$

$$nP_1 + E_2 \underset{k_{42r}}{\overset{k_{42}}{\Leftarrow\Rightarrow}} I_2$$

$$nP_2 + E_1 \underset{k_{41r}}{\overset{k_{41}}{\Leftarrow\Rightarrow}} I_1$$

$$(A_2) \xrightarrow{J_{a2}} A_2 + E_2 \underset{k_{12r}}{\overset{k_{12}}{\Leftarrow\Rightarrow}} B_2 \xrightarrow{k_{22}} E_2 + P_2 \xrightarrow{k_{32}} *$$

We assume that substrates A_1 and A_2 diffuse into the reaction volume at constant rates J_{a1} and J_{a2}, respectively. A_1 and A_2 combine with enzyme/catalysts E_1 and E_2, respectively, and are reversibly transformed into complexes B_1 and B_2. The complexes next decompose into free enzymes along with products. The free products then disappear with first-order kinetics as well as combine reversibly with n molecules of the complementary free enzyme to form inactive complexes, I_1 and I_2. We further assume that the two enzymes are conserved. That is:

$$e_{01} = e_1 + b_1 + i_1 \rightarrow e_1 = e_{01} - b_1 - i_1$$
$$e_{02} = e_2 + b_2 + i_2 \rightarrow e_2 = e_{02} - b_2 - i_2$$

Where e_{01} is the total enzyme #1 in the system, e_1 is the free enzyme #1, b_1 is the amount of enzyme #1 complexed with A_1, and i_1 is the amount of enzyme #1 complexed with n molecules of P_2 in storage reaction #1, etc. The running concentrations of reactants are: a_1 for A_1, b_1 for B_1, e_1 for E_1, i_1 for I_1, etc.

a. Write the 8, nonlinear, mass-action ODEs for the system. They are for: $\dot{a}_1, \dot{b}_1, \dot{p}_1, \dot{i}_1, \dot{a}_2, \dot{b}_2, \dot{p}_2$, and $\dot{i}_2$. Note that the #1 storage reaction ODE is:

$$\dot{i}_1 = k_{41} e_1 p_2^n - k_{41r} i_1$$

Note the exponentiation of p_2.

b. Now use a simulation program such as Simnon™ or Simulink® to see whether the system oscillates in a bounded manner. (Simnon allows you to algebraically enter the eight ODEs and the two enzyme conservation equations directly.) Use the following parameters [Northrop, 2000, p. 51]: $J_{a1}=3$, $J_{a2}=1$, $k_{11}=0.1$, $k_{11r}=0.05$, $k_{21}=1$, $k_{31}=0.3$, $k_{12}=0.1$, $k_{12r}=0.05$, $k_{22}=1$, $k_{32}=0.3$, $k_{42}=0.5$, $k_{42r}=0.5$, $k_{41}=0.5$, $k_{41r}=0.5$, $n=2$. Non-zero initial conditions: $b_1(0)=4$, $b_2(0)=4$, $e_{o_1}=5$, $e_{o_2}=5$.
Use a vertical scale of 0 to 30 and a time scale of 0 to 3000. To prove a stable limit cycle exists, plot $\dot{p}_1$ vs. p_1 and $\dot{p}_2$ vs. p_2.

9.6 A simplified feedback system model for the reduction of mean arterial pressure by IV infusion of the drug *sodium nitroprusside* (SNP) is shown in Figure P9.6 [Northrop, 2000]. The controller is an ON/OFF drug infuser; the system is to be designed to limit cycle around a set point of 110 mmHg $\overline{\text{MAP}}$. If no SNP is infused, the MAP rises to MAP_o = 200 mmHg. The MAP reduction plant parameters are $K_p=2$, and $a=1, b=0.2$ and $\delta=0.5$ minutes.

a. Find the u_{max} required to give a 50% duty cycle oscillation around the setpoint (i.e., $\overline{E}=0$).

b. Use the vector solution of $\mathbf{N}^{-1}(E)$ and $-\mathbf{G_p}(j\omega)$ to find the frequency of the limit cycle, f_o, in cycles/min. and the peak value of E for SP = 110 mmHg.

c. Using the system parameters above, *simulate the system with* Simulink®/Matlab®, or Simnon™. Plot u, SP and MAP(t). Step the SP

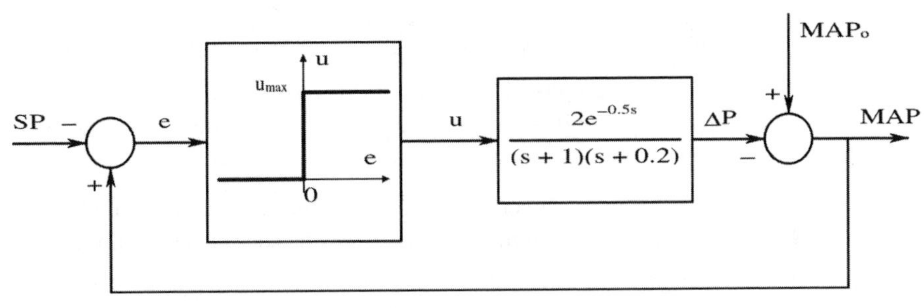

FIGURE P9.6

from 110 to 130 to 90 mmHg. Allow about 30 min at each SP level (model time) for the system to reach steady-state. Does the frequency of the limit cycle oscillations change with SP? Show what happens to MAP if the infuser is jammed on.

9.7 Figure P9.7 illustrates five Nyquist plots (steady-state, sinusoidal frequency response) of SISO feedback system loop gains, $A_L(s)$. The frequency response has been plotted for all complex **s**-values ranging from $\mathbf{s} = \varepsilon$ to $\mathbf{s} = j\varepsilon$, and up the $j\omega$ axis to $\mathbf{s} = j\infty$, thence around to $\mathbf{s} = +\infty$. (In practice, only $\mathbf{s} = j\omega$ values would be considered from 0 to $+\infty$.)

For each plot, tell whether the closed-loop system is stable as the figure is drawn, and whether it can become unstable for any positive K of the loop gain transfer function. Tell whether the system will oscillate or saturate without oscillation if the system is unstable. (Hint: draw the $\mathbf{A_L(s)}$ locus for **s** traversing the bottom half of the contour of text Figure 9.6 for each of the five plots shown.) For plot (e), discuss the stability characteristics of the closed-loop system as the loop gain K is varied.

9.8 Figure P9.8a illustrates a linear drug infusion controller with input infusion rate saturation. In order to use the DF method of analysis, we must convert the nonlinearity to an odd function, as shown in Figure P9.8b. In this system, the linear infuser gain is $K_i = u_m/v_m$. The system poles and zeros are: $a = 4$ r/hr, $b = 1$ r/hr, $c = 10$ r/hr (pharmacokinetic systems are not fast). The plant gain, K_p, is fixed, and the controller gain and infuser gain, K_c and K_i, can be varied as part of the design process. If the gain product, $K_pK_cK_i$, exceeds a certain value, the closed-loop system will break into a bounded oscillation (limit cycle).

a. Make a polar (Nyquist) plot of the linear loop gain, $\mathbf{A_L(s)}$ for **s** traversing the complete contour C_1 in the s-plane shown in text Figure 9.6.

b. Find the numerical value for ω_o where $\mathbf{A_L}(j\omega_o)$ crosses the $-360°$ axis. This will require an iterative trial and error solution. ω_o will be in radians/hour.

c. Find the DF for the odd nonlinearity shown in Figure P9.8b. Plot $\mathbf{N^{-1}}(v')$ on the polar plot of $\mathbf{A_L(s)}$. Let $K_i = 1$.

d. Find the range of $K_pK_cK_i$ over which the closed-loop system is stable.

e. If $\mathbf{A_L}(j\omega_o)$ intersects $\mathbf{N^{-1}}(v')$, find the system oscillation frequency, and the peak amplitude of the oscillations in y. (This question can be solved by simulation or analytically.)

9.9 The frequency response function of an LTI system is to be identified by its cross-power density spectrum, given a zero-mean Gaussian noise input. Text Equation 9.58 is used:

$$\mathbf{H}(j\omega) = \frac{\mathbf{\Phi_{xy}}(\omega)}{\mathbf{\Phi_{xy}}(\omega)}$$

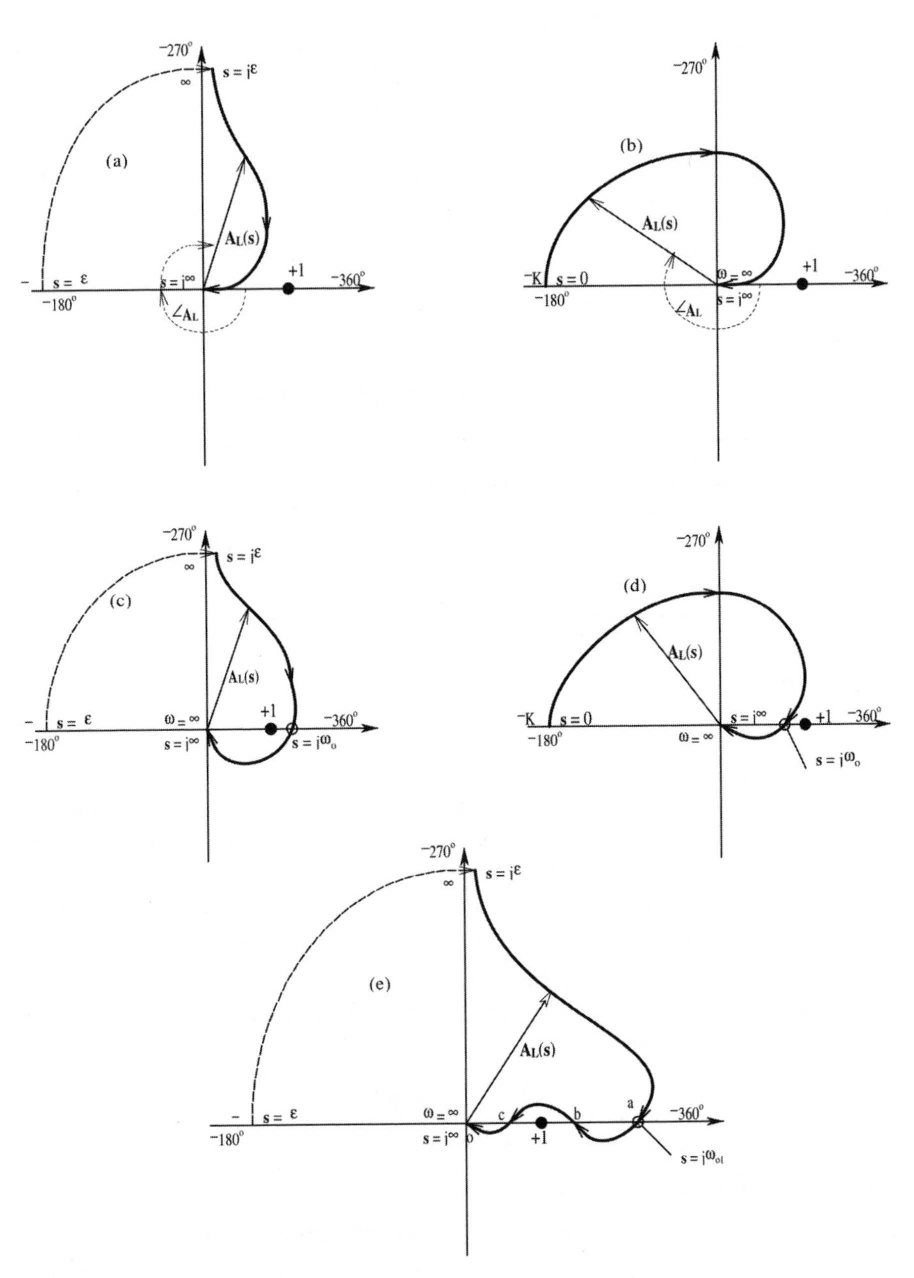

(a)
−270°
s = iε
∞
A_L(s)
s = ε
s = i∞
+1
−360°
−180°
∠A_L
(b)
−270°
A_L(s)
−K
s = 0
ω = ∞
s = i∞
+1
−360°
−180°
∠A_L
(c)
−270°
s = iε
∞
A_L(s)
s = ε
ω = ∞
s = i∞
+1
−360°
−180°
s = iω_o
(d)
−270°
A_L(s)
−K
s = 0
s = i∞
ω = ∞
+1
−360°
−180°
s = iω_o
(e)
−270°
s = iε
∞
A_L(s)
s = ε
ω = ∞
s = i∞
a
b
c
+1
−360°
−180°
s = iω_ol

FIGURE P9.7

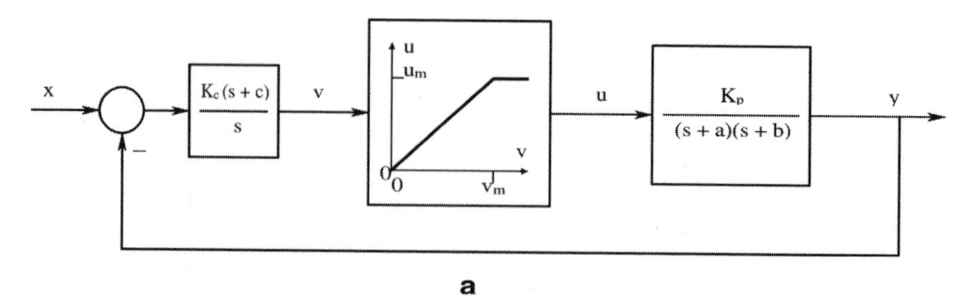

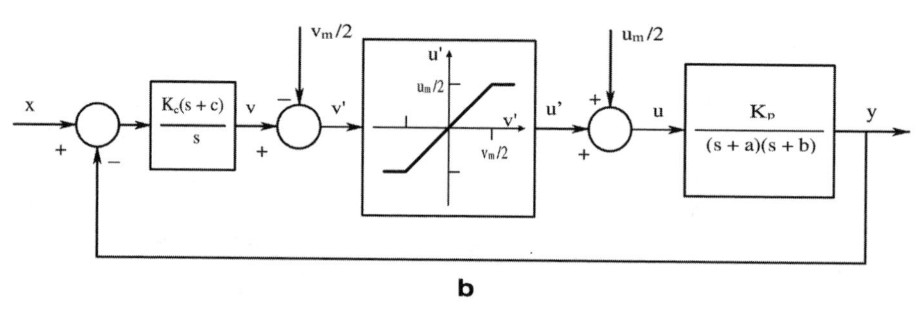

FIGURE P9.8

$\Phi_{xx}(\omega)$ is known to be of the form, $2\alpha\sigma_x^2/(\alpha^2+\omega^2)$, where σ_x^2 is the variance of the zero-mean Gaussian noise, and α is the half-power frequency of the noise autopower spectrum in radians/sec. The cross-power spectrum is found to be of the form: $\mathbf{\Phi}_{\mathbf{xy}}(\omega) = \beta/(j\omega+\beta)$. Find an algebraic expression for $|\mathbf{H}(j\omega)|$ and $\angle\mathbf{H}(j\omega)$. Assume $\alpha >> \beta$.

9.10 Broadband Gaussian noise having the autocorrelation function, $\varphi_{xx}(\tau) = \sigma_x^2 \exp(-a|\tau|)$ is the input to an LTI quadratic bandpass filter having the frequency response function,

$$\mathbf{H}(j\omega) = \frac{j\omega(K2\varepsilon/\omega_n)}{\{[j\omega/j\omega_n]^2 + (j\omega)(2\xi/\omega_n) + 1\}}$$

a. Find an expression for $\Phi_{xx}(\omega)$.

b. Find an expression for the filter output autopower spectrum, $\Phi_{yy}(\omega)$.

c. Plot and dimension $\Phi_{yy}(\omega)$ for $0 \leq \omega \leq 10$ r/sec. Let: $\sigma_x^2 = 1$, $a = 100$ r/sec, $\omega_n = 1$ r/sec, $\xi = 0.05$, $K = 10$.

9.11 Figure P9.11 illustrates a SISO LTI system. The inputs are two independent and uncorrelated Gaussian variables having zero means.

a. Write an expression for $y(t)$ in the time domain using real convolutions.

b. Write an expression for the output autopower spectrum, $\Phi_{yy}(\omega)$, in terms of the transfer functions and input autopower spectra.

c. Show that: $\mathbf{H_1}(j\omega) = \mathbf{\Phi_{xy}}(\omega)/\Phi_{xx}(\omega)$ and $\mathbf{H}_2(j\omega) = \Phi_{uy}(\omega)/\Phi_{uu}(\omega)$.

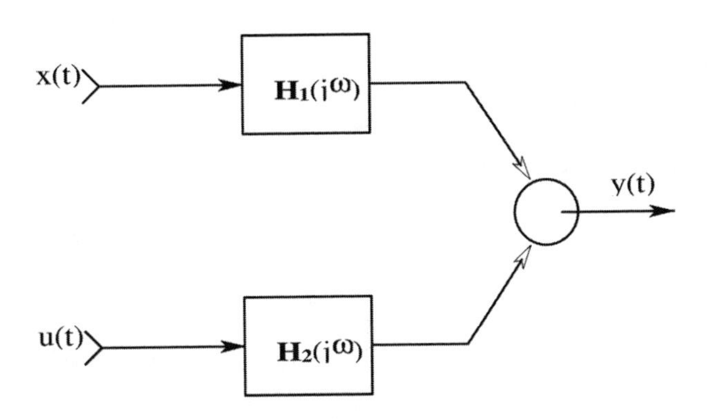

FIGURE P9.11

10

The Mathematics of Tomographic Imaging

10.1 Introduction

This chapter is *not* about the technology of the various means of medical tomographic imaging, but rather describes the mathematical tools common to many imaging modalities that permit the construction of tomographic sections of the body. In particular, we will consider the basic *algebraic reconstruction algorithm,* the *Radon transform,* the *Fourier slice theorem,* and the *filtered back-projection algorithm* (FBPA). With the exception of source-moving film and analog x-ray tomography, all other tomographical imaging is done numerically by computer. You will see that, in certain cases, it is expedient to use continuous calculus to introduce and describe certain tomographic imaging algorithms.

Most medical imaging seeks to resolve noninvasively the internal anatomy of the body — its organs and cells. A number of different modalities, each with its own advantages and disadvantages, are used in noninvasive medical imaging [Northrop, 2002]. The etymology of the word *tomography* comes from the Greek *tomos,* a cut or slice, and -graphy from the Greek *graphein*, to write. Different tomographic algorithms have been applied to a number of imaging modalities in order to reconstruct images of internal "slices" of body parts; the brain, lungs, intestines, skeletal structures, etc. The slices can then be stacked to produce a high-resolution 3-D image, characterized by volume elements called *voxels.*

There are basically three types of tomographic imaging systems: *emission tomography, transmission tomography,* and *magnetic resonance imaging* (MRI). In the first class are those imaging techniques that count γ photons emitted randomly from radioisotopes or radionuclides from within the body, e.g., positron emission tomography (PET) and single photon emission tomography (SPECT). In the second class are x-ray, microwave and ultrasound imaging systems in which the absorption of beams of radiation directed through the body is processed to give a tomographic image. In MRI, transient radio-frequency pulses emitted by certain molecules excited by a strong pulsed magnetic field are measured and used to measure the density of the responding atoms in the tissue slice [Northrop, 2002].

The central problem in any method of tomography is to generate, within the boundaries of the slice, a discrete 2-D pixel array that describes either the γ-ray or x-ray absorption properties of the different classes of tissues within the slice, or the radioactivity density (of γ-ray emitting molecules), or the density of RF-emitting molecules (in MRI) within the slice. The pixels are generally given gray density or can have pseudo-color.

In PET and SPECT, the basic measurement leading to a complete tomogram is the photon count over a preset time interval or radiation intensity with a sensor with a narrow acceptance angle. A sensor's *directional selectivity* (acceptance angle) defines a *line of response* (LOR) (one of many) through the plane of the slice along which the x- or γ-radiation photons pass and are absorbed. Alternately, the sensor is a collimated radiation counter that responds to radioactive decay photons arriving along its LOR in the plane of the slice. Many lines of response are required at many angles to completely characterize the radio density of pixels in a slice. Several complex discrete mathematical algorithms can be used to construct the pixels in the tomographic slice from the LOR geometry and the sensor responses. Two of them are introduced in the following sections.

Almost everyone is familiar with x-rays; no less important for visualizing the details of internal soft tissues is *ultrasound.* Injected or ingested radionuclides and radioisotopes that have affinity for particular types of internal tissues are used in SPECT, in PET and also in *scintimammography.* Another major imaging modality is MRI. In MRI, the patient ingests or is injected with compounds containing the magnetically sensitive atoms incorporated into synthetic biomolecules that have affinities to certain tissues. Microwaves have also been used to explore internal body structures; to-date, microwave tomography has given poor resolution, and is difficult to implement, requiring immersion of the patient, or a patient's body part, in a tank of distilled water, surrounded by water-covered antennas [Northrop, 2002].

In its simplest form, a radiation tomogram is generated by computer calculations done on photon sensor outputs when a source (e.g., x-ray) sends electromagnetic (photon) radiation through the body to sensors on the opposite side. Of consideration in the computation is the radiation pattern of the source, the radiation absorption characteristics of body organs in the total path a ray takes from source to sensor, the *directional sensitivity function* of the sensors, and the angle of the source and sensors with respect to the body's axis. As you will see below, there are several possible geometric forms for scanning the object slice in order to obtain data to compute a tomographic image. In SPECT and PET, an isotope-tagged biochemical within the body is concentrated by biochemical affinity to certain organs or cell structures such as cancers. The radioactive decay of the isotope is random in time and direction. By positioning collimated γ- ray sensors around the body in the plane of the desired tomogram and counting the radioactive photons emitted in each sensor position over a set time span, it is possible to mathematically construct a map of isotope density in the tomographic plane. Resolution in SPECT and PET is generally not as good as other imaging modalities because of the randomness of radioactive decay and the relatively poor collimation of the high-energy photon sensors.

X-ray tomography also has the problem of beam and sensor collimation. In x-ray computed tomography (also known as CAT), it is technically difficult to make a collimated, nearly mono-chromatic, x-ray source. The intensity of an emergent x-ray beams depends on the total energy absorption by all of the tissues in the path the photons travel, and x-ray scattering from within the tissues. By making many x-ray beam paths and rotating them around the circumference of the tomographic slice, it is possible to calculate the absorption in a small area element (pixel) in the tomographic slice. Modern CAT scanners use a flat, fan-shaped beam of x-rays of nearly constant intensity. The fan-shaped beam is rotated around the center (axis) of the slice; on the opposite side of the x-ray source an arc-shaped array of collimated x-ray photon sensors follows the rotation of the source. See Figure 10.1 for an illustration of this system.

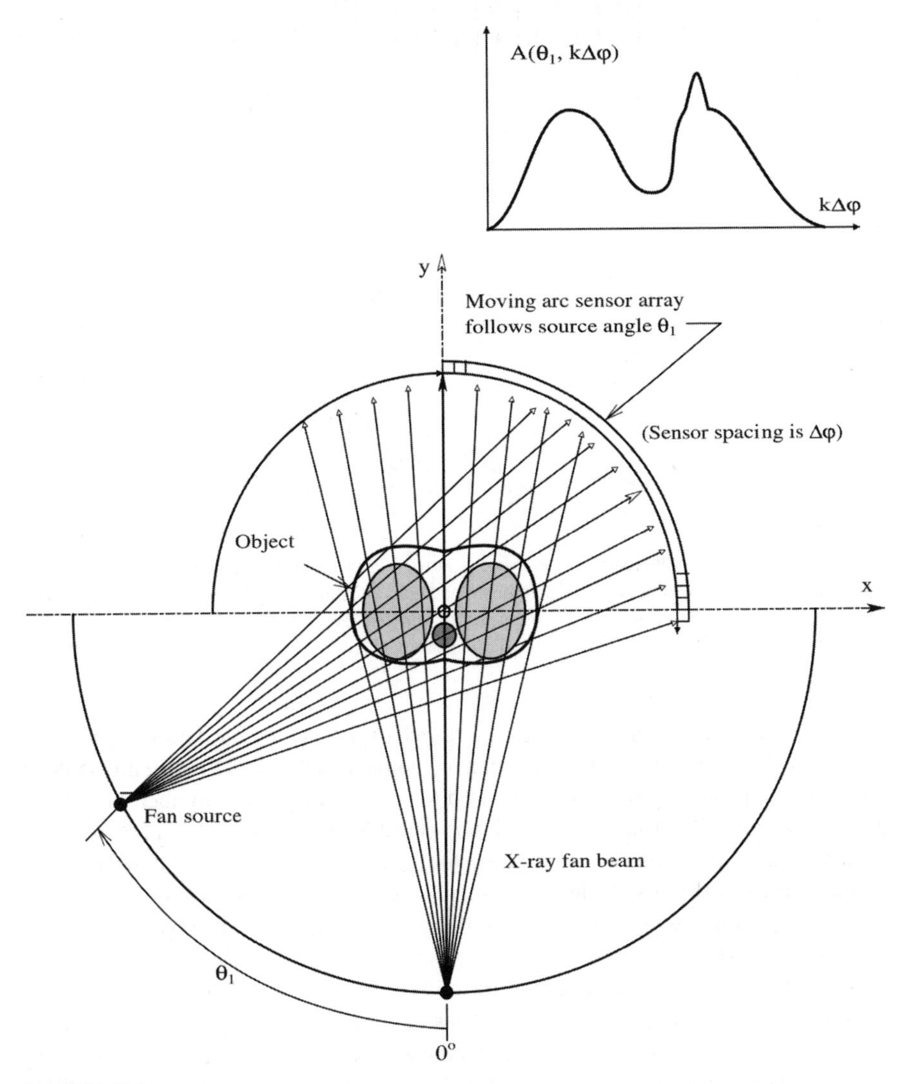

FIGURE 10.1

Schematic illustration of the fan-beam geometry used in modern x-ray computed tomography. The x-ray absorbance measured by the sensors in the array for source angle, θ_1, is shown in the inset diagram. $k\Delta\varphi$ is the sensor position in the array.

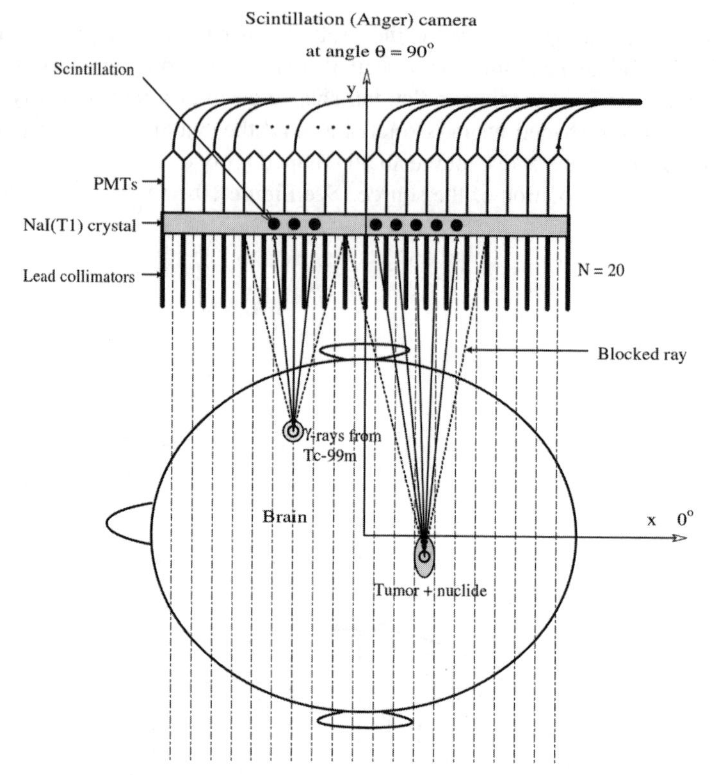

FIGURE 10.2
Schematic of a flat, scintillation-type gamma camera used to measure the location of radioisotope "hot spots" in tissues such as brain, breasts (scintimammography), and liver. (Northrop , R.B. 2000. *Endogenous and Exogenous Regulation and Control of Physiological Systems.* CRC Press, Boca Raton, With permission.)

In SPECT and scintimammography, a curved or flat-plate scintillation-type γ camera is used to count the photons produced by radioactive decay of the labeling isotope. Figure 10.2 illustrates such a camera used to sense brain tumors by their concentration of radioactivity. Tumor localization is possible by the lead collimators that pass nearly on-axis γ photons to the sensors. Obliquely directed (e.g., scattered) gamma photons are absorbed by the lead and do not reach the scintillation crystal. When an on-axis γ photon interacts with the scintillation crystal, a burst of visible photons is produced, some of which are detected by one of the sensitive photomultiplier tubes (PMTs) on the back of the collimator/scintillator/PMT assembly. The γ camera can be moved around the head to give a series of "views" of the radioactive volumes, providing 3-D localization. The information provided by the γ camera is the intensity of the radiation on a line from the center of a given collimator/scintillator/PMT cell. Range to the emitting isotope cannot be determined from one counting period at one angular position. Range to the center of the radioactivity can be obtained only by moving the camera around the head in the tomographic plane, stopping at various angular positions, and counting photons. Assuming negligible absorption and scattering of emitted γ photons, the various lines (actually vectors) from a given collimator/scintillator/PMT cell at various angular positions will intersect in the source volume of radioactivity. The exact shape and extent of the radio volume can then be calculated by one of several mathematical algorithms.

The next section describes the basic *algebraic reconstruction algorithm* that has been used to localize radioactivity in a tomographic slice, or to determine the x-ray density of small pixels in the slice. For high pixel resolution, the *algebraic reconstruction technique* (ART) is computationally intense.

10.2 Algebraic Reconstruction

To introduce the ART to form tomograms in SPECT, consider a very simple 2-D-model γ-ray emitter, shown in Figure 10.3. Four regions (pixels), each having a different radioactive density, μ_k, are shown. The γ-ray counts per second (CPS) is assumed to be the sum of the radioactivity in the two pixels in the acceptance line (LOR). Hence, the total CPS of emerging beam $j=2$ is $C_2=(\mu_1+\mu_2)$, and the total CPS of the diagonal beam $j=3$ is $C_3=(\mu_1+\mu_4)$, etc. The problem is to compute the $\{\mu_k\}$ in the slice from the counts $C_1 \ldots C_6$. Since six beams can be passed through the four-pixel absorber in a unique manner, six equations are available to solve for the four unknown pixel radioactivities, $\{\mu_k\}$:

$$C_1=\mu_3+\mu_4 \tag{10.1A}$$

$$C_2=\mu_1+\mu_2 \tag{10.1B}$$

$$C_3=\mu_1+\mu_4 \tag{10.1C}$$

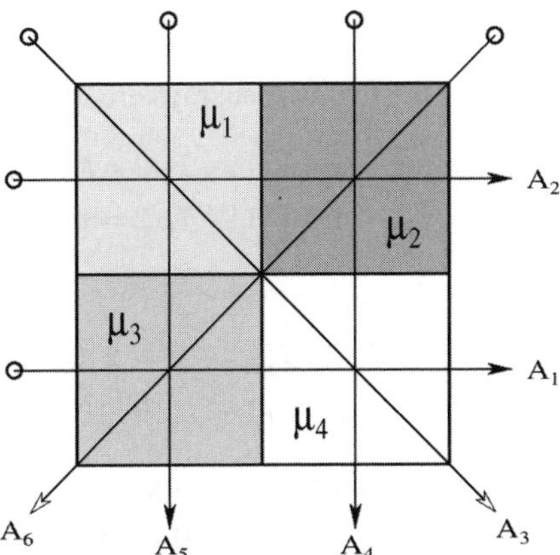

FIGURE 10.3

A simple four-pixel model of radioisotope density used to illustrate the algebraic reconstruction technique. (Northrop, R.B. 2000. *Endogenous and Exogenous Regulation and Control of Physiological Systems.* CRC Press, Boca Raton, With permission.)

$$C_4 = \mu_2 + \mu_4 \quad (10.1D)$$

$$C_5 = \mu_1 + \mu_3 \quad (10.1E)$$

$$C_6 = \mu_2 + \mu_3 \quad (10.1F)$$

With six equations and four unknowns, it appears that the system is overdetermined (four equations should be required to solve for four unknowns). However, solution for the $\{\mu_\mathbf{k}\}$ by using Cramer's rule to solve linear algebraic equations is impossible because the system determinant, $\Delta, \equiv 0$. Macovski (1983) showed that the $\{\mu_\mathbf{k}\}$ can be estimated by an iterative linear ART algorithm, illustrated below:

$$^{q+1}\mu_k = {}^q\mu_k + \left[C_j - \sum_{k=1}^{N} {}^q\mu_k\right] / N \quad (10.2)$$

Here, $^{q+1}\mu_k$ is the estimated radioactivity (in counts per minute, *cpm*) of the kth pixel in the jth ray path after the qth iteration, N is the number of pixels in the jth ray path, $\sum_{k=1}^{N} {}^q\mu_k$ is the sum of the estimated radioactivity for the pixels in the jth ray path, q is the iteration number, and C_j is the *measured* count over the jth ray path.

Let us do a numerical example, following the procedure as described in Makovski: Let $\mu_1 = 1$, $\mu_2 = 10$, $\mu_3 = 2$, $\mu_4 = 1$. Thus $C_1 = 3$, $C_2 = 11$, $C_3 = 2$, $C_4 = 11$, $C_5 = 3$, $C_6 = 12$. To obtain the q = 1 estimates, Macovski sets all the (initial) $q=0$, $\{^0\mu_k\}$ estimates to zero, and considers the two horizontal rays. For $q=1$ and C_1:

$$^1\mu_3 = {}^1\mu_4 = 0 + [3 - 0]/2 = 1.5 \quad (10.3)$$

For C_2:

$$^1\mu_1 = {}^1\mu_2 = 0 + [11 - 0]/2 = 5.5 \quad (10.4)$$

Thus the $q=1$ pixel estimates are:

$$\begin{matrix} 5.5 & 5.5 \\ 1.5 & 1.5 \end{matrix}$$

In the next (q = 2) iteration, the two vertical rays are used. For C_4:

$$^2\mu_2 = 5.5 + [11 - 7]/2 = 7.5 \quad (10.5A)$$

$$^2\mu_4 = 1.5 + [11 - 7]/2 = 3.5 \quad (10.5B)$$

For C_5:

$$^2\mu_1 = 5.5 + [3 - 7]/2 = 3.5 \quad (10.5C)$$

$$^2\mu_3 = 1.5 + [3 - 7]/2 = -0.5 \quad (10.5D)$$

Now the $q=2$ trial absorbance values are:

$$\begin{matrix} 3.5 & 7.5 \\ -0.5 & 3.5 \end{matrix}$$

Do not worry about the negative count in μ_3 in an intermediate step. For the third iteration, Macovski uses the two diagonals: For C_3:

$$^3\mu_1 = 3.5 + [2 - 7]/2 = 1.0 \quad (10.6A)$$

$$^3\mu_4 = 3.5 + [2-7]/2 = 1.0 \tag{10.6B}$$

For C_6:

$$^3\mu_2 = 7.5 + [12-7]/2 = 10 \tag{10.6C}$$

$$^3\mu_3 = -0.5 + [12-7]/2 = 2 \tag{10.6D}$$

Thus, we see that in only three iterations for this simple example, the exact $\{\mu_k\}$ values are obtained. When j, N and k are large, convergence on the exact $\{\mu_k\}$ values can be very slow. Exact convergence may be impractical in terms of computation time; convergence can be tested by examining the magnitude of the normalized error for the jth path at the qth iteration:

$$^q\varepsilon_j = \left| \left[C_j - \sum_{k=1}^{N} {}^q\mu_k \right] / C_j \right| \tag{10.7}$$

The linear ART process can be halted when the largest $^q\varepsilon_j$ reaches a preset minimum. Note that other nonlinear estimation techniques for the $\{\mu_k\}$ exist based on criteria such as the least MS error, etc, however, their description is beyond the scope of this chapter.

Note that the ART can also be used to calculate the x-ray absorbance in pixels. In this case, instead of counting γ photons from radioactive decay, the sensor output is proportional to the intensity of the emergent x-ray beam. Each pixel the beam traverses absorbs some of the entering beam's intensity according to the Beer's law rule for the jth beam:

$$I_{jo} = I_{in} \exp\left[-\sum_{k=1}^{N} \alpha_k \right] \tag{10.8}$$

The total absorbance along the jth path is just:

$$A_j = \ln[I_{in}/I_{jo}] = \sum_{k=1}^{N} \alpha_k \tag{10.9}$$

Now the ART can be applied using A_j instead of C_j, and solving for the $\{\alpha_k\}$ instead of pixel radioactivity, $\{\mu_k\}$.

10.3 The Radon Transform

The Radon transform was devised in 1917 by mathematician Johann Radon as a means of reconstructing an image from linear projections. Like many discoveries in mathematics and science, it did not find serious early application until the development of the x-ray CAT scanner in the early 1970s in England by G.N. Hounsfield and A. McCormack [Northrop, 2002].

To examine the use of the *Radon transform* in tomographic imaging, we first assume a continuous 2-D object slice that has either has a 2-D radioactivity density, $\mu(x,y)$, or an x-ray absorption density, $\alpha(x,y)$ in the tomographic slice being studied in the X, Y plane. In a discrete emission system, we consider $\mu_{jk} = \mu(j\Delta x, k\Delta y)$ in the j, k^{th} pixel, of area $(\Delta x \ \Delta y)$ etc. In practice, we must use discrete mathematics in tomography, although it is pedagogically sweeter to use continuous functions and integrals when introducing the mathematics of the Radon transform. Also, in describing the Radon transform, the mathematics are easier if we consider an array of *parallel* emitted γ-ray paths or x-ray beams, and a linear array of collimator/detectors (even though modern x-ray tomography uses fan beams).

Before we present the Radon transform and discuss its use, let us examine the simple geometry of a rotation of cartesian coordinates, preserving the origin. (See Figure 10.4.) Let us rotate the new (x', y') coordinates counter-clockwise by an

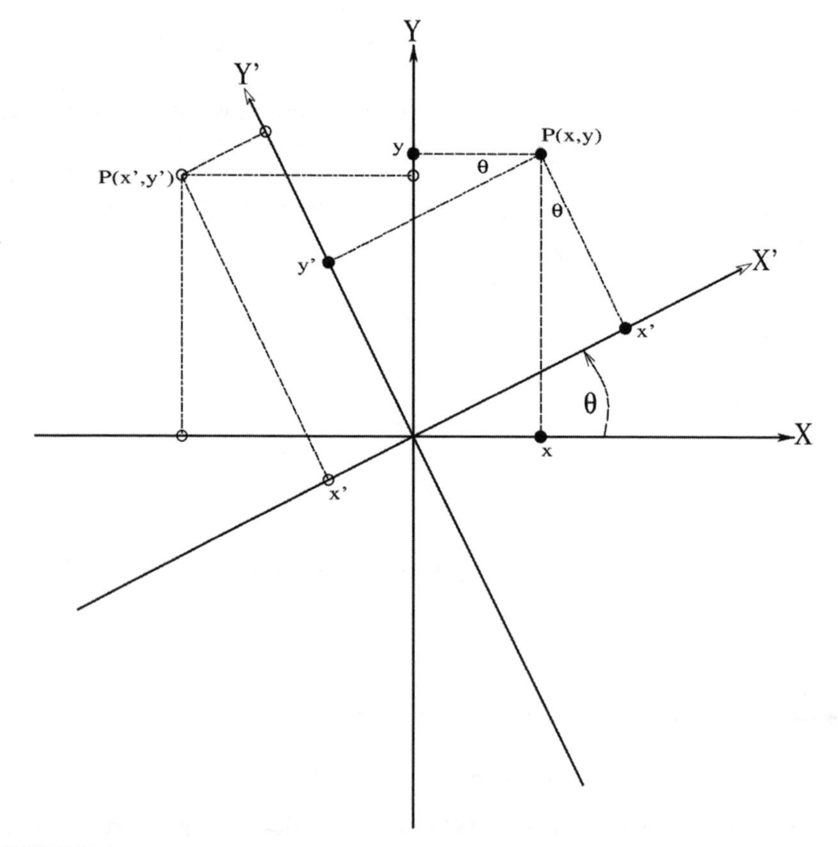

FIGURE 10.4
Geometric relations in simple rotation of cartesian coordinates around the origin.

angle θ. Consider a point $P(x,y)$ in the X, Y plane. In the rotated X′, Y′ plane, this point can be shown by simple trigonometry to project to:

$$x' = x\cos\theta + y\sin\theta \tag{10.10A}$$

$$y' = -x\sin\theta + y\cos\theta \tag{10.10B}$$

in the X′, Y′ plane. Similarly, a point at x', y' in the X′, Y′ plane is located at

$$x = x'\cos\theta - y'\sin\theta \tag{10.11A}$$

$$y = x'\sin\theta + y'\cos\theta \tag{10.11B}$$

in the original X,Y plane.

Now consider a 2-D object slice undergoing tomography, lying in the X, Y plane. The object can have either a radioactivity density, $\mu(x,y)$, or an x-ray absorption density, $\alpha(x,y)$. For an arbitrary straight path going from (x_i,y_i) to (x_o,y_o) as shown in Figure 10.5, the net radioactive decay count will be:

$$c_P = \int_{y_i}^{y_o}\int_{x_i}^{x_o} \mu(x,y)\,dx\,dy \tag{10.12}$$

Because it is required to estimate $\mu(x,y)$ from a finite set of straight paths, $\{P\}$, a systematic approach using the Radon transform was developed. See Figure 10.5 for the parallel scan geometry. Parallel beams or rays have been assumed for convenience. The Radon transform can be written to describe the net radioactive count along a *projection line* (PL) which lies at an angle θ with the Y axis and is parallel to the Y′ axis. The sifting property of the delta function is used to define the integration path. Liley (2001) used a vector dot product notation to define the PL over which $\mu(x,y)$ is integrated. **n** is a *unit vector* directed from the origin along the x' axis perpendicular to the PL. From Figure 10.5, we see that the angle of **n** with respect to the X axis is θ. ρ is a vector connecting the origin to any point P on the PL. Thus, $\mathbf{n}\cdot\rho = |\rho|\cos(\gamma) = \sigma$ is the scalar distance from the origin along the X′ axis to a point on the PL. (The X′ axis is always made $\perp$ to the PL.) Thus the polar parameters θ and ρ define the PL. Liley writes the Radon transform in vector form as:

$$c(\theta,x') = \int_{-\infty}^{\infty} \mu(\rho)\,\delta(\mathbf{n}\cdot\rho - x')\,d\rho \tag{10.13}$$

If the vector form is intimidating, we can write the argument of the delta function to define the PL in the more generally-used, cartesian form below:

$$c(\theta,\sigma) = \int_{-\infty}^{\infty}\int_{-\infty}^{\infty} \mu(x,y)\,\delta[x\cos(\theta) + y\sin(\theta) - \sigma]\,dx\,dy \tag{10.14}$$

Note that the Radon transform is a projective transformation of a two-dimensional function onto the polar coordinate space (θ,x'). σ is simply the distance a given PL is offset along the X′ axis from the origin. From another viewpoint, the RT is simply a definite line integral (a functional) that returns a real numerical value for a given

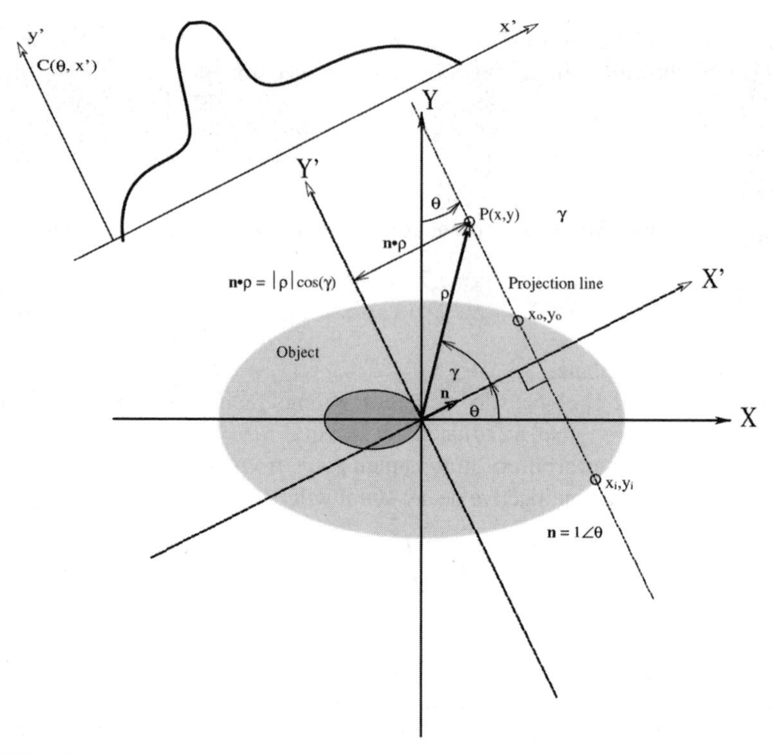

FIGURE 10.5
Schematic illustration of parallel scan geometry used in the development of the Radon transform. Scan lines are parallel to the X' axis, which is rotated by angle θ with respect to the X axis. A point $P(x',y')$ on a scan line can be located in polar coordinates by a vector ρ with length ρ from the origin and at an angle γ with the X' axis. $P(x',y')$ is at a distance $\sigma = \rho \bullet \mathbf{n} = x'$ from the Y' axis. (**n** is a unit vector pointing along the X' axis.)

object, rotation angle θ, and PL displacement, σ, from the X' axis. For a particular PL integration path as shown, x ranges from x_i to x_o, and y ranges from y_i to y_o. Clearly, these limits are a function of the object's geometry. In practice, a number of integration paths parallel to the y' axis are used, each spaced $\sigma(k) = k\Delta x'$ apart. The angle θ is also changed in finite increments: $\theta(j) = j\Delta\theta$. A total span of $0 \le \theta \le \pi$ is required. As a result, a huge, discrete, 2-D array of values for $c(j,k)$ approximating the continuous $c(\theta,\sigma)$ is obtained. This array is called the *sinogram* of the image. The sinogram is called that because the sinograms of simple objects (points, lines, etc.) appear to be a superposition of many sections of sine waves of different amplitudes and phases, but all having the same period. A sinogram of the well-known Shepp-Logan x-ray phantom is shown in Figure 10.6. Note that the sinogram must be processed further to construct an estimate of $\mu(x,y)$.

Sinograms by themselves have been used as an elementary form of feature detector. A linear object (straight line) in x,y space can be shown to have a point Radon transform in sinogram (θ,σ) space. An object of black-and-white lines on a gray

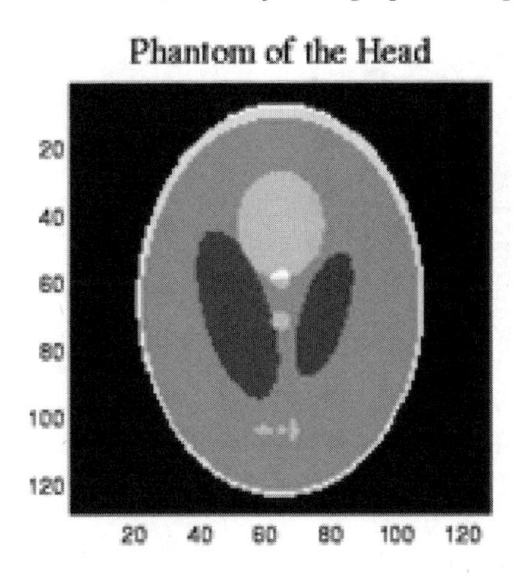

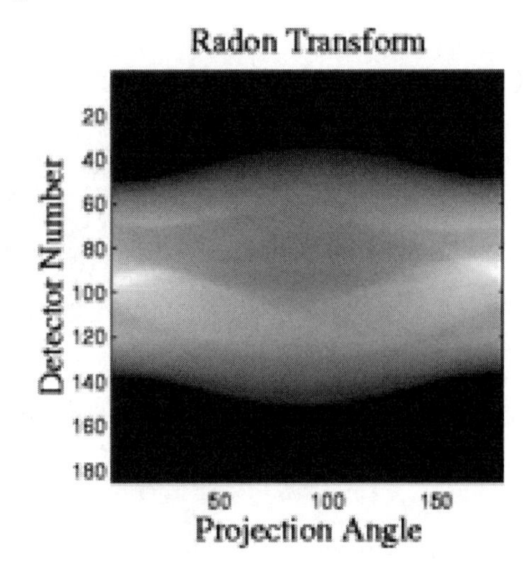

FIGURE 10.6

(Left) A Shepp-Logan x-ray phantom (x-ray-absorbing test object) of a head. (Right) The sinogram of the head phantom constructed from many Radon transforms taken at many values of θ and σ. (Amini, W., et al. 1997. *Tomographic Reconstruction of SPECT Data.* At URL: www.owlnet.rice.edu/˜elec539/Projects97/cult/report.html)

background is shown in x,y space in Figure 10.7. The sinogram for these lines is shown in Figure 10.8; note that the black lines produce black points and the white lines, white points in the sinogram. The intensity of a point is proportional to line length. The Radon transform sinogram is effective in detecting lines in a noisy background, as shown in Figures 10.9 to 10.12. The longer the line, the better the signal-to-noise ratio (SNR) will be in the sinogram. (A longer line gives a more intense spot in the sinogram, and there is a greater length over which the noise is

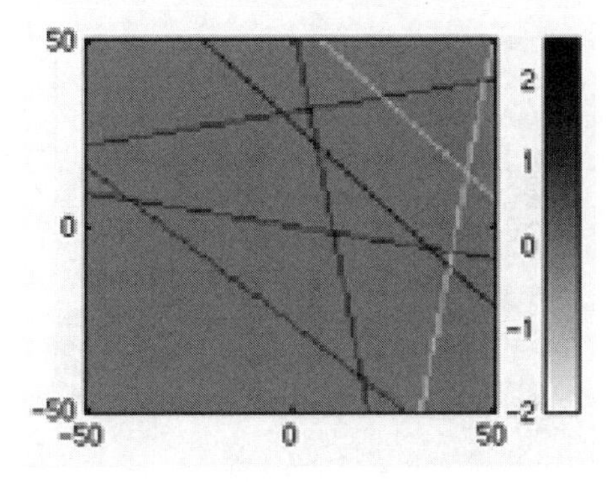

FIGURE 10.7

A radiographic test object containing black and white lines at various angles on a uniform gray field. (Toft, Peter. *The Radon Transform,* http://eivind.imm.dtu.dk/staff/ptoft/Radon/Radon.html. With permission.)

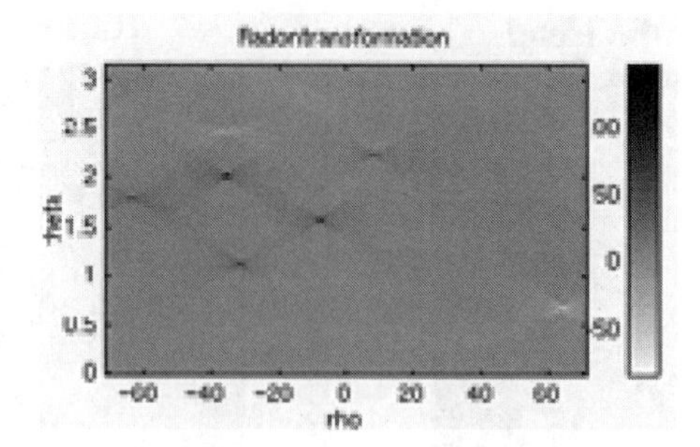

FIGURE 10.8
Sinogram for the lines of Figure 10.7. The Radon transform is seen to act as a line detector. (Toft, Peter. *The Radon Transform,* http://eivind.imm.dtu.dk/staff/ptoft/Radon/Radon.html. With permission.)

averaged.) Note that DSP techniques such as nonlinear thresholding can be used to reduce the noise components in the sinogram, so that when the image of the scanned object is reconstructed, it, too, will have a better SNR.

Let us now return to the 2-D continuous $c(\theta, \sigma)$ sinogram, and consider how $\mu(x, y)$ can be found from it.

10.4 The Fourier Slice Theorem

The *Fourier slice theorem* (FST) will now be examined. The FST states that the 1-D, CFT of a parallel projection of a 2-D real function, $\mu(x,y)$, taken at an angle θ, gives a slice of the 2-D transform, $\mathbf{M}(u,v)$, subtending an angle θ with the u frequency

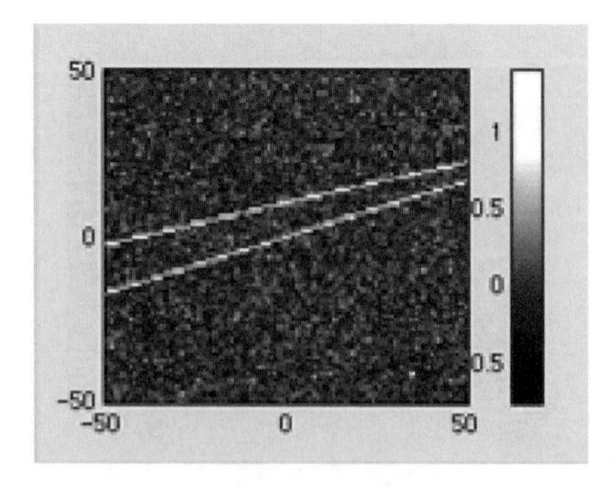

FIGURE 10.9
A test object having two lines on a noisy gray field. (Toft, Peter. *The Radon Transform,* http://eivind.imm.dtu.dk/staff/ptoft/Radon/Radon.html. With permission.)

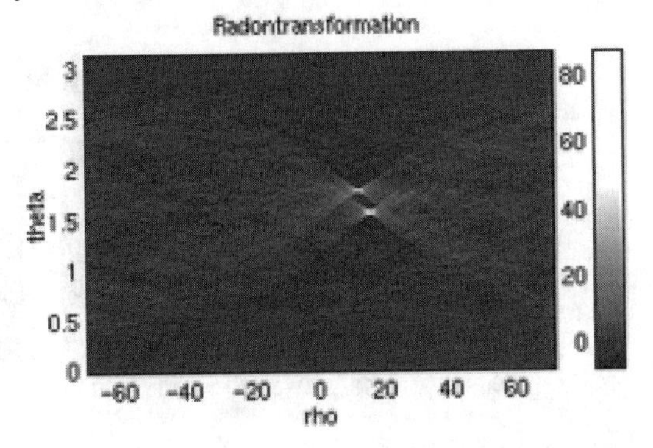

FIGURE 10.10
Sinogram for the two lines shown in Figure 10.9. Note that the Radon transform effectively averages out the high spatial frequency background noise. (Toft, Peter. *The Radon Transform,* http://eivind.imm.dtu.dk/staff/ptoft/Radon/Radon.html. With permission.)

axis. This theorem indicates that, as the number of projections, $\mathbf{C}(\theta, \mathrm{w})$, approaches infinity, $\mathbf{M}(\mathrm{u,v})$ is known at all points in the u,v frequency space. In the limit, the original radio-density image function, $\mu(\mathrm{x,y})$, can then be recovered by taking the 2-D IFT of $\mathbf{M}(\mathrm{u,v})$. Recall that the 2-D spatial CFT of a non-negative real 2-D function, $\mu(\mathrm{x,y})$, is given by:

$$\mathbf{M}(\mathrm{u,v}) = \mathbf{F}\{\mu(\mathrm{x,y})\} = \int_{-\infty}^{\infty}\int_{-\infty}^{\infty} \mu(\mathrm{x,y})\exp[-\mathrm{j}(\mathrm{xu}+\mathrm{yv})]\mathrm{dxdy} \quad (10.15)$$

In general, $\mathbf{M}(\mathrm{u,v})$ is a complex function of the spatial frequencies u and v which have the dimensions of radians per mm. If the image, $\mu(\mathrm{x,y})$, is rotated by an angle θ with respect to the X-axis, its 2-D CFT, $\mathbf{M}(\mathrm{u,v})$, will be correspondingly rotated by θ with respect to the u spatial frequency axis. Thus, it can be shown that the 1-D CFTs

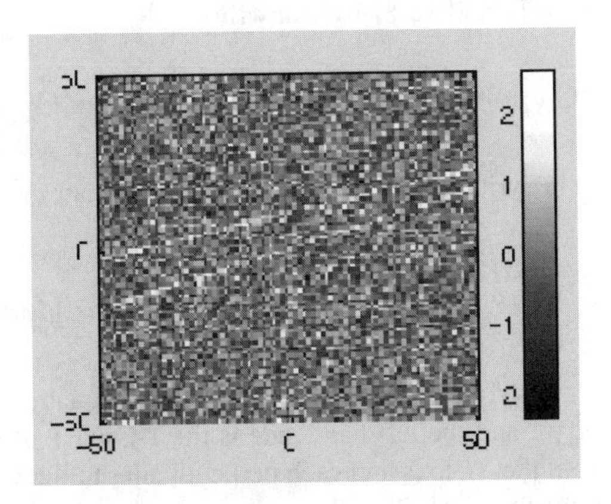

FIGURE 10.11
The same test lines as in Figure 10.9, but much more noise. (Toft, Peter. *The Radon Transform,* http://eivind.imm.dtu.dk/staff/ptoft/Radon/Radon.html. With permission.)

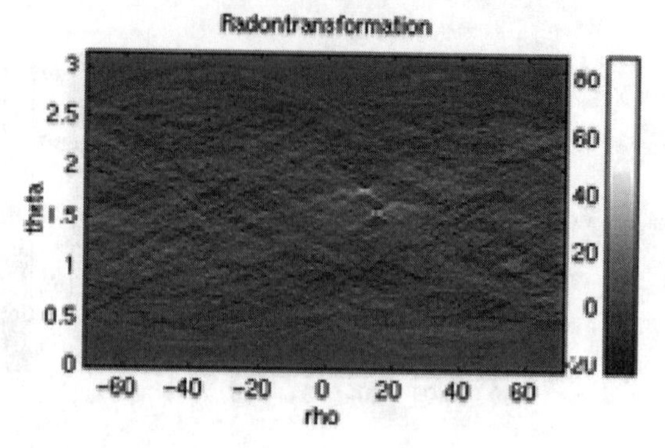

FIGURE 10.12
The sinogram corresponding to Figure 10.11 is also noisier, but the "bow-tie" signatures of the lines are still clear. (Toft, Peter. *The Radon Transform,* http://eivind.imm.dtu.dk/staff/ptoft/Radon/Radon.html. With permission.)

of projections along lines that make an angle of $(\theta+90°)$ with the X-axis (e.g., lines parallel with the Y′-axis) depict the FTs of $\mu(\text{x,y})$ along the radial line that makes an angle θ.

Let us now take the 1-D CFT of the real Radon function, $\text{c}(\theta,\sigma)$:

$$\mathbf{C}(\theta,\text{w})=\int_{-\infty}^{\infty}\text{c}(\theta,\sigma)\exp[-\text{j}\sigma\text{w}]\text{d}\sigma,\quad 0\leq\theta\leq\pi \tag{10.16}$$

Here, w is spatial frequency in radians/mm. Recall that σ is a distance in the x′ direction. As above, we define the X′, Y′ coordinate system by the linear transformation:

$$\begin{bmatrix}\text{x}'\\ \text{y}'\end{bmatrix}=\begin{bmatrix}\cos\theta & \sin\theta\\ -\sin\theta & \cos\theta\end{bmatrix}\begin{bmatrix}\text{x}\\ \text{y}\end{bmatrix} \tag{10.17}$$

From Equations 10.16 and 10.17 we can write:

$$\mathbf{C}(\theta,w)=\int_{-\infty}^{\infty}\left\{\int_{-\infty}^{\infty}\mu(\text{x}',\text{y}')\exp[-\text{j}w\text{x}']\text{dy}'\right\}dx' \tag{10.18}$$

$\mathbf{C}(\theta,w)$ can also be written in terms of the X,Y coordinates of the object. Equation 10.17 is used:

$$\mathbf{C}(\theta,w)=\int_{-\infty}^{\infty}\int_{-\infty}^{\infty}\mu(\text{x,y})\exp[-\text{j}w\text{x}']dx\,dy \tag{10.19}$$

Where: $\text{x}'=\text{x}\cos\theta+\text{y}\sin\theta$. The right-hand side of Equation 10.19 represents the 2-D CFT of $\mu(\text{x,y})$, and the left-hand side is the 1-D CFT of the projections, each spaced $\text{x}'=\sigma$ from the Y′-axis and each perpendicular to the X′-axis.

Therefore, taking the 1-D CFT of the projections of an object at angle θ is equivalent to obtaining the 2-D CFT of $\mu(\text{x,y})$ along the line σ inclined at an angle θ with the X-axis. Thus, if we consider these projections at many angles θ and for many

σ values, and the 2-D CFT is taken for the many θ and σ values, the 2-D, ICFT of these transforms will allow us to estimate the actual radioactive density, $\mu(\mathrm{x,y})$, with $\widehat{\mu}(\mathrm{x,y})$: In the limit,

$$\widehat{\mu}(\mathrm{x,y}) \cong \frac{1}{4\pi^2}\int_{-\infty}^{\infty}\int_{-\infty}^{\infty} \mathbf{C}(\theta,w)\exp[+j(\mathrm{ux}+\mathrm{vy})]\mathrm{dxdy} \tag{10.20}$$

represents the *back-projection* of the line σ, where:

$$\mathbf{C}(\theta,w) = \mathbf{M}(w\cos\theta, w\sin\theta) = \mathbf{M}(\mathrm{u,v}) \tag{10.21}$$

Note that $\mathbf{C}(\theta, w)$ is really not 2-D; it is a single-argument function defined on a set of $\{\theta_k\}$. The ICFT of $\mathbf{M}(\mathrm{u,v})$ yields $\widehat{\mu}(\mathrm{x,y})$. While we have illustrated this development with continuous integrals, the reader should remember that, in practice, finite discrete data are used, as are the DFT and IDFT to estimate $\mu(\mathrm{x,y})$.

10.5 The Filtered Back-Projection Algorithm

The goal of back projection is to estimate the 2-D radioactive density $\mu(\mathrm{x,y})$, from measurements characterized by the polar coordinate parameters, θ and distance σ along the X′-axis.

Let us transform the rectangular spatial frequency parameters, u and v, to *polar spatial frequencies.* We make the substitutions below into Equation 10.20:

$$\mathrm{u} = w\cos\theta \tag{10.22A}$$

$$\mathrm{v} = w\sin\theta \tag{10.22B}$$

$$\mathrm{dudv} = w\,dw\,d\theta \tag{10.22C}$$

The w term in Equation 10.22c comes from the Jacobian determinant used in the change of variables from rectangular to polar. That is:

$$w = \begin{vmatrix} \partial \mathrm{u}/\partial w & \partial \mathrm{v}/\partial w \\ \partial \mathrm{u}/\partial \theta & \partial \mathrm{v}/\partial \theta \end{vmatrix} \tag{10.23}$$

This gives:

$$\widehat{\mu}(\mathrm{x,y}) = \frac{1}{4\pi^2}\int_{0}^{2\pi}\int_{-\infty}^{\infty} \mathbf{M}(w,\theta)\exp[+jw(\mathrm{x}\cos\theta+\mathrm{y}\sin\theta)]\,w\,dw\,d\theta \tag{10.24}$$

Equation 10.24 can be further simplified by first breaking the integral on θ into two parts: 0 to π, and π to 2π. Thus:

$$\widehat{\mu}(x,y)=\frac{1}{4\pi^2}\int_0^{\pi}\int_{-\infty}^{\infty}\mathbf{M}(w,\theta)\exp[+jw(x\cos\theta+y\sin\theta)]w\,dw\,d\theta$$
$$+\frac{1}{4\pi^2}\int_{\pi}^{2\pi}\int_{-\infty}^{\infty}\mathbf{M}(w,\theta+\pi)$$
$$\times\exp\{+jw[x\cos(\theta+\pi)+y\sin(\theta+\pi)]\}w\,dw\,d\theta \quad (10.25)$$

It is known from Fourier transform theory that:

$$\mathbf{M}(w,\theta+\pi)=\mathbf{M}(-w,\theta) \quad (10.26)$$

Equation 10.26 can thus be used to simplify Equation 10.25:

$$\widehat{\mu}(x,y)=\frac{1}{2\pi}\int_0^{\pi}\int_{-\infty}^{\infty}\{\mathbf{M}(w,\theta)|w|\exp[+jw(x\cos\theta+y\sin\theta)]dw\}d\theta \quad (10.27)$$

From Equations 10.16 and 10.18, we can assert that $\mathbf{M}(w,\theta)=\mathbf{C}(\theta,w)$. So finally, we can write the FBP integral as:

$$\widehat{\mu}(x,y)=\int_0^{\pi}\left\{\frac{1}{2\pi}\int_{-\infty}^{\infty}\mathbf{C}(\theta,w)|w|\exp[+jw(x\cos\theta+y\sin\theta)]dw\right\}d\theta \quad (10.28)$$

Quoting Rao et al. (1995):

> "In the Equation [10.28] above, the terms inside the brackets (the operation indicated by the inner integral) represents a filtering operation and evaluate[s] the filtered projections, and the operation being performed by the outer integral evaluate[s] the back-projections, which basically represents a smearing of the filtered projections back onto the object and then finding the mean over all the angles."

The FBP algorithm can be subdivided into three steps:

1. Find the FT in 1-D of each of the projections.
2. Find the filtered projections. This means multiplying the results of step 1 with a response function that looks like that in Figure 10.13 in the spatial frequency domain, and then finding the IFT. This step is the same as carrying out convolution in the time domain. It can be represented by the IFT:

$$q(\theta,x')=\frac{1}{2\pi}\int_{-\infty}^{\infty}\mathbf{C}(\theta,w)|w|\exp(+jwx')dw \quad (10.29)$$

3. Find the back projections. This step is the smearing of the filtered projections back onto the object space, and is given mathematically by:

$$\widehat{\mu}(x,y)=\int_0^{\pi}q(\theta,x')d\theta=\int_0^{\pi}q(\theta,x\cos\theta+y\sin\theta)d\theta \quad (10.30)$$

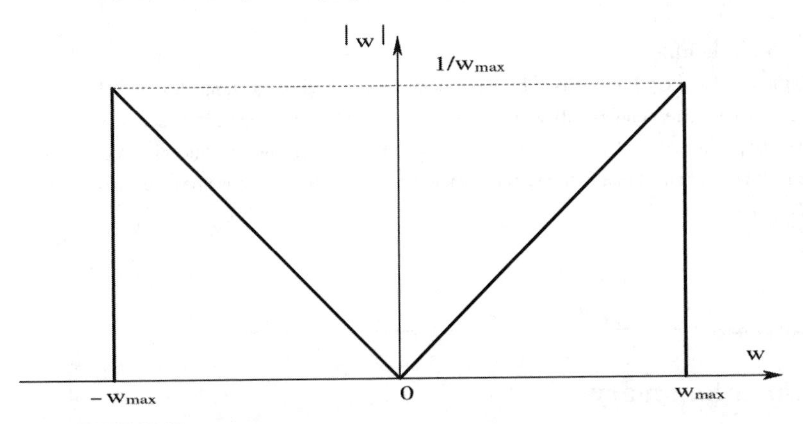

FIGURE 10.13
Spatial frequency response of the truncated spatial high-pass filter used in the filtered back-projection integral.

As a continuous integral, the FBPA looks simple, but in practice, done discretely, it is computationally intensive, even when the FFT and IFFT are used. Computational effort increases with the total number of pixels in $\widehat{\mu}(x,y)$. The $|w|$ factor in the FBP integral, Equation 10.28, acts like a spatial high-pass filter that accentuates the noise present in $c(\theta,\sigma)$. Consequently, to reduce the noise, $|w|$ can be replaced with an even filter function that rises linearly for $0 \leq |w/w_s| < 0.15$, then reaches a peak at about $|w/w_s| \cong 0.5$, then drops to zero at $|w/w_s| = 0.5$. (w_s is the spatial sampling frequency. $w = 0.5w_s$ is the (spatial) Nyquist frequency used in the discrete calculation of $\widehat{\mu}(x,y)$.)

As we have noted, in practical situations, the data is always discrete and finite. The discrete FBP algorithm proceeds as follows [Rao et al., 1995]:

1. Find the 1-D DFT of the projections for each angle. Attention must be given to the choice of Nyquist frequency and the windowing function.
2. Multiply the results of step 1 above with the response [filter] function in the frequency domain (equivalent to convolving with the response function in the time domain). In the actual simulations, the response function is simply a ramp [or other filter as described above] with a unity slope and a duration of $\pm\frac{1}{2}$ the sampling frequency.
3. Find the IFFT of the results in step 2 This gives us the filtered projections in the discrete domain and corresponds to $q(n)$, where the q's are taken at the various angles, θ_i, at which the projections were taken, and n is the ray number at which the line projection was taken.
4. Back project. The integral of the continuous time system now becomes a summation:

$$\widehat{\mu}(x,y) = \sum_{i=0}^{K} q(\theta_i, x\cos\theta_i + y\sin\theta_i) \tag{10.31}$$

Quoting Rao et al. again:

"It should be noted that (x,y) are chosen by the program while back-projecting. So the value of $x\cos\theta + y\sin\theta$ may not correspond exactly to a value of "n" for the filtered projection which may have been calculated in the previous step. Therefore interpolation has to be done, and usually linear interpolation is quite sufficient. It may be noted that in terms of computational time, this step consumes the maximum time (about 80%)."

10.6 Chapter Summary

In all the developments above, we have considered a tomographic slice with a radioisotope source. The 2-D quantity being estimated is the distribution of the radioactivity in the slice, $\mu(x,y)$. Because certain isotope-tagged biochemicals have affinities to certain tissue types, including cancers, $\widehat{\mu}(x,y)$ can be used to locate tumors, as in scintimammography. In SPECT and PET, the projection lines are determined by the angular position of the scintillation sensor array and the sensor spacing and collimation. The exact same mathematics apply for FBP when a transmission source (e.g., x-ray) is used. In this case, we are trying to map $\alpha(x,y)$, the 2-D distribution of x-ray absorption in a slice. Recall that:

$$A(\theta_n,j) = \ln[I_{in}/I_{o\theta nj}] = \sum_{k=1}^{N} \alpha_{\theta njk} \tag{10.32}$$

Where: $A(\theta_n,j)$ is the absorbance calculated for the jth line at angle θ_n, and I_{in} is the x-ray source intensity, $I_{o\theta nj}$ is the x-ray intensity of the beam emerging from tissue on the jth line, ln[*] is the natural logarithm, and $\alpha_{\theta njk}$ are the discretized x-ray absorption coefficients on the jth line at angle θ_n. When a radioactive source is used, the conditioned sensor output is a discrete count of scintillation events over a fixed counting time. When x-rays are used, the x-ray sensor output is also integrated over a short (exposure) time. Thus, the Radon transform can be written for x-rays:

$$a(\theta,\sigma) = \int_{-\infty}^{\infty}\int_{-\infty}^{\infty} \alpha(x,y)\,\delta[x\cos(\theta) + y\sin(\theta) - \sigma]\,dx\,dy \cong A(\theta_n,j) \tag{10.33}$$

Note that the summation line is selected by θ and σ in the continuous case.

It is understood that medical imaging is an enormous technical field, but underlying nearly all forms of tomography is one or more of the four algorithms described above. It is hoped that when the reader does delve into the technology of tomographic imaging, they will be mathematically forearmed from this chapter.

Problems

10.1 Consider an idealized tomogram slice with a radioactive density given by a point source at $x=x_o$ and $y=y_o$. Mathematically, this object is:

$$f(x,y)=\delta(x-x_o)\delta(y-y_o)$$

Its Radon transform (RT) can be written in simplified form using the notation for the line of response in the X,Y plane, $y=mx+b$. b is the LOR intercept with the Y axis, and m is its slope. Normally, b and m would be varied to scan the object, f(x,y).

$$C(x,y)=\int_{-\infty}^{\infty}\int_{-\infty}^{\infty}\delta(x-x_o)\delta(y-y_o)\delta[y-(mx+b)]dxdy$$

Derive a mathematical expression for C(x,y) from the Radon transform above. (Hint: Note that a delta function can be expressed as the inverse Fourier transform (IFT) of a constant.) That is:

$$\delta(x)=\frac{1}{2\pi}\int_{-\infty}^{\infty}(1)e^{+j\omega x}d\omega$$

Use this relation to substitute for $\delta[y-(mx+b)]$ in the RT, separate terms, perform the integrals on x and y, then take the IFT.

10.2 In this problem, you will calculate the *sinogram* of the impulse object, $f(x,y)=\delta(x-x_o)\delta(y-y_o)$. We will use the more commonly used form of the RT; see Equation 10.14 and Figure 10.5. As we have seen, the sinogram is simply the values of the RT calculated for various σ values along the X′ axis, for values of θ ranging between 0 and π. The RT is:

$$c(\theta,\sigma)=\int_{-\infty}^{\infty}\int_{-\infty}^{\infty}\delta(x-x_o)\delta(y-y_o)\delta[x\cos(\theta)+y\sin(\theta)-\sigma]dxdy$$

a. Derive an expression for $c(\theta,\sigma)$. (Use the approach in the hint for the first problem.) Note that $c(\theta,\sigma)$ only is defined for zero argument.

b. Let $x_o=1$, $y_o=1$. Let $\theta=0°$, 45°, 90°, 135°, and 180°. Plot and dimension the sinogram, $c(\theta,\sigma)$.

c. Repeat b for $x_o=-1$, $y_o=1$, and the same θ values.

d. Repeat b for $x_o=-1/2$, $y_o=-1/2$ and the same θ values.

10.3 In this problem, you will calculate the Radon transform of a straight line segment object in the X,Y plane. Refer to Figure P10.3a. The line object lies on the line, $y=mx+b$, extending from $x=x_1$ to $x=x_2$. To detect the

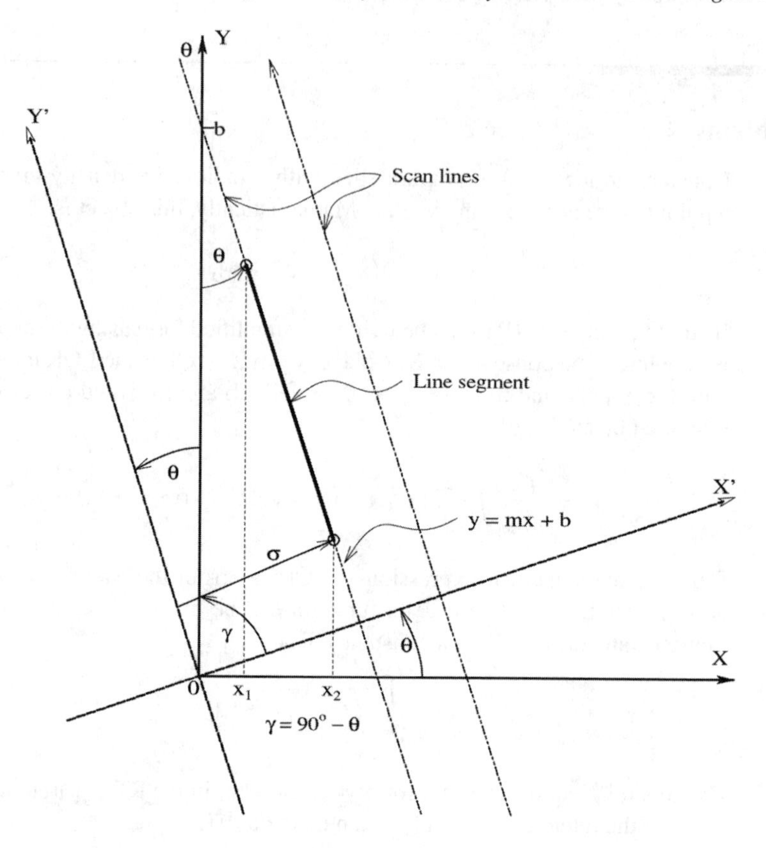

FIGURE P10.3a

line maximally, we must pass a Radon scan line, specified by θ,σ, through the line object. The RT can be written:

$$c(\theta,\sigma) = \int_{x_1}^{x_2} \int_{-\infty}^{\infty} \delta[y - (mx + b)]\delta[x\cos(\theta) + y\sin(\theta) - \sigma]dydx$$

We wish the slope m to be the same as the scan line. From the geometry of the Figure, we see that, for the scan line to be parallel to the object, $m = -\tan(\gamma) = -\tan(90° - \theta) = -\cot(\theta)$. Recall that $\cot(\theta) = \cos(\theta)/\sin(\theta)$. (Hint: eliminate the $\delta[y - (mx + b)]$ term first and substitute $(mx + b)$ for y in the second delta function argument, then integrate with respect to x.)

a. Find an expression for $c(\theta,\sigma)$ for the case where the scan line is coincident with the object line. Assume b and θ are known. Plot the sinogram.

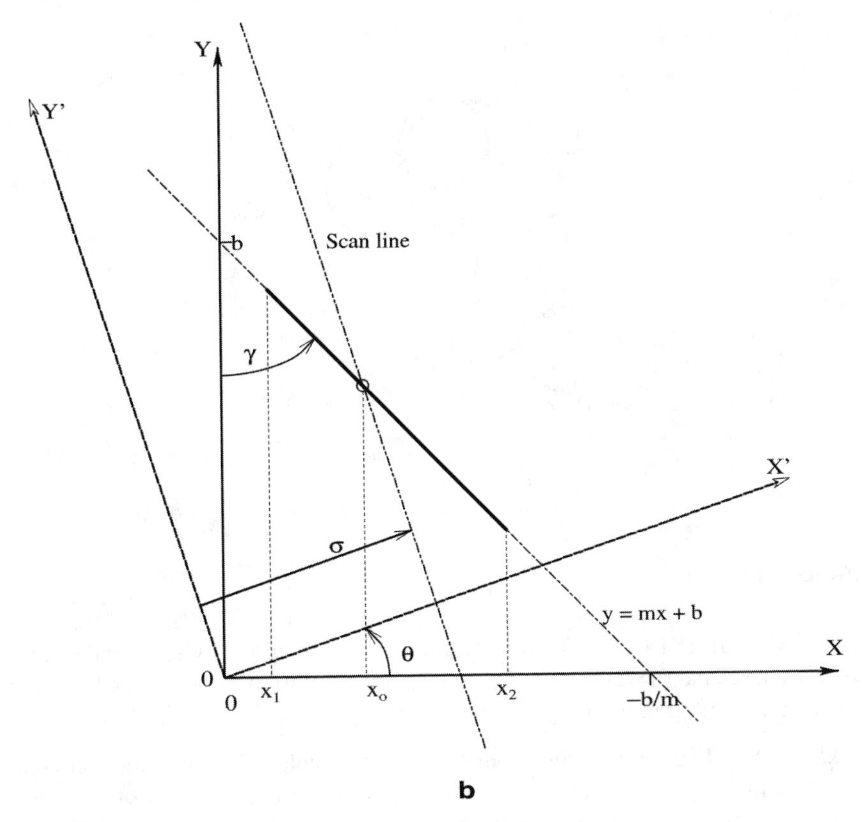

FIGURE P10.3b

b. When the scan line is not parallel with the object line, it can either intersect the object or not, depending on θ, σ, b, and m. Obviously, if the scan line and the object line do not intersect, $c(\theta,\sigma)=0$. Find an expression for $c(\theta,\sigma)$ when the lines are not parallel but intersect at a point, as shown in Figure P10.3b. Note that $x_1 \leq x_o \leq x_2$ when there is an intersection. Take $b=10$, $m=-1$, $x_1 = 2$, $x_2 = 8$, set $\theta=0°$. Find the σ values over which intersection occurs. Repeat for $\theta=30°$.

10.4 Figure P10.4 illustrates the 2-D spatial distribution of radioactivity in a hexagonal approximation to a tomographic slice. There are seven pixels, each with a radioactivity of μ_k kilocounts/second. A collimated counter makes counts C_1, C_2 and C_3 at angle $\theta=0°$, then counts C_4, C_5, and C_6 at angle $\theta=60°$, then counts C_7, C_8 and C_9 at angle $\theta = 120°$.

Use the ART process iteratively to find the $7\{\mu_k\}$ values given numerical values for C_1–C_9. For simplicity, take the true $\{\mu_k\}$ values as $\mu_k=k$. Thus the measured counts are $C_1=11$, $C_2=12$, $C_3 = 5$, $C_4 = 7$, $C_5 = 14$, $C_6=7$, $C_7 = 3$, $C_8 = 16$, $C_9 = 9$ kilocounts. Carry your calculations through q = 10 iterations. Show the intermediate estimates for the $7\{\mu_k\}$ values for each q

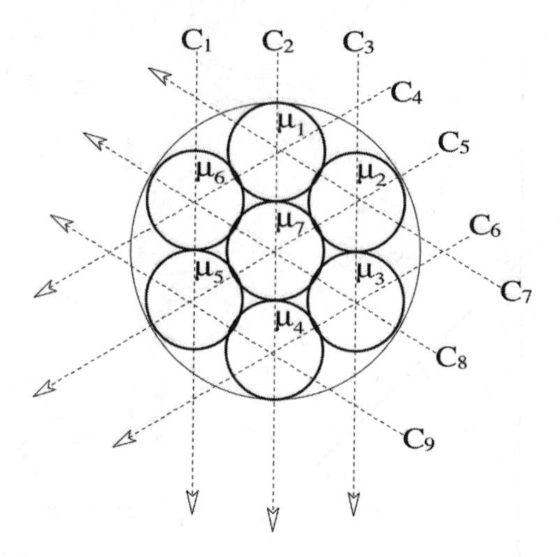

FIGURE P10.4

value from 1 to 10. The first iteration (q = 1) should use C_1, C_2 and C_3, for the second (q= 2) use C_4, C_5 and C_6, for the third use C_7, C_8, and C_9. For the fourth, return to C_1, C_2 and C_3; the fifth uses C_4, C_5 and C_6, etc.

10.5 Figure P10.5 illustrates a radioactive tomographic slice with ideal circular symmetry. The circle in the center has a linear radio-density of $(\mu_c + \mu_b)$ counts/sec/cm; the annular periphery has a radio-density of μ_b counts/sec/cm line length. The case for $\theta = 0°$ is shown in the figure for simplicity. σ is the displacement of a scan line along the X = X' axis. From simple geometry, the length of a scan line (SL) through the large circle can be expressed by $l = 2\sqrt{R^2 - \sigma^2}$ for $|\sigma| \leq R$, and clearly $l = 0$ for $|\sigma| > R$. (The scan lines are chords.)

a. Find and plot to scale the Radon transform of the object, $c(\theta, w)$. Let R = 3, r = 1, $\mu_b = 0.3$, and $\mu_c = 3.0$. (Hint: $c(\theta,\sigma)$ is proportional to the length of the scan lines through each part of the object. Note that the Radon transform of this object is independent of θ because it has circular symmetry.)

b. Find an algebraic expression for the CFT of $c(\theta,\sigma)$, $\mathbf{C}(\theta, w)$. Use the CFT pair:

$$g(x) = s\sqrt{1-(x/a)^2} \overset{F}{\longleftrightarrow} G(w) = (\pi a/2)\frac{J_1(wa)}{(wa)}$$

(A semicircle of radius a)

$g(x) = 0$ for $|x| > a$.

(J_1 is a Bessel function and w is frequency in r/cm.)

Plot $\mathbf{C}(\theta,w)$ vs. w to scale.

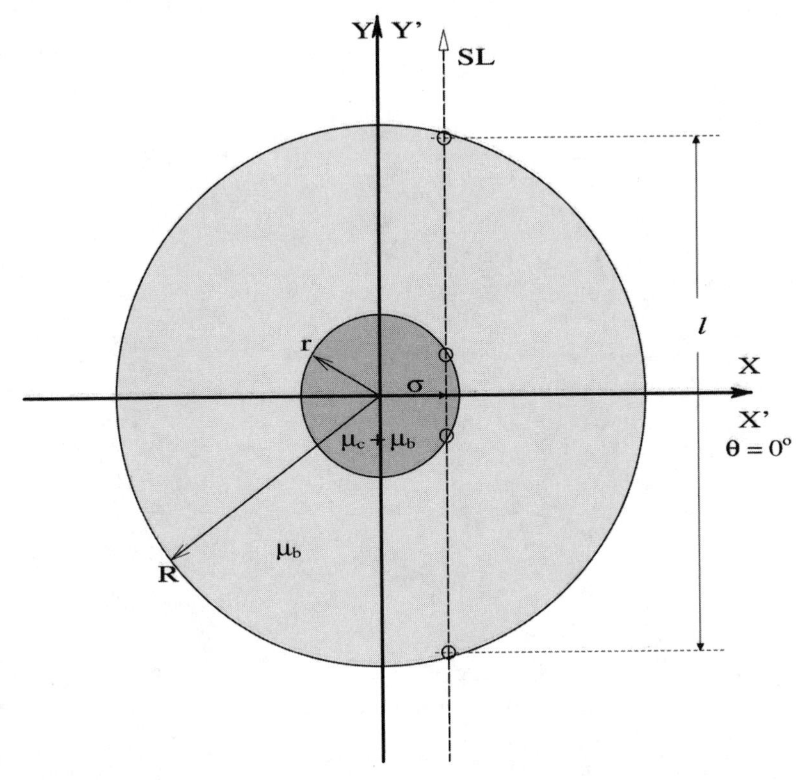

FIGURE P10.5

10.6 In this problem, you will examine the effect of finite spatial frequency bandwidth in estimating the tomographic image of an ideal radioactive point source using the filtered back-projection algorithm. You will calculate and plot the image. The radioactive object is $\mu(\mathrm{x,y}) = \mu_o \delta(\mathrm{x})\delta(\mathrm{y})$.

a. Use Equation 10.19 in the text to find $\mathbf{C}(\theta,\sigma)$, the 1-D CFT of the Radon transform of the object. Note that $\mathbf{C}(\theta,\sigma)$ is independent of θ and has circular symmetry.

b. Now use text Equation 10.29 to find $\mathrm{q}(\theta,\sigma)$. For practical purposes, $|w|$ is defined as $|w|$ for $-w_o \leq w \leq w_o$, and 0 for $|w| > w_o$. Hint: Of help will be the integral, $\int \mathrm{xe^{ax}dx} = \mathrm{e^{ax}(ax-1)/a^2}$, the Euler relations for $\sin(\mathrm{x})$ and $\cos(\mathrm{x})$, and the trig identity, $1-\cos(\mathrm{x}) = 2\sin^2(\mathrm{x}/2)$.

c. Now use Equation 10.28 to calculate the estimate of $\mu(\mathrm{x,y})$, $\widehat{\mu}(\sigma,w_o)$. Plot and dimension $\widehat{\mu}(\sigma,w_o)$ for w_o= 1, 3 and 10. Let $0 \leq \sigma \leq 8\pi/w_o$. Note that $\widehat{\mu}(\sigma,w_o)$ is even and has circular symmetry. Note that, curiously, $\widehat{\mu}(\sigma,w_o)$ has negative values. What significance do they have? Note that $\widehat{\mu}(\sigma,w_o)$ is the *point spread function* of the filtered back-projection algorithm [Papoulis, 1968].

Appendices

Appendix A Cramer's Rule

Cramer's rule is a quick, systematic algebraic routine for solving for the N unknowns in a set of N independent LTI simultaneous algebraic equations. The use of Cramer's rule can be demonstrated by solving a set of three general LTI algebraic equations. $[u_k]$ are the independent variables (inputs), $[a_{jk}]$ are the constant coefficients, and $[x_k]$ are the three unknowns (k = 1, 2, 3). The simultaneous equations are:

$$u_1 = a_{11}x_1 + a_{12}x_2 + a_{13}x_3 \tag{A1A}$$

$$u_2 = a_{21}x_1 + a_{22}x_2 + a_{23}x_3 \tag{A1B}$$

$$u_3 = a_{31}x_1 + a_{32}x_2 + a_{33}x_3 \tag{A1C}$$

Solution of $[x_k]$ proceeds as follows:

1. The system's A matrix is N X N, N = 3):

$$\mathbf{A} = \begin{bmatrix} a_{11} & a_{12} & a_{13} \\ a_{21} & a_{22} & a_{23} \\ a_{31} & a_{32} & a_{33} \end{bmatrix} \tag{A2}$$

We now find the system determinant, Δ:

$$\Delta \equiv \det[\mathbf{A}] = a_{11}(a_{22}a_{33} - a_{32}a_{23}) - a_{21}(a_{12}a_{33} - a_{32}a_{13}) + a_{31}(a_{12}a_{23} - a_{22}a_{13}) \tag{A3}$$

2. To solve for x_1, replace the *first column* in the matrix **A** with $[u_k]$. This matrix is now called Δx_1.

$$\Delta x_1 = \begin{bmatrix} u_1 & a_{12} & a_{13} \\ u_2 & a_{22} & a_{23} \\ u_3 & a_{32} & a_{33} \end{bmatrix} \tag{A4}$$

Now

$$x_1 = \frac{\det[\Delta \mathbf{x_1}]}{\Delta} \tag{A5}$$

Similarly, to find x_2, we replace the *second column* in **A** with $[u_k]$.

$$\Delta x_2 = \begin{bmatrix} a_{11} & u_1 & a_{13} \\ a_{21} & u_2 & a_{23} \\ a_{31} & u_3 & a_{33} \end{bmatrix} \tag{A6}$$

So

$$x_2 = \frac{\det[\Delta \mathbf{x_2}]}{\Delta} \tag{A7}$$

x_3 is found in the same way after replacing the third column in **A** with $[u_k]$. That's all there is to it. Cramer's rule is easy to apply to systems of order $N = 2$, or 3 in algebraic or numerical, pencil and paper solutions. Solutions of systems of order > 3 should be done with Matlab^{TM}.

Appendix B Signal Flow Graphs and Mason's Rule

Signal flow graphs (SFGs) are an LTI systems tool that enables one to take a set of ODEs describing a dynamic LTI system, put them in graphical form, and then, using *Mason's gain formula,* easily find the I/O transfer function for the system. The SFG approach is ideally suited for pencil-and-paper work because it replaces tedious, error-prone matrix inversion algebra as a necessary step to finding the state system's transfer function. SFGs were developed in 1953 by S.J. Mason, who published his gain formula in 1956. SFGs were developed in an era before desktop PCs running systems analysis applications such as Matlab™ and Simulink™. They have had application in electronic circuit analysis and, of course, the analysis of linear feedback systems.

An SFG has two components: *unidirectional branches* that condition a signal and *signal nodes.* Signals from branches sum algebraically at nodes. The signal at a node is multiplied by the *transmission* or *gain* of a branch leaving it; the input at a node from a branch is the product of the branch's transmission times the source node's signal. All signals are assumed to be in the frequency domain. As a first example of signal manipulation in SFGs, consider Figure B1a. Here, $y_1 = T_1 x_1$, $y_2 = T_2 x_1$ and $y_3 = T_3 x_1$. In Figure B1b, $y_1 = x_1 T_1 + x_2 T_2 + x_3 T_3$. When several branches are in series, as in Figure B1c, $x_4 = T_1 T_2 T_3 x_1$. When they are in parallel, as in Figure B1d, $y_1 = x_1(T_1 + T_2 + T_3)$.

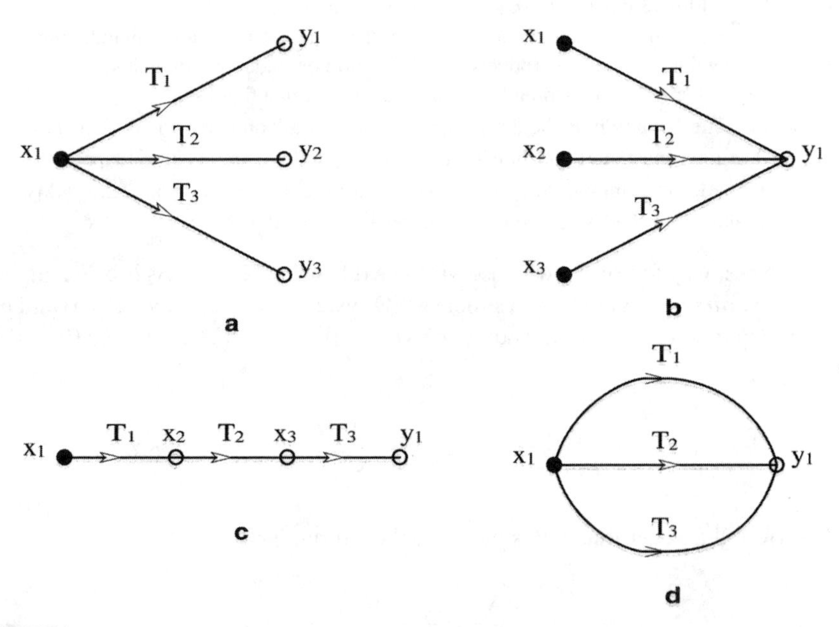

FIGURE B1

Four feed-forward signal flow graph topologies: (a) fan-out; (b) converging; (c) serial; (d) parallel.

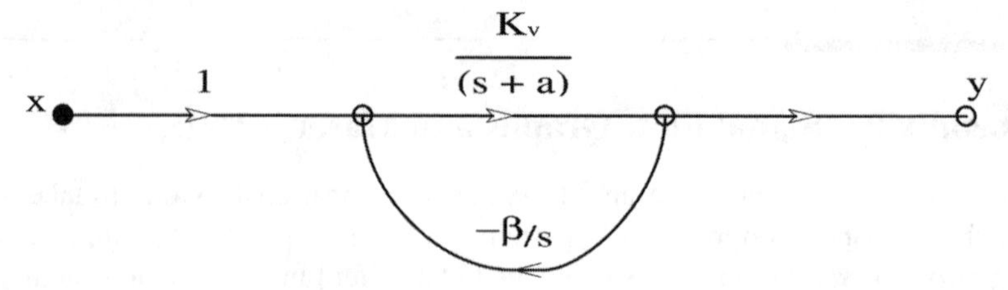

FIGURE B2
A simple single-loop LTI feedback system's SFG.

The systematic gain formula for SFGs developed by Mason in 1956 is deceptively simple. It does require some interpretation, however. It is written:

$$\frac{V_{ok}}{V_{ij}} = H_{jk} = \frac{\sum_{n=1}^{N} F_n \Delta_N}{\Delta_D} \tag{B1}$$

Where:

H_{jk} is the net transmission from the jth (input) node to the kth (output) node. F_n is the transmission of the nth *forward path.* The nth forward path is a connected path of branches beginning on the jth (input) node and ending on the kth (output) node along which no node is passed through more than once. A SFG can have several forward paths that can share common nodes.

Δ_D is the SFG denominator or determinant. $\Delta_D \equiv 1-$ [sum of all individual loop gains] + [sum of products of pairs of all nontouching loop gains] − [sum of products of nontouching loop gains taken three at a time] + $\cdots$.

The *Loop gain* is the net gain around a closed loop one or more branches. The loop must start and finish on a common node. *Nontouching* loops share no nodes in common. Δ_n is the *cofactor* for the nth forward path. $\Delta_n \equiv \Delta_D$ evaluated for nodes that do not touch the nth forward path.

The best way to learn how to use Mason's rule on systems SFGs is by example. In the *first example,* Figure B2 is a simple SISO system. There is only one forward path. The loop touches two of its nodes, so $\Delta_1 = 1$. F_1 is seen to be $1 \times K_v/(s+a) \times a$, and

$$\Delta_D = 1 - \left[\frac{-K_v \beta}{s(s+a)}\right] \tag{B2}$$

The overall transfer function is put in Laplace form. Thus:

$$\frac{V_o}{V_1} = \frac{sK_v a}{s^2 + sa + K_v \beta} \tag{B3}$$

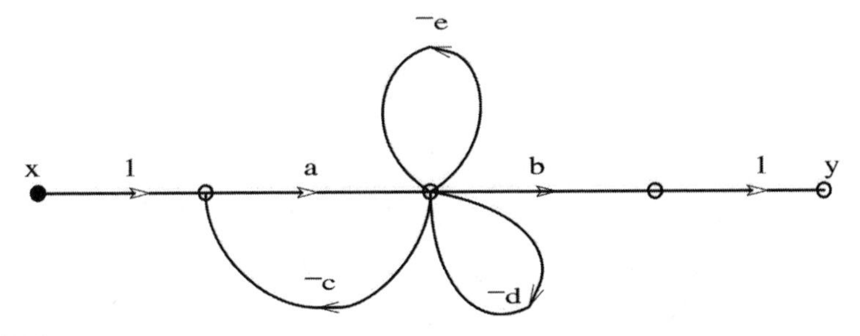

FIGURE B3

An SFG topology with three touching loops and one forward path.

In the *second example,* the SFG is shown in Figure B3. Now $n=1$, $F_1=ab$, $\Delta_D=1-[-ac-e-d]+0$, and $\Delta_1=1$. From which we have:

$$\frac{V_o}{V_1}=\frac{ac}{1+ac+e+d} \tag{B4}$$

In the *third example,* shown in Figure B4, the SFG is more complex: $n=3$, $F_1=abc$, $F_2=def$, $F_3=-akf$, $\Delta_D=1-[-bh-ge]+[(-bh)(-ge)]-0$, $\Delta_1=1+ge$, $\Delta_2=1+bh$, $\Delta_3=1$. The transfer function is thus:

$$\frac{V_o}{V_1}=\frac{abc(1+ge)+def(1+bh)-akf}{1+bh+ge+bhge} \tag{B5}$$

In a *fourth example*, Figure B5 illustrates a state-variable form SFG: Here $n=4$, $F_1=b_3$, $F_2=b_2/s$, $F_3=b_1/s^2$, $F_4=b_0/s^3$, all $\Delta_k=1$, $\Delta_D=1-[-a_1/s-a_2/s^2-a_3/s^3]+0$. The SFG's transfer function is easily seen to have a cubic polynomial in the numerator and denominator:

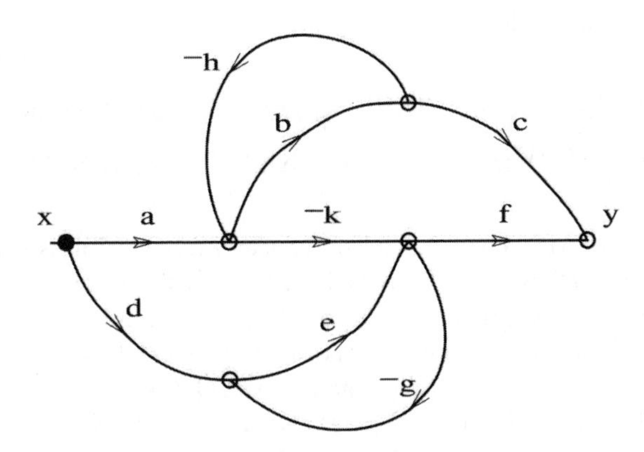

FIGURE B4

An SFG topology with three forward paths and two nontouching feedback loops.

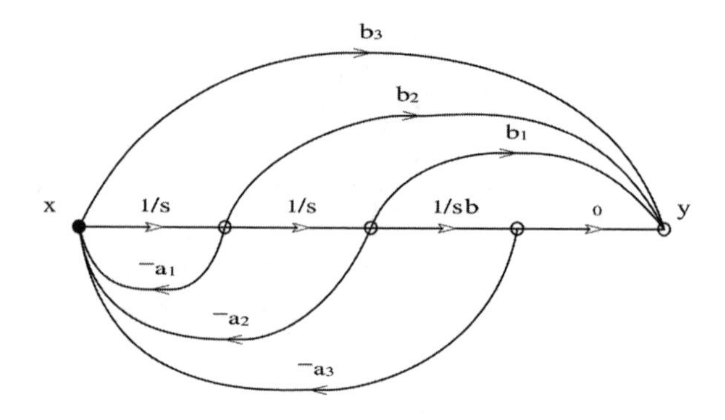

FIGURE B5

An SFG for a system described by the cubic state-variable format. There are four forward paths and three touching feedback loops.

$$\frac{V_o}{V_1} = \frac{b_3 s^3 + b_2 s^2 + b_1 s^1 + b_0}{s^3 + a_1 s^2 + a_2 s^1 + a_3} \tag{B6}$$

In a *fifth and final example*, a chemical, C, is synthesized in the mitochondria of a cell at a rate $\dot{\mathbf{Q}}_o$. Its concentration is $C_m \mu g/l$ in the mitochondria. It diffuses out of the mitochondria into the cytoplasm, where its concentration is C_c. It next diffuses through the cell membrane to what is basically zero concentration outside of the cell. The two compartments are (1) the mitochondria, and (2) the cytoplasm around the mitochondria. The compartmental state equations are based on simple diffusion (Fick's first law). V_m and V_c are compartment volumes.

$$V_m \dot{C}_m = \dot{Q}_o - K_{12}(C_m - C_c) \quad \mu g/\text{min.} \tag{B7A}$$

$$V_c \dot{C}_c = K_{12}(C_m - C_c) - K_2 C_c \quad \mu g/\text{min.} \tag{B7B}$$

Written in state form, we have:

$$\dot{C}_m = -C_m(K_{12}/V_m) + C_c(K_{12}/V_m) + \dot{Q}_o/V_m \quad \mu g/(\text{liter min.}) \tag{B8A}$$

$$\dot{C}_c = C_m(K_{12}/V_c) - C_c(K_2 + K_{12})/V_c \quad \mu g/(\text{liter min.}) \tag{B8B}$$

Note that mass diffusion rates depend on *concentrations* or mass/volume, so the diffusion rate constants K_{12} and K_2 must have the dimensions of liters/minute.

From the ODEs, we see that the system is linear, and can be described by a signal flow graph as shown in Figure B6. The signal flow graph can easily be reduced by Mason's rule to find the transfer function, $C_c/\dot{Q}_o(s)$: In this example, $n = 1$, $F_1 = (1/V_m)(1/s)(K_{12}/V_c)(1/s)$, $\Delta_1 = 1$, and $\Delta_D = 1 - [(-K_{12}/sV_m) + (-(K_2 + K_{12})/sV_c) + (K_{12}^2/s^2 V_m V_c)] + [(-K_{12}/sV_m)(-(K_2 + K_{12})/sV_c)] - 0$. This somewhat involved denominator is only a quadratic. After some algebra:

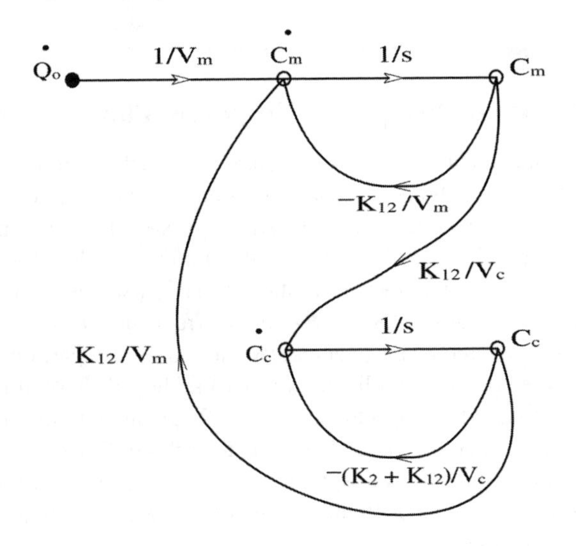

FIGURE B6

SFG for a second-order linear biochemical system. There is one forward path to C_c, and three feedback loops; two nontouching and one that touches the two nontouching loops. The Vs are compartment volumes.

$$\frac{C_c}{\dot{Q}_o} = \frac{K_{12}/V_m V_c}{s^2 + s[K_{12}/V_m + (K_{12}+K_2)/V_c] + K_2 K_{12}/V_m V_c} = \frac{K}{(s+a)(s+b)} \quad \text{(B9)}$$

Thus, the two-compartment system governed by diffusion is seen to have linear second-order dynamics with two real poles after factoring. Matlab's *Roots* utility can be used to numerically factor the denominator.

Appendix C Bode (Frequency Response) Plots

The steady-state sinusoidal frequency response is a widely used technique for characterizing LTI systems. The *Bode plot* is the standard means of displaying an LTI system's steady-state frequency response. An LTI system is given a pure sinusoidal input of constant amplitude and frequency; this input is applied for a long time to ensure the system's output is in the steady state. What is displayed in a Bode plot is the system's amplitude response (AR) vs Hz (input) frequency, and its phase response (PR) vs. frequency. Frequency is generally plotted on a logarithmic (horizontal) scale and the phase and AR on a linear (vertical) scale. We have already discussed the frequency response of LTI systems in Section 2.4.5, and introduced Bode plots in Section 2.4.6. This Appendix will elaborate on the rules of Bode plotting by presenting several examples of the use of asymptotes. The object of the asymptote method is, when doing pencil-and-paper studies, to avoid the need for extensive calculations to make an accurate Bode plot

Example 1: Consider the transfer function of a simple high-pass filter:

$$H(s) = \frac{-Ks}{s + \omega_o} \tag{C1}$$

To make a Bode plot, this filter's transfer function must be put in *time-constant form;* we also let $s \to j\omega$, where ω is the applied sinusoidal frequency in radians/sec.

$$\mathbf{H}(j\omega) = \frac{-(K\omega_o)j\omega}{j\omega/\omega_o + 1} \text{ (time constant form)} \tag{C2}$$

The phase angle of the transfer function, $\mathbf{H}(j\omega)$, is the phase of the output sinusoid, assuming the input (reference) sinusoid has zero phase. The phase of $\mathbf{H}(j\omega)$ is the phase of its numerator vector, minus the phase of its denominator vector. This is:

$$\varphi = (-180° + 90°) - \tan^{-1}(\omega/\omega_o) \tag{C3}$$

The $-180°$ comes from the minus sign in the numerator, the $+90°$ is from the j factor in the numerator, and the $-\tan^{-1}(\omega/\omega_o)$ term is from the angle of the denominator vector (real part $= 1$, imaginary part $= +\omega/\omega_o$). Now the Bode AR is found from taking $20\times$ the logarithm to the base 10 of the magnitude of the transfer function. The magnitude is:

$$|\mathbf{H}(j\omega)| = \frac{(K/\omega_o)\omega}{\sqrt{[(\omega/\omega_o)^2 + 1]}} \tag{C4}$$

The vector magnitude of the denominator term is found using the Pythagorean theorem. Taking the logarithms, the amplitude response (AR) is:

$$AR(\omega) = 20\log_{10}|\mathbf{H}(j\omega)| = 20\log_{10}(K/\omega_o) + 20\log(\omega) - 10\log[(\omega/\omega_o)^2 + 1]\text{dB} \tag{C5}$$

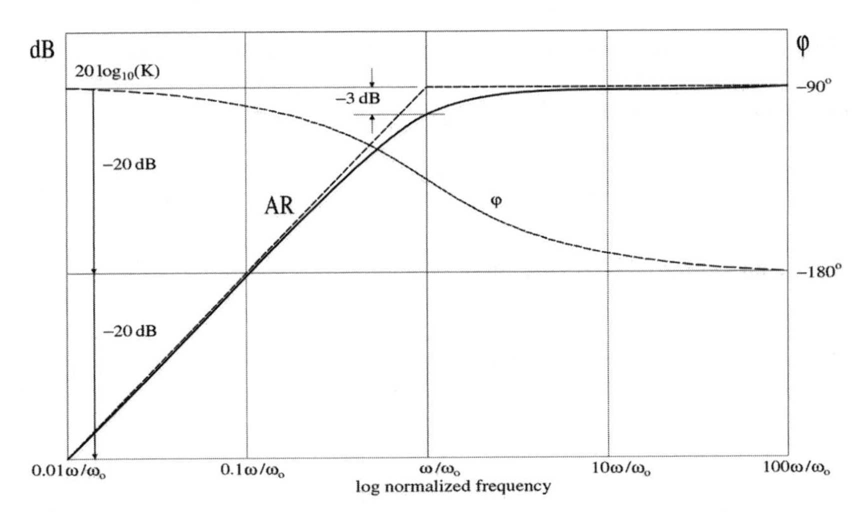

FIGURE C1
Bode plot for the simple highpass filter.

To make a pencil-and-paper Bode plot without resorting to tedious calculations, we consider the *Bode asymptotes* for three ranges of radian frequency: $\omega >> \omega_o$, $\omega = \omega_o$, and $\omega << \omega_o$. For $\omega >> \omega_o$, we can write the AR as:

$$\mathrm{AR(hi)} \cong 20\log(\mathrm{K}) - 20\log(\omega_o) + 20\log(\omega) - 20\log(\omega) + 20\log(\omega_o) = 20\log(\mathrm{K}) \tag{C6}$$

In other words, the high-frequency asymptote has $0°$ slope and is at $20\log(\mathrm{K})$ dB. The low-frequency behavior of the AR is given by:

$$\mathrm{AR(lo)} \cong 20\log(\mathrm{K}) - 20\log(\omega_o) + 20\log(\omega) + \log[1] \tag{C7}$$

Thus, the low-frequency Bode plot is *increasing in amplitude* from $-\infty$ with a slope of +20 dB/decade or 6 dB per octave of ω. Where $\omega = 1$ (assuming $\omega_o >> 1$), the $\mathrm{AR} = 20\log(\mathrm{K}/\omega_o)$ dB. Thus, the low-frequency asymptote of this $\mathbf{H}(\mathrm{j}\omega)$ has a slope of +20 dB/decade, and meets the high-frequency horizontal asymptote at $\omega = \omega_o$. The AR at $\omega = \omega_o$ is simply:

$$\begin{aligned} \mathrm{AR}(\omega_o) &= 20\log(K) - 20\log(\omega_o) + 20\log(\omega_o) - 10\log[2] \\ &= 20\log(K) - 10\log[2] dB \end{aligned} \tag{C8}$$

Note that, at the break frequency, ω_o, the actual AR is down -3 dB from the high-frequency level. It is also found that for $\omega = 2\omega_o$, the actual AR is down c. -1 dB from $20\log(\mathrm{K})$, and for $\omega = \omega_o/2$, the AR is down c. -1 dB from the low-frequency asymptote. The Bode plot for this simple high-pass $\mathbf{H}(\mathrm{j}\omega)$ is shown in Figure C1.

Unfortunately, there are no handy asymptotic tricks to plot $\varphi(\omega)$. Do realize, however, that the angle of the denominator vector is $45°$ when $\omega = \omega_o$.

Example 2: A lag/lead filter is used to attenuate high-frequency components in a signal, and also, in some cases, to compensate feedback control systems. The transfer function of a typical lag/lead filter is:

$$H(s) = K\frac{s+\omega_{HI}}{s+\omega_{LO}}, \quad \omega_{HI} > \omega_{LO} \tag{C9}$$

In time constant form, for Bode plotting:

$$\mathbf{H}(j\omega) = K(\omega_{HI}/\omega_{LO})\frac{j\omega/\omega_{HI}+1}{j\omega/\omega_{LO}+1} \tag{C10}$$

and

$$|\mathbf{H}(j\omega)| = K(\omega_{HI}/\omega_{LO})\frac{\sqrt{[(\omega/\omega_{HI})^2+1]}}{\sqrt{[(\omega/\omega_{LO})^2+1]}} \tag{C11}$$

In this example, there are *three* frequency regions in which we determine Bode asymptotes. For $\omega >> \omega_{HI}$, we can write for the AR,

$$\begin{aligned} AR(hi) &\cong \{20\log(K) + 20\log(\omega_{HI}) - 20\log(\omega_{LO})\} + 20\log(\omega) - 20\log(\omega_{HI}) \\ &\quad - 20\log(\omega) + 20\log(\omega_{LO}) \end{aligned}$$

$$\downarrow$$

$$AR(hi) \cong 20\log(K) \tag{C12}$$

Thus, the high-frequency asymptote is a line of zero slope at $20\log(K)$ dB. And for $\omega << \omega_{LO}$,

$$AR(lo) \cong 20\log(K) + 20\log(\omega_{HI}) - 20\log(\omega_{LO}) + 10\log(1) - 10\log(1) \tag{C13}$$

The last two terms are zero. So the low-frequency asymptote is flat at $20\log[K(\omega_{HI}/\omega_{LO})]$ dB; connecting the low- and high-frequency asymptotes in the frequency range, $\omega_{LO} \le \omega \le \omega_{HI}$, is an asymptote line with slope -20 dB/decade. This can be demonstrated by assuming that $\omega_{LO} << \omega << \omega_{HI}$ (even if the inequality does not strictly hold). Thus the numerator in Equation C11 $\cong 1$, and the denominator $\cong \omega/\omega_{LO}$.

$$\begin{aligned} AR(mid) &\cong \{20\log(K) + 20\log(\omega_{HI}) - 20\log(\omega_{LO})\} + 10\log(1) - 20\log(\omega) \\ &\quad + 20\log(\omega_{LO}) \end{aligned}$$

$$\downarrow$$

$$AR(mid) \cong 20\log[K\omega_{HI}] - 20\log(\omega) \tag{C14}$$

The Bode plot for the lag/lead filter is shown in Figure C2.

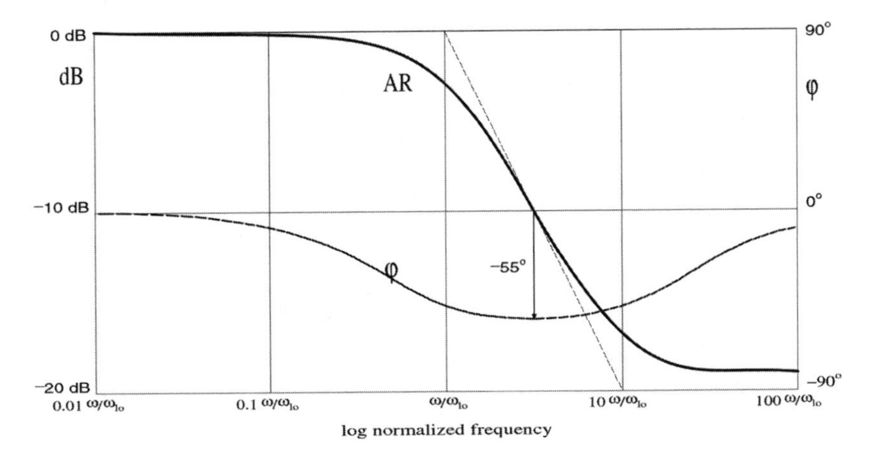

FIGURE C2
Bode plot for a two real-pole lad/lead filter.

Example 3: In the third example, we examine a transfer function for a bandpass system, typical of an ECG amplifier. The transfer function in Laplace form is:

$$H(s) = \frac{-Ks}{(s+\omega_{LO})(s+\omega_{HI})} \tag{C15}$$

In time-constant frequency response form this is:

$$\mathbf{H}(j\omega) = \frac{-K/(\omega_{LO}\omega_{HI})j\omega}{(j\omega/\omega_{LO}+1)(j\omega/\omega_{HI}+1)} \tag{C16}$$

The algebraic expression for the phase of this FR function is:

$$\varphi = (-180° + 90°) - \tan^{-1}(\omega/\omega_{LO}) - \tan^{-1}(\omega/\omega_{HI}) \text{ degrees} \tag{C17}$$

Note that the $-180°$ comes from the minus sign in the frequency response function, and the $+90°$ comes from the j operator in the numerator. The two $-\tan^{-1}(*)$ terms come from the factored denominator vectors.

To plot its AR asymptotes, we must consider three frequency ranges: $0 < \omega << \omega_{LO}$, $\omega_{LO} << \omega << \omega_{HI}$, and $\omega >> \omega_{HI}$. Following the treatment above, the AR(lo) can be written:

$$AR(lo) \cong 20\log(K) - 20\log(\omega_{LO}) - 20\log(\omega_{HI}) + 20\log(\omega) \text{ dB} \tag{C18}$$

The low-frequency asymptote rises from $-\infty$ dB with a slope of $+20$ dB/decade and intersects the mid-frequency asymptote at ω_{LO}. The zero-slope mid-frequency asymptote is found to be at:

$$AR(mid) \cong 20\log(K) - 20\log(\omega_{LO}) - 20\log(\omega_{HI}) + 20\log(\omega) - 20\log(\omega) + 20\log(\omega_{LO})$$

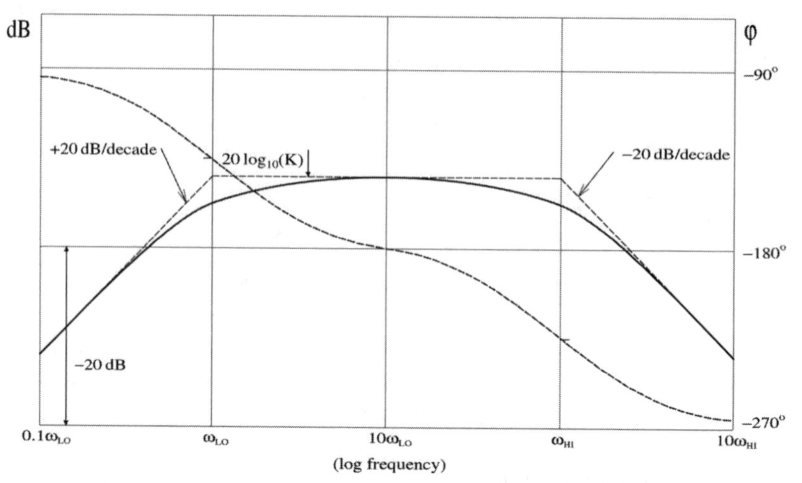

FIGURE C3
Bode plot for a two real-pole bandpass filter with a broad mid-band frequency range.

$$\downarrow$$

$$\text{AR(mid)} \cong 20\log(\text{K}/\omega_{\text{HI}})\ \text{dB} \tag{C19}$$

And the high-frequency asymptote is found from:

$$\begin{aligned}\text{AR(hi)} \cong \{&20\log(\text{K}) - 20\log(\omega_{\text{LO}}) - 20\log(\omega_{\text{HI}})\} + 20\log(\omega) - 20\log(\omega)\\ &+ 20\log(\omega_{\text{LO}}) - 20\log(\omega) + 20\log(\omega_{\text{HI}}) = 20\log(\text{K}) - 20\log(\omega)\ \text{dB}\end{aligned} \tag{C20}$$

It is seen to have a slope of -20 dB/decade, and begins for $\omega \geq \omega_{\text{HI}}$. The Bode plot for this transfer function is shown in Figure C3. Note that the actual plot is down -3 dB at both corner frequencies, provided $\omega_{\text{HI}} >> \omega_{\text{LO}}$.

Example 4: In this example, we consider a quadratic (two-pole) low-pass filter with an underdamped denominator. The transfer function in time-constant frequency response form is:

$$\mathbf{H}(\text{j}\omega) = \frac{\text{K}}{(\text{j}\omega)^2/\omega_{\text{n}}^2 + 2\xi(\text{j}\omega)/\omega_{\text{n}} + 1} \tag{C21}$$

The phase of $\mathbf{H}(\text{j}\omega)$ is:

$$\varphi(\omega) = -\tan^{-1}\left[\frac{2\xi/\omega_{\text{n}}}{1 - \omega^2/\omega_{\text{n}}^2}\right] \tag{C22}$$

There are two Bode AR plot asymptotes; one for $\omega << \omega_{\text{n}}$, and the other, for $\omega >> \omega_{\text{n}}$. ω_{n}, is the system's undamped natural frequency in r/s, and ξ is the system's damping factor. When $0 < \xi \leq 1$, the quadratic denominator is said to be *underdamped* and has

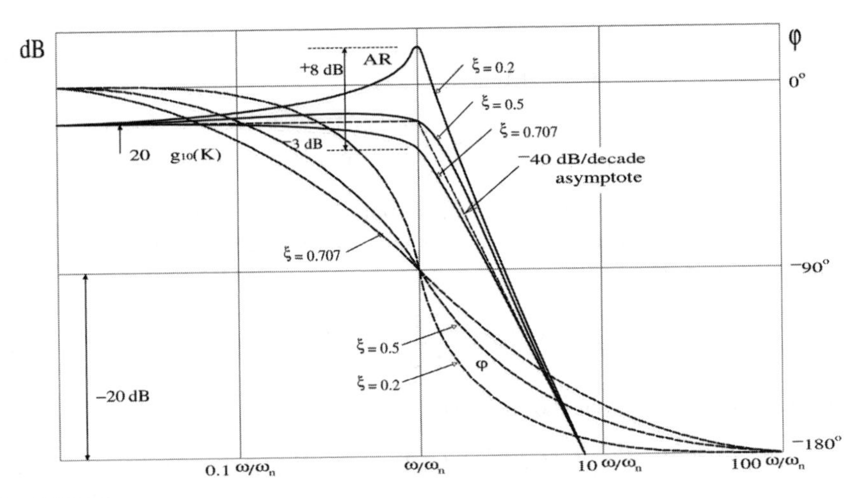

FIGURE C4
Bode plots for a low-pass filter with complex-conjugate poles. AR and phase are shown for damping factors of $\xi = 0.2$, 0.5 and 0.707.

complex-conjugate roots. If $\xi > 1$, the system is said to be *overdamped;* its roots are real and negative. The filter's AR is:

$$AR(\omega) = 20\log(K) - 10\log[(1-\omega^2/\omega_n^2)^2 + (2\xi\omega/\omega_n)^2] \text{ dB} \tag{C23}$$

The actual frequency response AR at ω_n is:

$$AR(\omega_n) = 20\log(K) - 20\log[2\xi] \text{ dB} \tag{C24}$$

So if $\xi = 1$, the actual $AR(\omega_n) \cong 20\log(K) - 6$ dB; if $\xi = 1/\sqrt{2} = 0.7071$, then $AR(\omega_n) \cong 20\log(K) - 3$ dB; and if $\xi = 0.5$, $AR(\omega_n) \cong 20\log(K)$ dB, exactly. When $0 < \xi < 0.5$, the peak AR at ω_n is $> 20\log(K)$.

Now, let us examine the asymptotes of the quadratic LPF. For $\omega << \omega_n$, the AR is:

$$AR(lo) \cong 20\log(K) \text{ dB} \tag{C25}$$

And when $\omega >> \omega_n$,

$$AR(hi) \cong 20\log(K) - 20\log[\omega^2/\omega_n^2] = 20\log(K) - 40\log(\omega) + 40\log(\omega_n) \text{ dB} \tag{C26}$$

Thus, the low-frequency asymptote has zero slope and is at $20\log(K)$ dB, the dc gain of the filter. The high frequency asymptote begins at $\omega = \omega_n$, and has a slope of −40 dB/decade. The exact behavior of the AR at $\omega = \omega_n$ was described above. The normalized Bode plot for the quadratic LPF is shown in Figure C4 for certain ξ values.

Example 5: In this example, we examine the frequency response of a non-minimum-phase *all-pass filter* with transfer function:

$$H(s) = \frac{K(s - \omega_o)}{(s + \omega_o)} \tag{C27}$$

Note that this transfer function has a stable pole in the left-half s-plane and a zero at the same $|\mathbf{s}|$ value in the right-half s-plane. Written in time-constant form, the frequency response is:

$$\mathbf{H}(j\omega) = \frac{K(j\omega/\omega_o - 1)}{(j\omega/\omega_o + 1)} \tag{C28}$$

The phase of $\mathbf{H}(j\omega)$ is what is of interest:

$$\varphi(\omega) = \{180^\circ - \tan^{-1}(\omega/\omega_o)\} - \tan^{-1}(\omega/\omega_o) \text{ radians} \tag{C29}$$

The angle in brackets is the angle of the numerator vector; the second term is from the denominator vector. The all-pass filters AR is simply:

$$AR(\omega) = 20\log(K) + 10\log[(\omega/\omega_o)^2 + 1] - 10\log[(\omega/\omega_o)^2 + 1] = 20\log(K) \text{ dB} \tag{C30}$$

That is, the AR is flat. Normally, several all-pass filters are cascaded to obtain a desired phase shift in a restricted range of frequencies.

Example 6: In this last example, we examine the frequency response of a simple low-pass filter with a *time delay:* The transfer function is:

$$H(s) = \frac{K\omega_o e^{-\delta s}}{s + \omega_o} \tag{C31}$$

The frequency-response function in time-constant form is:

$$\mathbf{H}(j\omega) = \frac{Ke^{-j\omega\delta}}{(j\omega/\omega_o + 1)} \tag{C32}$$

The phase function is:

$$\varphi(\omega) = -\omega\delta - \tan^{-1}(\omega/\omega_o) \text{ radians} \tag{C33}$$

The AR is:

$$AR(\omega) = 20\log(K) - 10\log[(\omega/\omega_o)^2 + 1] \text{ dB} \tag{C34}$$

Note that the magnitude of the phase delay vector is unity; i.e., $|e^{-j\omega\delta}| = 1$.

All circuit analysis programs, such as SPICE (many different "flavors"; try Beige Bag's B2-SPICE^{TM}), MicroCap 6, and APLAC contain routines that automatically calculate a circuit's frequency response and present Bode AR and phase plots vs. Hz frequency. This appendix was included to encourage the reader to develop skills in finding or predicting the frequency response of simple LTI systems on paper before a design is finalized by computer simulation and breadboarding.

Appendix D Computational Tools for Biomedical Signal Processing and Systems Analysis

D.1 Introduction

In this appendix, we will describe some of the computer applications (software) currently available to characterize stationary and nonstationary biomedical signals, and to analyze and describe the dynamic properties of LTI systems described by sets of first-order linear ODEs, as well as nonlinear and time varying systems found in medicine and biology. A danger in writing such a description (and also in reading it) is that such applications are continually evolving and new versions of programs are continually being released, hence what is described below will probably not be state of the art in 2 years.

Note that university and other websites exist where one can download free "tool boxes" for specialized applications such as joint time-frequency analysis. Such JTFA software is often written as *.m files compatible with the ubiquitous Matlab™ programs and toolboxes. One URL where one can download free Matlab-compatible JTFA programs is: `http://crttsn.univ-nantes.fr/~auger/tftb.html`.

Below we will describe three popular software applications that have great application in the analysis, simulation and modeling of biomedical systems and signals. These programs are Simnon™, Matlab™, and LabVIEW™. Each program has its strengths and weaknesses, and is best suited for a particular approach to systems and signal analysis.

D.2 Simnon™

Simnon is a time-domain differential equation solver. It was developed at the Department of Automatic Control at the Lund Institute of Technology, Sweden, in the late 1980s. The program in its early versions (V1.0 to V3.2) was written to run on PCs under nonWindows MS-DOS. A simple, algebraic input script was used. In 1988, the author found that Simnon was particularly well suited for simulation of *compartmental pharmacokinetic systems, biochemical kinetic systems* and nonlinear *physiological systems*. Because its input modality is in the form of the algebraic first-order linear, nonlinear and time-variable ODEs that arise naturally from the analysis and modeling of these three classes of systems, there is no need to put the sets of nonliear ODEs in transfer function (block-diagram) form. Simnon also allows the simultaneous simulation of a discrete controller along with a nonlinear analog system when it is desired to simulate a complete exogenous closed-loop control system. One can also model systems described by sets of linear or nonlinear difference equations. I have effectively used Simnon 3.2 to model the dynamic behavior of closed-loop nonlinear physiological systems [Northrop, 2000] and to model the behavior of neurosensory systems [Northrop, 2001].

The latest Windows™ version, Simnon 3.0/PCW, is well suited to solve sets of stiff nonlinear ODEs. The user has the choice of one of four integration algorithms: Runge-Kutta/Fehlberg 2nd/3rd order, Runge-Kutta/Fehlberg 4th/5th (4th order has variable or fixed step size), Euler, and Dormand-Prince 4th/5th. Simnon 3.0/PCW can handle up to: 10,000 states (ODEs), 100 subsystems, 50 pure time delays, 50 function tables, 32 plot variables and up to 100 stored variables. Noise can also be included in simulations. Calculations are performed with double precision. Simnon uses a user-friendly interactive GUI, and it has quality graphic outputs on monitors and to color laser and bubble jet printers. Solutions of sets of nonlinear ODEs by Simnon can be displayed in the time domain, or parametrically as phase-plane plots. Simnon data files can also be exported to Matlab. Matlab can then be used to do frequency- and JTF-domain operations not found in Simnon.

I have run the DOS Simnon V3.2 on a Pentium PC with the Windows NT4® operating system. Simnon V3.2 has color graphics that can be printed out as such with a suitable color printer. Simnon V3.2 cost about $750 in the early 1990s, the student version was $95.

The current Windows version of Simnon (v3.0/PCW), is available from SSPA Maritime Consulting, Göteborg, Sweden, email URL simnon@sspa.se. Its price is ECU 99 from SSPA (about US $86 in 02/02). It is truly a bargain. The well-written user manual is on the CD with the program.

D.3 National Instruments' LabVIEW™ Signal Processing Tools

National Instruments™(NI) software was originally developed for the control of real-time signal acquisition and display, and signal outputs by PC accessory cards with analog-to-digital and digital-to-analog converters. NI interface cards come in a wide variety of configurations; data is handled in 12 or 16 bit streams, in addition to multiple-channel real-time analog I/O signals; cards also have direct digital I/O channels. Basic DSP operations on acquired data were also provided (e.g., bandpass filter the acquired signal, compute its rms value, etc.). Operations were set up with a GUI using block diagram icons. At present, NI LabVIEW v 6.1 software has evolved into a sophisticated suite of proprietary DSP "toolsets" for processing acquired signals. User-defined graphical icons are used to control data I/O and signal processing (SP).

NI also offers a line of SCXI ("scuzzy") plug-in modules to condition signals from various types of sensors such as strain gauge bridges, thermocouples and LVDTs. The outputs from the *Signal Conditioning Modules* are passed to a multiplexer on the plug-in DAQ card in the computer.

Of particular interest to biomedical engineers, biophysicists, physiologists and medical researchers is NI's BioBench™, a low-cost turnkey software application that runs with a special NI multichannel interface board (PC-LPM-16 A/D DAQ). A Human Physiology Lab Kit is offered by NI that runs with the BioBench system. (The human physiology teaching kit was developed for NI by CB Sciences, Inc.) The lab kit includes a two-channel, "student-safe" ECG/EMG differential amplifier that is used in all the measurements. The BioBench employs various sensors that use the same amplifier including a grip force sensor, a pneumotach, a pulse sensor, etc.

The lab manual details 13 experiments and 50 exercises that can be done with this apparatus. There is no reason that other sensor systems cannot be used with the BioBench system; for example, the audio output of a Doppler ultrasound system or the output of a pulse oximeter.

NI has developed sophisticated DSP tools for use with LabVIEW, for example, the versatile *JTFA Toolkit* for the description of nonstationary signals. In addition to the JTFA Toolkit, NI software offers: A *Digital Filter Design Component,* a *Wavelet and Filter Bank Design Component* and a *Super-Resolution Spectral Analysis Component.* The object of much DSP software is to de-noise (improve the SNR) of acquired signals.

D.4 Matlab, Simulink, and Toolkits

Of all the software used for the analysis and characterization of biomedical signals and systems, the Matlab^{TM} family of object programs is the most ubiquitous. Most engineering schools introduce their students to Matlab early in their academic careers. It is used to solve home problems and is the designated software of certain systems engineering textbooks. Matlab and its associated toolboxes and programs are products of The MathWorks, Inc., Natick, MA. Historically, Matlab started out as a set of linkable object programs used for linear state-variable matrix operations on LTI systems. To satisfy the need for specialized applications, the Math-Works has developed some 30 different Toolboxes for Matlab. Each toolbox includes a collection of *m-files* dedicated to some specialized aspect of signal processing, system analysis or simulation. The toolboxes that may have the greatest application to biomedical signals and systems include: *Communications, Control Systems, Curve Fitting, Data Acquisition, Image Processing, Instrument Control, Neural Networks, Nonlinear Control Design, Partial Differential Equations, Signal Processing, Statistics, System Identification,* and *Wavelets.*

Of particular interest are the *Data Acquisition* and *Instrument Control* toolboxes. These object files permit real-time data acquisition through certain standard A/D I/O cards, such as made by NI, Agilent Technologies, Keithley Instruments, Measurement Computing Corporation (formerly ComputerBoards Inc.) and PC-compatible soundboards. The sampling frequency and acquired epoch length (record duration) are specified for each sampled analog signal, along with a start signal. The instrument control toolbox allows signals to be acquired via standard bus architectures (e.g., GPIB and VXI) from compatible instruments and passed to Matlab for analysis and display.

These two toolboxes provide real-time entry of sampled experimental data into the powerful Matlab environment, providing a direct challenge to the NI LabVIEW interface and DSP systems. Matlab DSP object files can then be applied to the acquired data to filter, de-noise, find frequency spectra, do JTFA analysis, etc.

Simulink^{TM} is a GUI modeling and simulation program that runs with Matlab (Simulink is now at v4.1.1 (02/02). Different flavors of Matlab and Simulink run on PCs with Windows 95, 98 NT4.0, Me, 2000, or on Macs or Unix platforms). Simulink is an icon-driven dynamic simulation package that allows the user to represent a dynamic system with a graphical block diagram. The blocks fall into the categories of: *Sources, Sinks, Discrete LTI Transfer Functions* (including delays and holds), *Continuous LTI Transfer Functions* (including time derivatives, integration, LTI state-variable systems, and delays), *Nonlinear Function Blocks* (including switching, hysteresis, etc.), *Mathematical and Matrix Operations* (including Matlab and toolbox functions), *Signal and Systems, and user-defined Subsystems operations.* Simulink blocks are also organized by application; for example, there is a *Communications Blockset v2, DSP Blockset v4, FixedPoint Blockset v3, Power Systems v2.1, Real-Time Workshop v4,* etc.

As a system's block diagram is built, the user has to specify numerical values for the parameters in the blocks, and, of course, the interconnections between them. Before the simulation is run, the user specifies the integration routine to be used, the stepsize and start and stop times. A diverse selection of integration routines includes: R-K 2-3, R-K 4-5, Euler, Gear, Adams, and "Linsim" (plain vanilla for purely linear state systems). Gear is recommended for stiff nonlinear systems. Because Simulink runs in the Matlab "shell," it can make use of all of the many features of Matlab and its various toolboxes.

Although extremely versatile for the simulation of analog or discrete systems whose subsystems are describable as rational polynomial transfer functions or sets of state equations, Simulink does not shine in the simulation of systems of functionally nonlinear ODEs, such as found in physiology, chemical kinetics or neural modeling. Its block diagram format becomes unwieldy, and it is clear that a program such as Simnon that accepts the algebraically written ODEs directly is easier to set up for running a simulation. Simulink is best used for systems engineering modeling and design verification.

The reader interested in learning more about Simulink and Matlab can visit the URL `http://www.mathworks.com/products/simulink`.

D.5 Summary

Simnon^{TM} is a powerful inexpensive program specialized to simulate systems made up from large sets of algebraic nonlinear first-order ODEs (which can be time-variable) in the time domain. There is no need to make a block diagram. In the biomedical area, Simnon is well suited to model chemical kinetic systems; physiological systems, including those under exogenous (digital) control (such as glucoregulation by controlled insulin injection) and neural model simulation (such as the Hodgkin-Huxley equation, cf. Northrop, 2001).

National Instruments^{TM} LabVIEW^{TM} hardware and software is designed for real-time data acquisition and subsequent signal processing and display. Once a LabVIEW system has been developed, it runs expeditiously in a turnkey manner controlled by a GUI. *BioBench* is an NI product specifically designed to acquire physiological signals. A unique feature of NI is its easy-to-use JTFA Toolkit (cf. National Instruments^{TM} 1998 *LabView^{TM} Joint Time-Frequency Analysis Toolkit Reference Manual.* Part No. 320544D-01. Available online).

Matlab^{TM} offers an enormous collection of object programs or executable *.m files, which enable an wide range of system simulation and signal analysis of LTI systems and signals. *.m files are organized by application into collections known as "toolboxes." To facilitate system analysis, the MathWorks developed Simulink,^{TM} which uses a block diagram approach to model systems. Simulink is best in modeling LTI systems where known component transfer functions, linear matrix operations and signal nonlinearities can be put into the interconnected blocks. Simulink is not well suited to simulate sets of algebraically nonlinear time-variable ODEs. For example, take the well-known Hodgkin-Huxley model for nerve spike generation. It is tedious to put the four H-H ODEs and auxiliary equations into Simulink form. Using Simnon, one need only write the four ODEs as given in algebraic form, etc., to complete the model.

Of significance to biomedical engineers are the new *Data Acquisition* and *Instrument Control* toolboxes in Matlab. As described above, these object files permit Matlab to use DAQ interface cards to acquire analog signals in real time and then pass the data to other specialized objects, for example, in the *Signal Processing Toolbox,* or in the *Time-Frequency Toolbox* [Auger et al., 2002]. It appears that Matlab is now competitive with LabVIEW for real-time data acquisition and signal analysis.

Bibliography and References

[1] Ackerman, E. 1962. *Biophysical Science.* Prentice-Hall. Englewood Cliffs, NJ.

[2] Amini, W., M. Björklund, R. Dror and A. Nygren. 1997. Tomographic Reconstruction of SPECT Data. `www.owlnet.rice.edu/~elec539/Projects97/cult/report.html`.

[3] Anasstasiou, D. 2000. Frequency-domain analysis of biomolecular sequences. *Bioinformatics.* 16(12): 1073–1081.

[4] Arnison, M.R., C.J. Cogswell, N.I. Smith, P.W. Fekete and K.G. Larkin. 2000. Using the Hilbert transform for 3D visualization of differential interference contrast microscope images. *J. Micros.* 199, 79–84.

[5] Auger, F., P. Flandrin, O. Lemoine and P. Goncalvès. 2002. *Time-Frequency Toolbox for Matlab.* free Matlab m-file software, `http://crttsn.univ-nantes.fr/~auger/tftb.html`.

[6] Bastiaans, M.J. 1997. Application of the Wigner distribution function in optics. In: *The Wigner Distribution–Theory and Applications in Signal Processing.* W. Mecklenbräuker and F. Hlawatsch, Eds. Elsevier Science.

[7] Bendat, J.S. and A.G. Piersol. 1966. *Measurement and Analysis of Random Data.* John Wiley and Sons, New York.

[8] Bentley, P.M., P.M. Grant and J.T.E. McDonnell. 1998. Time-frequency and time-scale techniques for the classification of native and bioprosthetic heart valve sounds. *IEEE Trans. Biomed. Eng.* 45(1): 125–128.

[9] Beyer, W.H., Ed. 1968. *CRC Handbook of Tables for Probability and Statistics,* 2nd ed. The Chemical Rubber Co., Cleveland, OH.

[10] Birds. 2001. What is a Sound Spectrogram? Cornell Bioacoustics Research Program. `http://birds.cornell.edu/BRP/spgdef.html`.

[11] Boashash, B. and M. Mesbah. 2001. A time-frequency approach for newborn seizure detection. *IEEE Eng. Med. Biol. Mag.* 20(5): 54–64.

[12] Carter, T. 2001. An Introduction to Information Theory and Entropy: Applications to Biology. On-line class notes for the Complex Systems Summer School, June, 2001. `http://astarte.csustan.edu/~tom/DFI-CSSS/info-theory/info-lec.html`.

[13] Celka, P., B. Boashash and P. Colditz. 2001. Preprocessing and time-frequency analysis of newborn EEG seizures. *IEEE Eng. Med. Biol. Mag.* 20(5): 30–39.

[14] Chandra, et al. 2002.

[15] Chandra, C., M.S. Moore and S.K. Mitra. 1998. An efficient method for the removal of impulse noise from speech and audio signals. *Proc. IEEE International. Symposium on Circuits and Systems.* Monterey, CA. 206 –209.

[16] Chirlian, P.M. 1981. *Analysis and Design of Integrated Electronic Circuits.* Harper and Row, New York.

[17] Choi, H. and W.J. Williams. 1989. Improved time-frequency representation of multicomponent signals using exponential kernels. *IEEE Trans. Acoust,. Speech Signal Proc.* 37: 862–871.

[18] Clarke, K.K. and D.T. Hess. 1971. *Communications Circuits: Analysis and Design.* Addison-Wesley, Reading, MA.

[19] Cohen, L. 1966. Generalized phase-space distribution functions. *J. Math. Phys.* 7: 781–806.

[20] Cooley, J.W. and J.W. Tukey. 1965. An algorithm for the machine computation of complex Fourier series. *Math. Comp.* 19: 297–301.

[21] Craig, E.J. 1964. *Laplace and Fourier Transforms for Electrical Engineers.* Holt, Rinehart and Winston, New York.

[22] Cunningham, E.P. 1992. *Digital Filtering: An Introduction.* Houghton-Mifflin Co., Boston.

[23] de Marchi, J.A. and K.C. Craig. 1999. Comments on natural frequencies and damping identification using wavelet transform: application to real data. *J. Mech. Syst. Signal Proc.* 4.

[24] Duchêne, J., D. Devedeux, S. Mansour and C. Marque. 1995. Analyzing uterine EMG: tracking instantaneous burst frequency. *IEEE Eng. Med. Biol. Mag.* March/April. 125–132.

[25] Durka, P.J. and K.J. Blinowska. 2001. A unified parametrization of EEG. `http://brain.fuw.edu.pl/~durka/papers/unification/unification.html`.

[26] ELIS. 2001. Time-Frequency Analysis of EEG Signals. Web paper, University of Ghent, `www.elis.rug.ac.be/ELISgroups/mbv/sigproc/timefreq/timefreq.html`.

[27] Feldman, M. 1997. Nonlinear free vibration identification via the Hilbert transform. *J. Sound Vib.* 208(3): 475–489.

[28] Finch, S. 2001. Favorite mathematical constants. `http://pauillac.inria.fr/algo/bsolve/constant/constant.html`

[29] Gabor, D. 1946. Theory of communication. *J. IEEE.* London. 93: 429–457.

[30] Genomes. 2001. The Human Genome. `http://exobio.ucsd.edu/Space_Sciences/genomes.htm`.

[31] Godfrey, K. 1983. *Compartmental Models and their Application.* Academic, London.

[32] Graps, A. 2000. Amara's Wavelet Page. `www.amara.com/current/wavelet.html`.

[33] Guillemin, E.A. 1949. *The Mathematics of Circuit Analysis.* John Wiley and Sons, New York.

[34] Guyton, A.C. 1991. *Textbook of Medical Physiology.* 8th ed. W.B. Saunders, Philadelphia.

[35] Hardman, J.G., L.E. Limbird, P.B. Molinoff, R.W. Ruddon and A.G. Gilman, Eds. 1996. *Goodman and Gilman's The Pharmacological Basis of Therapeutics.* McGraw-Hill, New York.

[36] Hultquist, P.A. 1988. *Numerical Methods for Engineers and Computer Scientists.* Benjamin Cummings, Menlo Park, CA.

[37] Jeong, J. and W.J. Williams. 1992. Kernel design for reduced interference distributions. *IEEE Trans. Sig. Proc.* 40(2): 402–412.

[38] Jones, R.W. 1973. *Principles of Biological Regulation.* Academic, New York.

[39] Jones, D.L. and T.W. Parks. 1992. A resolution comparison of several time-frequency representations. *IEEE Trans. Sig. Proc.* 40(2): 413–420.

[40] Kaplan, Ian. 2001. Applying the Haar Wavelet Transform to Time Series Information. `www.bearcave.com/misl/misl_tech/wavelets/haar.html`.

[41] Karchin, R. 1999. Hidden Markov Models and Protein Sequence Analysis. Web paper (17pp) `www.cse.ucsc.edu/research/compbio/ismb99.handouts/KK185FP.html`.

[42] Kollár, I. 1986. The noise model of quantization. *Proc. IMEKO TC4 Symposium, Noise in Electrical Measurements.* Como, Italy. June 19–21, 1986. OMIKK-Technoinform, Budapest. 1987. 125–129.

[43] Koren, N. 2001. Understanding Image Sharpness–Part 1: Resolution and MTF Curves in Film and Lenses.www.normankoren.com/Tutorials/MTF.html.

[44] Kraegen, E.W. and L. Lazarus. 1973. Feedback control of blood glucose. In *Regulation and Control in Physiological Systems.* Iberall, A.S. and A.C. Guyton, Eds. Instrument Society of America, Pittsburgh. 470–474.

[45] Krattenthaler, W. and F. Hlawatsch. 1993. Time-frequency design and processing of signals via smoothed Wigner distributions. *IEEE Trans. Sig. Proc.* 41(1): 278–287.

[46] Kuo, B.C. 1967. *Linear Networks and Systems.* McGraw-Hill, New York.

[47] Lathi, B.P. 1974. *Signals, Systems and Controls.* Harper and Rowe, New York.

[48] Laughlin, P., M. Redfern and J. Furman. 1996. Time-varying characteristics of visually induced postural sway. *IEEE Trans. on Rehab. Eng.* 4(4): 416–424.

[49] Lee, Y.W. 1960. *Statistical Theory of Communication.* John Wiley and Sons, New York.

[50] Leonhard Research. 2001. *Measuring the Instantaneous Energy in Signals.* `www.leonhardresearch.com/download/application.PDF`.

[51] Liley, D. 2001. Lecture Notes. Medical Imaging HET408. Swinburne University of Technology, Australia. `http://marr.bsee.swin.edu.au/~dtl/het408.html`.

[52] Lin, J. and L. Qu. 2000. Feature extraction based on Morlet wavelet and its application for mechanical fault diagnosis. *J. Sound Vib.* 20002864. `www.idealibrary.com`.

[53] Lindorff, D.P. 1965. *Theory of Sampled-Data Control Systems.* John Wiley and Sons, New York.

[54] Macovski. 1983.

[55] Maienschein, J. 2001. What's in a name? Embryos, clones and stem cells. *Am. J. Bioethics.* 2(1): `www.ajobonline.com/StemCells/excerpts_maienschein.html`.

[56] Marmarelis, P.Z. 1972. Nonlinear Dynamic Transfer Functions for Certain Retinal Neuronal Systems. Ph.D. dissertation. California Institute of Technology, Pasadena.

[57] Marmarelis, P.Z. and V.Z. Marmarelis. 1978. *Analysis of Physiological Systems.* Plenum, New York.

[58] Maron, S.H. and C.F. Prutton. 1958. *Principles of Physical Chemistry.* MacMillan, New York.

[59] Mason, S.J. 1953. Feedback theory–some properties of signal flow graphs. *Proc. IRE.* 41(9): 1144–1156.

[60] Mason, S.J. 1956. Feedback theory–further properties of signal flow graphs. *Proc. IRE.* 44(7): 920–926.

[61] Masum, H., F. Oppacher and G. Carmody. Spring, 2001. Genomic algorithms: Metaphors from molecular genetics. *Carleton J. Comp. Sci.* Carleton University, Ottawa.

[62] Mathews, C.K. and K.E. van Holde. 1990. *Biochemistry.* Benjamin/Cummings, Redwood City, CA.

[63] MathWorks, 2001. *Wavelet Toolbox 2.1.* `www.mathworks.com/products/wavelet/`.

[64] MCB 411. 2000. Module 15. *Post-Transcriptional Events: RNA Splicing.* Lecture notes. `www.blc.arizona.edu/marty/411/Modules/mod15.html`.

[65] Moore, M.S., M. Gabbouj and S.K. Mitra. 1999. Vector SD-ROM filter for removal of impulse noise from color images. *Proc. EURASIP Conference ECMCS '99.* June. Kraców, 24–26.

[66] National Instruments. 1998. *LabView^{TM} Joint Time-Frequency Analysis Toolkit Reference Manual.* Part No. 320544D-01. Available online.

[67] Nise, N.S. 1995. *Control Systems Engineering,* 2nd ed. Benjamin Cummings, Redwood City, CA.

[68] Northrop, R.B. 1990. *Analog Electronic Circuits: Analysis and Applications.* Addison-Wesley, Reading, MA.

[69] Northrop, R.B. 1997. *Introduction to Instrumentation and Measurements.* CRC, Boca Raton, FL.

[70] Northrop, R.B. 2000. *Endogenous and Exogenous Regulation and Control of Physiological Systems.* CRC, Boca Raton, FL.

[71] Northrop, R.B. 2001. *Introduction to Dynamic Modeling of Neuro-Sensory Systems.* CRC, Boca Raton, FL.

[72] Northrop, R.B. 2002. *Noninvasive Instrumentation and Measurements in Medical Diagnosis.* CRC, Boca Raton, FL.

[73] Ogata, K. 1970. *Modern Control Engineering.* Prentice-Hall, Englewood Cliffs, NJ.

[74] Ogata, K. 1990. *Modern Control Engineering,* 2nd ed. Prentice-Hall, Englewood Cliffs, NJ.

[75] Oppenheim, A.V. and A.S. Willsky. 1983. *Signals and Systems.* Prentice-Hall, Englewood Cliffs, NJ.

[76] Papoulis, A. 1965. *Probability, Random Variables, and Stochastic Processes.* McGraw-Hill, New York.

[77] Papoulis, A. 1968. *Systems and Transforms with Applications to Optics.* McGraw-Hill, New York.

[78] Papoulis, A. 1977. *Signal Analysis.* McGraw-Hill, New York.

[79] Parks, T.M. 1991. *Time-Frequency Analysis of Periodic Signals.* (Student paper for EE290t.) `http://ptolemy.eecs.berkeley.edu/~parks/papers/ee290t-s91/-2k`.

[80] Pearson, R. 2002. Scrub data with scale-invariant nonlinear digital filters. *EDN.* 24 Jan. 71–78.

[81] Peshkin, L. and M.S. Gelfand. 1999. Segmentation of yeast DNA using hidden Markov models. *Bioinformatics.* 15(12): 980–986.

[82] Phillips and Nagle. 1984.

[83] Polikar, R., M.H. Greer, L. Udpa and F. Keinert. 1997. Multiresolution wavelet analysis of ERPs for the detection of Alzheimer's disease. *Proc. 19th International. Conference IEEE/EMBS.* 30 Oct.–2 Nov. Chicago. 1301–1304.

[84] Polikar, R. 1998. *The Wavelet Tutorial* (Parts I–IV). `www.public.iastate.edu/%7erpolikar/WAVELETS/WTtutorial.html`.

[85] Proakis, J.G. and D.G. Manolakis. 1989. *Introduction to Digital Signal Processing.* Macmillan, New York.

[86] Qian, S. and D. Chen. 1996. *Joint Time-Frequency Analysis.* Prentice-Hall PTR, Upper Saddle River, NJ.

[87] Rabiner, L.R. and B.H. Juang. 1986. An introduction to hidden Markov models. *IEEE ASSP Mag.* June, 4–16.

[88] Rabiner, L.R. 1989. A tutorial on hidden Markov models and selected applications in speech recognition. *Proc. IEEE.* 77: 257–286.

[89] Ragazzini and Franklin. 1958.

[90] Rao, R.P.V., R.D. Kriz, A.L. Abbott and C.J. Ribbens. 1995. Parallel Implementation of the Filtered Back Projection Algorithm for Tomographic Imaging. `www.sv.vt.edu/xray_ct/parallel/Parallel_CT.html`.

[91] Rockmore, D.N. 1999. The FFT–an algorithm the whole family can use. `www.cs.dartmouth.edu/~rockmore/cse-fft.pdf`.

[92] Schneider, T.D. 2001. Molecular Information Theory and the Theory of Molecular Machines. `www.lecb.ncifcrf.gov/~toms`.

[93] Schneider, T.D. 2000. Information Theory Primer. `www.lecb.ncifcrf.gov/~toms/paper/primer`.

[94] Schneider, T.D. 1994. Sequence Logos, Machine/Channel Capacity, Maxwell's Demon, and Molecular Computers: A Review of the Theory of Molecular Machines. *Nanotechnology.* 5(1): 1–18.

[95] Schwartz, M. 1959. *Information, Transmission, Modulation and Noise.* McGraw-Hill, New York.

[96] Schwartz, M. and L. Shaw. 1975. *Signal Processing: Discrete Spectral Analysis, Detection, and Estimation.* McGraw-Hill, New York.

[97] Selesnick, I.W. 2001. Hilbert transform pairs of wavelet bases. *IEEE Signal Proc. Lett.* 8(6): 170–173.

[98] Serres, M.H., S. Gopal, L.A. Nahum, P. Liang, T. Gaasterland and M. Riley. 2001. A functional update on the *E. coli* K-12 genome. *Genome Biology.* 2(9): 35.1–35.7. genomebiology.com/2001/2/9/research/0035.1.

[99] Shannon, C. and W. Weaver. 1949. *The Mathematical Theory of Communication.* University of Illinois Press, Urbana.

[100] Spangler and Snell. 1961. *Nature* 191(4787): 457–458.

[101] Sikiö. 1999.

[102] Spring, K.R. and M.W. Davidson. 2001. *Modulation Transfer Function.* Web tutorial. `www.microscopyu.com/articles/optics/mtfintro.html`.

[103] Stark, L. 1968. *Neurological Control Systems.* Plenum, New York.

[104] Steeghs, P. 1997. *Local Power Spectra and Seismic Interpretation.* Ph.D. dissertation, Delft University of Technology. Ch.2. Time-Frequency Analysis and the Wigner Distribution: `www.ta.tudelft.nl/TG/local/section/Publications/publications.html`.

[105] Stern, R.M. 2000. Fast Fourier Transform Inverses and Alternate Implementations. EE791 Lecture Notes, Carnegie-Mellon University `www.ece.cmu.edu/~ee791/L16/FFTstructures.pdf`.

[106] Theussl, T. 1999. On Windowing for Gradient Estimation in Volume Visualization. Web paper. Institute of Computer Graphics, Vienna University of Technology. www.cg.tuwien.ac.at/studentwork/CESCG99/TTheussl/paper.html .

[107] Toft, Peter. The Radon Transform, `http://eivind.imm.dtu.dk/staff/ptoft/Radon/Radon.html`.

[108] Tomoviç, R. 1966. *Introduction to Nonlinear Automatic Control Systems.* Wiley, London.

[109] Tompkins, W.J., Ed. 1993. *Biomedical Digital Signal Processing.* Prentice-Hall, Englewood Cliffs, NJ.

[110] Torrance, C. and G.P. Compo. 1998. A practical guide to wavelet analysis. *Bull. Amer. Meteorol. Soc.* 79(1): 61–78.

[111] Truxall, J.G. 1955. *Automatic Feedback Control System Synthesis.* McGraw-Hill, New York.

[112] UCSD. 2001. *The Genetic Code.* Web notes. `http://exobio.ucsd.edu/Space_Sciences/genetic_code.htm`.

[113] University of Leeds, (UK). 1997. Notes on Hidden Markov Models. `www.comp.leeds.ac.uk/scs-only/teaching-materials/HiddenMarkovModels/htm_dev/main.html`.

[114] University of Strathclyde. 2001. Fourier and the Frequency Domain. (Online lecture notes with good section on FFT calculation by time decimation.) `www.spd.eee.strath.ac.uk/~interact/fourier/fourier.html`.

[115] Van Hoey, G., W. Phillips and I. Lemahieu. 1997. Time-frequency analysis of EEG signals. *Proc. ProRISC Workshop on Circuits, Systems and Signal Processing*. 549–553.

[116] Watson, J.D. and F.H.C. Crick. 1953. Molecular structure for nucleic acids: A structure for deoxyribose nucleic acid. *Nature*. 171: 737–738.

[117] Widrow, B. and S.D. Stearns. 1985. *Adaptive Signal Processing*. Prentice-Hall, Englewood Cliffs, NJ.

[118] Williams, C.S. 1986. *Designing Digital Filters*. Prentice-Hall, Englewood Cliffs, NJ.

[119] Williams, W.J., H.P. Zaveri and J.C. Sackellares. 1995. Time-frequency analysis of electrophysiology signals in epilepsy. *IEEE Eng. Med. Biol. Mag.* March/April. 133–143.

[120] Wood, J.C., A.J. Buda and D.T. Barry. 1992. Time-frequency transforms: A new approach to first heart sound frequency dynamics. *IEEE Trans. Biomed. Eng.* 39(7): 730–739.

[121] Wood, J.C. and D.T. Barry. 1995. Time-frequency analysis of the first heart sound. *IEEE Eng. Med. Biol. Mag.* March/April. 144–151.

[122] Yates, F.E., D.J. Marsh et al. 1973. Modeling metabolic systems and the attendant data handling problem. In *Regulation and Control in Physiological Systems*. Iberall, A.S. and A.C. Guyton, Eds. Instrument Society of America, Pittsburgh. 464–468.

[123] Yockey, H.P., R.L. Platzman and H. Quastler. 1958. *Symposium on Information Theory in Biology*. Gatlinburg, TN. 29–31 Oct. 1956. Pergamon, New York.

[124] Zhang, J-W, J-R Liu et al. 2000. Noninvasive early detection of focal cerebral ischemia. *IEEE Eng. Med. Biol. Mag.* Nov./Dec. 74–81.

[125] Zhao, Y., L.E. Atlas and R.J. Marks. 1990. The use of cone-shaped kernels for generalized time-frequency representations of nonstationary signals. *IEEE Trans. Acous. Speech and Sig., Proc.* 38(7): 1084–1091.

[126] Ziemer, R.E. and W.H. Tranter. 1990. *Principles of Communications: Systems, Modulation and Noise*. Houghton-Mifflin, Boston.

Index

G

H

I

J

L

M

N

O

P

Q

R

S

T

V

W

Z